Occupational Therapy
practice skills for physical dysfunction

Occupational Therapy

practice skills for physical dysfunction

LORRAINE WILLIAMS PEDRETTI, M.S., O.T.R.

Associate Professor, Department of Occupational Therapy,
San Jose State University, San Jose, California

SECOND EDITION

with 604 illustrations

The C. V. Mosby Company

ST. LOUIS • TORONTO • PRINCETON   1985

MOSBY

A TRADITION OF PUBLISHING EXCELLENCE

Editor: Rosa L. Kasper
Assistant editor: Connie Leinicke
Editing supervisor: Judi Wolken
Manuscript editors: Marybeth Engelhardt, Melissa Neves
Book design: Nancy Steinmeyer
Cover design: Tom Zigrang; Original graphic design by Linda Higgins
Production: Carol O'Leary, Barbara Merritt, Nancy Steinmeyer

SECOND EDITION

Previous edition copyrighted 1981

Printed in the United States of America

The C.V. Mosby Company
11830 Westline Industrial Drive, St. Louis, Missouri 63146

Library of Congress Cataloging in Publication Data

Pedretti, Lorraine Williams, 1936-
  Occupational therapy.

  Bibliography: p.
  Includes index.
  1. Occupational therapy. 2. Physically handicapped—
Rehabilitation. I. Title. [DNLM: 1. Occupational
Therapy. WB 555 P371]
RM735.P34 1985   615.8′5152   84-14733
ISBN 0-8016-3824-0

C/VH/VH 9 8 7 6 5 4   02/B/294

Contributors

ELIZABETH BIANCHI, O.T.R.

Occupational Therapist, Stanford University Hospital, Stanford, California

HELEN BOBROVE, O.T.R.

Occupational Therapist, Stanford University Hospital, Stanford, California

SHIRLEY W. CHAN, O.T.R.

Occupational Therapist, St. Francis Memorial Hospital, San Francisco, California

JAN ZARET DAVIS, O.T.R.

Formerly Director of Occupational Therapy, Baderklinik, Valens, Switzerland; Consultant, Neurodevelopmental Treatment, San Jose, California

DENISE FODERARO, O.T.R.

Senior Occupational Therapist, Santa Clara Valley Medical Center, San Jose, California

MARY C. KASCH, O.T.R.

Formerly President, American Society of Hand Therapists; Director of Hand Therapy, Hand Surgery Associates, Sacramento, California

GUY L. McCORMACK, M.S., O.T.R.

Associate Professor, Department of Occupational Therapy, San Jose State University, San Jose, California

SHARON PASQUINELLI-ESTRADA, M.S., O.T.R.

Occupational Therapist, Fairmont Hospital, San Leandro, California

KAREN PITBLADDO, O.T.R.

Occupational Therapist, Stanford University Hospital, Stanford, California

JAN POLON, O.T.R.

Occupational Therapist, Stanford University Hospital, Stanford, California

SALLY ABELE ROOZEE, M.S., O.T.R.

Formerly Director of Occupational Therapy, St. Francis Memorial Hospital, San Francisco, California; Private Practice, Walnut Creek, California

DIANE MEEDER RYCKMAN, O.T.R./L.

Chief Occupational Therapist, Occupational Therapy Division, Kettering Medical Center, Kettering, Ohio

GREGORY STONE, M.Ed., B.F.A., C.O.T.A.

Assistant Professor, Department of Occupational Therapy, San Jose State University, San Jose, California

NANCY D. THOMPSON, R.P.T.

Physical Therapist, Sacramento, California

BARBARA B. ZOLTAN, M.A., O.T.R.

Education Supervisor, Department of Occupational Therapy, Santa Clara Valley Medical Center; Lecturer, Department of Occupational Therapy, San Jose State University; A.O.T.A. appointed Specialty Resource Person for Head Injury and CVA Special Interest Sections, San Jose, California

Preface
to second edition

This book was designed for use by occupational therapy students in baccalaureate and entry-level master's degree programs. Its purpose is to support the preparation of the student for practice in occupational therapy for adults with acquired physical dysfunction. It is assumed that the readers of this text have knowledge of general psychology, anatomy and physiology, neuroanatomy and neurophysiology, kinesiology, orthopedic and neurological dysfunction, medical terminology, human growth and development, and theories of occupational therapy.

The content of the book is arranged according to the occupational therapy process. Part 1 is concerned with the foundations for treatment and includes a frame of reference for practice, psychosocial aspects of physical disabilities, and treatment planning. Part 2 covers evaluation procedures commonly used in occupational therapy for physical dysfunction and gives explicit instructions for their administration. Treatment methods most frequently used in physical disabilities practice are included in Part 3. This section covers therapeutic activities (including principles of therapeutic exercise), activities of daily living, four sensorimotor approaches to treatment and their neurophysiological basis, wheelchairs and wheelchair transfers, mobile arm supports and suspension slings, and hand splinting. Directions for many specific treatment procedures can be found in these chapters. The final part of the book, Part 4, is concerned with the application of treatment principles, evaluation procedures, and treatment methods to specific dysfunctions. These includes amputations, burns, arthritis, acute hand injuries, cardiac conditions, low back pain, hip fractures, lower motor neuron dysfunction, spinal cord injury, cerebral vascular accident, and head injury. These disabilities were selected because they are frequently encountered in practice and because principles that apply to them may be applied to other similar disabilities.

Each chapter concludes with review questions to assist the student to master content, achieve learning objectives, and prepare for evaluation of learning. Instructors may wish to use these questions for preparation of examinations or assignments.

Sample case studies and treatment plans are presented in each of the chapters in Part 4. These are *not* intended to present the only approach to the treatment of the particular dysfunction or to imply that there is a stereotyped method of treating the dysfunction. Rather, they are intended to serve as models for the novice from which to build diverse and alternate treatment plans for real or hypothetical clients encountered in their academic preparation. The terms *patient* and *client* have been used interchangeably in this book to designate the individual who is the consumer of occupational therapy services.

The chapter contributors are gratefully acknowledged for their willingness to share their expertise in the production of this text. My appreciation is extended to the artists, Karen Donaldson, Shirley W. Chan, Jan Zaret Davis, Gregory Stone, and Daryle Webb, and to the photographer Steven Sloan.

Appreciation is also extended to those who modeled for photographs: Joseph Brown, Janet Faubion, Roselle Fliesler, Guy L. McCormack, Morag Paterson, Julie Rasczewski, Deborah Stephany, Gregory Stone, Michael Swanson, and Norma Tanaka.

Those who served as consultants and to whom I wish to express my personal appreciation are Lela Llorens, Ph.D., O.T.R.; Amy Killingsworth, M.A., O.T.R.; Gregory Stone, M.Ed., B.F.A., C.O.T.A.; Vaunden Nelson, M.A.; and Peter I. Edgelow, R.P.T./ O.T. All my colleagues in the Department of Occupational Therapy at San Jose State University are acknowledged with appreciation for their support and encouragement.

Finally, my husband Robert and my son Mark are lovingly appreciated for their unending patience, support, and assistance.

Lorraine Williams Pedretti

Preface
to first edition

This book was designed for use by students of occupational therapy at the baccalaureate level. Its purpose is to help prepare the student for entry-level practice in occupational therapy for adults with acquired physical disabilities.

The arrangement of content is based on the occupational therapy process. Methods of evaluation and treatment planning and descriptions of frequently used treatment methods are presented. This foundation is followed by chapters on the application of occupational therapy to several specific physical disabilities. These were selected because they are often encountered in practice, and each is considered representative of a major classification of physical dysfunction. A chapter that includes principles of hand splinting and a self-instruction program on splint construction is designed for independent study. Its purposes are to introduce students to the elements of hand splinting and to direct them in the construction of a basic splint. Each chapter concludes with review questions to assist the student to master content, achieve learning objectives, and prepare for evaluation of learning.

Congenital and acquired physical disabilities of childhood have not been included. The sample case studies and treatment plans presented are not intended to present the only approach to the treatment of the particular dysfunction. Rather, they are designed to provide students with guidelines to treatment from which to build diverse and more specific treatment plans for hypothetical or real clients encountered in their academic preparation.

For clarity and ease of reading in this book clients or patients will be referred to in the masculine gender and therapists in the feminine gender.

This book evolved out of a manual that was first printed in 1972 as a collection of teaching materials and lecture outlines for use in the occupational therapy curriculum at San Jose State University. The original manual underwent several revisions and in 1977 was printed and distributed under the title *Basic Practice Skills in Occupational Therapy for Physical Dysfunction.*

It is assumed that the readers of this text have prior knowledge of anatomy, physiology, kinesiology, neuroanatomy, neurophysiology, orthopedic and neurological dysfunctions, medical terminology, human growth and development, and basic occupational therapy theory.

It is the nature of human beings to be active. Mental and physical activity is essential to personal health and to the health and progress of the culture or society in which individuals exist. Conversely, inactivity can lead to mental or physical deterioration and can be a deterrent to the progress of the culture or society in which human beings live.

At any age or stage in a person's life there is a desirable pattern and balance of optimum occupational performance for the maintenance of the health of the individual and the society. Disruptive forces, such as illness, injury, developmental disorders, and genetic defects, can alter the pattern and balance of occupational performance and place the organism in the state of disorder or imbalance so that it cannot achieve or maintain a desirable balance and pattern of occupational performance.

On these premises occupational therapy is viewed as an intervention agent whose roles are as follows:

1. Assess past and present patterns of occupational performance
2. Identify dysfunctions in occupational performance
3. Identify the dysfunctional performance components and their effect on occupational performance
4. Remedy or compensate for dysfunctions in occupational performance and performance components
5. Facilitate the structuring or restructuring of a pattern and balance in occupational performance that is suitable and optimal for the age, stage, and current life roles of the individual

Occupational therapy uses standardized testing procedures, clinical observations, and purposeful, goal-directed activity to achieve these objectives.

The chapter contributors, Mary C. Kasch, Jan Zaret Davis, Guy L. McCormack, Gregory Stone, Barbara A. Baum, and Diane L. Meeder, are gratefully acknowledged for their willingness to share in the production of this text. My appreciation is extended to Linda Higgins for the cover design and illustrations and to Bart Favero for the photographs.

My gratitude is extended to those who modeled for photographs—my students Catherine Oberschmidt and Marianne Woodall, my niece Ramona Fournier, and my colleagues Morag Paterson and Gregory Stone, San Jose State University—and to Jana Hostetter, Rehabilitation Center of Los Gatos—Saratoga, for the loan of assistive devices to be photographed.

Manuscript reviewers and consultants to whom I wish to express my personal appreciation are Joyce Gorham, Santa Clara Valley Medical Center; Amy Killingsworth, Associate Professor, San Jose State University; Dr. William Lages, Santa Clara Valley Medical Center; and John G. Russell, Jr. Carol Feinour is gratefully acknowledged for typing the manuscript so expertly and for accommodating to my schedule and special needs.

All of my colleagues in the Department of Occupational Therapy at San

Jose State University, especially Amy Killingsworth, Associate Professor, and Gregory Stone, Lecturer, are acknowledged with appreciation for their support and encouragement.

Last but not least, my husband Robert Leland Pedretti is lovingly appreciated for his unending patience, assistance, support, and encouragement. I thank my son Mark Samuel Pedretti,

age 4, who frequently wondered when the "book" would be finished, for never touching my materials, and for waiting patiently for my attention.

Lorraine Williams Pedretti

Contents

PART 1

FOUNDATIONS FOR TREATMENT OF PHYSICAL DYSFUNCTION

CHAPTER 1

A frame of reference for occupational therapy in physical dysfunction

LORRAINE WILLIAMS PEDRETTI

SHARON PASQUINELLI-ESTRADA

A frame of reference is a conceptual structure around which a program, organization, or project is developed and organized.[1] A frame of reference delineates a particular aspect of a profession and provides a central theme to which to refer for decisions regarding the appropriateness of the program design and content.[1,26] The frame of reference within which occupational therapy occurs influences the practitioner's choices and approach to treatment and thus gives unity, balance, and direction to the treatment program.[1,26]

The practice of occupational therapy in physical dysfunction needs to be guided by a unifying conceptual system that is in concert with the definition of occupational therapy,[27] the philosophical base of occupational therapy,[14] and the position of the American Occupational Therapy Association on purposeful activities.[15] It is proposed that "occupational performance" is a frame of reference that can serve as this unifying system and that treatment of physical

disabilities can be carried out in its context. Occupational performance is the frame of reference for this textbook.

OCCUPATIONAL PERFORMANCE

Occupational performance is

. . . the individual's ability to accomplish the tasks required by his or her role and related to his or her developmental stage. Roles include those of a "preschooler," student, homemaker, employee, and retired worker. Occupational performance includes self-care, work and play/leisure time performance.[1]

Self-care includes feeding, hygiene, dressing, grooming, mobility, and object manipulation. Work activities include school, home, and family management and employment. Play and leisure activities are games, sports, hobbies, and social activities.[1]

Performance components are "the learned developmental patterns of behavior which are the substructure and foundation of the individual's occupational performance."[1] The performance

components include (1) sensory-integrative functioning, (2) motor functioning, (3) social functioning, (4) psychological functioning, and (5) cognitive functioning. These elements of human function affect a person's ability to perform occupational tasks or performance skills.

The sensory-integrative component refers to the body scheme, posture, body integration, reflex and sensory functions, visual perception, and sensorimotor integration. The motor component refers to joint motion, muscle strength and tone, functional use of limbs and body, and gross and fine motor skills. The social component includes dyadic and group interaction skills. Emotional states, feelings, coping behaviors, defense mechanisms, self-identity, and self-concept are the elements of the psychological component. The cognitive component consists of written and verbal communication, concentration, problem solving, time management, conceptualization, and integration of learning.[1]

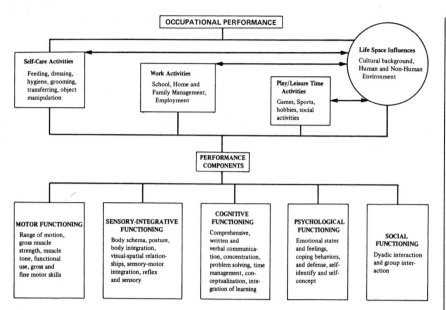

Fig. 1-1. Occupational performance frame of reference. (Reprinted with permission of The American Occupational Therapy Association, Inc., © 1974, A curriculum guide for occupational therapy educators, p. 12.)

Occupational performance requires learning and practice experiences with the role and developmental state-specific tasks, and the utilization of all performance components. Deficits in task learning experiences, performance components, and/or life space, may result in limitations in occupational performance.[1]

Life space refers to "the individual's cultural background and human and non-human environment"[29] (Fig. 1-1).

In this frame of reference the concerns of occupational therapy are the performance skills (self-care, work, and play and leisure activities) and the performance components that enable performance skills.[1,31] Therefore at any given time the occupational therapy program may include treatment methods designed for the remediaton of deficits or for the compensation for deficits in performance skills and performance components.[1] When working on a performance component (for example, motor skill development), it is essential that the methods be directed ultimately to the client's ability to master performance skills, if the methods are to be considered occupational therapy, because functional independence is a core concept of occupational therapy theory

and the goal of the occupational therapy process.[31] The occupational therapy program, then, must reflect a balance and a continuum of treatment methods that have as their purpose the maximal occupational performance of the client. Procedures that prepare the client for occupational performance but are preliminary to the use of the performance skills in treatment are necessarily the concerns of occupational therapy.[2] These procedures are regarded as "enabling" activities. Examples of enabling activities in occupational therapy are repetitive practice of a particular motor pattern, such as a skateboard activity (which can enable dressing or home-making activities), exercise for muscle strengthening (which could enable the use of a dynamic splint for writing and feeding), and balance training (which can enable transfers and dressing skills). It is important for occupational therapists to plan the progression of treatment so that performance skills are the ultimate outcome of enabling activities and are an integral part of the occupational therapy program. It is frequently possible to coordinate therapies so that the physical therapist guides the client through the major share of the

enabling aspect of treatment. The occupational therapist, aware of the client's physical therapy program and knowledgeable about the specific approach and principles of treatment being used, can reinforce and use available subskills during occupational performance activities. Examples of such an application would be the use of neurodevelopmental treatment techniques by the physical therapist and the application of the same patterns of motion to dressing training by the occupational therapist, as described in Chapter 16 of this text.

DEFINITION OF OCCUPATIONAL THERAPY

Occupational therapy is the art and science of directing man's participation in selected tasks to restore, reinforce and enhance performance, facilitate learning of those skills and functions essential for adaptation and productivity, diminish or correct pathology, and to promote and maintain health. Its fundamental concern is the development and maintenance of the capacity throughout the life span, to perform with satisfaction to self and others, those tasks and roles essential to productive living and to the mastery of self and environment.[27]

Relationship to occupational performance

In the definition just quoted *occupation* refers to the goal-directed use of time, energy, and interest.[27] The concept of occupation, then, includes all of the performance skills outlined in the occupational performance frame of reference: self-care, work, and play and leisure. Another key phrase in the definition of occupational therapy is "participation in selected tasks." This implies that the client's active involvement in his or her own treatment is essential to the effectiveness of the occupational therapy process and treatment outcomes. *Selected tasks* refers not only to those tasks that will best facilitate the achievement of the therapeutic objectives but to those that will have meaning to the client in terms of life roles and influences, which are also significant factors in the occupational performance frame of reference. The performance of tasks and roles essential to productive living throughout the lifetime is another central concept of the definition of occupational therapy. The occupational performance frame of reference has role performance as its unifying theme. The influence of the developmental process on occupational performance as a component of the frame of reference must always be considered when planning treatment programs. From these comparisons it is concluded that occupational performance as a frame of reference is compatible with the definition of occupational therapy.

THE PHILOSOPHICAL BASE OF OCCUPATIONAL THERAPY

In 1979 the Representative Assembly of the American Occupational Therapy Association adopted a philosophical base for occupational therapy.[14] The philosophical base of occupational therapy states:

Man is an active being whose development is influenced by the use of purposeful activity. Using their capacity for intrinsic motivation, human beings are able to influence their physical and mental health and their social and physical environment through purposeful activity. Human life includes a process of continuous adaptation. Adaptation is a change in function that promotes survival and self-actualization. Biological, psychological and environmental factors may interrupt the adaptation process at any time through the life cycle. Dysfunction may occur when adaptation is impaired. Purposeful activity facilitates the adaptive process.

Occupational therapy is based on the belief that purposeful activity (occupation) including its interpersonal and environmental components, may be used to prevent and mediate dysfunction, and to elicit maximum adaptation. Activity as used by the occupational therapist includes both intrinsic and therapeutic purpose.[14]

In addition to the adoption of this philosophical base, the Representative Assembly affirmed that

. . . there be universal acceptance and implementation of the common core of occupational therapy as the active participation of the patient/client in occupation for the purposes of improving performance [and that] the use of facilitating procedures is only acceptable as occupational therapy when used to prepare the patient/client for better performance and prevention of disability through self-participation in occupation.[14]

The philosophical base states that people can improve or influence their health through participation in purposeful activity (occupation). The term *purposeful activity* is a central theme of this philosophical base and was apparently used to mean *occupation*, as defined previously. It also implies that purposeful activity characterizes the tools of occupational therapy. The affirmations accompanying the philosophical base emphasized that the active participation of the client in purposeful activity is the core of occupational therapy and placed facilitating procedures in perspective as preparatory for purposeful activity. It is clearly stated that facilitating procedures are not acceptable as occupational therapy if they are used as ends unto themselves rather than the means to the ultimate goal of occupational therapy, functional independence.

Position paper on purposeful activities

When this philosophical base was presented, the American Occupational Therapy Association had not yet adopted an official definition of *purposeful activity*. The term had been used and defined by many experts.[12,20,26] Each of their definitions described purposeful activity as possessing goals independent of therapeutic goals and as facilitating function, achievement, competence, and spontaneous action.[28]

In April 1983 the Representative Assembly of the American Occupational Therapy Association adopted a position paper on purposeful activities. In this paper purposeful activity is defined as

. . . tasks or experiences, in which the person actively participates. . . . Engagement in purposeful activity requires and elicits coordination between one's physical, emotional and cognitive systems. An individual who is involved in purposeful activity directs attention to the task itself, rather than to the internal processes required for achievement of the task. . . . Purposeful activities, influenced by the individual's life roles, have unique meaning to each person.[15]

The authors of the position paper on purposeful activities described the role of the occupational therapist in the following way:

Occupational therapists evaluate clients to determine an individual's activity goals, the capacity to plan and perform purposeful activities, and the ability to meet the functional demands of the environment. Based on this evaluation, the occupational therapist designs activity experiences that offer the client opportunities for effective action. These activities are purposeful in that they assist and build upon the individual's abilities and lead to achievement of personal goals.[15]

In both the philosophical base statement and the position paper on purposeful activities a key theme is the active participation of the client. This seems to be the essential factor that differentiates purposeful activity from other types of activity. Other important factors for consideration in determining whether a particular activity is purposeful are whether it is meaningful to the client and whether it engages coordinated function of physical, emotional, and cognitive systems.

In describing the role of the occupational therapist the emphasis is on the evaluation of role dysfunction and remediation through purposeful activities.

Relationship to occupational performance

The definition and discussion of purposeful activity and the role of the occupational therapist as set forth in these important documents are in concert with the occupational performance frame of reference. Since the performance skills by their very nature are purposeful and meaningful, they serve as appropriate treatment modalities in the domain of occupational therapy. Treatment modalities to remediate or compensate for deficits in performance components can also be adapted to be purposeful in many instances.

The philosophical base and the occupational performance frame of reference take into account the human developmental process. The philosophical base also speaks to the biological, psychological, and environmental influences that may disrupt the adaptive process. These parallel the life space influences element in the occupational performance frame of reference. Thus development, adaptation, internal and external factors influencing adaptation, purposeful activity, and active participation in the recovery of health are common elements of both the occupational therapy philosophical base and the occupational performance frame of reference.

TREATMENT APPROACHES AND THEIR RELATIONSHIP TO THE OCCUPATIONAL PERFORMANCE FRAME OF REFERENCE
Biomechanical approach

The biomechanical approach to the treatment of physical dysfunction applies the mechanical principles of kinetics and kinematics to the movement of the human body.[37] These mechanical principles deal with forces acting on the body and the result of these forces on movement and equilibrium. Mechanics can be subdivided into (1) *statics*, which is concerned with the body in balance, and (2) *dynamics*, which is concerned with the body in motion. Dynamics is further subdivided into (1) *kinetics*, which deals with the forces that produce, arrest, or modify motion, and (2) *kinematics*, which is the geometry of motion. In biomechanics, equilibrium and motion are so closely interrelated that it is impractical to separate the static and dynamic aspects of human motion.[5] The biomechanical approach uses methods of treatment that employ principles of physics related to forces, levers, and torque.

The principles and methods of the biomechanical approach to treatment are appropriate for patients who have problems that directly affect range of motion (ROM), strength, and endurance but have an intact central nervous system (CNS). Therefore these clients possess control of isolated movement and specific movement patterns, although there is weakness, low endurance, or joint limitation.[37] Examples of such disabilities are orthopedic dysfunctions, such as rheumatoid arthritis, osteoarthritis, fractures, and amputations; hand trauma; burns; lower motor neuron disorders, such as peripheral nerve injuries, Guillain-Barré syndrome, and spinal cord injuries; and primary muscle diseases, such as muscular dystrophy.

The biomechanical approach includes those techniques of evaluation and treatment that use the application of forces to the body and employ principles of physics to select and direct those forces appropriately. Some examples are joint measurement, muscle strength testing, therapeutic activity for kinetic purposes, therapeutic exercise, and orthotics. The purposes of the biomechanical approach are (1) to assess specific physical limitations in range, strength, and endurance; (2) to restore function of range, strength, and endurance, and (3) to reduce deformity.

Although the concept of biomechanical treatment has long been used in occupational therapy, occupational therapists apply the principles of biomechanics perhaps more intuitively than scientifically. There is a great need for the study and analysis of a more scientific application of biomechanical principles to therapeutic activities.

RELATIONSHIP TO OCCUPATIONAL PERFORMANCE. Methods of evaluation and treatment that can be included in the biomechanical approach are primarily directed at restoration of motor function. Therefore this approach addresses the motor performance component in the occupational performance frame of reference. Many of the techniques and modalities that can be considered "enabling" methods, such as exercise, splints, and nonpurposeful kinetic activities, are biomechanical in nature. However, biomechanical principles can also be applied to purposeful activities and to performance skills. Biomechanical principles are used in activities, such as sawing wood, rolling out dough, and vacuuming a carpet. To place this approach appropriately within the frame of reference, it is important that the therapist use biomechanical methods to enable performance skills as a step in the progression of treatment toward functional independence. The exclusive use of biomechanical treatment methods for their physical restorative benefits would not be in concert with the occupational performance frame of reference.

Sensorimotor approaches

Historically, the biomechanical approach preceded the sensorimotor approaches to treatment.[37] Before the advent of the sensorimotor approaches to treatment, therapists tried to apply biomechanical principles to clients with a damaged CNS and met with many problems as a result. Since biomechanical treatment approaches demanded controlled voluntary movement, they were inappropriate for clients who lacked such control.

The sensorimotor approaches are used with clients who have CNS dysfunction. The normal CNS functions to produce controlled, well-modulated movement as a result of a balance between the inhibition and facilitation of motor responses.

In the damaged CNS the inhibition and facilitation of motor responses are out of balance and are not working together to produce smooth, well-modulated, controlled movement. The result can be too much facilitation, producing hypertonic, hyperkinetic, or rigid states of muscle, or too much inhibition, causing hypotonic or hypokinetic states of muscle.

In sensorimotor approaches to treatment it is assumed that specific, controlled sensory input can influence motor responses and that abnormal motor responses can be inhibited and more normal motor responses can be learned by the CNS. All sensorimotor approaches to treatment use proprioceptive stimuli, such as stretching and resistance, to influence thresholds for inhibition and facilitation of movement.[39] Cutaneous stimulation, which has been found to increase stretch receptor sensitivity, may be combined with proprioceptive stimulation to facilitate voluntary contraction of specific muscles. Exteroceptive stimuli, such as brushing to recruit touch receptors and icing to facilitate or inhibit muscle responses, are used. Reflex mechanisms may be used in some approaches. Some of these are the tonic neck and lumbar reflexes, righting and protective reactions, and associated reactions. The sequence in treatment may be based on the recapitulation of ontogenetic development, that is, the development of successive levels of CNS control—spinal, subcortical, then cortical control of movement.[35]

Chapters 13 through 17 of this text describe the sensorimotor approaches of Rood, Brunnstrom (movement therapy), Bobath (neurodevelopmental treatment), and Knott and Voss (proprioceptive neuromuscular facilitation). Treatment principles, some specific facilitation and inhibition techniques, and applications of the approach to purposeful activity are described.

RELATIONSHIP TO OCCUPA-TIONAL PERFORMANCE. All of the sensorimotor approaches use neuro-physiological mechanisms to elicit a specific motor response. There are many similarities and differences among the approaches, but they are all directed to motor recovery and improvement of motor performance. None of these approaches considers motivation, arousal, attention, role dysfunction, or temporal adaptation and the influence of these factors on motor behavior.[9]

The sensorimotor approaches are primarily directed toward the remediation of the motor and sensory-integrative performance components in the occupational performance frame of reference. However, occupational therapists have expressed concern about the direct application of the techniques of these approaches. If they are to be considered part of the armamentarium of the occupational therapist using this frame of reference, it will be important to apply the principles of these approaches to purposeful activity and performance skills, as described by Davis in Chapter 16, for example. In so doing it is possible to apply principles of sensorimotor approaches to performance skills. The direct application of the approach, not associated with activity, can be considered an enabling method "to prepare the client or patient for better performance and prevention of disability through self-participation in occupation."[14] Many occupational therapists have developed expertise in the application of these approaches. This is necessary if the approaches are to be scientifically applied during purposeful activity. The development of methods for their application to purposeful activity is limited at this time. These approaches need to be studied and their appropriate uses integrated into an occupational therapy framework. It is necessary to expand knowledge of the logical continuity beyond inhibition-facilitation techniques to activity and to the ways in which sensorimotor treatment principles can be applied during the performance of purposeful activity.[28] When used to precede and enable purposeful activity and as part of a purposeful activity, the sensorimotor approaches can be viable methods in the occupational performance frame of reference.

Rehabilitation approach

The term *rehabilitation* means a return to ability. This means the return to the fullest physical, mental, social, vocational, and economic usefulness that is possible for the individual. It means to be able to live and work with remaining capabilities.[16] Therefore the focus in the treatment program is on abilities rather than disabilities.

Rehabilitation is concerned with the intrinsic worth and dignity of the individual and with the restoration of a satisfying and purposeful life. In some sense the rehabilitation approach uses measures that enable a person to live as independently as possible with some residual disability. Its goal is to help the client learn to work around or compensate for physical limitations.

The rehabilitation approach is a dynamic process and requires that the client be a member of the rehabilitation team. It requires ongoing assessment and follow-up to maintain maximal function and therefore must keep pace with the scientific advances in methods and equipment (rehabilitation technology), social change, and community resources to provide the best services and opportunities for each client.[16]

RELATIONSHIP TO OCCUPA-TIONAL PERFORMANCE. In this approach occupational therapy focuses on performance skills more than on performance components. The aim of the occupational therapy program is to effect role performance and to minimize the barriers of residual disability to role performance. The occupational therapist must assess the client's capabilities and determine assets to facilitate the client's overcoming the effects of the disability on function. The treatment methods of the rehabilitation approach include:

1. Self-care evaluation and training
2. Acquisition and training in assistive devices
3. Use of adapted clothing
4. Homemaking and child care
5. Work simplification and energy conservation
6. Use of prevocational activities
7. Use of leisure activities
8. Prosthetic training
9. Wheelchair management
10. Home evaluation and adaptation
11. Transportation
12. Architectural adaptations
13. Acquisition and training in the use of communication aids and devices

INTEGRATION WITH OTHER APPROACHES. Frequently the methods of the rehabilitation approach are used in combination with the biomechanical or neurosensory approaches. First, biomechanical or neurosensory principles can be applied during rehabilitation activities to enhance and reinforce the restoration of the motor or sensory-integrative components. Second, in reality the treatment program often focuses on performance skills and performance components simultaneously. In this way the restoration of motor, sensory-integrative, cognitive, and psychosocial functions are combined to result in improvement of performance skills and thus role function.

Cognitive, psychological, and social performance components

In an examination of the treatment approaches described previously, the cognitive, psychological, and social performance components in the occupational performance frame of reference are not explicitly considered. The occupational performance frame of reference demands the consideration of life space influences, such as culture and human and nonhuman environment. These include genetic, biological, cultural, social, and environmental influences on the organism. Di Joseph[9] urges occupational therapists to consider not only motor control but motor behavior, that is, "a person acting purposefully within and upon his or her environment." She stated further that ignoring the emotive and cognitive aspects of motor behavior is a reductionistic approach that fails to consider all factors in the production of "purposeful action."[9] Treatment goals for clients must be based on a combination of mind, body, and environment; these goals should be reached through the use of activities that are compatible with the needs and values of the person and not necessarily with those of the therapist.[9] Interaction between the person and the environment is essential to the development of functional independence.[31] The person is mind and body, not just a motor system to be evaluated and "treated."

The occupational performance frame of reference is holistic in its application to the client and, as such, demands consideration of the cognitive, social, and psychological functions of the client for its application. These components must be assessed and included in the treatment program. Therapeutic use of self, individual, and group approaches described in Chapter 2 of this text is a way of dealing with these components. These approaches can often be integrated with methods for improvement of motor and sensory-integrative functions, such as the use of a woodwork group or a dance and exercise program for the improvement of motor function and the development of self-esteem and social skills.

CURRENT TRENDS

In the practice area of physical dysfunction there is evidence that the use of purposeful activity as occupational therapy has declined and the treatment methods that are used have changed significantly over the years.[3,8,11,24,33]

There has been a tendency toward reductionism in practice. The primary emphasis of reductionism is on a technique approach, and the focus of treatment is on one or more performance components and little integration with performance skills or vice versa. This continues to be a dominant influence in practice. Since the 1960s, there has been a growing awareness of the need to formulate a more adequate way to think about occupation and functional independence.[31]

Several authors contend that the occupational therapy profession is currently in a state of crisis.[6,11,19] The crisis is considered a result of the lack of a unified, systematic philosophy of occupational therapy practice. To appreciate the current crisis in occupational therapy it is necessary to review the historical development of the philosophy of occupational therapy.

Historical view

MORAL TREATMENT. Occupational therapy's philosophical roots extend to the period of moral treatment in early nineteenth-century America. The philosophy of moral treatment was derived from the cultural and political attitudes that dominated that time and was based on the idea that mentally ill individuals need to be engaged in creative and recreational activity with their fellow citizens. According to Bockoven[4]

The mentally deranged person best recovers his reason when accompanied by persons of sound mind and kindly nature who would help him by joining in the regimen of daily life. The regimen of daily life consisted of recreational and creative activity with others.[4]

The focus of moral treatment consisted of providing activity programs, such as ward work, craft shops, gardening, and outdoor game areas for the mentally ill. Adolf Meyer[23] summed up the philosophy of moral treatment by stating that the unique feature of people is their ability to organize time through activity. Meyer believed that even under difficulty people maintain a balance through actual doing or practice. Until the demise of moral treatment in 1900, activity was the fundamental medium of treatment for the neuropsychiatric patient.

1917 TO 1941. Occupational therapy formally began in 1917 as a result of the rebirth of moral treatment in psychiatry and the number of chronically disabled soldiers returning from World War I. Occupational therapy services were extended to include the treatment of the physically disabled. According to Woodside[40] the role of "occupational therapy in rehabilitation was one of using crafts to reactivate the minds and motivation of the mentally ill and the limbs of the veterans, starting them on the way to vocational training." Emphasis was placed heavily on craft and activity programs. The concept of activity was an effective philosophical base for the profession throughout the 1920s and 1930s. During that time, occupational therapy literature discussed activities as the fundamental treatment modality.[3] However, the depression years (1929 to 1941) had a substantial impact on the practice of occupational therapy. Budgets were cut and staff was limited. Therapists did not believe that occupational therapy could stand alone as a viable and independent profession. Occupational therapists sought alliance with the American Medical Association (AMA) to implement the Minimum Standards of Training to "establish standards for training institutions, and to accredit each new school . . . the powerful AMA came to the rescue."[30] The profession became a medical ancillary. Occupational therapy came under increasing pressure to think in reductionistic terms. The philosophy of activity was challenged by the medical community in both psychiatry and physiatrics.[19]

REHABILITATION MOVEMENT (1942 TO 1960). After World War II, occupational therapy joined the rehabilitation movement. As a result, the values, ideas, and activities related to the disabled were altered. According to Mosey[25]

Once involved, occupational therapists were uncomfortable with their simple operating principle that it was good for disabled people to keep active and busy doing things they enjoyed. Rather the occupational therapist borrowed techniques from other disciplines.

Emphasis was placed on acquiring techniques, such as progressive resistive exercises, neuromuscular facilitation, activities of daily living, prosthetic training, and making orthotic devices. The advantage of this trend was that physical disabilities therapists became proficient in the use of various treatment techniques. The disadvantage was that these techniques were practiced without integrating them into the concept of purposeful activity and without articulating a philosophical base. Emphasis was placed on technique acquisition rather than on development of a philosophical base.

1960 TO 1980. By the 1960s the profession recognized that occupational therapists had not only accepted reductionistic thinking but that this mode of thinking had replaced the original emphasis on purposeful activity or occupation. Reductionism had led to a precise and extensive technology for the treatment of a wide range of physical disabilities. This technical orientation resulted in a gradual erosion of the philosophical base underlying the profession. There was a shift in practice away from a broad philosophical base to a practice based on techniques.

Occupational therapy literature in the 1960s explored the need for change in the profession. There was and still is a growing concern over the inadequacies of the philosophical base supporting occupational therapy.[19]

1980 TO 1984. According to an article by Kielhofner[17] two different viewpoints regarding purposeful activity or occupation as the philosophical foundation of the profession currently exist. The first viewpoint sees the development of the occupational therapy profession as being in a process of continuous adaptation. In the process of adapting to meet the changing times and health-care needs, the profession has disavowed "activity . . . as a generic philosophy."[17] Proponents of this first perspective view purposeful activity or occupation as an impractical philosophical premise.

In contrast, proponents of the second viewpoint argue that the profession's earlier philosophical premise regarding purposeful activity or occupation offered a unique and accurate theoretical base to occupational therapy. Current occupational therapy practice is viewed as seriously deviating from the early philosophical premises of the field.[18,33] This last viewpoint acknowledges that current beliefs must be reunited with the earlier philosophy of occupational therapy. The term *occupation* is suggested as a concept that will enable the field to reestablish a continuity between current beliefs and the historical first beliefs of the profession.[17]

The acceptance and rejection of activity

The use of purposeful activity or occupation has characterized the profession throughout its history. Since its conception, occupational therapy has been founded on the idea that being engaged in activity (1) restores health in individuals suffering from either mental or physical dysfunction and (2) maintains the well-being of the healthy individual.[8] Activity is not only viewed as the core of occupational therapy but also as the unique feature of the profession.

In physical disabilities practice there is evidence of a decline in the use of activities and a concomitant increase in the use of other treatment modalities.[3,11,33] Shannon[33] called the profession's movement away from the traditional philosophy "the derailment of occupational therapy." He stated that a

new philosophy has developed that "views man as a mechanistic creature susceptible to manipulation and control via the application of techniques."[33] This "technique philosophy" contradicts the philosophy on which the profession was founded. According to Shannon the profession is now faced with two alternatives. The first alternative is to ignore the crisis between the traditional and the contemporary "technique philosophy." The second alternative is to reinstate the traditional "values and beliefs on which the profession was founded and thereby arrest the process of derailment."[33]

A study by Bissell and Mailloux[3] in 1981 explored the use of crafts in occupational therapy for the physically disabled. This study employed a survey of 250 occupational therapists in the United States who chose physical disabilities as their specialty section. The results of this study showed that 72% of the respondents used crafts as a treatment modality. Of these, 51% used some crafts 20% or less of the treatment time. The greatest percentage of treatment time was devoted to self-care activities and therapeutic exercise. The authors concluded that "if therapeutic crafts are no longer considered a central concept of occupational therapy, there may be a need to revise the curricula pertaining to craft use."[3]

Fidler[11] stated that occupational therapists have disclaimed activities and identified with the modalities of other professions to achieve credibility. These modalities "eliminate the self as the doer-agent and place the causative agent outside the self."[11] According to Fidler "when occupational therapists are comfortable labeling a significant part of their practice as 'unproductive activity,' the fundamental principles of occupational therapy are denied."[11]

During the past two decades, newer sensorimotor and neurophysiological approaches have developed. Clinical emphasis on these approaches has increased, whereas emphasis on activities has decreased. According to Cynkin[8] occupational therapists have incorporated these newer techniques into practice without looking at how they relate to an activity-oriented philosophical base for treatment. In the process of acquiring these techniques, occupational

therapists have disavowed the use of activities as the core of occupational therapy.[8]

Trend reversal

In an attempt to reestablish activities as the core of occupational therapy, the Representative Assembly of the American Occupational Therapy Association passed Resolution No. 531-79 in April 1979. The resolution stated that the Association shall adopt a single philosophical base of occupational therapy (cited previously).

Purposeful activity is the key concept in the philosophical base. Additionally, a survey of the professional literature from 1915 to 1977 revealed that purposeful activity was the second most frequently used term that consistently appeared in the literature.[13]

Despite the historical occurrence of the term, a definition of purposeful activity (cited previously) was not officially adopted by the profession until 1983.[15] Although open to interpretation, this definition of purposeful activity appears to be in concert with the traditional philosophy of occupational therapy and the concept of human occupation.

In response to the attempt of the American Occupational Therapy Association to promote the use of purposeful activity as the core of occupational therapy practice, several therapists expressed concern about the restrictions that purposeful activity would place on practice in physical disabilities.[7,10,36] These restrictions include, but are not limited to, (1) jeopardizing reimbursement, (2) negating the skills and knowledge achieved by experienced clinicians, (3) jeopardizing referrals, and (4) excluding techniques, such as exercise, range of motion, splinting, and inhibition-facilitation techniques. These issues stem from an unclear or unacceptable definition of purposeful activity that excludes exercise.[36] These therapists believe that tying treatment methods to purposeful activity is not always appropriate or effective. Many patients receiving occupational therapy are not yet at an appropriate level of motor activity to participate in purposeful activity. In these circumstances, it is argued, the clinicians must use "adjunctive" treatment techniques to assist in the development of motor ability needed to participate in purposeful activity. Adjunctive techniques, as described by Trombly,[36] include electrical stimulation, biofeedback, massage, whirlpool therapy, and thermal application. Therapists holding this viewpoint believe that the profession's history of purposeful activity should not be denied. However, they believe that the definition of purposeful activity needs to be expanded to incorporate contemporary treatment techniques. It is believed that, instead of attempting to redirect the focus of the profession, the profession needs to include current clinical practices that have proved effective on an empirical and practical basis.[36]

Concern has been expressed that, although purposeful activity may have been one of the unifying concepts of occupational therapy in the past, this philosophical base no longer promotes cohesiveness in the profession.[22,28] Pedretti[28] stated that purposeful activity "may have served to identify, define and articulate a disunity that has existed . . . for years." Lyons[22] reaffirmed this viewpoint in her statement that although purposeful activity "has been one of the unifying concepts of occupational therapy in the past, . . . today the use of this term seems more devisive than unifying."[22] She also stated that the phrase purposeful activity "has become an umbrella for a heterogeneous bag of human endeavors."[22] For some therapists the term *purposeful activity* means crafts, games, or activities of daily living. Other therapists include exercise and physical modalities in their own personal definitions of purposeful activity. Lyons warned that, by allowing the term to "mean all things to all people," purposeful activity is loosing "its power to direct and influence" the profession.[22]

Trombly[36] expressed the need for a clear definition of purposeful, goal-directed activity that takes into account theories of central motor control and motor acquisition. Such a definition would have to be a working one and tested by research.[36]

A definition of purposeful activity on a continuum that changes with the changing health status, values, and skills of the client and culminates in the performance of tasks essential to life roles[28] could be developed to include both the enabling or "adjunctive" treatment modalities and modalities that have been traditionally considered purposeful activity. Such a definition might satisfy both perspectives in the debate and would reflect the fact that occupational therapy has a service to offer at virtually every stage in the rehabilitation process. That service is one of the stimulation, integration, and continuous development of adaptive responses that enable and result in occupational performance.[28]

Rogers[31] contends that, although the current debate tends to center around the use of arts and crafts in treatment, the real issue is whether a skills or subskills approach is best for dealing with the problems of the physically disabled in managing activities of daily living. She proposes that the solution lies in the development of a philosophical base that will allow a synthesis of the skills and subskills approaches. The occupational performance frame of reference proposes such a synthesis with its emphasis on skills (self-care, work, and play and leisure) and subskills (motor, sensory-integrative, cognitive, social, and psychological components).

Yet the selection of appropriate treatment modalities (especially those that are directed to the remediation of the subskills) within this frame of reference continues to be debated.[38] In addition, lawful use of modalities and competency to practice certain modalities are being questioned[38]; they must be considered in the debate on treatment modalities appropriate for occupational therapy.

SUMMARY

A view of the individual as an environment that requires balance for adaptation was proposed by Llorens.[21] If occupational therapists hold such a view, "the biological, psychological, and intrapersonal environment components of sensory, motor, psychological, sociological, and cognitive functions that permit interaction with the familial and cultural environment" must be considered.[21] The use of purposeful activity for self-care, work, play, leisure, and learning promotes such interactions.[21]

The occupational performance frame of reference makes the performance components, performance skills, and occupational theory operational in relation to the sociocultural and the biological-psychological environments. Occupational theory "refers to the inherent factors or properties of activity that elicit intrinsic reinforcement."[21] This theory is operative when occupational therapists prescribe and administer purposeful activity to bring about change in the individual's internal or external environments.[21]

The intrinsic goal of purposeful activity is generated from its inherent quality to arouse sensations, require processing of sensation, and elicit effective cognitive and motor responses that feed back into the individual system to effect balance. That purposeful activity facilitates change in the individual environment has been shown over time; its effectiveness needs to be verified through research.[21]

Llorens[21] concluded that occupational therapy practice must be founded on a holistic philosophy that uses purposeful activity or occupation. She claims that "the philosophy, theory, process in practice and frames of reference must be compatible" and that the techniques and modalities of occupational therapy must be congruent with its philosophical base, the science of occupation, occupational theory, and occupational behavior-performance frames of reference. The evaluation process and methods of the profession must allow the diagnosis of occupational dysfunction. Llorens made several recommendations to her professional colleagues. Among these were a commitment to (1) "unity of the profession;" (2) "the science of occupation;" and (3) "the ownership of the meaning of occupation and activity and the responsibility to explain the phenomenon."[21]

Rogers[32] called for a study of human occupation. She stated that occupation is the medium of therapy and, if it is to be used effectively, the occupational therapist needs a deep understanding of the health-enhancing nature of occupation.[32]

A definition of occupation cited by Rogers[34] is that it is "volitional, goal-directed behavior aimed at the development of play, work, and life skills for optimal time management." The study of human occupation is an important professional skill, since applying knowledge of occupation to those whose occupational performance is at risk or dysfunctional is the mission of occupational therapy. Three general areas of knowledge needed for effective application are "knowledge of normal occupational fuctions; knowledge of ineffective performance in occupational functions; and knowledge of the therapeutic properties of occupation."[32] A precise knowledge of occupation will allow occupational therapists to refine the focus of their practice and of the science of occupational therapy and permit a more adequate definition of the unique contribution of occupational therapy to health care.[32]

West[38] summarized the positive and negative aspects of the current debate over a common philosophical base and appropriate treatment modalities. Furthermore, she reviewed the origins, history, and possible causes of the loss of the scope of some of the traditional intervention strategies of occupational therapy and looked at the influence of social change and future social trends on occupational therapy practice. According to West[38] futuristic trends toward a more humanistic and holistic approach to disability and health is a significant reaffirmation of traditional philosophical and practice modes of occupational therapy.

As a conclusion, several recommendations for the rerooting of occupational therapy in its philosophical traditions were proffered. These included[38]:

1. The consistent use and implementation of the concept and the term *occupation* as the common core of occupational therapy
2. Speaking of the profession as serving the *occupational need of human beings* rather than as "treating the whole person," a claim that can be made by any of the health professions
3. The definition and organization of occupational therapy around occupational performance dysfunction rather than in terms of disabilities
4. The renewed commitment to the *mind-body-environment interrelationships* activated through occupation, one of the early tenets of occupational therapy

There are many commonalities in the recommendations of these experts. They are committed to the concept of occupation as the core of occupational therapy practice. The consideration of internal and external environmental interrelationships and the effect of occupation on the facilitation of these interrelationships are common themes of their writings. There is a strong recommendation for the focus of the profession to be on the occupational needs, roles, and role dysfunctions of the individual and on the foundation of occupational therapy on a holistic philosophy. The philosophy needs to be organized around occupational performance dysfunction rather than in terms of disabilities. Such a philosophy would expand the horizons of occupational therapy beyond the remediation of illness and disabilities to community and home settings. Perhaps clients served by therapists in these settings have occupational performance dysfunction because of environmental and sociocultural problems rather than only health problems.[21]

Modalities thought of as necessary for enabling the performance of purposeful activity have become commonplace in occupational therapy practice.[21] In some instances they are used exclusively and not tied to purposeful activity (occupation) in any way. Much debate has centered on the use of various modalities and their appropriateness in occupational therapy practice. Neither the occupational performance frame of reference nor the philosophical base of occupational therapy and the affirmations that accompanied it (adopted in 1979) negate the use of such preliminary activities.[1,14] Both, however, view such preliminary activities in the perspective of occupational role performance and recommend that they be used in that context. The selection of appropriate modalities, then, would provide a continuum of treatment from preparation, to sheltered trial, to satisfying occupational role performance, a process that is in progress in many treatment facilities. The selection of enabling treatment modalities must be guided by appropriate competency of the practitioner, lawful use, and their integration and relationship to *occupation* as the core concern of occupational therapy.

REVIEW QUESTIONS

1. Define "frame of reference."
2. Why is a frame of reference necessary?
3. Briefly outline the elements in the occupational performance frame of reference.
4. What is the difference between a "performance skill" and a "performance component"? How are they related?
5. Define "enabling" activities?
6. What is a key concept in the definition of occupational therapy? How is it related to the occupational performance frame of reference?
7. Define "purposeful activity."
8. Which treatment modalities can be thought of as primarily biomechanical in nature?
9. With which diagnoses is a biomechanical approach most likely to be used? Why?
10. How does the biomechanical approach fit into the occupational performance frame of reference?
11. For which diagnoses are the sensorimotor approaches most likely to be effective?
12. How can the sensorimotor approaches be integrated in an occupational performance framework?
13. Define what is meant by "rehabilitation approach."
14. List six treatment modalities that would be considered within the rehabilitation approach?
15. How is the rehabilitation approach integrated with the other approaches to treatment discussed in this chapter?
16. Discuss the current trends in occupational therapy practice in physical disabilities.
17. Identify the current controversy regarding philosophies and modalities and suggest possible solutions.

REFERENCES

1. American Occupational Therapy Association: A curriculum guide for occupational therapy educators, Rockville, Md., 1974, American Occupational Therapy Association.
2. Ayres, A.J.: Basic concepts of clinical practice in physical disabilities, Am. J. Occup. Ther. **12**:300, 1958.
3. Bissell, J.C., and Mailloux, Z.: The use of crafts in occupational therapy for the physically disabled, Am. J. Occup. Ther. **35**:369, 1981.
4. Bockoven, J.S.: Legacy of moral treatment: 1800s to 1910, Am. J. Occup. Ther. **25**:223, 1971.

5. Brunnstrom, S.: Clinical kinesiology, ed. 3, Philadelphia, 1972, F.A. Davis Co.
6. Clark, P.N.: Human development through occupation: theoretical frameworks in contemporary occupational therapy practice. Part 1, Am. J. Occup. Ther. **33**:505, 1979.
7. Courtsunis, D.G., et al.: Purposeful activity restricts practice (Letters to the editor), Am. J. Occup. Ther. **36**:468, 1982.
8. Cynkin, S.: Occupational therapy: toward health through activities, Boston, 1979, Little, Brown & Co.
9. Di Joseph, L.M.: Independence through activity: mind, body, and environment interaction in therapy, Am. J. Occup. Ther. **36**:740, 1982.
10. English, C., et al.: On the role of the occupational therapist in physical disabilities (The Issue) Am. J. Occup. Ther. **36**:199, 1982.
11. Fidler, G.S.: From crafts to competence, Am. J. Occup. Ther. **35**:567, 1981.
12. Fidler, G.S., and Fidler, J.W.: Doing and becoming: purposeful action and self-actualization, Am. J. Occup. Ther. **32**:305, 1978.
13. Gillette, N., and Keilhofner, G.: The impact of specialization on the professionalization and survival of occupational therapy. Am. J. Occup. Ther. **33**:20, 1979.
14. Highlights of actions taken by the Representative Assembly during its recent meeting, Occupational Therapy Newspaper, p. 1, Rockville, Md., June 1979. The American Occupational Therapy Association.
15. Hinojosa, J., et al.: Purposeful activities, Am. J. Occup. Ther. **37**:805, 1983.
16. Hopkins, H.L., Smith, H.D., and Tiffany, E.G.: Rehabilitation. In Hopkins, H.L., and Smith, H.D., editors: Willard and Spackman's occupational therapy, ed. 6, Philadelphia, 1983, J.B. Lippincott Co.
17. Kielhofner, G.: A heritage of activity: development of theory, Am. J. Occup. Ther. **36**:723, 1982.
18. Kielhofner, G., and Burke, J.P.: Occupational therapy after 60 years: an account of changing identity and knowledge, Am. J. Occup. Ther. **31**:675, 1977.
19. Kielhofner, G., and Burke, J.P.: A model of human occupation. I. Conceptual framework and content, Am. J. Occup. Ther. **34**:572, 1980.
20. King, L.J.: Toward a science of adaptive responses, Am. J. Occup. Ther. **32**:429, 1978.
21. Llorens, L.: Changing balance: environment and individual, Am. J. Occup. Ther. **38**:29, 1984.
22. Lyons, B.G.: The issue is: purposeful versus human activity, Am. J. Occup. Ther. **37**:493, 1983.
23. Meyer, A.: The philosophy of occupational therapy, Am. J. Occup. Ther. **31**:630, 1977.
24. Moore, J.: Changing methods in the treatment of physical dysfunction, Am. J. Occup. Ther. **21**:18, 1967.
25. Mosey, A.C.: Involvement in the rehabilitation movement: 1942-1960, Am. J. Occup. Ther. **25**:234, 1971.
26. Mosey, A.C.: Occupational therapy: configuration of a profession, New York, 1981, Raven Press.
27. Occupational therapy: its definition and functions, Am. J. Occup. Ther. **26**:204, 1972.
28. Pedretti, L.W.: The compatibility of treatment methods in physical disabilities with the philosophical base of occupational therapy, Paper presented to the American Occupational Therapy Association National Conference, Philadelphia, May, 1982.
29. Project to delineate the roles and functions of occupational therapy personnel, Rockville, Md., 1972, American Occupational Therapy Association. Cited in A curriculum guide for occupational therapy educators, Rockville, Md., 1974, American Occupational Therapy Association.
30. Rerek, M.D.: The depression years: 1929 to 1941, Am. J. Occup. Ther. **25**:231, 1971.
31. Rogers, J.C.: The spirit of independence: the evolution of a philosophy, Am. J. Occup. Ther. **36**:709, 1982.
32. Rogers, J.C.: The foundation: why study human occupation? Am. J. Occup. Ther. **38**:47, 1984.
33. Shannon, P.D.: The derailment of occupational therapy, Am. J. Occup. Ther. **31**:229, 1977.
34. Shannon, P.D.: Project to identify the philosophy of occupational therapy, Rockville, Md., 1983, American Occupational Therapy Association (unpublished). Cited in Rogers, J.C.: The foundation: why study human occupation? Am. J. Occup. Ther. **38**:47, 1984.
35. Stockmeyer, S.A.: An interpretation of the approach of Rood to the treatment of neuromuscular dysfunction, Am. J. Phys. Med. **46**:900, 1967.
36. Trombly, C.A.: Include exercise in purposeful activity (Letters to the editor), Am. J. Occup. Ther. **36**:467, 1982.
37. Trombly, C.A., editor: Occupational therapy for physical dysfunction, ed. 2, Baltimore, 1983, The Williams & Wilkins Co.
38. West, W.: A reaffirmed philosophy and practice of occupational therapy for the 1980s, Am. J. Occup. Ther. **38**:15, 1984.
39. Willard, H.L., and Spackman, C.S., editors: Occupational therapy, ed. 4, Philadelphia, 1971, J.B. Lippincott Co.
40. Woodside, H.H.: The development of occupational therapy: 1910-1929, Am. J. Occup. Ther. **25**:226, 1971.

CHAPTER 2

Psychosocial aspects of physical dysfunction

LORRAINE WILLIAMS PEDRETTI

PSYCHOSOCIAL CONSEQUENCES OF PHYSICAL DYSFUNCTION

The experience of loss of any physical part or function involves not only the painful distortion of body image and the image of oneself as a physical being but also the image of self as a social being whose family and social roles and vocational and leisure occupations may be unalterably changed. Independence, self-sufficiency, and autonomy may have to be given up partially or totally, temporarily or permanently.[6]

The onset of physical dysfunction necessitates a sudden change in daily life. The individual is likely to be thrown into the new world and lifestyle of a health care facility where there is enforced passivity and dependence. The newly disabled person must adapt to a new environment, new personnel, new food, and new time schedules. Privacy must be surrendered and virtual strangers must be allowed to probe the body. The person may be devastated by the drastic interruption of familial, occupational, and social roles.[10] Previous roles may be slightly changed, seriously impaired, or completely eliminated as a result of the disability. The damage to previously held roles may be due directly to the disability or may indirectly result from changed life circumstances brought about by the disability.[15]

The onset of physical disability affects the person who has the disability and all of those with whom he or she comes in contact. The individual's particular response and the responses of others to the disability will have a significant impact on rehabilitation personnel and on the rehabilitation process.[17] The disabled adult is confronted with the task of survival, first, then with regaining essential physical skills, and finally, the greater goals of resuming meaningful life roles. These are monumental and formidable tasks that require managing many overwhelming personal problems and overcoming external blockades to readjustment.[15]

Personal reactions to physical dysfunction

As a result of the major life changes brought about by the onset of physical dysfunction, the individual's defense mechanisms are highly taxed as he or she attempts to deal with the changed social interactions and sexual patterns and the ability to direct his or her own life and to control the environment through physical action. Concomitantly the individual is dealing with fears, realistic and unrealistic, physical pain and suffering, and the symbolic meaning of the physical dysfunction. Changed attitudes of family and friends may provoke stress, fears, and expectations that others will react differently and reject him or her.[10,22]

Individual reactions to physical dysfunction depend on the previously held body image and compromise body image and the psychological meaning of the specific dysfunction in relation to the individual's personality.[22] Paraplegia may have a very different meaning to an athlete who defines self-worth in terms of physical performance and physique than to an office worker whose sense of self may be defined more in terms of use of head and hands, for instance.

Although it is commonly believed that physical dysfunction generates only negative and disruptive psychological reactions, it has been found that opportunities and gratification may be generated as well.[20] The dysfunction may be regarded as a well-deserved punishment, especially if it is associated with an unsuccessful suicide attempt, asocial behavior, or the death of another. This attitude could gratify masochistic wishes and paradoxically lead to a greater sense of well-being.[10,22] The dysfunction may be seen as the final confirmation of a lack of self-worth and could precipitate a suicide or psychotic reaction.[22] The gratification of longed for dependency on a caring person leading to relative comfort may be satisfied by the dysfunction. Conversely the reawakening of intolerable dependency longings and rage related to a lack of satisfaction of early dependency needs can result in marked anxiety or a paranoid reaction.[10,22] Exhibitionistic wishes and the need to manipulate and control others may also be satisfied through the physical dysfunction. The dysfunction may be used as a means of expressing hostility or avoiding responsibilities by some individuals.[10] Conversely the onset of dysfunction may lead to constructive, alternative life roles and offer social and career opportunities that were not contemplated by the individual before the onset of the physical dysfunction.

Great emphasis and value are placed on productivity and on physical attractiveness in the American culture. To not have achieved them or be in the process of achieving them may evoke feelings of self-devaluation. Feelings of low worth tend to be all-or-none in quality. They may be evoked by consideration of only one characteristic out of many by the disabled person, yet the person may conceive of self as all worthless. The feelings of low self-worth also tend to extend into the past and into the future so that the person can neither conceive of self as ever having been productive or attractive nor contemplate the possibility of future change.

The conclusions of worthlessness are in a sense true, since they are based on a self-definition in terms of degree of productivity and attractiveness. This is a distortion, since it bases the self-worth on deficits and overlooks the remaining assets and intrinsic worth. Although the concept of intrinsic worth, that is, the person is valued for self alone without external comparisons, is desirable and ideal, it is probably difficult or impossible to achieve for most people. In general, people in American society value themselves according to external standards of attractiveness, productivity, and achievements.

Disabled persons may conclude that they are worthless and of negative value and therefore that they are "awful" as well. They may expect and think that they deserve the rejection of others based on that notion. If they are not of any value to themselves, then others will not see them as valuable and therefore will reject them. This kind of thinking can persist for long periods of time and may account for withdrawal behavior or an intense search for approval and love. Some persons will draw this thinking process to what seems like a logical conclusion, which is they are worth nothing to self or to others, therefore life is meaningless and empty and they should not exist. This feeling may be especially strong in those who have intense guilt feelings.[7]

It has been assumed by many that a certain type of personality or adjustment pattern is associated with a specific physical disability or that the degree and type of dysfunction will cause psychological maladjustment. These premises have been refuted by research. It has been concluded that particular personality types or characteristics are not associated with specific dysfunctions nor is there evidence to support the notion that the severity or type of disability is correlated with the degree of psychological adjustment.[20]

Societal reactions to physical dysfunction

Attitudes of others toward physical disability affect attitudes toward oneself. A physically handicapped individual reflects attitudes of self-depreciation. In the newly disabled, devaluing attitudes toward the disabled, once an out-group, may now be directed to the self with very serious consequences.[20] Physical dysfunction was once considered divine punishment or evidence of sinfulness. This is still the belief of some individuals. It is more likely to be viewed as ugly, loathsome, or, at the very least, discomforting. Few people are really comfortable with disabled or deformed individuals. Their presence constitutes a threat to the nondisabled about their own vulnerability. To avoid the threatening feeling the nondisabled reject or avoid disabled or

deformed persons.[22] The appearance of the injury or disability also engenders nonacceptance. If the disability is unsightly, this tends to be overestimated by the nondisabled and is a factor that prompts rejection or avoidance. The nondisabled may display unwarranted pity or excessive curiosity. The disabled person feels set apart from most "normal" people and is constantly striving to fight the negative implications of the physical dysfunction and gain genuine social acceptance. Nonacceptance resides in the nondisabled and stems from negative attitudes. It is a resistance or a reluctance to enter into various degrees of social interchange with the disabled person and carries an aura of ostracism.

Disabled individuals perceive a lack of patience on the part of the nondisabled toward performance ease and speed. Whether this attitude is maintained by the nondisabled or is projected by the disabled, it engenders the same feeling of nonacceptance in the disabled person.

The disabled person may perceive an apparent rather than a genuine social acceptance by the nondisabled. The latter may be perceived as motivated by pity or duty and may offer empty gestures of acceptance devoid of meaning or real pleasure in the interchange. Apparent acceptance is not more desirable than nonacceptance. In each the disabled see the underlying inability or unwillingness on the part of the nondisabled to know them as they really are.

Another tendency of the nondisabled is to judge the disabled not only in terms of the apparent physical limitation but also in terms of psychological factors assumed to be concomitant to the disability.[16] The nondisabled may treat the physically disabled as if they were limited mentally and emotionally as well.[5] The evaluation of the visible disability is spread to other characteristics that are not necessarily affected. The frequent assumption that a person who has cerebral palsy is also mentally retarded and the practice of speaking loudly to a blind person as if also deaf are examples of this phenomenon. It is generally a devaluing process, and the disabled person is thereby stigmatized and considered of lower social status and unworthy of acceptance.[16]

Words exist in the language of

American culture that have a stigmatizing effect on the disabled. Expressions such as "retard," "crip," and "psycho" are examples. Within the language of the medical and allied health professions these terms become formalized to "mentally retarded," "physically disabled," and "mentally ill." These terms have value for the classification of persons into diagnostic categories, but they stigmatize as well.[5] It follows that when rehabilitation workers refer to their clients as a diagnosis or disability (for example, "quad" or "hemi"), they are contributing to the stigmatization of those who they set out to help.

Stigma may be considered as negative perceptions or behaviors of normal people toward the physically disabled or toward all persons different from themselves. Physically disabled persons are regarded in much the same way as other minority groups in the population. They are subject to stereotyping and a reduced social status. Stigmatization is a basic fact of life for nearly all disabled persons. Interpersonal relationships between the nondisabled and the disabled tend to follow a superior-inferior pattern or to not exist at all. The nondisabled tend to demonstrate stereotyped, inhibited, and overcontrolled behavior in interactions with disabled persons. They tend to show less variable behavior, terminate interactions sooner, and express opinions less representative of their actual beliefs.

There is a substantial amount of segregation of the physically disabled. Although some of this segregation is necessary (for example, institutionalization or special schools) and designed to assist disabled persons, it nevertheless sets them apart psychologically and evokes feelings of inferiority in relation to nondisabled peers. This kind of segregation should be minimized. The fact that restrictive legislation exists in reference to disabled persons testifies to the systematized stigmatization of the disabled within American society.[5]

The health care facility can be considered a microcosm of society. There is a tendency for health care workers to believe that societal prejudices toward the disabled do not exist in the facility. The assumption is that rehabilitation personnel are immune from discriminatory attitudes and that clients are accepted as persons when they are accepted as clients.[8]

The clients view themselves as disabled and unable to perform and perceive themselves as applicants asking the knowledgeable, powerful, and authoritative others if they can regain the characteristics and skills of nondisabled persons. The clients confront a closed, self-sufficient subculture with an unfamiliar value system and are, in fact, outsiders in the facility seeking acceptance from omnipotent persons in authority. The clients occupy the lowest level in the status hierarchy of the institution and are manipulated by many forces over which they have no control. Individual life goals may be partly or completely determined by others and choices and decisions imposed under a facade of personal involvement and self-determination. There is segregation of staff and clients throughout the facility that parallels the exclusion of disabled persons by nondisabled persons in the real world, and the physical impairment is the symbol of that exclusion.[8]

Although the staff may hold the view that prejudice does not exist in the facility, in reality, the view of the staff is that the client is one to be helped, a malleable individual who can be shaped and educated into a specific health status and behavior. Convictions of superiority are reinforced by the emergence of a teacher-student relationship, a superior-inferior pattern.[8] This pattern is further reinforced by the segregated dining areas, the uniforms of the staff, and the organizational hierarchy of the institution.

To change this, it is necessary for the rehabilitation worker to shed the role of a teacher and authority and to assume the role of a facilitator and guide. Segregation in the facility needs to be abandoned to the extent possible, perhaps in the dining and recreation areas. The recognition and respect for different needs, goals, and value systems other than their own can change the attitudes of health care workers toward their clients. Real involvement of the client in the decision-making process for treatment and in patient government can also be helpful in reducing the prejudice and equalizing the status of the residents of the health care facility.

ORIGINS OF ATTITUDES TOWARD DISABILITY. Some of the origins of negative attitudes toward the physically disabled can be found in the way they have been represented in the media and literature.[2] Another source can be traced to scripture.[14]

Traditional children's literature contributes to the stereotyping of the disabled. Physical deformity, illness, and, at the very least, unattractiveness often symbolize inner defects, evil natures, and villainous behavior in children's literature.[23] Some of the oldest and best known children's stories convey prejudices and stereotype the disabled. These stories can be a subtle form of teaching children scorn for the handicapped. Examples of such characters are Cinderella's stepsisters who were obese and unattractive or Captain Hook of *Peter Pan* who wore a prosthesis. The wicked witch of *Hansel and Gretel* was aged, arthritic, and had a kyphosis.[2] Gigantism affected the character whom Jack met at the top of the beanstalk in *Jack and the Beanstalk*.

An examination of these and other well-known stories reveals that physical attractiveness, health, and intactness of the body are usually features of the heroes and heroines, the noble and the good, while the villains are often portrayed with some infirmity or unattractive features, such as large noses, wrinkles, and warts. The association of moral character and personality is thus made with the external appearance.[23]

Some stories show physical disability as a consequence of a misdeed. Pinocchio's nose grew as a result of his failure to tell the truth, whereas pirates lost eyes and limbs as a result of their violent behavior.[23]

There have been almost no average ordinary physically abnormal individuals in children's stories in the past. More recently several children's books that portray the disabled in a more favorable and matter-of-fact manner have been published.[1,4,18,19,23]

This same type of stereotyping occurs in television programs, movies, cartoons, comic strips, and adult fiction. Although it is not possible to eliminate classical children's literature, it is possible for parents and others reading this literature to children to be aware of the biases that may be conveyed and to discuss and reflect on

them with the children to minimize the unquestioned acceptance of these portrayals.[23] Fortunately, children today are much more matter-of-fact about handicaps, since they are likely to have handicapped classmates, and there is open discussion of handicaps in the classroom.[2]

The question still must be asked how it came about that these characters were portrayed in these ways.[2] Thurer[23] believes that the stereotyping in literature reflects the subtle prejudice of the Judeo-Christian ethic that fosters the notion that God has smiled on those who are whole and successful, whereas those who are wrongdoers are rewarded with suffering and physical defects.[23] In the pagan world suffering was regarded as a result of the god's displeasure with man.

Many people have grown up with the notion that God is all wise, all loving, and all powerful. He is seen as a parent figure who rewards for obedience and who disciplines for disobedience. He protects those in His favor from harm and arranges for each person to get what he deserves in life.[14] If this premise is accepted, then the question must be considered: "Why do bad things happen to good people?"[14] This question is raised when personal tragedy is experienced and when there are daily media confrontations with seemingly senseless tragedies that occur everywhere and to all types of people. It is troubling to know that suffering is distributed unfairly in the world. For many, this awareness raises questions about the goodness and even the existence of God. Kushner[14] outlines various popular explanations of suffering based on this notion of God and then discusses the faulty reasoning in each.[14]

Some of the most common notions of the causes of suffering that are based on scripture are that (1) suffering is punishment for sin (Isaiah 3:10-11 and Proverbs 3:7-8[3]), (2) suffering is for personal growth or testing of spiritual strength (Genesis 22[3]), and (3) suffering is a cure for personality flaws (Proverb 3:11-12[3]).[14]

The New Testament introduces the concept of suffering as a share in the glory of Jesus Christ (Romans 8:17[3]). Illness and disability are also sometimes shown as associated with the presence of demons (Matthew 8:16 and 8:28; Luke 9:37-43, 11:14, and 13:10-14[3]). However, there are also many accounts of healings in which there is no association with sin or evil spirits (Matthew 8:8-13, Mark 8:22-26, and Luke 17:11-18[3]).

Someone who believes that suffering is punishment for sin will believe that the suffering have gotten what they deserve. The difficulty arises when the individual cannot find a misdeed that deserves the punishment and may become angry at God or repress that anger to protect the perceived reputation of God as the fair and just parent.[14]

If the notion that suffering is for the enoblement of people to repair faulty aspects of the personality is accepted, then it follows that suffering is for the individual's own good, that God teaches a lesson with suffering, and that everything happens for a purpose, although that purpose may be obscure and known only to God. Another explanation of suffering is that God tests only those whom He knows are strong of spirit.[14] This generates the idea that those with afflictions are priviledged or chosen by God for a special role and may cause the believer to perceive the sufferer in an elevated status in God's sight. This idea does not explain all of those who break under the strain of their suffering and indeed who do not appear strong enough to deal with it.[14]

If the presence of demons as a cause of illness and disability is accepted, it may follow that there is some spiritual illness or defect, and if the demons are driven out with prayers of healing, the sufferer will surely get well. Although there are documented accounts of sudden and unexplained healings, it is not possible to say that there is a "formula" that works in every instance.

All of these responses or attempts at explaining tragedy assume that God is the cause of suffering. They attempt to explain why God would mete out suffering. Is it for the individual's own growth, is it divine punishment, or is it that God does not care what happens to human beings? Some approaches lead the believer to self-blame and foster the denial of reality and repression of true feelings. Kushner[14] asks his readers to consider the possibility that God does not cause suffering and that maybe it occurs for reasons other than the will of God. Perhaps God does not cause bad things to happen and the question is not "Why me?" but rather, "God see what is happening to me, can you help?" (Psalm 121:1-2[3]).[14] There may be some things God does not control. Some of the misfortunes that are visited on humanity may be the result of "bad luck," bad people, human weakness, random events, and the inflexible laws of nature.[14] Any health care worker or client who is wrestling with this question is well advised to read Kushner's book, *When Bad Things Happen To Good People*.[14]

Spiritual counseling is a necessary aspect of the treatment program for many clients. Therapists should recognize this need and make the appropriate referrals.

ADJUSTMENT TO PHYSICAL DYSFUNCTION

Since there is no direct relationship between the type of physical dysfunction and personality structure, physical injury or illness resulting in disability should be regarded as one of several life stresses to which the individual brings a unique repertoire of coping mechanisms and response patterns.[21] There is usually little or no prolonged effect on personality that results from physical dysfunction. Personality structure may be temporarily disordered by the crisis of physical change but appears to be capable of drawing on its resources and integrating the crisis experience into the self to become reestablished.[20]

The individual with physical dysfunction is faced with the problem of coping with fears and anxieties and maintaining a balance between conflicting needs and tendencies at a time when it is most difficult to cope and defenses are weakened. These anxieties may be dealt with by using a variety of defense mechanisms. Denial may be manifested by cheerfulness and an unrealistic lack of concern about the disabling condition. Undue involvement in hospital routines may be a sign of overactivity used to cope with underlying anxiety. Overdependency may be manifested by keeping family and personnel close by and having more attendant care than is realistically needed.

Bravado and aggressiveness may be used to cover helplessness and dependency and to hide deep fears and anxieties. Excessive talking may be a mechanism used to discharge emotional tension. Some individuals may be unusually cooperative and demonstrate considerable interest in details of the illness and treatment as a means of coping with fears and anxieties. Most of these defense mechanisms are not in the conscious awareness of the person employing them.[10]

According to Simon[22] the ultimate adjustment to the physical dysfunction is intimately related to the process of developing a new "compromise body image." The body image consists of multiple perceptions about the body based on past experience, current sensations, and personal investment in the body. The development of the body image is influenced by the attitudes and values of the culture and the views, values, and fantasies of the significant others in one's life. Parental attitudes about body parts and body functions are important factors in the development of the body image. All of the experiences and attitudes may result in an overvaluation of particular body parts and the perception of the body as good or bad, handsome or repugnant, lovable or unlovable. One may compare one's body to the bodies of others and develop derogatory attitudes toward the body or its parts. One may also develop mechanisms of compensation to obscure perceived stigma.

The ego may feel anxiety, shame, or disgust in relation to the body image and may develop defenses to avoid the unpleasant effect of an unacceptable body image. By using such defenses as denial, sublimation, repression, and overcompensation the person comes to accept the "compromise body image" that incorporates and modifies some of the unacceptable features. The compromise body image is an important factor in considering the emotional effects of physical dysfunction.

Most people who incur physical disability will initially experience worry and anxiety about the dysfunction. Old anxieties and fears about illness and disability will be evoked. The individual will experience realistic fears about the loss of security or loss of love from spouse, family, and friends. There is a loss of the fantasied future and a serious concern that the future may be dramatically altered.

Sadness and depression are to be expected for periods as long as 1 year. Depression is a mourning for the lost part or function. The lost part, function, and former body image are gradually surrendered, and there is resolution of anger. Psychic energy can then be freed for new activity, often for wholehearted involvement in rehabilitation efforts. The individual may compensate or even overcompensate for the loss in a healthy manner, and a new compromise body image emerges.[22]

Stages in adjustment to physical dysfunction

Kerr[12] described the adjustment to physical dysfunction as progressing through five stages. It is necessary to remember that the stages are points on a continuum and that all stages are not inevitable for all disabled persons. It is also important to understand the adjustment process, since there appears to be a relationship between the person's attitude toward the physical disability and the success of rehabilitation.

The stages are identified and described as follows:

1. Shock: "This isn't me."
2. Expectancy of recovery: "I'm sick but I'll get well."
3. Mourning: "All is lost."
4. Defensive A—healthy: "I'll go on in spite of it." Defensive B—pathological: Marked use of defenses to deny the effects of the disability.
5. Adjustment: "It's different but not bad."

SHOCK. The shock stage occurs during the early diagnostic and treatment period. The person lacks understanding that the body is ill or of the extent of the seriousness of the illness or injury. Because of these factors there may be an apparent lack of anxiety that appears to be unrealistic. As the reality of the situation becomes more apparent to the person, the reaction is ".This can't be me. It's a bad dream. I'll wake up, and this will all be gone." The disabled person is likely to blame the hospital and medical personnel for the lost ability to function. The feeling is "If I could only get out of here, I'd be all right." Psychologically the person is still a normal, able-bodied person, pursuing the same goals and doing the same things as before the onset of the disabling condition.

There is an incompatibility between the person's real physical situation and the mental image. This incompatibility may account for the person's apparently inappropriate references to the disability, situation, recovery, and future performance. At this stage body image is more potent than perceptions. Perceptions that are incompatible with the self-image are rejected.

There is also an inevitable testing of reality that occurs after the onset of disability, and when the fact of changed function comes into focus, the psychological situation changes. A pathological "denial of illness" may occur and some persons previously considered psychologically healthy remain in this stage.

EXPECTANCY OF RECOVERY. In this stage the person recognizes the illness but believes he or she will get well. Initially the individual *knows* he or she will recover. The client may make frequent references to getting well or being whole again and may discuss future plans in which full recovery or a normally functioning body is essential.

The individual's only goal is to get well. This may lead to the search for a cure and "shopping" from one physician or health agency to another. There is a preoccupation with the physical condition. Small improvements may be overestimated or misinterpreted. The person will do anything perceived as aiding recovery, since this is the primary goal. To the extent that it is believed that recovery will take place, motivation toward learning to function with a disability will be minimal.

The person believes realistically that the disability is a barrier to everything in life that is important and worthwhile. A whole body is needed to attain important personal goals. Therefore full recovery must be achieved before anything else can be undertaken.

A change in this belief system or movement toward the next stage comes about when the person is moved toward a condition more similar to normal living than to the state of being temporarily ill. Being transferred from an acute care setting to the rehabilitation unit, being sent home in a wheelchair, having therapy terminated, redirecting therapy to teaching the person to live with the disability, or being told that full recovery will not occur are some of the events that may precipitate mourning.

MOURNING. Mourning occurs when there is a shift from expectancy of recovery to the realization that the disability is permanent. This realization may be overwhelming and may require the intervention of specialists in psychiatry or psychology.

This stage is one of acute distress. All seems lost, and all former goals seem unattainable. Motivation to cope with the disability is gone. The person wants to give up and may contemplate suicide. If the individual is not allowed to express grief for the lost function or part because of the reprimands and attitudes of rehabilitation personnel and significant others, discussion of these feelings may be avoided and hostility toward those who forbid the expression of feelings may be demonstrated. The result is a "problem patient" who will not work and who spends much time complaining about the health agency procedures and personnel.[12]

The person may become resigned to this fate, believing that he or she is worthless and inadequate, and may remain at this stage in the process. The person may adopt the role of the invalid and become a permanent resident of a health care institution.[15] He or she simply lives and remains dependent and possibly hostile.

The disability is now seen as an impenetrable barrier to important life goals, and unlike the hope for recovery that characterized the previous stage, the goal of recovery is now seen as unrealistic.

To effect progress to the next stage the barrier imposed by disability must be decreased. To the degree that this is possible progress in adjustment and rehabilitation can be made. It may be possible to create situations in which previously held goals can be attained. However, since self-care activities were probably taken for granted, their accomplishment may not be seen as a positive goal by adults.

The person in this stage may also begin to mourn the loss of some psychological characteristics. The client may believe he or she has lost his "fight," "pride," or "faith," which can be more distressing than the physical loss. When this occurs it may be important to expose the person to situations in which disabled persons can be observed demonstrating these qualities. The person can then begin to realize that the disability is irrelevant for the attainment of some more basic goals.

DEFENSIVE A—HEALTHY. The defensive stage may be considered healthy if the person begins to deal with the disability and goes on in spite of it. Motivation to learn to function with the disability increases significantly. The person is pleased with his or her accomplishments and takes an active interest in being as normal as possible.

The disability barrier is being reduced and becomes less impenetrable. The person realizes the attainment of some goals that were held as a normal person. Some treasured experiences, albeit small, are still possible. The barrier is still present, however, but there is the discovery of ways to circumvent it. The person learns to achieve previously held goals by other routes. Other goals may remain unattainable, and the person may remain distressed by the areas perceived to be unachievable.

The movement toward adjustment comes through a changed need system. The need for a whole or normal body may be relinquished when important goals can be attained in spite of the disability. The goals are attainable, therefore the disability becomes less relevant. When physical impairment does in fact interfere with goal attainment, the person must relinquish the goals and discover equally satisfying ways of meeting important needs.

DEFENSIVE B—PATHOLOGICAL. The defensive stage may be considered pathological if the person uses defense mechanisms to deny the continued existence of a partial barrier imposed by the disability. Diverse behavior may be displayed, depending on the defense mechanisms used. The person may try to conceal the disability; may rationalize and say he or she does not want the things that are unattainable; may project negative feelings to others, claiming they cannot accept the disability although he or she has; and may try to convince others that he or she is well-adjusted. The existence of barriers imposed by the disability is denied.[12] A new compromise body image that can be accepted both consciously and unconsciously fails to develop. Psychotic reactions may result. Passive, dependent reactions may be manifested by a complete loss of motivation and a surrendering of all ambition. Psychological regression may become apparent. Pathological denial may be manifested by an inability to express negative feelings and a repression of anger.[22]

Under some additional stress the person may regress to an earlier stage and remain there permanently or may progress to adequate adjustment after a temporary regression.

ADJUSTMENT. If an adequate adjustment is attained, the person considers the disability as merely one of many personal characteristics. The disability is no longer considered a major barrier to be overcome. It is regarded as one of many assets or liabilities, and satisfying ways to meet personal needs and goals have been found.

It cannot be assumed that teaching the disabled person to do things will automatically lead to an adequate adjustment. Two other goals, held by many people, will need to be attained before adjustment is possible. The first goal lies in religion or personal philosophy. The person with religious beliefs must feel "right with God." All of the beliefs about the role of suffering in relation to God's influence on life must be worked through. The disability will be a barrier between the person and God as long as it is regarded as a punishment or the person believes that God surely will heal those who love Him. Second is the goal of achieving a feeling of personal adequacy. Because of the tendency in our society to relegate the disabled to an inferior status, the disabled person must be helped to discriminate between adequate and inferior on the basis of characteristics rather than on physique and productivity. The person must be helped to reach these more abstract goals before adjustment is attained.[12]

Analogy of adjustment to physical dysfunction to the grief process

The stages of adjustment to physical dysfunction are somewhat analogous to the grief process described by Kübler-Ross.[13] The five stages in the grief process are (1) denial and isolation, (2) anger, (3) bargaining, (4) depression, and (5) acceptance.[13]

The "shock" and "expectancy of recovery" stages described previously are similar to the first stage of the grief process, "denial and isolation." Kübler-Ross characterizes this stage with the statement, "No, not me, it cannot be true."[13] She stated that denial can be a healthy way of dealing with a painful situation. It serves as a buffer for shocking and unexpected news and gives the client time to mobilize his or her defenses. This denial is usually temporary, and it is a state from which most persons recover.

The "expectancy of recovery stage" may also be characterized by some elements of the second stage of the grief process, "anger." There may be much searching for a cure or another prognosis for recovery. Medical personnel, treatments, and the hospital are to blame for the client's plight, and the client may express many grievances against those who are responsible for his or her care. Anger during this stage can be displaced toward others. It is important that family and personnel not take this anger personally and retaliate with their own anger. Rather, the client needs to be respected and understood and given some time and attention. The client needs to feel that he or she is a valuable human being.[13] The third stage of the grief process is "bargaining." This is a wish to be rewarded for good behavior or special services. Most bargains are made with God and are usually not shared with many others. For the dying patient the wish is for an extended life.[13] For the disabled client, surely the wish is for a full recovery or at least a better recovery than the one that has been prognosticated. This bargaining process is likely to take place during the stage of "expectancy of recovery."

The "mourning stage" in the adjustment process is similiar to the fourth stage of the grief process, "depression."

The reality of the situation is acknowledged, anger subsides, and a deep sense of loss sets in.[13] For the physically disabled, the loss is not only the loss of a body part or physical function but also the loss of finances, loss of job, and loss of previous roles.

The fifth stage of the grief process is "acceptance." When there is acceptance, the client is no longer depressed or angry about his or her state. The previous stages have been worked through successfully.[13] In these ways, Kübler-Ross's stage of acceptance is similar to the defensive A stage and the stage of adjustment described previously. The process of acceptance of death, however, is quite different from adjustment to a disability in that the latter has an acceptance in which interests are increased and there is a forward mobilization of life, whereas the former is characterized as being "almost void of feelings," "the final rest before the long journey," and is accompanied by diminishing interests and detachment from important relationships.[13]

PSYCHOSOCIAL CONSIDERATIONS IN TREATMENT OF PHYSICAL DYSFUNCTION

In the treatment of physical dysfunction the client must be regarded as a whole person. The individual's capabilities, problems, interests, experiences, needs, fears, prejudices, beliefs, cultural influences, and reactions to the physical dysfunction are as important as the physical considerations in planning interaction strategies and the treatment program.[25]

The meaning of the disability to the client is the crucial factor in planning a sound approach in treatment and in aiding with the adjustment process. Therefore treatment directed to aid psychosocial adjustment must be based on individual reactions to the circumstances rather than on reactions and characteristics assumed to be similar among clients with the same physical disability or the same degree of severity of disability.[20]

Interpersonal relationships

The client will reflect attitudes of personnel and family. The psychological reactions and relationships between personnel and clients will affect the client's reaction to the disability and often the degree of participation in the rehabilitation program. The client must have someone who cares and someone who waits for him or her, or the individual may lose the will to live.[10] One or several of the rehabilitation workers dealing with the client may assume this role.

Becoming disabled alters a person's life situation not only in terms of functional performance but in social interactions with others as well. The newly disabled person knows that there has not been a change in selfhood because of the disability, yet that person may be assigned to an inferior status by the nondisabled and by professional "helpers." Customary behavior may stimulate responses very different from those that are usual or anticipated by the disabled individual. This may cause questioning of personal identity, appropriate roles, and expectations in performance ability. The early answers to such questions come from the rehabilitation personnel in everyday treatment situations. By their words and actions personnel may communicate answers to critical and perhaps unspoken questions of the disabled person.[11]

One of the problems in interpersonal relationships frequently encountered by disabled persons is the tendency of nondisabled persons to assess the limitations as more severe and restrictive than they actually are. Frequently when the nondisabled judge that the physical dysfunction precludes participation in a given activity or social situation, the disabled person knows that some level of participation is possible. The degree of difference between their assessments may make the difference between nonparticipation and nonacceptance. Since it is not possible for the nondisabled person to know the capabilities of the disabled person in a given situation, it is wise for the nondisabled to invite the participation of the disabled thus leaving him or her to determine whether or not performance is feasible. Even if participation appears patently impossible to the nondisabled, the invitation should still be made to avoid rejection and allow for the possibility of the disabled to participate in an alternative role from the ones most participants

will be assuming. The disabled person may be willing to restructure the situation so that participation is possible. The changes devised to allow participation may be simple or complex, but should be left to the discretion of the disabled person and not structured by the preconceived notions of the nondisabled. The role of the nondisabled is to provide opportunities for participation in social interchange for the disabled.[16]

Interpersonal approach in treatment

The reactions of personnel can be positive or negative. Negative reactions will result in a negative response in the client. Such reactions increase the client's suffering and may result in negativistic behavior demonstrated by an apparent loss of motivation and uncooperative behavior.[10]

Behavior of personnel that connotes respect for the rights, capabilities, and ability of the disabled person to make judgments and be involved in the rehabilitation process communicates their belief in the disabled individual as a human being and a fully functioning adult. It is important for rehabilitation personnel to not automatically assign clients to an inferior status or treat them as dependent children. The communication of a belief in the capacities of the disabled is essential. An attitude of helping the disabled person to explore and discover possibilities in performance skills and social interchange is much more helpful than preconceived notions and conclusions about their capacities by the "experts." Involvement of the client on the rehabilitation team to the extent possible is a critical factor in communicating the belief that the disabled person can be a self-determining agent in the rehabilitation process.[11]

The focus of rehabilitation should be on helping the person to reformulate an approving self who wishes to continue with life despite important discontinuity with past identity. This means the development of a new self-image based on a sense of worth rather than on deficiency and self-contempt.

The goal of rehabilitation then is to promote ego integrity and feelings of self-worth. Early rehabilitation efforts should be directed toward shaping basic life goals, and later efforts should shift to the emotional, physical, and technical resources necessary for their accomplishment.

The job of rehabilitation workers is to help the disabled person feel that he or she, as a personality, still continues. Functional aid should be seen in the larger context of enhancing self-respect. Functional and physical progress can be ego builders and aid in the adjustment process. However, functional efforts in the early stages of rehabilitation should be strategies designed to help the client see that performance is possible and should serve as a promise for the future. Emphasis on functional achievements as ends in themselves for specific skill development can serve as a means of avoiding the affective implications of physical dysfunction that must be manifested and worked through.

Therefore the proper role of the rehabilitation worker is that of assistant to the client. Unfortunately most rehabilitation settings are founded on the medical model. The professionals are in the expert and authoritarian role whereas the clients are in a passive, dependent, and compliant role. Passivity and authoritarian direction are inappropriate for persons with chronic, permanent conditions. Their role is the principal investment, and the roles of personnel are secondary.

The client's self-enhancement is supported when rehabilitation workers abandon their sense of omnipotence and see themselves as assistants to the client as he or she goes about the job of reconstituting his or her life. The roles of the professional must shift from active authoritarian to a more passive mode of professional behavior. The role of the client must shift from passive recipient of services to active doer. The rehabilitation approach is more suitable than the medical model approach when treating physically disabled persons. Except for the period of acute illness or injury and the subsequent maintenance of good health, the problems to be faced are social, emotional, functional, and vocational performance problems, for which the medical model is not suitable.[21]

Adverse or negative reactions of rehabilitation workers toward clients may stem from a variety of reasons. Personality incompatibility or prejudicial reactions to a particular age, sex, ethnic group, or physical dysfunction are some of the factors that can evoke a negative reaction. Awareness and admission of adverse reactions are the first steps in coping with them constructively. Some signs of adverse reactions to clients are (1) failure to keep appointments; (2) cutting treatment time short; (3) frequently arranging for the client to be treated by an aide, student, or other therapist; (4) unnatural and excessive politeness and service to the client; (5) a feeling of boredom when the client is present; (6) a tendency to ignore the client when others are present; (7) unrealistic optimism or pessimism about the client's prognosis or potential achievements; and (8) giving the client sketchy answers and inadequate instructions.[10]

To deal with adverse reactions to clients rehabilitation personnel who become aware of these reactions may undergo a self-analysis or analysis with the aid of peers or a psychological counselor to identify the underlying cause of the negative reaction, if it is not readily apparent. Discussion of such reactions with the client who evokes them is sometimes appropriate. If the reaction is caused by an asocial or inappropriate behavior that is within the client's capacity to change and if changed would aid acceptance by others, discussion of the feeling with the client may be helpful. Personnel may be able to change their reactions and reconstruct interaction with the client more positively through ongoing counseling with peers or a professional counselor. If these measures fail and the negative reactions cannot be dealt with and resolved, transferring the client to the care of another is essential to progress.

Pathological reactions in adjustment may be prevented if personnel can recognize the stage of adjustment that the client is experiencing and structure approaches and activities to accommodate the client's particular emotional needs at that point in the adjustment process. Clients should be encouraged to express their fears, anxieties, worries, and sense of loss. This must be done with tact and understanding. Personnel must expect that strong emotions exist in the client and must be prepared to invite the expression of these emotions and to cope with them. Personnel should not minimize the problems or enter into the client's denial. Attitudes of acceptance of the individual with the physical dysfunction will help his self-acceptance. A cheerful and optimistic attitude is useful, but the appropriate expression of irritation and anger by personnel may help the client realize that expressions of emotion are allowed and the acceptance of personnel will not be lost if such feelings are expressed.[10,22]

Early recognition of pathological reactions by personnel trained in personality development and the use of mental defense mechanisms is important. Personnel should observe for deep depression, suicidal tendencies, undue guilt or preoccupation with symptoms, bizarre behavior, confusion, paranoid symptoms, or schizophrenic behavior.[10]

Personnel should share their observations for reality testing and for referral of problems to the appropriate specialists with other members of the rehabilitation team. There should be a concerted effort of the team to deal with the normal adjustment process and minor problems. Assistance and special treatment by psychiatric or psychological specialists may be required to deal with pathological reactions. Evaluation and treatment of the client and counsel of personnel by these specialists may be helpful in dealing effectively with the client, coping with feelings toward the client, and helping the client progress toward a healthy adjustment. All professionals dealing with the client, then, need to be aware of the client's perception of self and of the immediate and extended interpersonal environment. The focus of rehabilitation should be on helping the client reconstruct the body image in accepting and approving terms.[21]

Geis[7] stresses self-definition and a sense of personal worth as critical factors in successful rehabilitation and suggests some methods for helping clients to value themselves positively. If the disabled person is to achieve successful adjustment and adaptation, he or she cannot continue to value the self in terms of a self-image that can never be.

The individual's definition of self is the crucial factor, determining the degree of sense of worth and self-satisfaction that can be achieved. Things outside of the client do not satisfy him or her, rather, satisfaction is derived in terms of these things. The client determines which things will bring satisfaction in terms of personal definition and conception of self. If this is the case, what kind of self-definition must be achieved for success, and how can rehabilitation personnel help the client achieve a positive and worthwhile definition of self?

The goal of rehabilitation is to aid the client to change a self-defeating definition to one that is self-enhancing. When the client's standards for attractiveness, productivity, or achievement are fixed and he or she can only define self and measure individual value in terms of these standards, then problems are encountered in the rehabilitation process and adjustment. Therapy involves helping the client to experience the fact that a person does not have to achieve a certain standard of productivity to be worthwhile and that his or her need to do this is only a fixed belief. The client needs to be directed to satisfactions that are attainable and helped to value goals and self preferentially rather than by some absolute standard.

In treatment the traditional focus has been on helping the client develop better modes of "doing." An emphasis on doing only or becoming efficient at reaching performance goals may focus self-valuation on an extrinsic standard of productivity. What is needed is to add to treatment modalities techniques for helping the client to simply "be" and to value things in themselves. Geis[7] describes "being" as a spontaneous expressive activity that may be purposeless and nonstriving. It exists during such pursuits as fiestas, ballet, dancing, and leisure activities and witnessing theatrical performances, comic events, and sports events, where gratification is intrinsic and linked with the process rather than the goal or end result of the activity. In contrast, "doing" activity has its satisfaction linked with the effect or ultimate achievement of the end goal of the activity process. Before the onset of physical disability the client's self-

definition and sense of personal worth, in most cases, have been based largely on "doing" behavior. With the onset of physical dysfunction there is a major loss of the self-satisfaction derived from "doing." This may evoke a reduced sense of self-worth, which can be improved by helping the client derive gratification, and increase value to self as a result, from "being" experiences. Treatment methods that emphasize the client's exploration, manipulation, personal interests and choices, enjoyment, delight, and play can facilitate self-satisfaction from "being."[7]

Group approaches

Besides the interpersonal interaction strategies to facilitate adjustment to physical dysfunction just cited, several group approaches have been proposed that can be applied in occupational therapy. Therapeutic communities, self-help groups, milieu therapy, and sensitivity training may be helpful ways to facilitate adjustment and the development of a positive self-image in the client.[21]

Kutner[15] states that "in the diagnostic work-up and medical treatment plan of the recently disabled patient, it is rather rare to include a listing of 'role disorders' accompanying the illness or injury. . . . They require not the cursory attention typically accorded them but specific and purposeful therapy." This statement has important implications for occupational therapy. The occupational therapist, concerned with the client's occupational performance in self-maintenance, work, play, and leisure roles, is the expert in role definition, role analysis, and role change. Indeed a list of "role disorders" should appear in the medical record contained in the occupational therapy reports. Kutner[15] suggests that milieu therapy may offer a solution for acquiring new roles, readapting old ones, and gaining the social and physical skills necessary to reach goals.

Milieu therapy is particularly appropriate for use by occupational therapists, since it uses environmental or residential settings as training ground for clients to practice social, interpersonal, and functional skills and to test their ability to deal with problems commonly encountered in the community.

This approach to treatment has always been fundamental to occupational therapy practice.

The milieu therapy program engages the client in a variety of social encounters, both group and individual, and exposes the client to increasingly challenging problems. This same gradation can be applied to performance skills concomitantly. The experiences are structured to test social competence, judgment, problem-solving ability, and social responsibility.

The major therapeutic objective of milieu therapy is the maintenance of the achievements acquired in the rehabilitation program. It attempts to provide the client with the necessary social, psychological, and performance skills to overcome frustration, to deal effectively with new or risky social situations, to cope with rebuff or rejection, and to remain independent.

Most therapeutic efforts have been concentrated on physical restoration with the assumption that personal and social readjustment follow automatically when physical integrity is restored. When adjustment difficulties occur, it has been customary to call on social, psychological, and psychiatric services to deal with these special problems. In contrast, milieu therapy deals with the problems of adjustment to new or changed roles by structuring situations and environments to allow the client to adopt and test roles as part of the treatment process.[15]

The self-help group model is another approach to dealing with psychosocial adjustment to physical dysfunction. Jaques and Patterson[9] reviewed the growth and development of self-help groups in this country and describe their effectiveness in the aid and rehabilitation of their members. The self-help group is one that provides aid for each group member around specific problems or goals. Positive benefits to members of self-help groups include (1) gaining information and knowledge about the dysfunction or the problem, (2) learning coping skills from group members who are living successfully with the condition, (3) gaining motivation and support through communication with others who have similar experiences, (4) modeling the successful problem-solving behaviors of group members, (5) evaluating one's own progress, (6) belonging to and identifying with a group, and (7) finding self-help in a situation of mutual concern. The mutual aid or self-help group is an excellent means of maintaining rehabilitation gain and preventing deterioration of function. It provides modeling by members who are coping with stigma and problems of functioning and reintegrating life roles.

Certain operational assumptions are characteristic of the self-help approach. Individuals with shared problems come together. All group members maintain the status of peer relationships. Peers come together expecting to help themselves or one another. Behavior change is expected in each person at his own pace. Group members identify with the program, are committed to it, and practice its principles in daily life. There are regularly scheduled group meetings, but peers are avilable to one another as needed outside of group meetings. This allows for both individual and group modes of contact. The group process consists of acknowledging, revealing, and relating problems; receiving and giving feedback; and sharing hopes, experiences, encouragement, and criticism. Members are responsible for themselves and their behavior. Leadership develops and changes within the group on the basis of giving and receiving help. Status comes from giving and receiving help effectively.

Many persons who were not helped in professional relationships and experiences turned to and received aid in self-help groups, which arose to meet needs that professionals could not meet. The professional process and self-help group models can share experiences with one another under certain conditions. The professional must meet the conditions of common problems, peer relationship, and mutual aid, and those professionals who cannot meet these conditions can only act as visitors or observers. A professional can act as a consultant or speaker to self-help groups if invited to do so by the group. However, professional therapeutic skills cannot be used as such inside the self-help group.[9]

The self-help group model or some modification of it has application in occupational therapy. It may have most potential for use in long-term rehabilitation programs, extended care facilities, or community day-care programs. Self-help groups could be initiated out of the common needs of the clients in the program. The focus on solving problems in functional performance can provide a safe area for sharing. Ultimately as group relationships are cemented and mutual support is achieved, group members may move freely to emotional and social concerns and problems of community reintegration. The occupational therapist and other concerned professionals could act as consultants, invited speakers, or group members if the necessary conditions outlined previously are met.

SUMMARY

The occupational therapy program for clients with physical dysfunction must include objectives and methods designed to facilitate psychosocial adjustment. The treatment approaches include using therapeutic relationships, structuring a therapeutic environment, and using group and dyadic interpersonal experiences. Activities selected should aid the client in adjusting to the physical dysfunction and restructuring his or her life-style to achieve the maximal independence possible.

Occupational therapy uses methods that demand the action and involvement of the client in the rehabilitation process. In the initial stages of rehabilitation when depression and denial are present and ego strength is poor, formal teaching or discussion groups fail because the client cannot integrate verbal material that deals with psychological exploration. Therefore social, recreational, special interest, and activity groups can be used to facilitate participation in rehabilitation tasks.

The group process may include discussion of needs and feelings, mutual support, and learning skills for dealing with the health care agency, its personnel, and the community. In dealing with those with physical dysfunctions the therapist should plan and structure group experiences that enhance the development of social skills, allow opportunities to test interaction strategies, discover assets and new or modified roles, and practice problem-solving behavior.

The occupational therapist can facilitate a collaborative treatment program through the use of individual and group processes. The client's involvement in treatment planning is critical because the client who uses individual skills in planning, sharing, playing, socializing, and making judgments is more likely to want to pursue daily living skills and other modalities for physical and functional improvements.

If the client is involved in this kind of programming, it will not be necessary to point out that all skills have not been lost and that there are still assets and capabilities that can be used. There is usually a concomitant and gradual increase in self-esteem and progress toward healthy adjustment and accommodation to the physical dysfunction.[24]

REVIEW QUESTIONS

1. List some of the life changes that occur with the onset of physical dysfunction.
2. Describe the physical and psychological suffering that may be caused by illness or injury.
3. What are some of the negative and positive secondary gains that may result from physical dysfunction?
4. How do body image and self-valuation affect the process of adjustment to physical dysfunction?
5. How does personality structure or adjustment pattern correlate with specific types of physical disabilities?
6. Describe two typical attitudes of the nondisabled toward the disabled.
7. Describe how rehabilitation workers may be demonstrating prejudice and reduced social status to their clients.
8. Define "stigma."
9. Describe how the health care facility is a microcosm of the society in which the disabled individual will emerge? What can be done to minimize this phenomenon?
10. List and discuss two possible origins of negative attitudes toward the disabled.
11. List and briefly describe the steps in the process of adjustment to physical dysfunction.
12. How is the process of adjustment to physical dysfunction similar to the grief process outlined by Kübler-Ross?

13. List the defense mechanisms that the disabled person may use to cope with physical dysfunction, and describe how they may be manifested.
14. What are the psychosocial factors that the therapist must consider in treatment planning?
15. How do the reactions of family, friends, and rehabilitation personnel affect treatment?
16. What is the role and helping pattern that rehabilitation workers should assume to facilitate the adjustment process?
17. List four signs of adverse reactions of personnel to clients.
18. Describe at least two ways adverse reactions of personnel to clients can be handled.
19. List signs of pathological adjustment to physical dysfunction.
20. What are some steps that should be taken if pathological reactions are recognized?
21. List three types of group approaches to treatment, and describe how each can aid in the psychosocial adjustment to physical dysfunction.

EXERCISE

This is an empathy experience that is designed to help the student experience some of the personal and interpersonal reactions outlined in this chapter.

1. Select a wheelchair, walker, crutches, arm sling, or training arm prosthesis, and use the device as you would if you were so disabled.
2. Use the device for a minimum of 2 hours to tolerance.
3. Perform all of your usual daily living activities, and appear in public, perhaps to shop, eat in a restaurant, or look for an apartment during the experiential period.
4. During the experience take notes and write a brief report describing your personal responses to people and objects, your affect and attitudes while performing daily living skills, and while in public, reactions of others to you, your attitude toward dependency, if and how others offered assistance, and architectural barriers and how they foster dependency.

REFERENCES

1. Blume, J.: Deenie, Scarsdale, N.Y., 1973, Bradbury Press, Inc.
2. Burtoff, B.: Fairy tale stereotypes can harm, San Jose Mercury News, p. 1C, January 26, 1980.
3. Catholic Biblical Association of America, The Bishops' Committee of the Confraternity of Christian Doctrine: The New American Bible, Nashville, Tenn., 1971, Thomas Nelson, Inc.
4. Corcoran, B.: A dance to still music, New York, 1974, Atheneum Publishers.
5. English, R.W.: Correlates of stigma toward physically disabled persons. In Marinelli, R.P., and Dell Orto, A.E., editors: The psychological and social impact of physical disability, New York, 1977, Springer Publishing Co., Inc.
6. Garner, H.H.: Somatopsychic concepts. In Marinelli, R.P., and Dell Orto, A.E., editors: The psychological and social impact of physical disability, New York, 1977, Springer Publishing Co., Inc.
7. Geis, H.J.: The problem of personal worth in the physically disabled patient. In Marinelli, R.P., and Dell Orto, A.E., editors: The psychological and social impact of physical disability, New York, 1977, Springer Publishing Co., Inc.
8. Gellman, W.: Roots of prejudice against the handicapped, excerpted from J. Rehabil. **25:**4, 1959. In Stubbins, J., editor: Social and psychological aspects of disability, Baltimore, 1977, University Park Press.
9. Jaques, M.E., and Patterson, K.: The self help group model: a review. In Marinelli, R.P., and Dell Orto, A.E., editors: The psychological and social impact of physical disability, New York, 1977, Springer Publishing Co., Inc.
10. Jeffress, E.J.: Psychological implications of physical disability, Videotape no. ITV 86 A and 86 B, San Jose State University, Instructional Resources Center.
11. Kerr, N.: Staff expectations for disabled persons: helpful or harmful. In Marinelli, R.P., and Dell Orto, A.E., editors: The psychological and social impact of physical disability, New York, 1977, Springer Publishing Co., Inc.
12. Kerr, N.: Understanding the process of adjustment to disability. In Stubbins, J., editor: Social and psychological aspects of disability, Baltimore, 1977, University Park Press.
13. Kübler-Ross, E.: On death and dying, New York, 1969, Macmillan Publishing Co., Inc.
14. Kushner, H.S.: When bad things happen to good people, New York, 1981, Avon Books.
15. Kutner, B.: Milieu therapy. In Marinelli, R.P., and Dell Orto, A.E., editors: The psychological and social impact of physical disability, New York, 1977, Springer Publishing Co., Inc.
16. Ladieu-Leviton, G., Adler, D.L., and Dembo, T.: Studies in adjustment to visible injuries: social acceptance of the injured. In Marinelli, R.P., and Dell Orto, A.E., editors: The psychological and social impact of physical disability, New York, 1977, Springer Publishing Co., Inc.
17. Marinelli, R.P., and Dell Orto, A.E., editors: The psychological and social impact of physical disability, New York, 1977, Springer Publishing Co., Inc.
18. O'Dell, S.: Sing down the moon, Boston, 1970, Houghton Mifflin Co.
19. Robinson, V.: David in silence, Philadelphia, 1956, J.B. Lippincott Co.
20. Shontz, F.: Physical disability and personality. In Marinelli, R.P., and Dell Orto, A.E., editors: The psychological and social impact of physical disability, New York, 1977, Springer Publishing Co., Inc.
21. Siller, J.: Psychological situation of the disabled with spinal cord injuries. In Stubbins, J., editor: Social and psychological aspects of disability, Baltimore, 1977, University Park Press.
22. Simon, J.I.: Emotional aspects of physical disability, Am. J. Occup. Ther. **15:**408, 1971.
23. Thurer, S. cited by Burtoff, B.: Fairy tale stereotypes can harm, San Jose Mercury News, January 26, 1980.
24. Versluys, H.: Psychological adjustment to physical disability. In Trombly, C.A., and Scott, A.D., Occupational therapy for physical dysfunction, Baltimore, 1977, Williams & Wilkins.
25. Willard, H.S., and Spackman, C.S., editors: Occupational therapy, ed. 4, Philadelphia, 1971, J.B. Lippincott Co.

CHAPTER 3

Treatment planning

LORRAINE WILLIAMS PEDRETTI

A treatment plan is the design or proposal for a therapeutic program. It includes specific treatment objectives and methods for reaching those objectives and indicates how the program should progress.

The importance of writing a treatment plan cannot be overstated. It is necessary to have specific objectives set down in an orderly and sequential manner. These, then, will be clear to the therapist, the client, and other concerned personnel. The treatment plan helps the therapist know how to proceed efficiently and provides a standard for measuring the progress of the client and thus the effectiveness of the plan of action.

Therapists who do not write treatment plans may be working in a trial and error manner, wasting precious time and money. They may be poorly prepared to defend their course of action to themselves, the client, or the rehabilitation team. They may tend to lack confidence in reporting about the clients assigned to their care. The failure to have a well-written treatment plan available will also present many problems to other staff members who may have to apply treatment in the absence of the assigned therapist. Even experienced therapists who think they no longer need to write treatment plans may find that their mental plans are not as clear or as comprehensive as they imagined when they attempt to set them on paper.

Perhaps one of the most important purposes for writing a treatment plan, then, is that it allows the therapist to plan and analyze the proposed course of action. In so doing the therapist should ask many questions. Some of these are (1) What are the client's capabilities and assets? (2) What are the client's limitations and deficits? (3) What does occupational therapy have to offer this client? (4) What are specific short-range objectives? (5) What are some long-range objectives? (6) Are the treatment objectives consistent with the client's needs and personal objectives? (7) If objectives are not compatible, how do they need to be modified? (8) What treatment methods are available to meet these objectives? (9) What is the best theoretical framework for treatment of this client? (10) When should the client have met the objectives? (11) What standards shall be used to determine when the client has reached an objective? (12) How shall the effectiveness of the treatment plan be evaluated?

The treatment plan affirms therapist's competence and the professionalism of occupational therapy. It can provide a systematic method for gathering research data and documents the purposes and effectiveness of occupational therapy services. The treatment plan can enhance the quality of service and its effectiveness.

THE TREATMENT PLANNING PROCESS
Data gathering

After the client is referred for occupational therapy services, the therapist must gather data to develop an appropriate treatment plan. Sources for these data are the referral form; the medical record; social, educational, vocational, and play histories; interview of the client or family and friends; and the results of evaluation procedures completed by occupational therapy and other services.

Data analysis and problem identification

After data have been gathered, they are analyzed to identify functions and dysfunctions, and it is determined if occupational therapy can be employed to alleviate the problems. From a careful analysis of all of the data gathered,[6] a list of problems should be developed, which forms the basis of the treatment plan. Those physical, psychosocial, cognitive, and performance skills deficits that may be amenable to occupational therapy intervention should be noted. Limitations that require intervention by other professional services should be communicated through the appropriate referral process.

Selecting and writing treatment objectives

The next step in the treatment planning process is the setting down of objectives. Following the data gathering process, the therapist may conceptualize one or more treatment approaches and some general kinds of treatment methods that would facilitate the client's rehabilitation. For example, following evaluation it might be apparent that the client could benefit from training in activities of daily living or from one of the sensorimotor approaches to treatment for influencing muscle tone and movement patterns. Having ideas for such methods can facilitate the selection and writing of specific treatment objectives. The writing of objectives and selection of treatment methods actually are concurrent and mutually dependent processes.

Objectives should reflect the client's needs and should be consistent with the more general objectives stated on the referral, although they need not be limited to these, if the referral agent approves. The occupational therapy objectives should complement objectives of ancillary services. Whenever possible the therapist should select objectives and plan the treatment program in conjunction with the client.

A treatment objective is a statement of intent describing a proposed change in a client. The statement conveys clearly the physical function, performance skill, or behavior pattern the client will demonstrate when the treatment procedure or program has been successfully completed.

The therapist must select objectives that the client is to reach by the end of a treatment program so that treatment procedures relevant to those objectives may also be selected. Progress and evaluation of the client's performance will be based on the objectives selected.

When no clearly defined objectives have been stated, there is no sound basis for selecting appropriate treatment methods, and it is impossible to evaluate the effectiveness of the treatment program. It is important to state objectives to be able to evaluate the degree to which the client is able to perform in the desired manner.

A meaningful objective conveys to others a picture of what the client will be like when the objective has been achieved. The picture conveyed is identical to the one the therapist has in mind. Thus it succeeds in communicating the therapist's intent and describes the terminal behavior of the client well enough to preclude misinterpretation. A comprehensive treatment objective has the following three qualities:

1. Statement of terminal behavior. The physical changes, kind of behavior, or performance skill that the client is expected to display.
2. Conditions. The circumstances that will allow terminal behavior to take place, for example, environment, special devices, data, or degree of training and assistance required for the client to perform the desired terminal behavior.
3. Criteria. The level of acceptable performance and or degree of competence the client is expected to achieve to have successfully accomplished the terminal behavior.

The following are examples of comprehensive treatment objectives and their analysis:

Given instruction, daily practice, and assistive devices the client's performance of dressing and feeding skills will be improved so that they are performed independently in no more than twice the time it takes nondisabled individuals to perform the same activities.
CONDITIONS: Given instruction, daily practice, and assistive devices.
TERMINAL BEHAVIOR: The client's performance of dressing and feeding skills will be improved.
CRITERIA: Independently in no more than twice the time it takes nondisabled individuals.
Given demonstration, instruction, and practice in principles of joint protection and energy conservation the client will use these principles in self-care, school, and play activities so that deformity is prevented and activity tolerance is increased from 2 to 4 hours.
CONDITIONS: Given demonstration, instruction, and practice in principles of joint protection and energy conservation.

TERMINAL BEHAVIOR: The client will use these principles in self-care, school, and play activities.
CRITERIA: So that deformity is prevented and activity tolerance is increased from 2 to 4 hours.
After guided participation in a structured activity group the client will be able to initiate and sustain social interaction in an activity program 50% of the time.
CONDITION: After guided participation in a structured activity group.
TERMINAL BEHAVIOR: The client will be able to initiate and sustain social interaction in an activity program.
CRITERION: 50% of the time.
Given a program of daily exercise and activity the range of motion (ROM) of right shoulder flexion will increase from 110° to 160°.
CONDITIONS: Given a program of daily exercise and activity.
TERMINAL BEHAVIOR: The ROM of right shoulder flexion will increase.
CRITERION: From 110° to 160°.

There are many variables and unknown factors in the growth and development or recovery of clients with physical dysfunction. Therefore the degree to which they can benefit from or participate in or succeed in rehabilitation programs cannot be predicted with certainty. This often makes it difficult for therapists to write comprehensive treatment objectives. However, the therapist should attempt to write such objectives, using past experience with similar clients and knowledge gained from gathering pertinent data to describe desired terminal behavior, conditions, and criteria for each treatment objective. If this is not possible, it is recommended that a specific statement of terminal behavior should suffice until applicable conditions and criteria become apparent. The stated terminal behaviors can then be modified to become comprehensive objectives as treatment progresses.

The following are examples of specific statements of terminal behavior:

1. The joint ROM of the left elbow will increase.
2. The client will be able to operate the control systems of the left above-elbow prosthesis.
3. The client will be able to dress.
4. The strength of the client's left deltoid and biceps muscles will increase.

5. The client will be able to use the mobile arm supports.
6. The client will develop feelings of self-worth and acceptance of disability.

Selecting treatment methods

When objectives have been selected, the treatment methods that will help the client achieve them are chosen. This is probably one of the most difficult steps in the treatment planning process. A treatment principle or assumption that is applied to the cause of an identified problem should underlie the selection of an appropriate treatment method.[3] For example, after peripheral nerve injury and repair, when nerve regeneration is progressing, a principle would be that use of reinnervated muscles will maintain or increase their tone and strength. Therefore graded therapeutic activity or exercise may be the method of choice to effect the desired goals. Many other factors will affect the selection of treatment methods. Some of the factors that should be considered in the selection of treatment methods are (1) What is the goal for the client? (2) What are the precautions or contraindications that affect the occupational therapy program? (3) What is the prognosis for recovery? (4) What were the results of evaluations in occupational therapy and other services? (5) What other treatment is the client receiving? (6) What are the goals of other treatment programs, and are the occupational therapy goals consonant with these? (7) How much energy does the client expend in other therapies? (8) What is the state of the client's general health? (9) What are the client's interests, vocational skills, and psychological needs? (10) What roles will the client assume in the community? (11) What kinds of activities or exercise will be most useful and meaningful to the client?[11] (12) How can treatment be graded to meet the client's changing needs as progression or regression occurs? (13) What special equipment or adaptations of therapeutic equipment are needed for the client to perform maximally?

When treatment methods are selected, it should be clear to others reading the treatment plan exactly how the methods will be used to reach specific objectives. Sometimes several methods may be needed to achieve one objective, or it may happen that the same methods may be used to reach several objectives.

Implementing the treatment plan

When at least one objective and one or more treatment methods have been selected, the treatment plan is implemented. The client engages in the procedures that have been designed to ameliorate the problems and capitalize on strengths and capabilities. A comprehensive treatment plan may evolve over a period of time. While a lengthy evaluation is in progress, for example, Activities of Daily Living assessment, the client may have commenced a program of therapeutic activity to strengthen specific muscle groups. Thus as a comprehensive evaluation is being completed, an increasing number of problems may be identified, and additional objectives and methods may be added to the treatment plan.

Reevaluating the client and the initial treatment plan

Once the treatment plan is implemented, its effectiveness is evaluated on an ongoing basis. The therapist must be an alert observer and ask (1) Are the objectives suitable to the client's needs and capabilities? (2) Are the methods the best ones for fulfilling the treatment objectives? (3) Does the client relate to the treatment methods and see them as worthwhile and meaningful? (4) Are the treatment objectives realistic, and are they consonant with the client's personal objectives?

Scrutinizing the treatment plan in this way will enable the therapist to modify the plan as the need arises. The criterion for determining the effectiveness of the plan is the progress of the client toward the stated objectives in the time set for reaching those objectives. Therefore periodic reevaluation of the client, using the same tests and observations that were used to determine baseline function, can provide objective evidence of maintenance or progress, which validates the treatment plan.

Revising the treatment plan

The information gained from observations and reevaluation of the client, as outlined earlier, may necessitate some revision or modification of the initial treatment plan. The client's progress may be significant enough to increase such factors as duration, complexity, or resistance of activity. In degenerative diseases where maintenance of optimal function is often a primary objective, resistance, duration, and complexity of activity may need to be decreased to accommodate the gradual inevitable decline of physical resources. The client's motivation or inability to see the therapeutic program as helpful or meaningful may necessitate change in treatment approaches and methods.

When the initial plan is revised according to the client's needs and progress, it is once again implemented. This process of reevaluation, revision, and reimplementation of the treatment plan is continuous throughout the course of the therapeutic program (Fig. 3-1).

A TREATMENT PLAN MODEL

The treatment plan model is an adaptation of one that was used at the Hartford Easter Seal Rehabilitation Center in Hartford, Connecticut.[4] It is useful for teaching treatment planning during academic preparation, and it may be modified for clinical use.

The student is presented with a hypothetical case study, or a real client if a practicum experience is available, and is directed to complete the treatment plan, using the Treatment Planning Guide. If given a hypothetical client the student is directed to complete the Results of Evaluation segment of the treatment plan according to his or her knowledge of the particular diagnosis and its resultant disability.

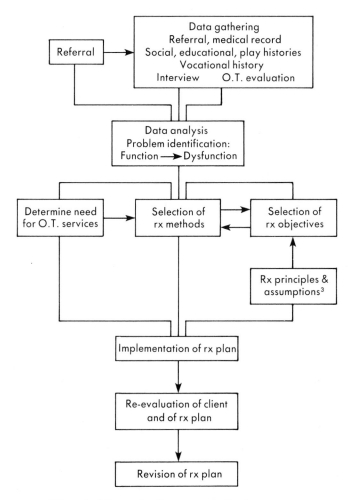

Fig. 3-1. Schematic of treatment planning process.

Treatment plan model[4]

Case _____

Refer to questions and information on the Treatment Planning Guide and fill out a treatment plan for the assigned case study. List information or use outline form only.

A. **Statistical data.**
   1. Name
      Age
      Diagnosis
      Disability
   2. Treatment aims as stated in referral.
B. **Other services.**
C. **OT evaluation.**
D. **Results of evaluation.** List function tested or observed in each category, and summarize the results of the OT evaluation.

1. Evaluation data
   a. Physical resources
   b. Sensory-perceptual functions
   c. Cognitive functions
   d. Psychosocial functions
   e. Prevocational potential
   f. Functional skills
2. Problem identification. List the problems that have been identified that require occupational therapy intervention.

E Specific OT objectives	F Methods used to meet objectives	G Gradation of treatment

E. **Special equipment.**
   1. Ambulation aids. List ambulation aids required by the client, and give a short statement of justification for each choice.
   2. Splints. List splints required by client with a short statement of justification for each choice. Describe how and when client is to use splints.
   3. Assistive devices. List devices needed for increased independence in self-care, home management, or travel, and give a short statement of justification for each choice.

Treatment planning guide

A. **Statistical data.** Fill in the requested information from the information given in the case study.
B. **Other services.** What other services would be active with this client? List and give a brief statement of the role of the services listed.
   Medical service
   Nursing
   Social service
   Speech therapy
   Physical therapy
   Vocational counseling
   Sheltered employment
   Psychology-psychiatry
   Community social groups
   Educational services
   Spiritual counselor
C. **OT evaluation.** From the list below select the performance components and performance skills that should be evaluated. Indicate whether assessment would be by testing or by observation.
   1. Physical resources.
      Muscle strength
      ROM
      Physical endurance
      Standing tolerance
      Walking tolerance
      Sitting balance
      Involuntary movement
      Speed of movement

Level of motor development
Equilibrium and protective
   mechanisms
Coordination—muscle control
Spasticity
Stage of recovery, synergy patterns (stroke patients only)
Postural reflex mechanism
Available functional movements
Hand function
   2. Sensory-perceptual functions.
      Sensation—touch, pain, temperature, smell, taste
      Body scheme
      Stereognosis
      Proprioception
      Visual perception
         Visual fields
         Spatial relations
         Position in space
         Figure-ground
         Perceptual constancy
         Visual-motor coordination
         Depth perception
         Verticality
      Motor planning—gross and fine
   3. Cognitive functions.
      Judgment
      Safety awareness
      Motivation
      Memory
      Sequencing
      Anticipation

Problem solving
Rigidity
Basic language skills for function
   Comprehension
   Expression
   Reading
   Writing
   4. Psychosocial functions.
      Maturity (development)
      Interpersonal skills
      Adjustment to disability
      Reality functioning
   5. Prevocational potential.
      Work habits and attitudes
      Potential work skills
      Work tolerance
   6. Functional skills.
      Self-care
      Homemaking
      Home evaluation
      Community travel
         Public transportation
         Private transportation
D. **Results of evaluation.** Summarize findings from tests and observations, and identify the problems that require occupational therapy intervention.
E. **Treatment objectives.** List specific objectives of treatment. Write them in comprehensive form as described on pp. 22 to 23.

Continued.

Treatment planning guide—cont'd

F. **Treatment methods.** List the activities or exercises that might be appropriate for this client. Show how they will fulfill stated treatment objectives. Describe them specifically enough so another student or therapist could carry out the procedures easily.

G. **Grading.** Describe or list ways in which methods have to be graded for this client.

H. **Special equipment.**
1. Ambulation aids. List ambulation aids required by the client, and give a short statement of justification for each choice.
2. Splints. List splints required by client with a short statement of justification for each choice. Describe how and when the client is to use splints.

3. Assistive devices. List devices needed for increased independence in self-care, home management, or travel, and give a short statement of justification for each choice.

Sample treatment plan

Case study

Mrs. R. is 49 years old. She has two sons. One is age 26 and married and the other is age 17. Mrs. R. is divorced. She and her younger son make their home with her married son, his wife, and 4-year-old son. Before the onset of her illness Mrs. R. lived in an apartment with her younger son.

Mrs. R. has had Guillain-Barré syndrome. She has been left with residual weakness of all four extremities. Leg strength is in the poor to fair plus range, and arm strength is fair to good. There may be some further recovery, but muscle strength is not expected to reach normal level. Mrs. R. can ambulate with the aid of a walker but often uses a standard wheelchair for safety and energy conservation.

Mrs. R. appears thin and frail. She speaks in a weak voice and appears to be passive and discouraged. She feels she cannot accomplish anything. The home situation is poor. Mrs. R. does not communicate with her daughter-in-law, and there are conflicts between the couple and Mrs. R. concerning the management of the teenaged son. Mrs. R. feels unable to assert her authority as his mother or to express her needs and feelings. The disability has brought about the loss of her independence and has changed her role in relation to her younger son.

Her daughter-in-law reported that Mrs. R. is dependent for self-care, never attempts to help with homemaking, and isolates herself in her room much of the time. She believes that her mother-in-law is capable of more activity "if only she would try." She says she is willing to allow Mrs. R. to do some of the household work.

Mrs. R. was referred for occupational therapy services as an outpatient for physical restoration (or maintenance) and training toward increased independence.

Treatment plan[2]

Refer to questions and information on the treatment planning guide, and fill out a treatment plan for the assigned case study. List information, or use outline form only.

A. **Statistical data.**
1. Name: Mrs. R.
Age: 49
Diagnosis: Guillain-Barré syndrome
Disability: Residual weakness, upper and lower extremities
2. Treatment aims as stated in referral:
Physical restoration or maintenance
Training toward increased independence

B. **Other services.**
Medical service: Medication prescription, supervision of rehabilitation program, general health maintenance
Physical therapy: Muscle strengthening
Social service: Family counseling and group therapy for psychological support
Group therapy: Psychological support

C. **OT evaluation.**
Muscle strength: Manual muscle test
Passive ROM: Test
Physical endurance: Observe
Walking tolerance (with walker): Observe
Sitting balance: Observe
Speed of movement: Observe
Coordination: Test and observe
Available functional movements:
Test and observe
Sensation: Test[1,5]
Motivation: Observe
Maturity, interpersonal skills, adjustment to disability: Observe
Self-care: Observe
Homemaking: Observe
Home evaluation: Observe[9]

D. **Results of evaluation.**
1. Evaluation data.
   a. Physical resources.
      (1) Strength: All muscles same grade bilaterally.
         Scapula: All muscles G
         Shoulder: All muscles G
         Elbow: Flexors F+, extensors F
         Forearm: Supinators F, pronators F+
         Wrist: Flexors F, extensors F
         Hand: All muscles F, except finger flexors F+
         Trunk: All muscles G
         Hip: All muscles F+, except adductors and external rotators F
         Knee: Extensors and flexors F
         Ankle: Dorsiflexors P+, plantar flexors F
         Foot: Invertors P, evertors F−
         Toes: Flexors F−, extensors P
      (2) ROM: All joints within functional to normal range.
      (3) Physical endurance, ambulation: Mrs. R.'s physical endurance is low. She can ambulate with a walker but fatigues quickly. For safety and

energy conservation she often uses a wheelchair. She has slight incoordination of her legs and cannot perform fine movements using the hands because of muscle weakness.

b. Sensory-perceptual functions.
  (1) Primary sensation
      Touch: Intact
      Pain: Intact
      Temperature: Intact
  (2) Somesthetic perception
      Proprioception: Intact
      Stereognosis: Intact

c. Cognitive functions. No cognitive deficits observed.

d. Psychosocial functions. Mrs. R. has not adjusted well to her disability. She appears to be passive and discouraged and feels she cannot accomplish anything. Much of each day she isolates herself in her room.

  The home situation is poor. Before the onset of her illness Mrs. R. lived in an apartment with her younger son, who is age 17. They now make their home with the older son, age 26, his wife, and 4-year-old son. Mrs. R. does not communicate with her daughter-in-law, and there are conflicts between the couple and Mrs. R. concerning the management of the teenage son. The disability has brought about the loss of her independence and has changed her role in relation to her younger son. She feels unable to assert her authority as his mother or to express her needs and feelings.

e. Prevocational potential. Not applicable because Mrs. R. is not a candidate for future employment.

f. Functional skills. Mrs. R. is dependent in self-care activities. She manages some light personal care, such as washing her face, brushing her hair, and brushing her teeth with an adapted toothbrush, but needs assistance in getting on and off the toilet, to and from the shower, and drying herself.

  Mrs. R. can put on a blouse, cardigan, and loose dress but cannot fasten buttons or zippers. She does not dress any part of the lower extremities except for putting on loose socks. Mrs. R. does not do any of the house cleaning, kitchen work, laundry, or gardening, although she is capable of some light activities such as dusting and folding clothes.

2. Problem identification.
   a. Self-care dependence
   b. Muscle weakness
   c. Low physical endurance
   d. Incoordination as a result of muscle weakness
   e. Home management dependence
   f. Depression
   g. Self-isolation
   h. Lack of self-assertiveness
   i. Reduced social interaction
   j. Poor family communication
   k. Changed role as mother

E Specific OT objectives	F Methods used to meet objectives	G Gradation of treatment

Given dressing training Mrs. R. will be able to dress herself within a half hour in most types of clothing	Putting on slacks, panties, stockings, skirts, shirts, blouses, pullover shirts, brassiere, and shoes
	Fastening buttons
	Teaching energy-saving techniques:
	    Button house dresses before slipping over head
	    Deciding which articles to put on before transferring to wheelchair, for example, socks or slacks
	    Placing these articles within reach of bed before retiring each night
	Teaching methods of dressing:
	    Rolling hips to put on slacks
	    Stabilizing body while standing to let dress fall over hips
		Start with easier tasks—house dresses, large pullover shirts, and loafers
		Go to more difficult tasks as muscle strength increases and client becomes proficient in easier tasks—stockings, slacks, tie, and shoes

Given home management training, observation of same by Mrs. R's daughter-in-law, and facilitated communication between the two women, Mrs. R. will be able to perform light household tasks and will perform them willingly at home	Dusting up to levels reachable from wheelchair Folding clothes and washing fine clothes in bathroom sink Washing dishes—sitting on high chair with legs under sink Setting napkins and silverware on table[1] Interacting more with daughter-in-law through planning together and dividing household tasks	

Continued.

Sample treatment plan—cont'd

E Specific OT objectives	F Methods used to meet objectives	G Gradation of treatment
Through exercise and activity muscle strength will increase in both hands and wrists from F to G (finger flexors, F+ to G) and coordination of the hands will improve so that Mrs. R. can perform homemaking activities in less time and with less fatigue	Teaching active isotonic exercise for F muscles and progressive resistive exercise for finger flexors through the following activities: Breaking up lettuce Washing small clothes Beating eggs Painting	Add weights; advance to progressive resistive isotonic exercise when muscles reach F+ Increase complexity of exercise as coordination increases Use activities requiring more strength and coordination: Cutting vegetables Wringing out clothes Sifting flour Watercolor with large brush; paint with acrylic paint using small brush
Through regular performance of daily activities muscle strength of shoulders, elbows, and forearms will increase so that activities can be performed more quickly and efficiently Shoulders: G to N Elbow extensors: F to G Flexors: F+ to G Supinators: F to G Pronators: F+ to G	Making orange juice (wheelchair side to side with waist-level table; use pronators and supinators; alternate sides) Washing glasses Rolling out pastry Wiping table and counter Setting plates and glasses on table Removing plates and glasses from cupboard where they are slightly above waist level Braid-weaving project	Client must remove more and more meat of oranges Use a heavier pin and heavier, more elastic dough Change to tasks requiring more strength—scrubbing wall Remove more plates at one time; placement of plates at higher level; add weight to upper arm
Given training and practice Mrs. R. will be independent in using the toilet and will not take more than 10 minutes to transfer on and off toilet	Teaching nonweight-bearing front transfer, not only using arms but also scooting hips and turning trunk[7]	Assistance in bringing body forward until elbow extensors F+; assistance in bringing body backwards until knee muscles F+ and elbow extensors F+; supervision until patient performs task in safest and easiest manner
Given improved physical endurance Mrs. R. will increase performance of ambulatory activities at home so that self-care independence will be achieved	Dressing—standing to pull slacks over hips and zipper up slacks instead of using bed Transferring to bed, toilet, tub, and car Using walker instead of wheelchair for self-care and household tasks	Balance of activities—watch for fatigue At start use returning lower extremity strength only for dressing and transferring Increase use of walker commensurately with returning strength
As a result of treatment, Mrs. R. will be a more active, participating member of the family, communicating freely with all members of the family so that she no longer isolates herself in her room and instead asserts herself without hesitation	Increasing confidence by becoming more independent Forming closer relationship with daughter-in-law resulting from change in attitude as client gains confidence and realizes potential Aiding family in understanding psychological aspects of client's disability and rehabilitation Family providing encouragement and praising client's accomplishments and attempts Encouraging client to express her feelings and needs Not letting client get away with statements such as "Yes, I'm doing fine," when she does not look it[10]	Less and less encouragement from therapist and family
As a result of treatment, adjustment to disability will improve so that Mrs. R. no longer depends on her family and therapies for social interaction, and instead initiates contact with friends and church group independently	Initially therapist will accompany Mrs. R. to a meeting or on a community outing; later recruit friend to accompany her until she is able to travel independently and is motivated to do so Evening strolls and interacting with neighbors Attending nearby church Visiting friends in former neighborhood Taking up old and new hobbies Watching grandson at park	Start with less demanding activities, such as evening strolls; build up to more demanding ones

Sample treatment plan—cont'd

H. Special equipment
1. Ambulation aids.
   Walker for support during ambulation
   Electric wheelchair or regular wheelchair accompanied by assistant for outings into community to conserve time and energy
2. Splints.
   None required
3. Assistive devices.

a. Button fastener and loops of ribbon on ends of zippers: To facilitate self-care activities
b. Installation of a low dowel in closet that is reachable from wheelchair to hang blouses: To make it possible for Mrs. R. to reach clothing from sitting position
c. Flannel mitt: To facilitate dusting by eliminating static grasp of dust cloth
d. Terry cloth mitt: For dish washing to eliminate static grasp of dishcloth

e. Large sponge: For gross grasp and ease of handling
f. Built-up handles on eggbeater and brush: For gross grasp and ease of handling
g. 2½-inch rounded guardrail at each side of toilet (on side of shower, on wall)[7]: For safety in transfers
h. Swinging, detachable footrests on wheelchair: To get as close as possible to toilet

REVIEW QUESTIONS
1. Define "treatment plan."
2. Why is it important to write a treatment plan?
3. List the steps in developing a treatment plan.
4. List and define the three qualities of a comprehensive treatment objective. Give an example of each.
5. If it is not possible to write a comprehensive objective, which one quality would be *most* important to set down first?
6. List at least six factors to consider when selecting treatment methods.
7. Is it necessary to develop a complete comprehensive treatment plan before treatment can commence? How is the plan developed?
8. Is it ever necessary to change the initial treatment plan?
9. How is a treatment plan evaluated for its effectiveness?
10. How does the therapist know when to modify or change the treatment plan?

EXERCISES
1. Analyze the following objectives by asking which characteristics of a comprehensive objective each contains and which ones each lacks. Then rewrite and state each one more comprehensively.
   a. Joint ROM at the left elbow will be improved from 40° to 135° to 15° to 135°.
   b. The client will become more self-assertive among her peers.
   c. The client will become proficient in control and use of the left below-elbow prosthesis.
2. Read the following case study and write three treatment objectives, relative to improving strength, for this

patient. Incorporate all of the qualities of a comprehensive treatment objective for each.

Case study

   Mr. P. is a 35-year-old electronics assembler. He completed the tenth grade in school. He is right-handed, married, and the father of two children under 8 years old. He suffered an injury of the right radial nerve at elbow level with minor involvement of the median nerve. The injury occurred 2 months ago and partial to full recovery is expected to occur within 10 months.
   Mr. P. is now supporting his family with insurance compensation payments but fears these will terminate before recovery has occurred, and he is back on the job. He is worried and depressed about this.
   The client is an outpatient and has been referred to occupational therapy for physical and functional restoration.
   Muscle grades
   Extensor carpi radialis brevis: F
   Extensor carpi ulnaris: P+
   Extensor digitorum communis: F
   Supinator: P+
   Extensor pollicis longus and brevis: P−
   Abductor pollicis longus and brevis: P
   Extensor indicis proprius: P−

3. Using the directions for writing a treatment plan and the Treatment Planning Guide, write a brief treatment plan for the client described in the case study with emphasis on improvement of muscle function.

REFERENCES
1. American Occupational Therapy Association: The objectives and functions of occupational therapy, New York, 1958, American Occupational Therapy Association.
2. Balwinski, C.M.: Treatment plan for lower motor neuron dysfunction. Unpublished paper presented in partial fulfillment of the requirements for OT 167, San Jose, Calif., Spring 1977, San Jose State University.
3. Day, D.: A systems diagram for teaching treatment planning, Am. J. Occup. Ther. 27:239-243, 1973.
4. Hartford Easter Seal Rehabilitation Center: Adaptation from Treatment plan model, 1968, Hartford, Conn. Unpublished.
5. Holvey, D.N., and Talbott, J.H.: The Merck manual of diagnosis and therapy, ed. 12, Rahway, N.J., 1972, Merck & Co., Inc.
6. Illinois Occupational Therapy Association Committee on Practice: Evaluation procedures in occupational therapy, New York, 1969, American Occupational Therapy Association.
7. Ince, L.: The rehabilitation medicine services, Springfield, Ill., 1974, Charles C Thomas, Publisher.
8. Mager, R.F.: Preparing objectives for programmed instruction, San Francisco, 1962, Fearon · Pittman Publishers, Inc.
9. Nichols, P.J.R.: Rehabilitation of the severely disabled, Borough Green, Sevenoaks, Kent, England, 1971, Butterworth & Co., Ltd.
10. Pedretti, L.W.: Manual for advanced physical disability procedures, San Jose, Calif., 1973, San Jose State University.
11. Willard, H.S., and Spackman, C.S., editors: Occupational therapy, ed. 4, Philadelphia, 1971, J.B. Lippincott Co.

PART 2

EVALUATION OF PATIENTS WITH PHYSICAL DYSFUNCTION

CHAPTER 4

Occupational therapy evaluation of physical dysfunction
PRINCIPLES AND METHODS

LORRAINE WILLIAMS PEDRETTI

Evaluation of physical dysfunction is a process of gathering data and assessing performance and performance components, that is, motor, sensory integrative, cognitive, emotional, and psychological functions, that underlie adequate performance. Its purpose is to aid the occupational therapist in developing treatment objectives and treatment strategies based on the problems identified in the evaluation process. Results of an evaluation may indicate a specific direction for occupational therapy intervention or that occupational therapy is inappropriate or not feasible for the particular client or at a given time.

The evaluation process includes collecting data from the client, medical record, other professionals, friends, and family members. The process continues with the administration of specific occupational therapy assessment tools and concludes with an analysis and summary of the results and the identification of problems and assets in the client's life situation. Treatment objectives and methods are then selected on the basis of this information. It is important that the client be involved, to the extent possible, throughout the evaluation and treatment planning processes.

As the treatment program progresses, periodic reevaluation is essential to assess the effectiveness of treatment and to modify it to suit current client needs. This may involve the deletion of unattainable goals, the modification of goals partially or completely achieved, and the addition of new goals as progress is made.

Evaluation also provides the therapist with a specific and concrete method of determining his or her own effectiveness as a planner and administrator of treatment. It provides specific information that can be communicated to other members of the rehabilitation team.

Further, careful evaluation can enhance the development of occupational therapy. If evaluation data are collected systematically, they may be used for the development of more standardized evaluation instruments and may contribute to a better understanding of which evaluation and treatment techniques are suitable and effective in occupational therapy practice.

To be an effective evaluator, the therapist must be knowledgeable about the dysfunction, its causes, course, and prognosis; be familiar with a variety of evaluation methods, their uses, and proper administration; and be able to select evaluation methods that are suitable to the client and the dysfunction. This means that an understanding of all the possible dysfunctional performance and performance components and the applicable treatment principles is essential. In addition the therapist must approach the client with openness and without preconceived ideas about his or her limitations or personality. The therapist must have good observation skills and be able to enlist the trust of the client in a short period of time.[6]

METHODS OF EVALUATION
Medical records

Data gathered from the medical record are an important part of the evaluation process. The medical record can provide information on the diagnosis, prognosis, current treatment regime, social data, psychological data, and other rehabilitation therapies. Daily notes from nurses and physicians can give information about current medications and the client's reactions and responses to the hospital, the treatment regime, and persons in the treatment facility.

Ideally the occupational therapist should have had the opportunity to study the medical record before seeing the client to begin specific evaluation. This is not always possible, however, and it may mean that the therapist has to begin the evaluation without benefit of the information gleaned from the medical record.

The information serves as a good basis for selecting methods of evaluation of and even approach to the client. It suggests the problem areas and helps the therapist focus attention on the relevant factors in the situation.[6]

Interview

The initial interview is a valuable step in the evaluation process. It is a time when the occupational therapist gathers information on how the client perceives his or her roles, dysfunction, needs, and goals and a time when the client can learn about the role of the occupational therapist and occupational therapy in the rehabilitation program.[6] An important outcome of the initial interview is the beginning development of rapport and trust between therapist and client.

The initial interview should occur in an environment that is quiet and ensures privacy. A specified period of time, known to interviewer and client at the outset, should be set aside for the interview. The first few minutes of the interview may be devoted to getting acquainted and orienting the client to the occupational therapy area as well as the role and goals of occupational therapy in the treatment facility.

The therapist should have the interview planned by knowing what information is to be acquired and having some specific questions prepared. As the interview progresses, there should be an opportunity for the client to ask questions as well. The therapist must have good listening and observation skills to glean the greatest amount of information from the interview.

During the initial or opening phase of the interview, the therapist should explain the role of the therapist, the purpose of the interview, and how the information is to be used. As the interview progresses, the therapist may seek the desired information by asking appropriate questions and guiding the responses and ensuing discussion so that they remain on relevant topics. The occupational therapist may wish to seek information about the client's family and friends, community and work roles, educational and work histories, leisure and social interests and activities, and the living situation to which the patient will return. Information about the way the client spends and manages time is important. This can be gleaned by using a tool such as the daily schedule described in the following section or the activity configuration described by Watanabe[7] and Cynkin.[2]

THE DAILY SCHEDULE. The therapist should interview the client to get a detailed account of the client's activities for a typical day (or week) in his or her life before the onset of physical dysfunction. Information that should be elicited is outlined as follows:

Rising hour
Morning activities with hours
  Hygiene
  Dressing
  Breakfast
  Work-leisure-home management
  Child care
  Luncheon
Afternoon activities with hours
  Work-leisure-home management
  Child care
  Rest
  Social activities
  Dinner
Evening activities with hours
  Leisure-social activities
  Preparation for retiring
Bedtime

The amount of time spent on each activity should be recorded carefully. During the interview the therapist should be careful not to allow the client to gloss over or omit any of the daily activities by cuing the client with appropriate questions.

The therapist might ask "What time did you get up?" "What was the first thing that you did?" "When did you eat lunch?" "Who fixed it for you?" The review of the former daily schedule may evoke many recollections of family, friends, and social, community, vocational, and leisure activities about which the client may share information freely. At times this digression from the schedule itself is desirable to elicit a well-rounded picture of the client's roles and relationships, as well as some ideas of his or her needs, values, and personal goals. In other instances tangential conversation should be limited or discouraged to focus the client's attention on the specific daily schedule.

If memory or communication disorders make the construction of the daily schedule impossible in the manner described, friends or family members may be consulted to get an approximation of the client's activities pattern that may be helpful for goal setting and activity selection.

A second daily schedule of present activities pattern in the treatment facility or at home, if the client is an outpatient, is then constructed. It is important during this interview to ask the client who helps him or her with each activity, and how much assistance the client believes he or she needs and receives. A discussion and comparative analysis of these two schedules between therapist and client should yield valuable information about the client's needs, values, satisfaction-dissatisfaction with the activities pattern, primary and secondary goals for change, interests, motivation, interpersonal relationships, and fears. On the basis of this information and the activity analysis it becomes possible to set priorities for treatment objectives according to the client's needs and values rather than the therapist's priorities. Activities that will be meaningful to the client as an individual and in his or her particular social group, and may be appropriate for use in the intervention plan, begin to emerge. Their potential for facilitation of change may be presented, and selection of therapeutic modalities to meet objectives that have been agreed on can be made.

Throughout the interview the therapist should sense the client's attitude toward the dysfunction, implicitly or explicitly. The client should have an opportunity to express what he or she sees as the primary problems and goals for rehabilitation. These may differ substantially from the therapist's judgment and must be given careful consideration when therapist and client reach the point of setting treatment objectives together.

The two essential elements for a successful interview are a solid knowledge base and active listening skills. These requirements necessitate study, practice, and preparation. The therapist's knowledge will underlie the selection of questions or topics to be covered in the interview. The interview should reflect the therapist's knowledge and cover the areas that are relevant to occupational therapy and the construction of a meaningful treatment plan. The interviewer who uses active listening demonstrates that he or she respects and is vitally interested in the client.[1] In active listening, the receiver (therapist) tries to understand what the sender (client) is feeling or the meaning of the message. The therapist then puts that understanding into his or her own words and feeds it back to the client for verification, that is, "This is what I believe you mean. Have I understood you correctly?" The therapist does not send a new message, such as an opinion, judgment, advice, or analysis. Rather the therapist sends back only what he or she thinks the patient meant.[3]

The interview can be concluded with a summary of the major points covered, information gained, an estimate of problems and assets, and plans for further occupational therapy evaluation. The occupational therapist will probably need to take notes of or record the initial interview. The client should be advised of this in advance, understand the reasons why, know the uses to which the material will be put, and be allowed to view or listen to the record if it is desired.[6]

Observation

Some aspects of the evaluation of the client will be based on the occupational therapist's observation of the client during the interview and the evaluation procedures that follow. As treatment commences, the occupational therapist will be basing some of the reevaluation of the client on observations during treatment. The occupational therapist can gain much information by observing the client as he or she approaches or is approached. What is the posture, mode of ambulation, and gait pattern? How is he or she dressed? Is there obvious motor dysfunction? Are there apparent musculoskeletal deformities? What is the facial expression, tone of voice, and manner of speech? How are the hands held and used?

Besides these observations that can be made during the first few minutes of the initial contact with the client, occupational therapists use observation to evaluate performance of activities of daily living, vocational potential, and cognitive functions. Evaluation of these skills is usually carried out by observing the client perform them in real or simulated environments to determine the client's level of independence, speed, skill, need for special equipment, and feasibility for further training.

The rapport and trust that develops between the client and the therapist will be based on the communication between them. The communication that occurs in the interview and observation phases of the evaluation will be critical to all subsequent interactions and thus the effectiveness of treatment. The client needs to have a sense that he or she has been heard and understood by someone who is empathetic and who has the necessary knowledge and skills to facilitate rehabilitation. The therapist needs to project self-confidence and confidence in the profession. This confidence will set the tone for all future transactions with the client. It will enhance the development of the client's trust in the therapist and in the potential effectiveness of occupational therapy.[6]

Formal evaluation procedure

Several formal modes of evaluation are used in occupational therapy. There are procedures with a systematic and widely accepted method of administration. Among these are the manual muscle test, joint range of motion (ROM) measurement, hand function evaluations, coordination tests, motor evaluation of hemiplegia, sensory evaluation, perceptual testing, cognitive evaluation, spasticity evaluation, reflex testing, and endurance evaluation.

Standardized tests are also used by occupational therapists. Examples of some of these are the Jebsen-Taylor Test of Hand Function,[4] the Minnesota Rate of Manipulation Test, the Lincoln-Oseretsky Motor Development Scale, the Marianne Frostig Development Test of Visual Perception, and the Southern California Sensory Integration Tests.[5] Smith[5] lists and describes these and several other standardized tests and their sources.

SUMMARY

The occupational therapy evaluation of the client with physical dysfunction includes an examination of medical records, interview, observation, and the administration of specific formal and informal evaluation procedures. The treatment program is based on an analysis of the data gathered from all of these methods, which results in the identification of problems and assets in the client's life. The evaluation process can help to determine if occupational therapy intervention is indeed appropriate.

Occupational therapists have developed many informal evaluation procedures that are useful to them in their particular treatment facilities. These include tests, batteries of tests, checklists, and rating scales. These are useful tools and many of them can be or have been developed into standardized tests. In recent years the need for reliable standardized tests has become more evident, and occupational therapists have recognized that they need to identify and employ tools that are commonly used to help establish their legitimacy. Some of the tests that are currently used by occupational therapists and that have standard protocols, such as the

Southern California Sensory-Integrative tests, require additional training and certification for proper use. It is important for therapists who need to use such tests to attain the necessary training and qualification.[6]

The selection of the appropriate evaluation procedures will depend on the client's diagnosis, medical history, lifestyle, interests, living situation, needs, and values. The information gleaned throughout the evaluation process will determine the selection of objectives, methods, and treatment progression in the construction of the treatment plan.[6] The remainder of Part 2 contains descriptions of a variety of nonstandardized evaluation procedures used for evaluation of physical dysfunction.

REFERENCES

1. Allen, C.: The performance status examination, Paper presented at the American Occupational Therapy Association Annual Conference, San Francisco, October 1976. Cited in Smith, H.D., and Tiffany, E.G.: Assessment and evaluation: an overview. In Hopkins, H.L., and Smith, H.D.: Willard and Spackman's occupational therapy, ed. 6, Philadelphia, 1983, J.B. Lippincott Co.
2. Cynkin, S.: Occupational therapy: toward health through activities, Boston, 1979, Little, Brown & Co.
3. Gordon, T.: P.E.T.: Parent effectiveness training, New York, 1970, The New American Library, Inc.
4. Jebsen, R.H., et al.: An objective and standardized test of hand function, Arch. Phys. Med. Rehabil. **50:**311, 1969.
5. Smith, H.D.: Assessment and evaluation: specific evaluation procedures. In Hopkins, H.L., and Smith, H.D.: Willard and Spackman's occupational therapy, ed. 6, Philadelphia, 1983, J.B. Lippincott, Co.
6. Smith, H.D., and Tiffany, E.G.: Assessment and evaluation: an overview. In Hopkins, H.L., and Smith, H.D.: Willard and Spackman's occupational therapy, ed. 6, Philadelphia, 1983, J.B. Lippincott Co.
7. Watanabe, S.: Regional institute on the evaluation process, Final Rep. RSA-123-T-68, New York, 1968, American Occupational Therapy Association.

CHAPTER 5

Evaluation of joint range of motion

LORRAINE WILLIAMS PEDRETTI

Joint measurement is a primary evaluation procedure for those physical dysfunctions that could cause limitation of joint motion, for example, arthritis, fractures, burns, and hand trauma. Range of motion (ROM) is the arc of motion through which a joint passes. Passive ROM is the arc of motion through which the joint passes when moved by an outside force. Active ROM is the arc of motion through which the joint passes when moved by the muscles acting on the joint. The instrument used for measuring ROM is the goniometer.

The purposes for measuring ROM are to (1) determine limitations that interfere with function or may produce deformity, (2) determine additional range needed to increase functional capacity or reduce deformity, (3) keep a record of progression or regression, (4) measure progress objectively, (5) determine appropriate treatment goals, (6) select appropriate treatment modalities, positioning techniques, and other strategies to reduce limitations, and (7) determine the need for splints and assistive devices.

PRINCIPLES OF JOINT MEASUREMENT

The evaluator should know the average normal ROM;[3] how the joint moves; and how to position self, client, and joints for measurement. Before measuring, the evaluator should ask the client to move the part through the available ROM, if muscle strength is fair or better, and observe the movement. The evaluator should move the part passively through the ROM to see and feel how the joint moves.

Formal joint measurement is *not* necessary with every client. When joint limitation is not a primary symptom or the disability is of recent onset with proper positioning and daily ROM exercises, limited ROM would not be anticipated. In such cases, however, ROM should be visually observed by using active ROM or by putting all joints

through passive ROM. Normal ROM varies from one person to the next. Establish norms for each individual by measuring the uninvolved part if possible.[3] If this is not possible, use average ranges listed in the literature. Check records and interview the client for the presence of fused joints and other limitations caused by old injuries. Do not try to force joints when resistance is met on passive ROM. Be aware that pain may limit ROM and crepitation may be heard on movement in some conditions.

METHODS OF JOINT MEASUREMENT
The 180° system

Using the 180° system of joint measurement, 0° is the starting position for all joint motions. For most motions the anatomic position is the starting position, and the 180° is superimposed as a semicircle on the body in the plane in which the motion will occur. The axis of the joint is the axis of the semicircle or arc of motion. All joint motions begin at 0° and increase toward 180°.[4] The 180° system is used later in this chapter to describe procedures for joint measurement.

The 360° system

Using the 360° system of joint measurement, movements occurring in the coronal and sagittal planes are related to a full circle. When the body is in the anatomic position, the circle is superimposed on it in the same plane in which the motion will occur with the joint axis as the pivotal point. "The 0° (360°) position will be overhead and the 180° position will be toward the feet."[4] Thus, for example, shoulder flexion and abduction are movements that proceed toward 0°, and shoulder adduction and extension proceed toward 360°.[4] The average normal ROM for shoulder flexion is 170°. Therefore using the 360° system the movement would start at 180° and progress toward 0° to 10°. The ROM recorded would be 10°. On the

other hand, shoulder extension that has a normal ROM of 60° would begin at 180° and progress toward 360° to 240°,[4] and 240° would be the ROM recorded. The total ROM of extension to flexion would be 240° minus 10°, that is, 230°.[4,5]

Some motions cannot be related to the full circle. In these instances a 0° starting position is designated, and the movements are measured as increases from 0°. These motions occur in a horizontal plane around a vertical axis. They are (1) forearm pronation and supination, (2) hip internal and external rotation, (3) wrist radial and ulnar deviation, and (4) thumb palmar and radial abduction (carpometacarpal extension).[4]

GONIOMETERS

Goniometers are used to measure the range of joint motion. They are made of metal or plastic, come in several sizes, and are available from medical and rehabilitation equipment companies.[4]

The goniometer consists of a stationary bar and a movable bar. Attached to the stationary bar is a small protractor (half circle) or a full circle printed with a scale of degrees from 0° to 180° for the half circle and 0° to 360° for the full circle goniometer.[3] The movable bar is attached at the center or axis of the protractor and acts as a dial. As the movable bar rotates around the protractor, the dial points to the number of degrees on the scale.

Two scales of figures are printed on the half circle. Each starts at 0° and progresses toward 180° but in opposite directions. Since the starting position in the 180° system is always 0° and increases toward 180°, the outer row of figures is read if the bony segments being measured are end to end, as in elbow flexion. By the same token the inner row of figures is read if the bony segments are being measured are alongside one another, as in shoulder flexion.

Fig. 5-1 shows five styles of goniometers. The first (Fig. 5-1, *A*) is a full circle goniometer that can be used for both the 360° and the 180° systems, since it has calibrations for both printed on its face. This goniometer has longer arms and is convenient for use on the large joints of the body. Fig. 5-1, *B*, is a half circle instrument used for the 180° system. This particular goniometer is radiopaque and could be used during x-ray examinations if necessary. Its dial is notched at two places so that an accurate reading of motion can be taken regardless of whether the convexity of the half circle is directed toward or away from the direction of motion. The advantage of this is that the examiner does not have to reverse the goniometer, obscuring the figures on the scale from view. A special finger goniometer is shown in Fig. 5-1, *D*. Its arms are short and flattened. It is designed to be used over the finger joint surfaces rather than on their lateral aspects, as in most of the larger joint motions. Small plastic goniometers are shown in Fig. 5-1, *C* and *E*. These are inexpensive and easy to carry about. They can be used with both large and small joints. The dials of goniometers that are transparent are also marked or notched in two places like the goniometer in Fig. 5-1, *B*. The smaller of these two goniometers is simply a larger one that has been cut to be adapted as a finger goniometer.

One important feature of the goniometer is the axis or fulcrum. The nut or rivet that acts as the fulcrum must move freely, yet it must be tight enough to remain where it was set when the goniometer is removed from the body segment following the joint measurement.[3] Some goniometers have a locking nut for the fulcrum. This nut is tightened just before removing the goniometer so that the reading can be easily and accurately made.[4]

There are other types of goniometers. Some use fluids with a free-floating bubble that provides the reading after the motion is completed.[4] Others can be attached to a body segment and have dials that register rotary motions, such as pronation and supination.

RECORDING RESULTS OF MEASUREMENTS

When using the 180° system, the evaluator should record the number of degrees at the starting position and the number of degrees at the final position after the joint has passed through the maximal possible arc of motion. Normal ROM always starts at 0° and increases toward 180°. A limitation is indicated if the starting position is not 0°. For example:
1. Elbow.
   Normal: 0° to 140°

Extension limitation: 15° to 140°
Flexion limitation: 0° to 110°
2. Abnormal hyperextension of the elbow may be recorded by indicating the number of degrees of hyperextension *before* the 0° starting position.
   Normal: 0° to 140°
   Abnormal hyperextension: 20° to 0° to 140°
3. There are alternate methods of recording ROM. The evaluator is advised to learn and adopt the particular method required by the health care facility. One method is to record limitations in minus degrees of motion. For example, elbow extension limitation would be recorded as −15°/140°.

A sample of a form for recording ROM measurements is shown in Fig. 5-2.

Average normal ROM is listed in Table 5-1. It should be noted that movements of the shoulder (glenohumeral) joint are accompanied by scapula movement as outlined. Glenohumeral joint motion is highly dependent on scapula mobility, which gives the shoulder its flexibility and wide ranges of motion. Although it is not possible to measure scapula movement with the goniometer, the evaluator should assess scapula mobility before proceeding with shoulder joint measurements. If the scapula musculature is in a state of spasticity or contracture and the shoulder joint is

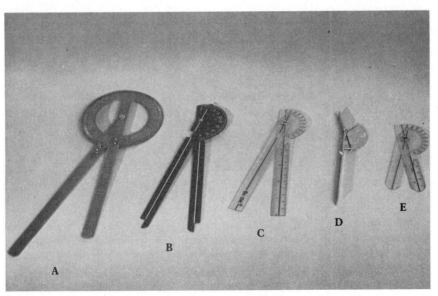

Fig. 5-1. Types of goniometers.

JOINT RANGE MEASUREMENTS

Patient's name _____ Chart no._____

Date of birth_____ Age_____ Sex_____

Diagnosis_____ Date of onset_____

Disability_____

3	LEFT 2	1	SPINE		1	RIGHT 2	3
			Cervical spine				
			Flexion	0-45			
			Extension	0-45			
			Lateral flexion	0-45			
			Rotation	0-60			
			Thoracic and lumbar spine				
			Flexion	0-80			
			Extension	0-30			
			Lateral flexion	0-40			
			Rotation	0-45			
			SHOULDER				
			Flexion	0 to 170			
			Extension	0 to 60			
			Abduction	0 to 170			
			Horizontal abduction	0-40			
			Horizontal adduction	0-130			
			Internal rotation	0 to 70			
			External rotation	0 to 90			
			ELBOW AND FOREARM				
			Flexion	0 to 135-150			
			Supination	0 to 80- 90			
			Pronation	0 to 80- 90			
			WRIST				
			Flexion	0 to 80			
			Extension	0 to 70			
			Ulnar deviation	0 to 30			
			Radial deviation	0 to 20			
			THUMB				
			MP flexion	0 to 50			
			IP flexion	0 to 80- 90			
			Abduction	0 to 50			
			FINGERS				
			MP flexion	0 to 90			
			MP hyperextension	0 to 15- 45			
			PIP flexion	0 to 110			
			DIP flexion	0 to 80			
			Abduction	0 to 25			
			HIP				
			Flexion	0 to 120			
			Extension	0 to 30			
			Abduction	0 to 40			
			Adduction	0 to 35			
			Internal rotation	0 to 45			
			External rotation	0 to 45			
			KNEE				
			Flexion	0 to 135			
			ANKLE AND FOOT				
			Plantar flexion	0 to 50			
			Dorsiflexion	0 to 15			
			Inversion	0 to 35			
			Eversion	0 to 20			

Fig. 5-2. Form for recording joint ROM measurement.

moved into ROMs that require scapula mobility (for example, above 90° of flexion or abduction), joint damage can result.

When joint measurements may be performed in more than one position, for example, as in shoulder internal and external rotation, the evaluator should note on the record in which position the measurement was taken.

RESULTS OF EVALUATION AS A BASIS FOR TREATMENT PLANNING

Common causes of joint limitation include skin contracture caused by adhesions or scar tissue, muscle weakness, spasticity, displacement of fibrocartilage or presence of other foreign bodies in the joint, bony obstruction or destruction, and soft tissue contractures,[6] such as tendon, muscle, or ligament shortening. Following joint measurement, the therapist should analyze the results in relationship to the client's life role requirements. The therapist's first concern should be to correct ROMs that fall below functional limits. Many ordinary activities of daily living (ADL) do not require full ROM. Functional ROM refers to the amount of joint range necessary to perform essential ADL without the use of special equipment.[6] The first concern of treatment, then, would be to try to increase ROMs that are limiting performance of self and home maintenance tasks to "functional range of motion."[6] For example, a significant limitation of elbow flexion would affect ability to eat and perform oral hygiene. Therefore it would be important to increase elbow flexion to nearly full ROM for function. Likewise, a severe limitation of forearm pronation would affect the performance of tasks, such as eating, washing the body, telephoning, child care, and dressing. To sit comfortably hip ROM must be at least 0° to 90°, so that if hip flexion is limited, a first goal might be to increase it to 90°. Of course, if additional ROM can be gained, the therapist should plan the progression of treatment to increase the ROM to the normal range.

In some instances the ROM limitations may be permanent, and it will not be possible to increase ROM. In such cases the role of the therapist is to work out methods to compensate for the loss of ROM. These may include assistive devices, such as a comb, brush, or shoe horn with long handles, device to apply stockings, or adapted methods of performing a particular skill. See Chapter 12 for further suggestions of ADL techniques for those with limited ROM. In many diagnoses, as with burns or arthritis, loss of ROM can be anticipated; the goal of treatment would be to prevent joint limitation before it occurs with splints, positioning, exercise, activity, and application of the principles of joint protecton.

Limitations of ROM, their causes, and the prognosis for increasing ROM will suggest treatment approaches. Some of the specific methods used to increase ROM are discussed elsewhere in this text. These include passive or active stretching exercise, resistive exercise, strengthening of antagonistic muscle groups, activities that require active motion of the affected joints through the full available ROM, splints, and positioning. To increase ROM the physician may perform surgery or may manipulate the part while the patient is under anesthesia. The physical therapist may employ manual stretching with heat and massage.[6]

PROCEDURE FOR JOINT MEASUREMENT

Average normal ROM for each joint motion is listed in Table 5-1, in Fig. 5-2, and before each of the following procedures for measurement. The reader should bear in mind that these are averages and there may be considerable variation in ROM from one individual to the next. Therefore the subject in the illustrations may not always demonstrate the average ROM listed for the particular motion.

The goniometer in the illustrations is shown so that the reader can most easily see its correct positioning. However, the examiner may not always be in the best position for the particular measurement. For the purposes of clear illustration the examiner is necessarily shown

off to one side and may have only one hand on the instrument. Many of the motions require that the examiner be squarely in front of the subject or that the examiner's hands obscure the goniometer. The manner in which the examiner holds the goniometer and supports the part being measured is determined by factors, such as degree of muscle weakness, presence or absence of joint pain, and whether active or passive ROM is being measured. The examiner should always position self and the subject for the greatest comfort, correct placement of the instrument, and adequate stability of the part being tested to effect the desired motion in the correct plane.

General procedure—180° method of measurement

1. Have client comfortable and relaxed in appropriate position.
2. Explain and demonstrate to client what you are going to do, why, and how you expect client to cooperate.
3. Uncover joint to be measured.
4. Stabilize joints proximal to joint being measured.
5. Have client move joint through ROM or move part passively through ROM to observe available ROM and get a sense of joint mobility.
6. At starting position place axis of goniometer over axis of joint. Place stationary bar on stationary bone and movable bar on moving bone. Avoid goniometer dial going off semicircle by always facing curved side away from direction of motion unless the goniometer can be read when it moves in either direction.
7. Record number of degrees at starting position and remove goniometer. Do not attempt to hold goniometer in place while moving joint through ROM.
8. Evaluator should hold part securely above and below joint being measured and *gently* move joint through available ROM to determine full *passive* ROM. *Do not force joints.* Watch for signs of pain and discomfort. Unless otherwise indicated, passive ROM should be measured.
9. Reposition goniometer and record number of degrees at final position.
10. Remove goniometer and gently place part in resting position.

Table 5-1

Average normal ROM (180° method)

Joint	ROM	Associated girdle motion	Joint	ROM
Cervical spine			**Wrist**	
Flexion	0° to 45°		Flexion	0° to 80°
Extension	0° to 45°		Extension	0° to 70°
Lateral flexion	0° to 45°		Radial deviation (abduction)	0° to 20°
Rotation	0° to 60°		Ulnar deviation (adduction)	0° to 30°
Thoracic and lumbar spine				
Flexion	0° to 80°		**Fingers***	
Extension	0° to 30°		MP flexion	0° to 90°
Lateral flexion	0° to 40°		MP hyperextension	0° to 15°-45°
Rotation	0° to 45°		PIP flexion	0° to 110°
Shoulder			DIP flexion	0° to 80°
Flexion	0° to 170°	Abduction, lateral tilt, slight elevation, slight upward rotation	Abduction	0° to 25°
			Thumb*	
Extension	0° to 60°	Depression, adduction, upward tilt	DIP flexion	0° to 80°-90°
			MP flexion	0° to 50°
Abduction	0° to 170°	Upward rotation, elevation	Adduction, radial and palmar	0°
Adduction	0°	Depression, adduction, downward rotation	Palmar abduction	0° to 50°
Horizontal abduction	0° to 40°	Adduction, reduction of lateral tilt	Radial abduction	0° to 50°
			Opposition	
Horizontal adduction	0° to 130°	Abduction, lateral tilt	**Hip**	
Internal rotation		Abduction, lateral tilt	Flexion	0° to 120° (bent knee)
Arm in abduction	0° to 70°		Extension	0° to 30°
Arm in adduction	0° to 60°		Abduction	0° to 40°
External rotation		Adduction, reduction of lateral tilt	Adduction	0° to 35°
			Internal rotation	0° to 45°
Arm in abduction	0° to 90°		External rotation	0° to 45°
Arm in adduction	0° to 80°		**Knee**	
Elbow			Flexion	0° to 135°
Flexion	0° to 135°-150°		**Ankle and foot**	
Extension	0°		Plantar flexion	0° to 50°
Forearm			Dorsiflexion	0° to 15°
Pronation	0° to 80°-90°		Inversion	0° to 35°
Supination	0° to 80°-90°		Eversion	0° to 20°

Data adapted from American Academy of Orthopaedic Surgeons: Joint motion: method of measuring and recording, Chicago, 1965, American Academy of Orthopaedic Surgeons, and Esch, D., and Lepley, M.,: Evaluation of joint motion: methods of measurement and recording, Minneapolis, 1974, University of Minnesota Press.

*DIP, Distal interphalangeal; MP, metacarpophalangeal; PIP, proximal interphalangeal.

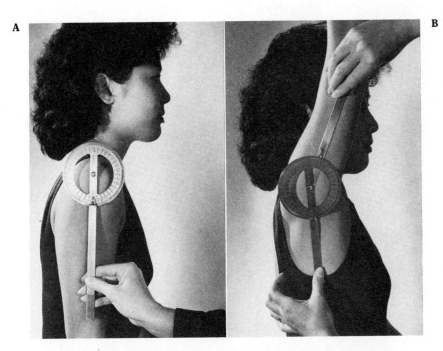

Fig. 5-3. Shoulder flexion. **A,** Starting position. **B,** Final position.

DIRECTIONS FOR JOINT MEASUREMENT—180° SYSTEM
Upper extremity[1,2,4,7]
Shoulder

Flexion—0° to 170° (Fig. 5-3)

POSITION OF THE SUBJECT: Seated or supine with humerus in neutral rotation.

POSITION OF GONIOMETER: Axis is in the center of humeral head just distal to the acromion process on the lateral aspect of humerus. Stationary bar is parallel to trunk, and moveable bar is parallel to humerus.

Extension—0° to 60° (Fig. 5-4)

POSITION OF SUBJECT: Seated or prone with no obstruction behind humerus and humerus in neutral rotation.

POSITION OF GONIOMETER: Same as for flexion.

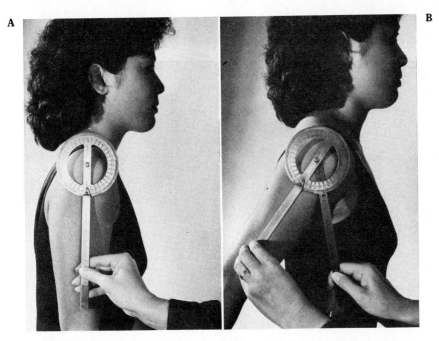

Fig. 5-4. Shoulder extension. **A,** Starting position. **B,** Final position.

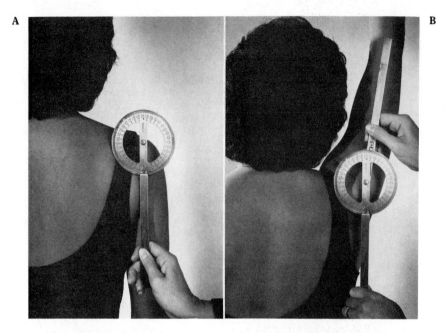

Fig. 5-5. Shoulder abduction. **A**, Starting position. **B**, Final position.

Abduction—0° to 170° (Fig. 5-5)

POSITION OF SUBJECT: Seated or prone with humerus in neutral rotation. Measure on posterior surface.

POSITION OF GONIOMETER: Axis is on acromion process on posterior surface of shoulder. Stationary bar is parallel to trunk, and movable bar is parallel to humerus.

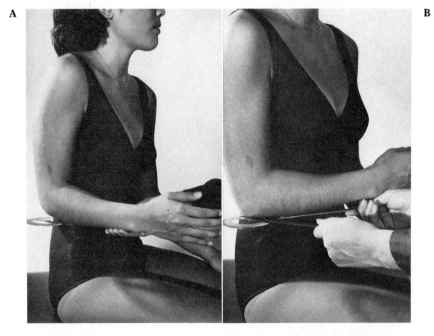

Fig. 5-6. Shoulder internal rotation, shoulder adducted. **A**, Starting position. **B**, Final position.

Internal rotation—0° to 60 ° (Fig. 5-6)

POSITION OF SUBJECT: Seated with humerus adducted against trunk, elbow at 90°, and forearm at midposition and perpendicular to body.

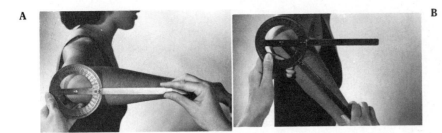

Fig. 5-7. Shoulder internal rotation, shoulder abducted. **A,** Starting position. **B,** Final position.

ALTERNATE POSITION: 0° to 70° (Fig. 5-7) seated with humerus abducted to 90°, elbow flexed to 90°, and forearm parallel to floor.

POSITION OF GONIOMETER: Axis on olecranon process of elbow and stationary bar and movable bar parallel to forearm.

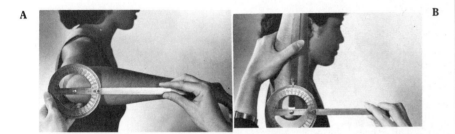

Fig. 5-8. Shoulder external rotation, shoulder abducted. **A,** Starting position. **B,** Final position.

External rotation—0° to 90° (Fig. 5-8) arm in abduction; 0° to 80° (Fig. 5-9) arm in adduction

POSITION OF SUBJECT AND GONIOMETER: Same as for internal rotation.

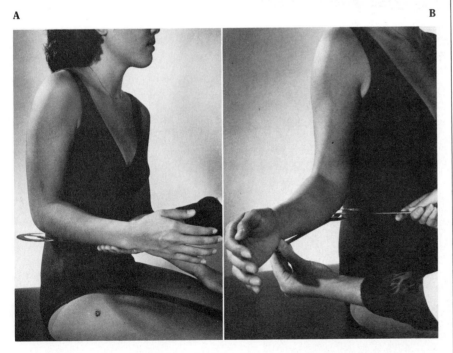

Fig. 5-9. External rotation, shoulder adducted. **A,** Starting position. **B,** Final position.

A 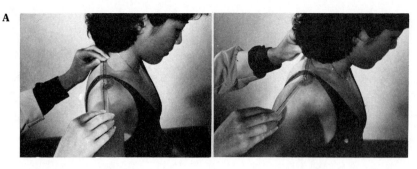 B

Fig. 5-10. Shoulder horizontal abduction. **A,** Starting position. **B,** Final position.

A 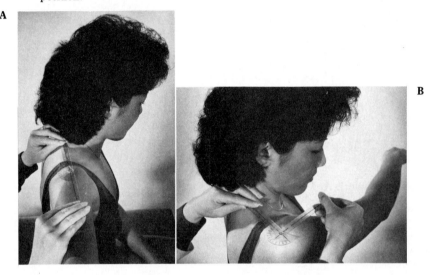 B

Fig. 5-11. Shoulder horizontal adduction. **A,** Starting position. **B,** Final position.

A 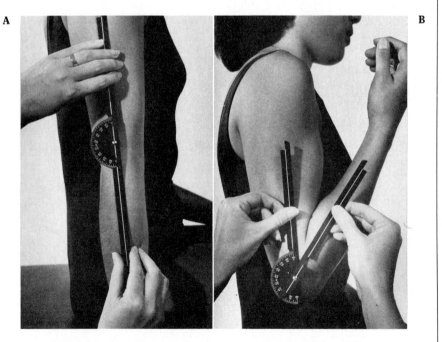 B

Fig. 5-12. Elbow flexion. **A,** Starting position. **B,** Final position.

Horizontal abduction—0° to 40° (Fig. 5-10)

POSITION OF SUBJECT: Seated erect with the shoulder to be tested abducted to 90°, elbow extended, and palm facing down.

POSITION OF GONIOMETER: The axis is centered over the acromion process. The stationary bar is parallel over the shoulder toward the neck, and the movable bar is parallel with the humerus.

Horizontal adduction—0° to 130° (Fig. 5-11)

POSITION OF SUBJECT AND GONIOMETER: Same as for horizontal abduction.

Elbow

Extension to flexion—0° to 135°-150° (Fig. 5-12)

POSITION OF SUBJECT: Standing, sitting, or supine with humerus adducted and externally rotated and forearm supinated.

POSITION OF GONIOMETER: Axis is placed over the lateral epicondyle of humerus at end of elbow crease. Stationary bar is parallel to midline of humerus, and movable bar is parallel to radius. After the movement has been completed, the position of the elbow crease changes in relation to the lateral epicondyle because of the rise of the muscle bulk during the motion. The axis of the goniometer should be repositioned so that it is over, although will not be directly on, the lateral epicondyle.

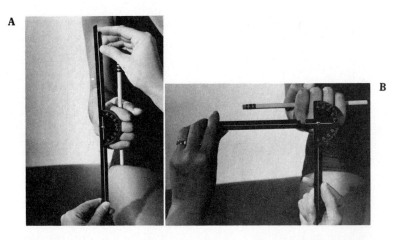

Fig. 5-13. Forearm supination. **A,** Starting position. **B,** Final position.

Forearm
Supination—0° to 80°-90° (Fig. 5-13)
POSITION OF SUBJECT: Seated or standing with humerus adducted, elbow at 90°, and forearm in midposition. Place pencil in hand so it is held by subject perpendicularly to floor.
POSITION OF GONIOMETER: Axis is over the head of third metacarpal, and stationary bar is perpendicular to floor. Movable bar is parallel to pencil.

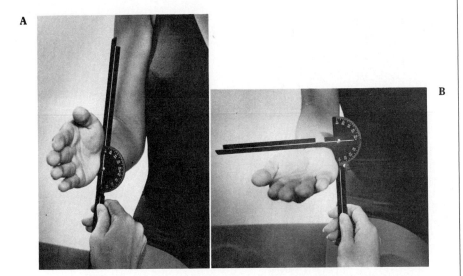

Fig. 5-14. Supination, alternate method. **A,** Starting position. **B,** Final position.

ALTERNATE METHOD: (Fig. 5-14). Subject is positioned same but without pencil in hand. Axis of goniometer is at ulnar border of volar aspect of wrist just proximal to the ulnar styloid. Movable bar is resting against volar aspect of wrist, and stationary bar is perpendicular to floor.

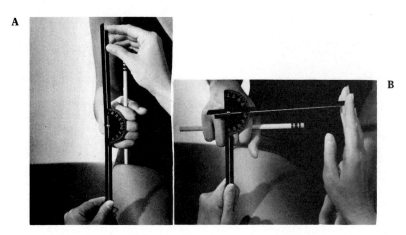

Fig. 5-15. Pronation. **A,** Starting position. **B,** Final position.

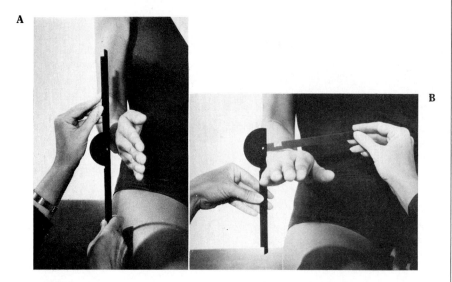

Fig. 5-16. Pronation alternate position. **A,** Starting position. **B,** Final position.

Pronation—0° to 80°-90° (Figs. 5-15 and 5-16)

POSITION OF SUBJECT AND GONIOMETER: Same as for supination.

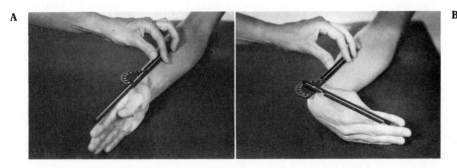

Fig. 5-17. Wrist flexion. **A,** Starting position. **B,** Final position.

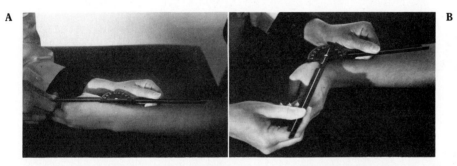

Fig. 5-18. Wrist extension. **A,** Starting position. **B,** Final position.

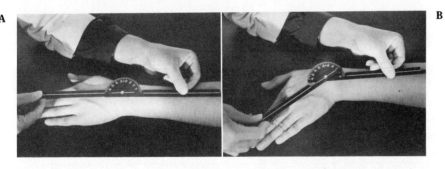

Fig. 5-19. Wrist ulnar deviation. **A,** Starting position. **B,** Final position.

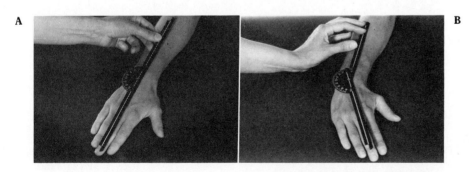

Fig. 5-20. Wrist radial deviation. **A,** Starting position. **B,** Final position.

Wrist

Flexion—0° to 80° (Fig. 5-17)

POSITION OF SUBJECT: Seated with forearm in midposition and hand and forearm resting on table on ulnar border.

POSITION OF GONIOMETER Axis is on lateral aspect of wrist just distal to radial styloid in anatomical snuff box. Stationary bar is parallel to radius, and movable bar is parallel to metacarpal of index finger.

Extension—0° to 70° (Fig. 5-18)

POSITION OF SUBJECT AND GONIOMETER: Same as for wrist flexion.

Ulnar deviation—0° to 30° (Fig. 5-19)

POSITION OF SUBJECT: Seated with forearm pronated and palm of hand resting flat on table surface

POSITION OF GONIOMETER: Axis is on dorsum of wrist at base of third metacarpal. Stationary bar is parallel to third metacarpal.

Radial deviation—0° to 20° (Fig. 5-20)

POSITION OF SUBJECT AND GONIOMETER: Same as for ulnar deviation.

A 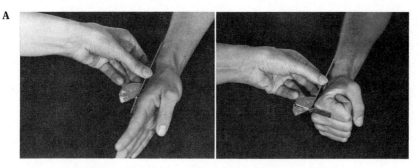 B

Fig. 5-21. MP flexion. **A,** Starting position. **B,** Final position.

A 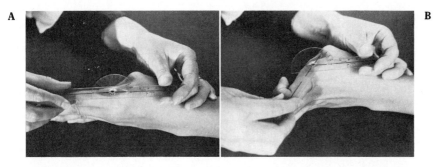 B

Fig. 5-22. MP hyperextension. **A,** Starting position. **B,** Final position.

A 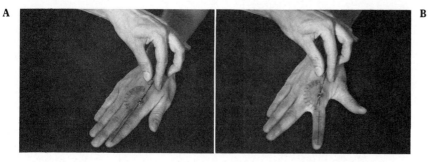 B

Fig. 5-23. MP abduction. **A,** Starting position. **B,** Final position.

A 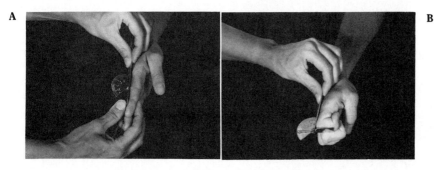 B

Fig. 5-24. PIP flexion. **A,** Starting position. **B,** Final position.

Fingers

Metacarpophalangeal (MP) flexion—0° to 90° (Fig. 5-21)

POSITION OF SUBJECT: Seated with forearm in midposition, wrist at 0° neutral, and forearm and hand supported on firm surface on ulnar border

POSITION OF GONIOMETER: Axis is centered on top of middle of MP joint. Stationary bar is on top of metacarpal, and movable bar is on top of proximal phalanx.

MP hyperextension—0° to 15°-45° (Fig. 5-22)

POSITION OF SUBJECT: Seated with forearm in midposition, wrist at 0° neutral, and forearm and hand supported on a firm surface on ulnar border.

POSITION OF GONIOMETER: Axis is over lateral aspect of MP joint of index finger. Stationary bar is parallel to metacarpal, and movable bar is parallel to proximal phalanx. Fifth finger MP joint may be measured similarly. ROM of third and fourth fingers can be estimated by comparison.

MP abduction—0° to 25° (Fig. 5-23)

POSITION OF SUBJECT: Seated with forearm pronated and hand palm down, resting on firm surface. Fingers straight.

POSITION OF GONOMETER: Axis is centered over MP joint being measured. Stationary bar is over corresponding metacarpal, and movable bar is over corresponding proximal phalanx.

Proximal interphalangeal (PIP) flexion—0° to 110° (Fig. 5-24)

POSITION OF SUBJECT: Seated with forearm in midposition, wrist at 0° neutral, and forearm and hand supported on a firm surface on ulnar border.

POSITION OF GONIOMETER: Axis is centered on dorsal surface of PIP joint being measured. Stationary bar is placed over the proximal phalanx, and movable bar is over distal phalanx.

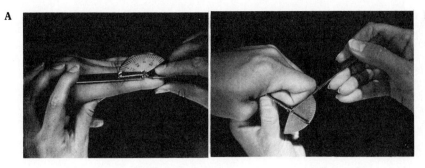

Fig. 5-25. DIP flexion. **A,** Starting position. **B,** Final position.

Distal interphalangeal (DIP) flexion—
0° to 80° (Fig. 5-25)

POSITION OF SUBJECT: Seated with forearm in midposition, wrist at 0° neutral, and forearm and hand supported on the ulnar border on a firm surface.

POSITION OF GONIOMETER: Axis is on dorsal surface of DIP joint. Stationary bar is over middle phalanx, and movable bar is over distal phalanx.

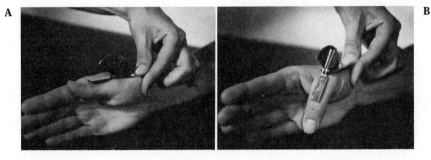

Fig. 5-26. Thumb MP flexion. **A,** Starting position. **B,** Final position.

Thumb

*MP flexion—*0° to 50° (Fig. 5-26)

POSITION OF SUBJECT: Seated with the forearm in 45° of supination, wrist at 0° neutral, and forearm and hand supported on a firm surface.

POSITION OF GONIOMETER: Axis is on dorsal surface of MP joint. Stationary bar is over thumb metacarpal, and movable bar is over proximal phalanx.

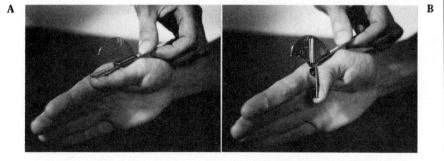

Fig. 5-27. Thumb IP flexion. **A,** Starting position. **B,** Final position.

*Interphalangeal (IP) flexion—*0° to 80°-90° (Fig. 5-27)

POSITION OF SUBJECT: Same as described for PIP and DIP finger flexion.

POSITION OF GONIOMETER: Axis is on dorsal surface of IP joint. Stationary bar is over proximal phalanx, and movable bar is over distal phalanx.

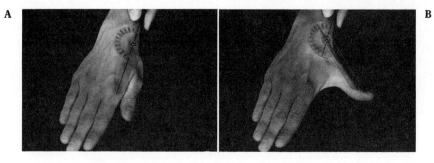

Fig. 5-28. Radial abduction. **A,** Starting position. **B,** Final position.

*Radial abduction (carpometacarpal [CMC] extension)—*0° to 50° (Fig. 5-28)

POSITION OF SUBJECT: Seated with forearm pronated and hand palm down, resting flat on firm surface.

POSITION OF GONIOMETER: Axis is over CMC joint at base of thumb metacarpal. Stationary bar is parallel to radius, and movable bar is parallel to thumb metacarpal.

A

B

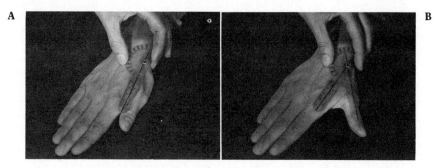

Fig. 5-29. Radial abduction, alternate method. **A,** Starting position. **B,** Final position.

ALTERNATE METHOD: (Fig. 5-29). Subject is positioned same as described in first method. Axis is over the CMC joint at the base of the thumb metacarpal. The stationary and movable bars are together and parallel to the thumb and the first metacarpals. Neither will be directly over these bones.

A

B

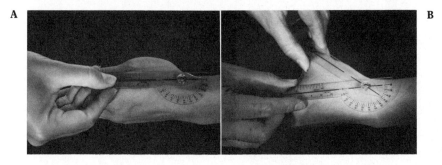

Fig. 5-30. Palmar abduction. **A,** Starting position. **B,** Final position.

Palmar abduction—0° to 50° (Fig. 5-30)
POSITION OF SUBJECT: Seated with forearm at 0° midposition, wrist at 0°, and forearm and hand resting on ulnar border. The thumb is rotated so that it is at right angles to the palm of the hand.

POSITION OF GONIOMETER: Axis is over CMC joint at base of thumb metacarpal. Stationary bar is over radius, and movable bar is over thumb metacarpal.

A

B

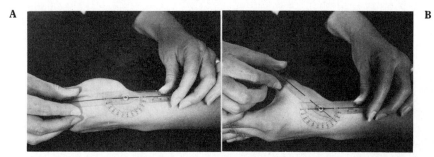

Fig. 5-31. Palmar abduction, alternate method. **A,** Starting position. **B,** Final position.

ALTERNATE METHOD: (Fig. 5-31). Subject is positioned same as described in first method. Axis is over the CMC joint at the base of the thumb metacarpal. The stationary and movable bars are lined up together parallel to the thumb and the first metacarpals.

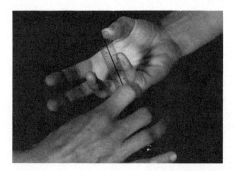

Fig. 5-32. Thumb opposition to fifth finger.

Opposition—(Fig. 5-32) Deficits in opposition may be recorded by measuring distance between pad of the thumb and pad of fifth finger with a centimeter ruler.

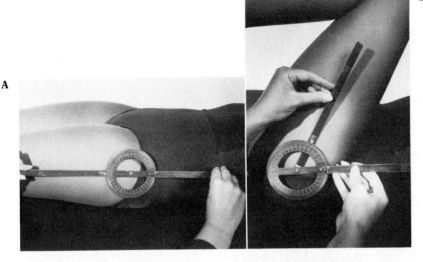

Fig. 5-33. Hip flexion. **A,** Starting position. **B,** Final position.

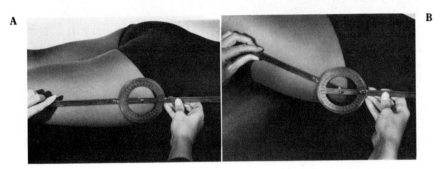

Fig. 5-34. Hip extension. **A,** Starting position. **B,** Final position.

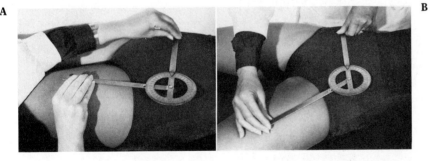

Fig. 5-35. Hip abduction. **A,** Starting position. **B,** Final position.

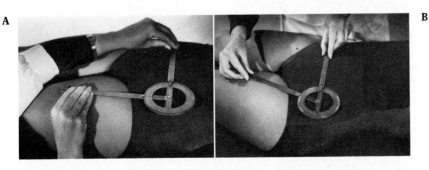

Fig. 5-36. Hip adduction. **A,** Starting position. **B,** Final position.

Lower extremity[4,5]

Hip

Flexion—0° to 120° (Fig. 5-33)

POSITION OF SUBJECT: Supine lying with hip and knee in extension.

POSITION OF GONIOMETER: Axis is on lateral aspect of hip over greater trochanter of femur. Stationary bar is at middle of lateral aspect of lower trunk, and movable bar is parallel to long axis of femur on lateral aspect of thigh.

Extension (hyperextension)—0° to 30° (Fig. 5-34)

POSITION OF SUBJECT: Prone lying with hip and knee at 0° neutral extension.

POSITION OF GONIOMETER: Same as for hip flexion.

Abduction—0° to 40° (Fig. 5-35)

POSITION OF SUBJECT: Supine lying with legs extended.

POSITION OF GONIOMETER: Axis is placed on anterior superior iliac spine. Stationary bar is placed on a line between two anterior superior iliac spines, and movable bar is parallel to longitudinal axis of femur over anterior aspect of thigh. Note that starting position is at 90° for this measurement, and recording of measurement should be adjusted to accommodate to this exception to usual positioning of goniometer by subtracting 90° from total number of degrees obtained in arc of joint motion.

Adduction—0° to 35° (Fig. 5-36)

POSITION OF SUBJECT AND GONIOMETER: Supine lying with hip and knee of the leg to be tested in extension and neutral rotation. The leg not being tested should be in hip abduction with the knee flexed over the edge of the table. The goniometer is positioned same as for hip abduction.

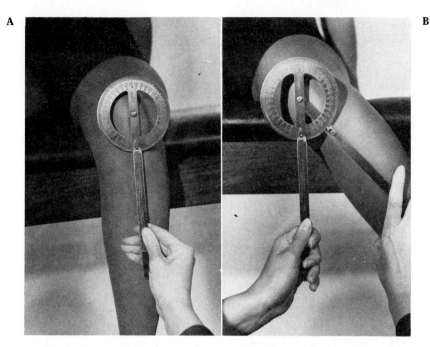

Fig. 5-37. Hip internal rotation. **A,** Starting position. **B,** Final position.

Internal rotation—0° to 45° (Fig. 5-37)
POSITION OF SUBJECT: Seated or supine with hip and knee flexed to 90°.

POSITION OF GONIOMETER: Axis is on center of patella of knee. Stationary and movable bars are parallel to longitudinal axis of tibia on anterior aspect of lower leg. Stationary bar remains in this position, perpendicular to floor, while movable bar follows tibia as hip is rotated.

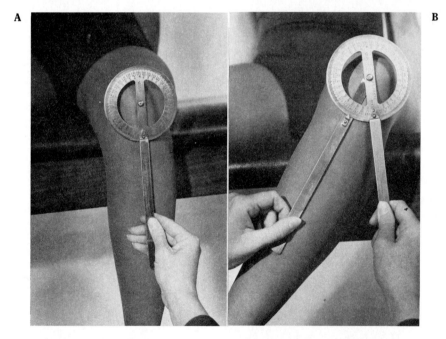

Fig. 5-38. Hip external rotation. **A,** Starting position. **B,** Final position.

External rotation—0° to 45° (Fig. 5-38)
POSITION OF SUBJECT AND GONIOMETER: Seated with hip and knee of leg to be tested flexed to 90°. The other leg should be (1) flexed at the knee so that the lower leg is back under the table or (2) flexed at the hip and knee so that the foot is resting on the table. This will allow the motion to take place without obstruction. The trunk should remain erect during the performance of the motion. The goniometer is positioned the same as for internal rotation.

A

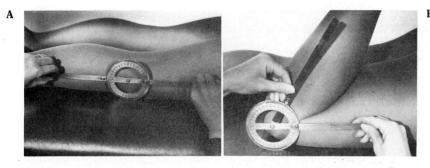

B

Fig. 5-39. Knee flexion. **A,** Starting position. **B,** Final position.

Knee
Extension-flexion—0° to 135° (Fig. 5-39)

POSITION OF SUBJECT: Prone lying with legs extended.

POSITION OF GONIOMETER: Axis is centered on lateral aspect of knee joint at tibial condyle. Stationary bar is on lateral aspect of thigh to parallel longitudinal aixs of femur. Movable bar is parallel to longitudinal axis of tibia on lateral aspect of leg.

A

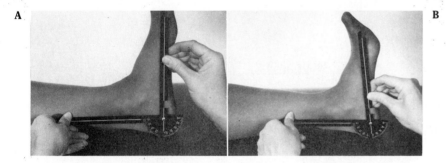

B

Fig. 5-40. Ankle dorsiflexion. **A,** Starting position. **B,** Final position.

Ankle
Dorsiflexion—0° to 15° (Fig. 5-40)

POSITION OF SUBJECT: Supine lying or seated with knee flexed. Ankle is at 90° neutral position.

POSITION OF GONIOMETER: Axis is placed approximately 1 inch below medial malleolus. Stationary bar is parallel to midline of lower leg and movable bar parallel with first metatarsal. Note that measurement begins at 90° so that this must be subtracted when recording joint measurement.

A

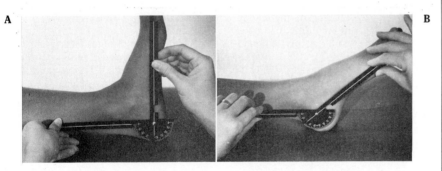

B

Fig. 5-41. Ankle plantar flexion. **A,** Starting position. **B,** Final position.

Plantar flexion—0° to 50° (Fig. 5-41)

POSITION OF SUBJECT AND GONIOMETER: Same as for dorsiflexion.

A

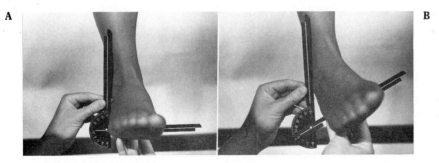

B

Fig. 5-42. Inversion. **A,** Starting position. **B,** Final position.

Inversion—0° to 35° (Fig. 5-42)

POSITION OF SUBJECT: Sitting or supine with knee flexed and ankle in 90° neutral position.

POSITION OF GONIOMETER: Axis is placed at lateral border of foot near heel. Stationary bar is parallel to longitudinal axis of tibia on lateral aspect of leg. Movable bar is parallel to plantar surface of heel.

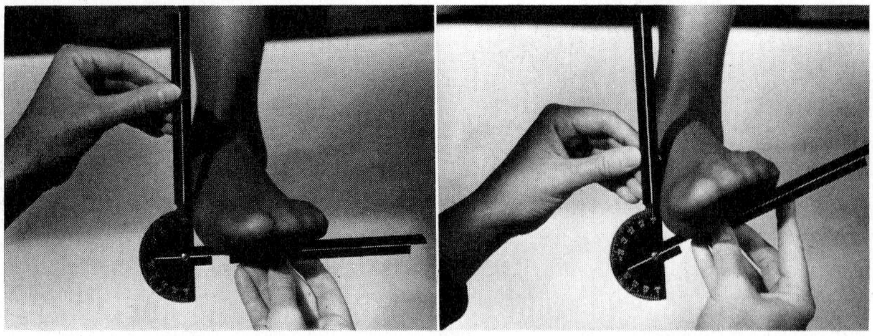

Fig. 5-43. Eversion. **A,** Starting position. **B,** Final position.

Eversion—0° to 20° (Fig. 5-43)

POSITION OF SUBJECT: Same as for inversion.

POSITION OF GONIOMETER: Axis is on medial border of foot just proximal to metatarsal-phalangeal joint. Stationary bar is parallel to longitudinal aspect of tibia on medial aspect of lower leg. Movable bar is parallel to plantar surface of sole. Note that measurements for inversion and eversion both begin at 90°. Therefore this amount must be subtracted from total when recording measurement.

REVIEW QUESTIONS

1. Describe general rules for positioning the goniometer when measuring joint ROM.
2. With which diagnoses would joint measurement be a primary evaluation procedure?
3. List and discuss four purposes of joint measurement.
4. Is formal joint measurement necessary for every client? If not, how may ROM be evaluated?
5. Describe the steps in the procedure for joint measurement.
6. How is joint ROM measurement recorded on the evaluation form?
7. List the average normal ROM for elbow flexion, shoulder flexion, finger MP flexion, hip flexion, knee flexion, and ankle dorsiflexion.
8. Describe how to read the goniometer when using the 180° system of joint measurement.
9. List three common causes of joint limitation.
10. Define what is meant by "functional range of motion."
11. Discuss two approaches to treatment of joint limitation in occupational therapy.
12. List six treatment methods that could be used by occupational and physical therapy to increase ROM.

REFERENCES

1. American Academy of Orthopaedic Surgeons: Joint motion: method of measuring and recording, Chicago, 1965, American Academy of Orthopaedic Surgeons.
2. Baruch Center of Physical Medicine: The technique of goniometry, Lynchburg, Va., Medical College of Virginia. Mimeographed.
3. Cole, T.: Measurement of musculoskeletal function: goniometry. In Kottke, F.J., Stillwell, G.K., and Lehmann, J.F.: Krusen's handbook of physical medicine and rehabilitation, ed. 3, Philadelphia, 1982, W.B. Saunders Co.
4. Esch, D., and Lepley, M.: Evaluation of joint motion: methods of measurement and recording, Minneapolis, 1974, University of Minnesota Press.
5. Hurt, S.P.: Considerations of muscle function and their application to disability evaluation and treatment: joint measurement, Am. J. Occup. Ther. **1:**69, 1947; **2:**13, 1948.
6. Killingsworth, A.: Basic physical disability procedures, Oakland, Calif., 1976, Cal-Syl Press.
7. Rancho Los Amigos Hospital: How to measure range of motion of the upper extremities, Downey, Calif., Rancho Los Amigos Hospital. Mimeographed.

CHAPTER 6

Evaluation of muscle strength

LORRAINE WILLIAMS PEDRETTI

Many physical disabilities cause muscle weakness. Loss of strength places slight to significant limitations on the performance of occupational roles, depending on the degree of weakness and whether the weakness is permanent or temporary. Therefore the occupational therapist must assess the weakness and plan treatment that will improve strength or compensate for the loss of strength if it is not expected to improve.

Causes of muscle weakness

Disabilities in which a loss of muscle strength is a primary symptom or direct result of the disease or injury include (1) the lower motor neuron disorders, such as peripheral neuropathies and peripheral nerve injuries, spinal cord injury (since those muscles innervated at the level(s) of the lesion generally have a lower motor neuron paralysis), Guillain-Barré syndrome, and cranial nerve dysfunctions; (2) primary muscle diseases, such as muscular dystrophy and myasthenia gravis; and (3) neurological diseases in which the lower motor neuron is affected, such as in amyotrophic lateral sclerosis or multiple sclerosis. Disabilities in which a loss of muscle strength is caused by disuse or immobilization rather than a direct effect of the disease process include burns, amputation, hand trauma (unless there is an accompanying nerve injury), arthritis, fractures, and a variety of other orthopedic conditions. In the final recovery stages of stroke or head injury when spasticity and synergy patterns have disappeared and the client has achieved isolated control of voluntary muscle function, some underlying residual weakness may be detected. In these instances some assessment of strength can be of value in designing a treatment program.

Limitations resulting from muscle weakness

Muscle weakness can restrict the performance of occupational roles and thus prevent pursuit of self-care, vocational, avocational, and social activities. These limitations are assessed through muscle testing combined with performance testing. Given good to normal endurance, the client with good (G) to normal (N) muscle strength will be able to perform all ordinary activities of daily living (ADL) without undue fatigue.[9] (Ordinary ADL are considered here to be all self-maintenance tasks, mobility, and vocational roles except strenuous labor.) The client with fair plus (F+) muscle strength usually has low endurance and will fatigue more easily than one with G to N strength. However, the client will be able to independently perform many ordinary ADL but may require frequent rest periods. The client with muscle grades of fair (F) will be able to move parts against gravity and perform light tasks requiring little or no resistance.[7,9] Low endurance is a significant problem and will limit the amount of activity that can be done. The client can probably feed himself or herself finger foods and perform light hygiene if given the time and rest periods needed to reach the goals.[9] If muscle strength in the lower extremities is only F, ambulation will not be possible.[7] Poor (P) strength is considered below functional range[7] but the client can perform some ADL with mechanical assistance and range of motion (ROM) can be maintained independently. Clients with muscle grades of trace (T) and zero (0) are completely dependent and can perform no ADL without externally-powered devices. Some activities are possible with special controls on equipment, such as the electric wheelchair, communication devices, and hand splints.[9]

Purposes for evaluating muscle strength

Muscle testing, particularly the evaluation of individual muscles, is essential for diagnosis in some neuromuscular conditions, such as peripheral nerve lesions and spinal cord injury. In peripheral nerve or nerve root lesions the pattern of muscle weakness may help determine which nerve or nerve roots are involved and whether the involvement is partial or complete. Careful evaluation can help determine the level or levels of spinal cord involvement.[8] Therefore muscle testing along with sensory evaluation can be an important diagnostic aid in neuromuscular conditions.

The purposes for evaluating muscle strength are (1) to determine the amount of muscle power available and thus establish a baseline for treatment; (2) to discern how muscle weakness is limiting performance of ADL; (3) to prevent deformities that can result from imbalances of strength; (4) to determine the need for assistive devices as compensatory measures; (5) to aid in the selection of activities within the client's capabilities; and (6) to evaluate the effectiveness of treatment.[9]

Methods of evaluation

Muscle strength can be evaluated in several ways. The most precise method is a test of individual muscles, as nearly as that is possible. In this procedure the muscle is carefully isolated through proper positioning, stabilization, and careful control of the movement pattern, and its strength is graded. This type of muscle testing is described by Kendall, Kendall, and Wadsworth.[8] Another and perhaps a more common method of manual muscle testing is to assess the strength of groups of muscles that perform specific motions at each joint. This type of testing was described by Daniels and Worthingham[7] and for the most part, is the form that is presented later in this chapter. Functional motion tests, functional muscle tests, or screening tests are also used to assess muscle strength. These tests are not as precise as manual muscle testing and their purpose is to quickly evaluate strength and determine areas of weakness and the need for more precise testing. Finally, muscle strength can be observed in the performance of ordinary activities.[7] During an ADL performance evaluation, for example, the therapist can observe for difficulties and movement patterns that may signal weakness, muscle imbalance, poor endurance for activity, and substitutions that the client uses for function. The performance evaluation should always be part of the assessment of strength.

Results of evaluation as a basis for treatment planning

When planning treatment for the maintenance or improvement of strength, the occupational therapist must consider several factors before determining treatment priorities, goals, and modalities. The results of the muscle strength assessment will suggest the progression of a strengthening program. What is the degree of weakness? Is it generalized or specific to one or more muscle groups? Are the muscle grades generally the same throughout, or is there significant disparity in muscle grades? If there is disparity, is there an imbalance of strength between the agonist and antagonist muscle that will require protection of the weaker muscles during treatment and ADL? Where there is significant imbalance between an agonist and antagonist muscle, treatment goals may be directed toward strengthening the weaker group while maintaining the strength of the stronger group. Muscle imbalance may also suggest the need for orthoses to protect the weaker muscles from overstretching while recovery is in progress. Devices such as the bed footboard to prevent

overstretching of the weakened ankle dorsiflexors and the wrist cock-up splint to prevent overstretching of weakened wrist extensors are examples. Muscle grades will suggest the level and type of therapeutic exercise and activity that can help to maintain or improve strength. Is the weakness mild (G range), moderate (F to F+), or severe (P to 0)?[9] Muscles graded F−, for example, could be strengthened by using active assisted exercise or activity against gravity. Muscles graded P likewise will require active exercise in a gravity-eliminated plane with little or no resistance to increase strength. Further discussion of appropriate exercise and activity for specific muscle grades appears in Chapter 11.

The endurance of the muscles (how many repetitions of the muscle contraction are possible before fatigue sets in) is an important consideration in treatment planning. Frequently, one of the goals of the therapeutic activity program is to increase endurance as well as strength. Since the manual muscle test does not measure endurance, the therapist should assess it by engaging the client in periods of exercise or activity graded in length to determine the amount of time that the muscle group can be used in sustained activity. There is usually a correlation between strength and endurance. Weaker muscles will tend to have less endurance than stronger ones. When selecting treatment modalities for increasing endurance, the therapist may elect not to tax the muscle to its maximal ability but rather emphasize repetitive action at less than maximal contraction to increase endurance and prevent fatigue.[9]

Sensory loss, which often accompanies muscle weakness, complicates the ability of the client to perform in an activity program. If there is little or no tactile or proprioceptive feedback from motion, the impulse to move is decreased or lost, depending on the severity of the sensory loss. Thus the movement may appear weak and ineffective even when strength is adequate for performance of a specific activity. With some diagnoses, a sensory stimulation program may be indicated to increase the client's sensory awareness and feedback from the part. In other instances, the therapist may elect to help the

client compensate for the sensory loss through visual devices, such as mirrors, video playback, and biofeedback. These can be used as adjuncts to the strengthening program.

Another important consideration is the diagnosis and expected course of the disease. Is strength expected to increase, decrease, or remain about the same? If it is expected to increase, what is the expected recovery period? What effect will exercise or activity have on muscle function? Will too much activity delay the progress of the recovery? If muscle power is expected to decrease, how rapid is the progression? Are there factors to be avoided that can accelerate the decrease in strength, such as a vigorous exercise program? If strength is declining, is special equipment practical and necessary? How much muscle power is needed to operate the equipment? How long will the client be able to operate a device before a decrease in muscle power makes it impracticable?[9]

The therapist should assess the affect of the muscle weakness on the ability to perform ADL. This can be observed during the ADL evaluation. Which tasks are most difficult to perform because of the muscle weakness? How does the client compensate for the weakness? Which tasks are most important for the client to be able to perform? Is special equipment necessary or desirable for the performance of some ADL, such as the mobile arm support for independence in eating?[9]

If the client is involved in a total rehabilitation program and receiving the services of several other professionals, the strengthening and activity programs must be synchronized and well balanced to meet the client's needs rather than the needs of the professionals, their schedules, and possibly their competition. The occupational therapist needs to be aware of the nature and extent of the programs in which the client is engaged in physical therapy, recreational therapy, and any other services being received. Ideally, the team should plan the exercise or activity program in concert to determine that the programs complement one another. Questions that might be asked are: What is the client doing in each of the therapies? How long is each treatment session? Are the goals of all of the therapies similar or complementary or are they divergent and conflicting? Is the client being overfatigued in the total program? Are the various treatment sessions in rapid succession or are they well spaced to meet the client's need for rest periods?

On the basis of these considerations and of others pertinent to the specific client, the occupational therapist can select enabling and functional activities designed to maintain or increase strength, improve performance of ADL, and enable the use of special equipment while protecting weak muscles from overstretching and overfatigue.

Relationship between joint ROM and muscle weakness

One criterion used to grade muscle strength is the excursion of the joint on which the muscle acts, that is, did the muscle move the joint through complete, partial, or no ROM. Another criterion is the amount of resistance that can be applied to the part once the muscle has moved the joint through the available ROM. In this context ROM is not necessarily the full average normal ROM for the given joint. Rather, it is the ROM available to the individual client. When measuring joint motion, discussed in an earlier chapter, it is the *passive* ROM that is the measure of the range available to the client. Passive ROM, however, is no indication of muscle strength. When performing muscle testing, the occupational therapist must know what the client's available passive ROM is to assign muscle grades correctly. It is possible that the passive ROM is limited or less than the average for that joint motion but the muscle strength is normal. Therefore it is necessary for the therapist to have either measured joint ROM or to move the joint passively through its ROM to assess the available ROM before administering the muscle test. For example,

the client's passive ROM for elbow flexion may be limited to 0° to 110° because of an old fracture. If the client can flex the elbow joint to 110° and hold against moderate resistance during the muscle test, the grade would be G. In such cases the examiner should record the limitation with the muscle grade, for example, 110°/G.[7] Conversely, if the client's available ROM for elbow flexion was 0° to 140°, and he or she flexed the elbow against gravity through only 110°, the muscle would be graded F −, since the part moved through only partial ROM against gravity. When the therapist determines the *client's* available ROM before performing the muscle test, the former is able to grade muscle strength on that basis rather than using the average normal ROM as the standard.

MANUAL MUSCLE TESTING

The manual muscle test is a means of measuring the maximal contraction of muscles or muscle groups. It is used to determine amount of muscle power and to record gains and losses in strength. The muscle test is a primary evaluation tool for clients with lower motor neuron disorders, primary muscle diseases, and orthopedic dysfunction, as cited previously. The criteria used to measure strength are evidence of muscle contraction, amount of ROM through which the joint passes, and amount of resistance against which the muscle can contract, including gravity as a form of resistance.[7] The limitations of the manual muscle test are that it cannot measure muscle endurance (number of times the muscle can contract at its maximal level), muscle coordination, or smooth rhythmic interaction of muscle function, or motor performance capabilities of the client (use of the muscles for functional activities).

Validity of the manual muscle test depends on careful observation of movement, careful and accurate palpation, correct positioning, consistency of procedure, and experience of the examiner.[7,8]

To perform manual muscle testing accurately the examiner should have a good working knowledge of muscles and their functions, the position of muscles, direction of muscle fibers, and their angle of pull on the joints. The

therapist should know the joints and their motions and the innervation of the muscles, be familiar with muscle testing procedures and know how to observe for and rule out substitutions during the test, and be able to palpate muscles accurately and estimate normal strength for each client.

The manual muscle test cannot be used accurately with clients who have spasticity caused by upper motor neuron disorders, such as a cerebrovascular accident or cerebral palsy. This is because in these disorders muscles are often hypertonic, muscle tone and ability to perform movements are influenced by primitive reflexes and the position of the head and body in space, and movements tend to occur in gross synergistic patterns that make it impossible for the client to isolate joint motions, which is demanded in the manual muscle testing procedures.[2,3,11] Methods for measuring motor performance of persons with upper motor neuron lesions will be reviewed in subsequent chapters.

General principles of manual muscle testing

GRAVITY FACTORS INFLUENCING MUSCLE FUNCTION. Gravity is a form of resistance to muscle power.[8] Therefore one criterion used to determine the muscle grade is whether or not a muscle can move the part against gravity. A gravity-assisted movement is toward the floor and is never used in the testing procedure. The gravity-eliminated position and movement are parallel to the floor and are used with 0, T, P, and P+ grades. Movements against gravity are away from the floor or toward the ceiling and are used with grades F, G, and N. Movements against gravity and resistance are performed away from the floor with added manual or mechanical resistance and are used with F+ to N grades. In many of the muscle tests the effect of gravity on the ability to perform the movement must be considered in grading muscle power. It is of lesser importance, however, in tests of the forearm, fingers, and toes because the weight of the part lifted against gravity is insignificant compared with the muscle strength.[2,4] Therefore the examiner may choose to do the tests for F to N in the gravity-eliminated plane. In other tests, positioning for movements in the gravity-eliminated position or the against-gravity position may not be feasible. For example, in the test for scapula depression, positioning to perform the movement against gravity would require the subject to assume an inverted position. In individual cases positioning for movement in the correct plane may not be possible because of generalized weakness, trunk instability, immobilization devices, and medical precautions. In these instances the examiner must adapt the positioning to the client's needs and modify the grading using clinical judgment.

If tests of the forearm, fingers, and toes are done against gravity rather than in the gravity-eliminated plane, the standard definitions of muscle grades can be modified when recording muscle grades. The partial ROM against gravity is graded P, and the full ROM against gravity is graded F.[7] Such modifications in positioning and grading should be noted by the examiner when recording results of the muscle test.

For consistency in procedure and grading, the gravity-eliminated positions and against-gravity positions have been used in the muscle testing procedures described later except where the positioning is not feasible or would be awkward or uncomfortable for the subject. Modifications in positioning and grading have been cited with the individual tests.

MUSCLE GRADES. Although the definitions of the muscle grades[7] are standard, the assignment of muscle grades during the manual muscle test depends on clinical judgment, knowledge, and experience of the examiner. This is especially true when determining "slight," "moderate," or "full" resistance. Age, sex, body type, occupation, and avocations all influence the amount of resistance that can be considered "slight," "moderate," or "full" for a subject. "Normal" strength for an 8-year-old girl will be considerably less

than for a 25-year-old man, for example. By the same token, strength tends to decline with age[7], and "full" resistance to the same muscle group will vary considerably from the 80-year-old man to the 25-year-old man. Therefore the amount of resistance that can be applied to grade a particular muscle group as N or G varies from one individual to another.[7]

The amount of resistance that can be given also varies from one muscle group to another.[7] For example, the flexors of the wrist take much more resistance than the abductors of the fingers. The examiner must consider the size and relative power of the muscles and the leverage used when giving resistance.[9] The amount of resistance applied should be modified accordingly. When only one side of the body is involved in the dysfunction causing the muscle weakness, the examiner can establish the standards for strength by testing the unaffected side first.

In manual muscle testing muscles are graded according to the following criteria:

SUBSTITUTIONS. When weakness exists, substitution movements occur.[8] Since the brain "knows" only the goal of the action rather than considering which muscle is the "correct" one to perform the motion, it seeks to reach the goal in whatever way possible. Therefore a functioning muscle or muscle group will attempt to compensate for the lack of function in a weak or paralyzed muscle. This is called *substitution*.[8] To test muscle strength accurately, it is necessary to eliminate substitutions in the testing procedure by correct positioning, stabilization, palpation of the muscle being tested, and careful performance of the test motion without extraneous movements. The correct position of the body should be maintained and movement of the part performed without shifting the body or turning the part to allow substitutions.[8] In the tests that follow the possible substitutions are described at the end of the directions for the test of each muscle group. It is wise for the examiner to become familiar with these at the outset, so that while observing the test

Number grade	Word/letter grade	Definition
0	Zero (0)	No muscle contraction can be seen or felt.
1	Trace (T)	Contraction can be felt, but there is no motion.
2−	Poor minus (P−)	Part moves through an incomplete ROM with gravity eliminated.
2	Poor (P)	Part moves through a complete ROM with gravity eliminated.
2+	Poor plus (P+)	Part moves through incomplete ROM (less than 50%) against gravity or through complete ROM with gravity eliminated against slight resistance.
3−	Fair minus (F−)	Part moves through an incomplete ROM (more than 50%) against gravity.
3	Fair (F)	Part moves through complete ROM against gravity.
3+	Fair plus (F+)	Part moves through a complete ROM against gravity and slight resistance.
4	Good (G)	Part moves through a complete ROM against gravity and moderate resistance.
5	Normal (N)	Part moves through complete ROM against gravity and full resistance.

movement possible substitutions can be detected and the procedure can be corrected. Detecting substitutions is a skill that is gained with time and experience in muscle testing.

PROCEDURE FOR MANUAL MUSCLE TESTING. Manual muscle testing should be performed according to a standard procedure to ensure accuracy and consistency of the examiner. The tests that follow are divided into four major steps. The first step is "position and stabilize." The second step is "palpate and observe." The third and fourth steps are "resist" and "grade," respectively. This format is used for conciseness and to avoid unnecessary repetition. However, it can be broken into more discrete components for the novice. First, the client should be positioned for the specific muscle test to be performed. Next the examiner (E) should position him or herself in relation to the subject (S). Then E stabilizes the part proximal to the part being tested to isolate the muscle group and eliminate substitutions. E should then demonstrate or describe the test motion to S and ask S to perform the test motion and return to the starting position. During this performance, E makes a general observation of the form and quality of movement, looking for substitutions or difficulties that may require adjustments in positioning and stabilization. E then places fingers for palpation of one or more of the prime movers, or its tendinous insertion, in the muscle group being tested and asks S to repeat the test motion. During the performance of the motion, E again observes the movement for possible substitution and the amount of range completed. When S has moved the part through the available ROM, S holds the position at the end of the available ROM and E resists in the opposite direction of the test movement. The muscle tests that follow use the "break test." That is, the resistance is applied *after* S has reached the end of the available ROM. S should be allowed to establish a maximal contraction (set the muscles) before the resistance is applied.[7,9] E applies the resistance after preparing S by giving the command to

"hold, don't let me pull it down or out." Resistance should be applied gradually in a direction opposite to the line of pull of the muscle or muscle group being tested. The "break test" should not evoke pain, and resistance should be released immediately if pain or discomfort occurs.[7] Finally, E grades the muscle strength according to the preceding standard definitions of muscle grades. This procedure is used for the tests of strength of grades F and above. Resistance is not applied for tests of muscles from P to 0. Slight resistance, however, is sometimes applied to a muscle that has completed the full available ROM in the gravity-eliminated plane to determine if the grade is P+. Fig. 6-1 is a sample form for recording muscle grades after specific manual muscle testing.

SEQUENCE OF MUSCLE TESTING. To avoid frequent repositioning of the client, the manual muscle test can be given in the sequence outlined so that all tests are performed in order of backlying position, facelying position, sidelying position, and finally sitting position.

Backlying (supine)
Grades N to F

Scapula abduction and upward rotation
Shoulder horizontal abduction
All tests for forearm, wrist, and fingers can be given in the backlying position if necessary

Grades P to 0

Shoulder abduction
Elbow flexion
Elbow extension
Hip abduction
Hip adduction
Hip external rotation
Hip internal rotation
Foot inversion
Foot eversion

Facelying (prone)
Grades N to F

Scapula depression
Scapula adduction
Scapula adduction and downward rotation
Shoulder extension
Shoulder external rotation
Shoulder internal rotation
Shoulder horizontal abduction
Elbow extension
Hip extension
Knee flexion
Ankle plantar flexion

Grades P to 0

Scapula elevation
Scapula depression
Scapula adduction

Sidelying
Grades N to F

Hip abduction
Hip adduction
Foot inversion
Foot eversion

Grades P to 0

Shoulder flexion
Shoulder extension
Hip flexion
Hip extension
Knee flexion
Knee extension
Ankle plantar flexion
Ankle dorsiflexion

Sitting
Grades N to F

Scapula elevation
Shoulder flexion
Shoulder abduction
Elbow flexion
All forearm, wrist, finger, and thumb movements
Hip flexion
Hip external rotation
Hip internal rotation
Knee extension
Ankle dorsiflexion with inversion

Grades P to 0

All forearm, wrist, finger, and thumb movements
Ankle dorsiflexion with inversion

LIMITATIONS OF INSTRUCTIONS FOR PROCEDURES. The directions for manual muscle testing that follow do not include tests for the face, neck, and trunk. The reader is referred to Kendall, Kendall, and Wadsworth,[8] or Daniels and Worthingham[7] for these tests.

MUSCLE EXAMINATION

Patient's name _____ Chart no. _____

Date of birth _____ Name of institution _____

Date of onset _____ Attending physician _____ MD

Diagnosis:

LEFT						RIGHT		
			Examiner's initials					
			Date					
			NECK	Flexors	Sternocleidomastoid			
			Extensor group					
			TRUNK	Flexors	Rectus abdominis			
			Rt. ext. obl. / Lt. int. obl.	Rotators	Lt. ext. obl. / Rt. int. obl.			
			Extensors		Thoracic group / Lumbar group			
			Pelvic elev.		Quadratus lumb.			
			HIP	Flexors	Iliopsoas			
			Extensors		Gluteus maximus			
			Abductors		Gluteus medius			
			Adductor group					
			External rotator group					
			Internal rotator group					
			Sartorius					
			Tensor fasciae latae					
			KNEE	Flexors	Biceps femoris / Inner hamstrings			
			Extensors		Quadriceps			
			ANKLE	Plantar flexors	Gastrocnemius / Soleus			
			FOOT	Invertors	Tibialis anterior / Tibialis posterior			
			Evertors		Peroneus brevis / Peroneus longus			
			TOES	MP flexors	Lumbricales			
			IP flexors (first)		Flex. digit. br.			
			IP flexors (second)		Flex. digit. l.			
			MP extensors		Ext. digit. l. / Ext. digit. br.			
			HALLUX	MP flexor	Flex. hall. br.			
			IP flexor		Flex. hall. l.			
			MP extensor		Ext. hall. br.			
			IP extensor		Ext. hall. l.			

Measurements:

Cannot walk   Date   Speech

Stands   Date   Swallowing

Walks unaided   Date   Diaphragm

Walks with apparatus Date   Intercostals

KEY

5	N	Normal	Complete range of motion against gravity with full resistance.
4	G	Good*	Complete range of motion against gravity with some resistance.
3	F	Fair*	Complete range of motion against gravity.
2	P	Poor*	Complete range of motion with gravity eliminated.
1	T	Trace	Evidence of slight contractility. No joint motion.
0	0	Zero	No evidence of contractility.
S or SS			Spasm or severe spasm.
C or CC			Contracture or severe contracture.

*Muscle spasm or contracture may limit range of motion. A question mark should be placed after the grading of a movement that is incomplete from this cause.

Fig. 6-1. Muscle examination. (Adapted with the express permission and authority of the March of Dimes Birth Defects Foundation.)

	LEFT						RIGHT		
				Examiner's initials					
				Date					
				SCAPULA	Abductor	Serratus anterior			
					Elevator	Upper trapezius			
					Depressor	Lower trapezius			
					Adductors	Middle trapezius			
						Rhomboids			
				SHOULDER	Flexor	Anterior deltoid			
					Extensors	Latissimus dorsi			
						Teres major			
					Abductor	Middle deltoid			
					Horiz. abd.	Posterior deltoid			
					Horiz. add.	Pectoralis major			
					External rotator group				
					Internal rotator group				
				ELBOW	Flexors	Biceps brachii			
						Brachioradialis			
					Extensor	Triceps			
				FOREARM	Supinator group				
					Pronator group				
				WRIST	Flexors	Flex. carpi rad.			
						Flex. carpi uln.			
					Extensors	Ext. carpi rad. 1. & br.			
						Ext. carpi uln.			
				FINGERS	MP flexors	Lumbricales			
					IP flexors (first)	Flex. digit. sub.			
					IP flexors (second)	Flex. digit. prof.			
					MP extensor	Ext. digit. com.			
					Adductors	Palmar interossei			
					Abductors	Dorsal interossei			
					Abductor digiti quinti				
					Opponens digiti quinti				
				THUMB	MP flexor	Flex. poll. br.			
					IP flexor	Flex. poll. 1.			
					MP extensor	Ext. poll. br.			
					IP extensor	Ext. poll. 1.			
					Abductors	Abd. poll. br.			
						Abd. poll. 1.			
					Adductor pollicis				
					Opponens pollicis				
				FACE					

Additional data:

Fig. 6-1, cont'd. Muscle examination.

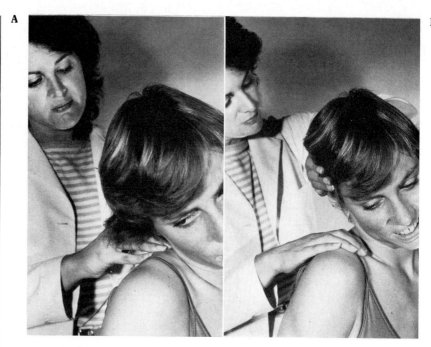

Fig. 6-2. Scapula elevation. **A,** Palpate and observe. **B,** Resist.

PROCEDURE FOR MANUAL MUSCLE TESTING OF THE UPPER AND LOWER EXTREMITIES
Manual muscle testing of the upper extremity

Motion

Scapula elevation, neck rotation, and lateral flexion

Muscles[5,7]	Innervation (nerve, nerve roots)[7,8]
Levator scapulae	Dorsal scapular nerve, C3-5
Upper trapezius	Accessory nerve (Cr. XI), C2-4

Procedure for testing grades N to F

POSITION AND STABILIZE: S is seated erect with arms resting at sides of body. The hands should not be allowed to rest on the supporting surface. E stands behind S toward the side to be tested. Stabilization is usually not necessary if S has good sitting balance and can maintain the erect posture. A chair back can offer stabilization to the trunk if necessary.

PALPATE AND OBSERVE: Before instructing S to perform the test movement, E places fingers for palpation of the upper trapezius parallel to the cervical vertebrae near the shoulder-neck curve.[7] The levator scapulae may be palpated on the lateral surface of the neck, anterior to the upper trapezius and posterior to the sternocleidomastoid if S has a hand on the lumbosacral region of the back while elevating the scapula.[4] S elevates the scapula by shrugging the shoulder toward the ear. At the same time S rotates and laterally flexes the neck toward the side being tested[8] (Fig. 6-2, *A*).

RESIST: E removes the palpating fingers and offers resistance with one hand on top of the shoulder toward scapula depression and the other hand on the side of the head toward derotation and lateral flexion to the opposite side[8] (Fig. 6-2, *B*).

Procedure for testing grades P, T, and 0

POSITION AND STABILIZE: S is lying prone with the head in midposition. E stands opposite the side being tested. Weight of the trunk on the supporting surface is adequate stabilization. E may support S's arm at the proximal end of the humerus to minimize the resistance of gravity and weight of the arm during scapula elevation.

PALPATE AND OBSERVE: E palpates the upper trapezius as previously described while observing S shrug the shoulder being tested toward the ear. Because of the positioning, the neck rotation and lateral flexion components are omitted for these grades.

GRADE: Grade strength according to standard definitions of muscle grades cited previously.

SUBSTITUTIONS: The rhomboid major and minor and levator scapulae can effect scapula elevation if the upper trapezius is weak or absent.[4] In the event of substitution some downward rotation of the acromion would be observed during the movement.[9]

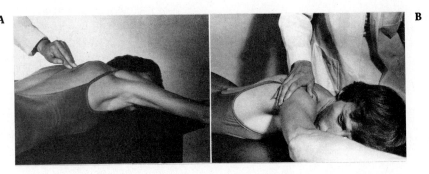

Fig. 6-3. Scapula depression. **A,** Palpate and observe. **B,** Resist.

Motion
Scapula depression, adduction, and upward rotation

Muscles[1,4]	Innervation[7]
Lower trapezius	Accessory nerve, spinal portion
Middle trapezius	Accessory nerve, spinal portion
Serratus anterior	Long thoracic nerve, C5-7

Procedure for testing grades N to F
POSITION AND STABILIZE: S is lying in a prone position. E stands next to S across from the side being tested. S's arm is positioned overhead in approximately 120° to 130° of abduction and resting on the supporting surface. If the posterior deltoid and triceps are weak, E may cradle the arm, supporting it at the elbow.[7] This test is given in the gravity-eliminated position, since it is not feasible to position S for the against-gravity movement (head down).

PALPATE AND OBSERVE: E places fingers for palpation of the lower trapezius distal to the medial end of the spine of the scapula and parallel to the thoracic vertebrae approximately at the level of the inferior angle of the scapula. S is asked to lift the arm up from the supporting surface. During this movement there is strong downward fixation of the scapula by the lower trapezius (Fig. 6-3, *A*).

RESIST: E removes the palpating fingers and gives resistance at the lateral angle of the scapula toward elevation and abduction.[7,8] Resistance may be given on the dorsum of the forearm in a downward direction if shoulder and elbow strength are adequate[8] (Fig. 6-3, *B*).

Procedure for testing grades P, T, and 0
POSITION AND STABILIZE: S and E are positioned as described previously. No stabilization is required unless it is necessary for E to support S's arm because of weak posterior deltoid and triceps.

PALPATE AND OBSERVE: Palpate and observe as described previously.

GRADE: Because it is not possible to position S for performance of the movement against gravity, grading criteria are modified.

F if full ROM was achieved
P if 50% ROM was achieved
P− if slight ROM was achieved[7]

SUBSTITUTIONS: If the arm is down at the side of the body, the latissimus dorsi acting on the humerus will pull the head of the humerus down, which will cause the scapula to be depressed. Observe for scapula motion with downward thrust of the humerus.[9] Since the test position is with the arm above the head, this substitution will not occur during the test but may be observed in performance of functional activities.

A

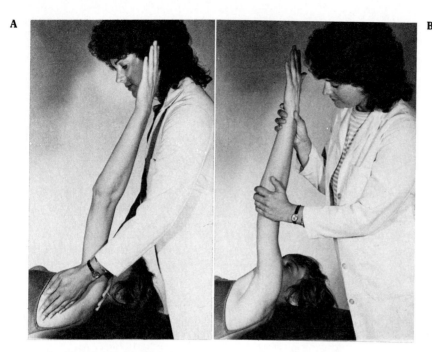

B

Fig. 6-4. Scapula abduction. **A,** Palpate and observe. **B,** Resist.

A

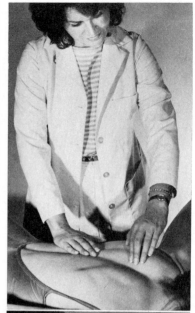

B

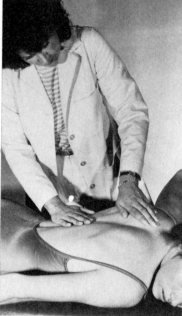

Fig. 6-5. Scapula adduction. **A,** Palpate and observe. **B,** Resist.

Motion

Scapula abduction and upward rotation

Muscles[7,8]	Innervation[7,8]
Serratus anterior	Long thoracic nerve, C5-7

Procedure for testing grades N to F

POSITION AND STABILIZE: S is lying supine with the shoulder flexed 90° and slightly abducted. The elbow is extended. E stands next to S on the side being tested. E stabilizes by placing a hand over S's shoulder to prevent trunk rotation or scapula elevation.

PALPATE AND OBSERVE: E places fingers for palpation of the digitations of the origin of the serratus anterior on the ribs, along the midaxillary line and just distal and anterior to the axillary border of the scapula. Muscle contractions may be difficult to detect on women and overweight clients. E asks S to reach upward as if pushing the arm toward the ceiling, abducting the scapula[7] (Fig. 6-4, *A*).

RESIST: E removes the palpating fingers, grasps around the elbow with one hand and the distal end of the forearm with the other, and pushes S's arm directly downward toward scapula adduction[7] (Fig. 6-4, *B*).

Procedure for testing grades P, T, and 0

POSITION AND STABILIZE: S is seated at a high table with the arm resting on it in 90° of shoulder flexion,[7] or E may support S's arm slightly above the table surface to eliminate resistance from friction and the weight of the arm. Stabilization is the same as described previously.

PALPATE AND OBSERVE: E palpates for the serratus anterior as previously described as S moves the arm forward. E observes for abduction of the scapula.[7]

GRADE: Strength is graded according to the definitions of muscle grades cited previously.

SUBSTITUTIONS: The pectoralis major may act to pull the scapula forward into abduction at its insertion on the humerus. E should observe for humeral horizontal adduction followed by scapula abduction to detect possible substitution.[9]

Motion
Scapula adduction

Muscles[7,8]	Innervation[7]
Middle trapezius	Spinal accessory nerve, C3-4
Rhomboid major and minor	Dorsal scapular nerve, C5

Procedure for testing grades N to F

POSITION AND STABILIZE: S is lying prone with the shoulder abducted 90° and externally rotated. The elbow is flexed 90°. The humerus should rest on the supporting surface. E stands on the side being tested. The weight of the trunk on the supporting surface is usually adequate stabilization. E may stabilize above the midthorax to prevent trunk rotation if necessary.

PALPATE AND OBSERVE: E places fingers for palpation of the middle trapezius between the medial end of the spine of the scapula and the adjacent vertebrae in a straight line with the abducted humerus. E asks S to lift the arm off the supporting surface while maintaining the position of the shoulder and elbow joints previously described. E observes movement of the vertebral border of the scapula toward the thoracic vertebrae (Fig. 6-5, *A*).

RESIST: E removes the palpating fingers when the motion is complete and uses the hand to resist at the vertebral border of the scapula toward abduction[7] (Fig. 6-5, *B*).

Procedure for testing grades P, T, and 0

POSITION AND STABILIZE: S and E are positioned as described previously, but E now supports the weight of the arm by cradling under the humerus and forearm.[8] S may also be positioned sitting erect with the arm resting on a high table with the shoulder midway between 90° flexion and abduction.[7] E stands behind S in this instance.

PALPATE AND OBSERVE: E palpates for the middle trapezius as previously described, then asks S to "bring the shoulders together" as if assuming an erect posture. E observes movement of the scapula toward the vertebral column.

GRADE: Grade strength according to standard definitions of muscle grades.

SUBSTITUTIONS[8]: The posterior deltoid can act on the humerus and produce scapula adduction because of the momentum effected. Observe for humeral extension being used to initiate scapula adduction.

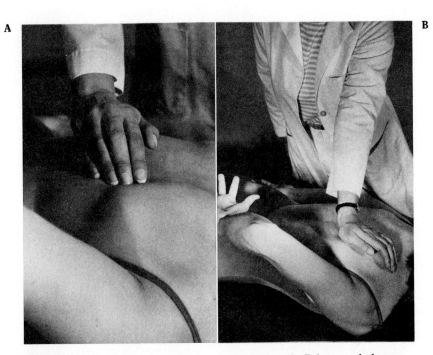

Fig. 6-6. Scapula adduction and downward rotation. **A,** Palpate and observe. **B,** Resist.

Motion
Scapula adduction and downward rotation

Muscles[7,8]	Innervation[7,8]
Levator scapulae	Dorsal scapular nerve, C3-5
Middle trapezius	Spinal accessory nerve, C3-4
Rhomboid major and minor	Dorsal scapular nerve, C5

Procedure for testing grades N to F

POSITION AND STABILIZE: S is lying in the prone position with the head rotated to the opposite side being tested. The arm on the side being tested is placed in shoulder adduction and internal rotation with the elbow slightly flexed and the dorsum of the hand resting over the lubosacral area of S's back. E stands opposite the side being tested.[7] The weight of the trunk on the supporting surface offers adequate stabilization.[8]

PALPATE AND OBSERVE: E places fingers for palpation of the rhomboid major and minor between the vertebral border of the scapula and the second to fifth thoracic vertebrae.[7,8] (They may be more easily discerned toward the lower half of the vertebral border of the scapula, since they lay under the trapezius muscle.) E asks S to raise the hand up from the back. During this motion E observes scapula adduction and downward rotation while the shoulder joint is in extension (hyperextension)[7] (Fig. 6-6, *A*).

RESIST: E removes the palpating fingers and resists on the vertebral border of the scapula toward abduction and upward rotation (Fig 6-6, *B*).

Procedure for testing grades P, T, and 0

POSITION AND STABILIZE: S is sitting erect with the arm positioned behind the back in the same manner described previously. E stands behind S and a little opposite the side being tested.[7] E stabilizes S's trunk by placing one hand over the shoulder opposite the one being tested to prevent trunk flexion and rotation.

GRADE: Grade strength according to the standard definition of muscle grades.

SUBSTITUTIONS: The middle trapezius can substitute for weak or absent rhomboid major and minor. The movement will not be accompanied by downward rotation. The posterior deltoid acting to perform horizontal abduction or glenohumeral extension can produce scapula adduction through momentum. Scapula adduction would be preceded by extension or abduction of the humerus.[9]

Motion

Shoulder flexion

Muscles[7]	Innervation[7]
Anterior deltoid	Axillary nerve, C5-6
Coracobrachialis	Musculocutaneous nerve, C6-7

Procedure for testing grades N to F

POSITION AND STABILIZE: S is seated with the arm relaxed at the side of the body and the hand facing backward. A straight-back chair may be used for trunk support. E stands on the side being tested and slightly behind S. E stabilizes the shoulder being tested to prevent scapula elevation, trunk rotation, or trunk flexion.

PALPATE AND OBSERVE: E places fingers for palpation of the anterior deltoid just below the clavicle on the anterior aspect of the humeral head. E then asks S to flex the shoulder joint by raising the arm horizontally to 90° of flexion (parallel to the floor) (Fig. 6-7, *A*).

RESIST: When S has reached 90° of flexion, E removes the palpating fingers and uses the hand to resist at the distal end of the humerus downward toward shoulder extension (Fig. 6-7, *B*).

Procedure for testing grades P, T, and 0

POSITION AND STABILIZE: S is lying on the side. The side being tested is superior. If S cannot maintain weight of the arm against gravity, it can be supported on a smooth board placed under it or by E. E stands behind S.[6] If the sidelying position is not feasible, S may remain seated and the test procedure described previously can be used with some modification in grading.[7]

PALPATE AND OBSERVE: Palpation and observation are the same as previously described. E asks S to move the arm forward toward the face, flexing the shoulder 90°.

GRADE: Grade strength according to standard definitions of muscle grades. If the seated position was used for the tests of grades P to 0, partial ROM against gravity should be graded P.[7]

SUBSTITUTIONS: The clavicular fibers of the pectoralis major can perform flexion through partial ROM while performing horizontal adduction. Biceps may flex the shoulder, but the humerus will first be rotated externally for the best mechanical advantage. The upper trapezius will assist flexion by elevating the scapula. Observe for flexion accompanied by horizontal adduction, external rotation, or scapula elevation.[9]

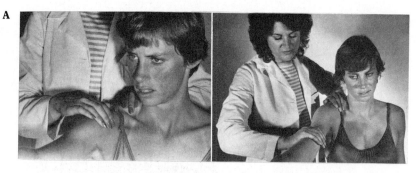

Fig. 6-7. Shoulder flexion. **A,** Palpate and observe. **B,** Resist.

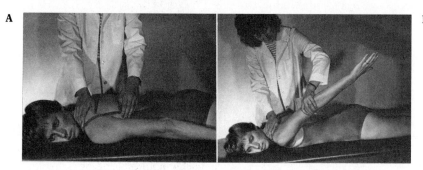

Fig. 6-8. Shoulder extension. **A,** Palpate and observe. **B,** Resist.

Motion

Shoulder extension (hyperextension)

Muscles[4,7,8]	Innervation[7]
Latissimus dorsi	Thoracodorsal nerve, C6-8
Posterior deltoid	Axillary nerve, C5-6
Teres major	Inferior subscapular nerve, C5-6

Procedure for testing grades N to F

POSITION AND STABILIZE: S is lying in prone position with the shoulder joint adducted and internally rotated so that the palm of the hand is facing up. E stands opposite the side being tested. E may stabilize above the scapula on the side being tested to prevent scapula elevation and trunk rotation.

PALPATE AND OBSERVE: E places fingers for palpation of the teres major along the axillary border of the scapula. The latissiumus dorsi may be palpated slightly below this point[7] or closer to its origins, parallel to the thoracic and lumbar vertebrae. The posterior deltoid may be found over the posterior aspect of the humeral head. When E has placed the fingers for palpation of one of these muscles, E asks S to lift the arm up from the table, extending the shoulder joint (Fig. 6-8, *A*).

RESIST: E removes the palpating fingers and offers resistance at the distal end of the humerus in a downward and outward direction, toward flexion and slight abduction[7,8] (Fig. 6-8, *B*).

Procedure for testing grades P, T, and 0

POSITION AND STABILIZE: S is placed in a sidelying position and E stands behind S. E stabilizes above S's scapula to prevent elevation and trunk rotation. If S cannot maintain the weight of the part against gravity, E should support S's arm or place a smooth board between the arm and the trunk.[6] If the sidelying position is not feasible, S may remain in the prone lying position and the test may be performed as described previously with modified grading.[7]

PALPATE AND OBSERVE: Palpation is done as previously described. E asks S to move the arm backward in a plane parallel to the floor.

GRADE: Grade strength according to the standard definitions of muscle grades. If the test for grades P to 0 were done in the prone lying position, completion of partial ROM should be graded P.[7]

SUBSTITUTIONS: Gravity will return the arm from flexion to extension when in the upright position. Momentum produced by the quick contraction and release of the shoulder flexors will cause the arm to swing backward. Scapula adduction will effect some shoulder extension. Observe for flexion of the shoulder or adduction of the scapula preceding extension of the humerus.[9]

Motion
Shoulder abduction

Muscles[7,8]	Innervation[7]
Middle deltoid	Axillary nerve, C5-6
Supraspinatus	Suprascapular nerve, C5

Procedure for testing grades N to F

POSITION AND STABILIZE: S is seated with the arms relaxed at the sides of body. The elbow on the side to be tested should be slightly flexed and the palms facing toward the body. E stands behind S. E stabilizes over the shoulder on the side to be tested to prevent scapula elevation and trunk movement.[7,8]

PALPATE AND OBSERVE: E places fingers for palpation of the middle deltoid over the middle of the shoulder joint from the acromion to the deltoid tuberosity,[7-9] then asks S to abduct the shoulder 90°. During the movement, S's palm should remain down and E should observe that there is no external rotation of the shoulder[7,8] or elevation of the scapula.[7,9] The supraspinatus may be difficult to palpate,[9] since it lays under the trapezius muscle, but it may be palpated in the supraspinatus fossa[7] (Fig. 6-9, *A*).

RESIST: E removes the palpating fingers and resists at the distal end of the humerus as if pushing the arm down toward adduction (Fig. 6-9, *B*).

Procedure for testing grades P, T, and 0

POSITION AND STABILIZE: S is lying in a supine position with the arm to be tested resting at the side of the body, palm facing in, and the elbow slightly flexed. E stands in front of the supporting surface toward the side to be tested. E places one hand over the shoulder to be tested to prevent scapula elevation.

PALPATE AND OBSERVE: Palpation is the same as described previously. E asks S to bring the arm out and away from the body, abducting the shoulder to 90°.

GRADE: Grade strength according to standard definitions of muscle grades cited earlier.

SUBSTITUTIONS: The long head of the biceps may attempt to substitute. Observe for external rotation accompanying the movement. The anterior and posterior deltoids can act together to effect abduction. The upper trapezius may attempt to assist. Observe for scapula elevation preceding the movement.[9]

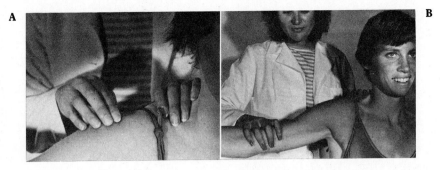

Fig. 6-9. Shoulder abduction. **A,** Palpate and observe. **B,** Resist.

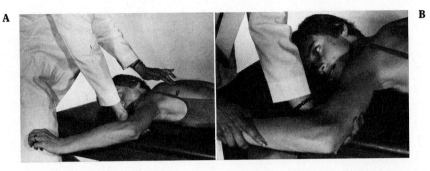

Fig. 6-10. Shoulder external rotation. **A,** Palpate and observe. **B,** Resist.

Motion
Shoulder external rotation

Muscles[4,7-9]	Innervation[4,7,8]
Infraspinatus	Suprascapular nerve, C5-6
Teres minor	Axillary nerve, C5-6

Procedure for testing grades N to F

POSITION AND STABILIZE: S is lying prone with the shoulder abducted to 90° and the humerus in neutral (0°) rotation. The elbow is flexed to 90°. The forearm is in neutral rotation, hanging over the edge of the table, and perpendicular to the floor. E stands in front of the supporting surface toward the side to be tested.[7,8] E stabilizes the humerus at the distal end by placing a hand under the arm on the supporting surface. This prevents adduction and abduction of the humerus and prevents pressure of S's arm into the table when resistance is given.[9]

PALPATE AND OBSERVE: E places fingers for palpation of the infraspinatus just below the spine of the scapula on the body of the scapula or for palpation of the teres minor along the axillary border of the scapula. E then asks S to rotate the humerus, moving the arm upward so that the back of the hand is moving toward the ceiling[7,8] (Fig. 6-10, *A*).

RESIST: E resists on the distal end of S's forearm toward the floor in the direction of internal rotation[7,8] (Fig. 6-10, *B*).

Procedure for testing grades P, T, and 0

POSITION AND STABILIZE: S is seated. The arm is adducted and in neutral rotation at the shoulder. The elbow is flexed 90° with the forearm in neutral rotation. E stands in front of S toward the side to be tested. E stabilizes S's arm against the trunk at the distal end of the humerus to prevent abduction and extension of the shoulder[5] and over the shoulder to be tested. This hand can be used to palpate the infraspinatus simultaneously.

PALPATE AND OBSERVE: E places fingers for palpation as previously described and asks S to move the forearm away from the body, rotating the humerus.

GRADE: Grade strength according to standard definitions of muscle grades cited previously.

SUBSTITUTIONS: If the elbow is extended and S supinates the forearm, the momentum could aid external rotation of the humerus. Scapular adduction can pull the humerus backward and into some external rotation. E should observe for scapular adduction and initiation of movement with forearm supination.[9]

Motion
Shoulder internal rotation

Muscles[7-9]	Innervation[4,5,7]
Latissimus dorsi	Thoracodorsal nerve, C6-8
Pectoralis major	Anterior thoracic nerve, C5 to T1
Subscapularis	Subscapular nerve, C5-6
Teres major	Subscapular nerve, C5-6

Procedure for testing grades N to F

POSITION AND STABILIZE: S is lying prone with the shoulder abducted 90° and the humerus in neutral rotation. The elbow is flexed 90°. The forearm is in neutral rotation, hanging over the edge of the table, and perpendicular to the floor. E stands in front of the supporting surface toward the side to be tested, just in front of S's arm. E stabilizes the humerus at the distal end by placing a hand under the arm and on the supporting surface as for external rotation.[7,8]

PALPATE AND OBSERVE: E places fingers for palpation of the teres major and latissimus dorsi along the axillary border of the scapula toward the inferior angle. The subscapularis is not palpable, and the pectoralis major will be difficult to reach with S in the prone position. E asks S to move the palm of the hand upward toward the ceiling, internally rotating the humerus[7] (Fig. 6-11, *A*).

RESIST: E resists over the volar surface of the distal end of the forearm anteriorly toward external rotation[7,8] (Fig. 6-11, *B*).

Procedure for testing grades P, T, and 0

POSITION AND STABILIZE: S is seated with the shoulder adducted and in neutral rotation. The elbow is flexed 90° with the forearm in neutral rotation next to S on the side to be tested. E stabilizes S's arm against the trunk at the distal end of the humerus to prevent abduction and extension of the shoulder.

PALPATE AND OBSERVE: E places fingers for palpation as described previously and asks S to move the palm of the hand toward the chest, internally rotating the humerus.

SUBSTITUTIONS: If the trunk is rotated, gravity will act on the humerus, rotating it internally. If the arm is in extension, pronation of the forearm can substitute. E should observe for trunk rotation during the test in sitting.[9]

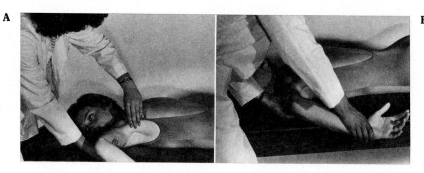

Fig. 6-11. Shoulder internal rotation. **A,** Palpate and observe. **B,** Resist.

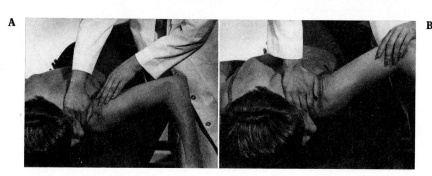

Fig. 6-12. Shoulder horizontal abduction. **A,** Palpate and observe. **B,** Resist.

Motion
Shoulder horizontal abduction

Muscles[4,7,9]	Innervation[7]
Infraspinatus	Suprascapular nerve, C5-6
Posterior deltoid	Axillary nerve, C5-6

Procedure for testing grades N to F[7,8]

POSITION AND STABILIZE: S is lying prone with the shoulder abducted 90° and in slight external rotation. The elbow is flexed 90° and the forearm is perpendicular to the floor. E stands on the side being tested. E stabilizes over the scapula to prevent scapula motion and trunk rotation.

PALPATE AND OBSERVE: E places fingers for palpation of the posterior deltoid below the spine of the scapula and distally toward the deltoid tuberosity on the posterior aspect of the shoulder. Then E asks S to lift the arm toward the ceiling, horizontally abducting the humerus (Fig. 6-12, *A*).

RESIST: E offers resistance just proximal to the elbow obliquely downward toward adduction and horizontal adduction[8] (Fig. 6-12, *B*).

Procedure for testing grades P, T, and 0

POSITION AND STABILIZE: S is seated with the arm in 90° abduction, the elbow flexed 90° and the palm down supported on a high table or by E. If a table is used, powder may be used on the surface to reduce friction.

PALPATE AND OBSERVE: Palpate as described previously. E asks S to pull the arm backward, horizontally abducting it.

GRADE: Grade strength according to standard definitions of muscle grades.

SUBSTITUTIONS: The latissimus dorsi and teres major may assist the movement if the posterior deltoid is weak. Movement will occur with more shoulder extension rather than at the horizontal level. Scapula adduction may produce slight horizontal abduction of the humerus.[9]

Motion
Shoulder horizontal adduction

Muscles[4,9]	Innervation[4,7]
Anterior deltoid	Axillary nerve, C5-6
Coracobrachialis	Musculocutaneous nerve, C6-7
Pectoralis major	Medial and lateral anterior thoracic nerves, C5-8, T1

Procedure for testing grades N to F

POSITION AND STABILIZE: S is lying in the supine position with the shoulder abducted 90°. The elbow can be flexed or extended. E stands next to S on the side being tested or behind S's head.[4,7] E stabilizes the trunk by placing one hand over the shoulder on the side being tested to prevent trunk rotation and scapula elevation.

PALPATE AND OBSERVE: E places fingers for palpation over the insertion of the pectoralis major at the anterior aspect of the axilla. Then E asks S to move the arm toward the opposite shoulder, horizontally adducting the humerus to a position of 90° of shoulder flexion.[8] If S cannot maintain elbow extension, E may guide the forearm to prevent the hand from hitting S's face (Fig. 6-13, *A*).

RESIST: E offers resistance at the distal end of the humerus in an outward direction toward horizontal abduction[7] (Fig. 6-13, *B*).

Procedure for testing grades P, T, and 0

POSITION AND STABILIZE: S is seated next to a high table with the arm supported in 90° of shoulder abduction and slight flexion at the elbow.[4] Powder may be sprinkled on the supporting surface to reduce the effect of resistance from friction during the movement or E may support the arm. E may stabilize the shoulder on the side being tested, using the stabilizing hand to simultaneously palpate the pectoralis major.

PALPATE AND OBSERVE: E places fingers for palpation as previously described, then asks S to move the arm toward the opposite shoulder, horizontally adducting it in a plane parallel to the floor.

SUBSTITUTIONS: The pectoralis major, anterior deltoid, and coracobrachialis may substitute for one another. If the pectoralis major is not functioning, the other muscles will perform the motion but it will be considerably weakened.[9]

Motion
Elbow flexion

Muscles[7-9]	Innervation[7]
Biceps	Musculocutaneous nerve, C5-6
Brachialis	Musculocutaneous nerve, C5-6
Brachioradialis	Radial nerve, C5-6

Procedure for testing grades N to F

POSITION AND STABILIZE: S is sitting with the arm adducted at the shoulder, extended at the elbow, and held against the side of the trunk. The forearm is supinated to primarily test for the biceps. (Forearm should be positioned in pronation to primarily test for the brachialis, and in midposition to primarily test for brachioradialis.[7]) E stands next to S on the side being tested or directly in front of S. E stabilizes S's humerus in adduction to prevent abduction and internal rotation at the shoulder.

PALPATE AND OBSERVE: E places fingers for palpation of the biceps over the muscle belly on the middle of the anterior aspect of the humerus. Its tendon may be palpated in the middle of the antecubital

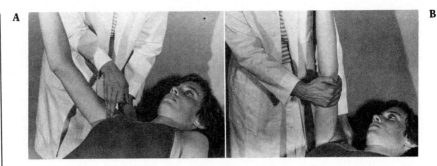

Fig. 6-13. Shoulder horizontal adduction. **A,** Palpate and observe. **B,** Resist.

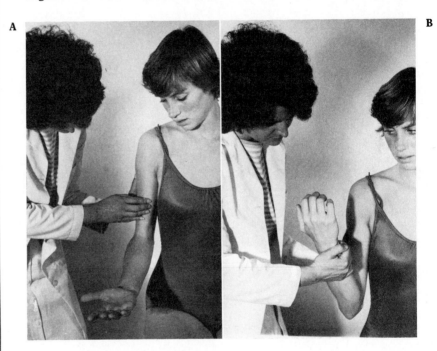

Fig. 6-14. Elbow flexion. **A,** Palpate and observe. **B,** Resist.

space.[7] The brachioradialis is palpated over the upper one third of the radius on the lateral aspect of the forearm just below the elbow. The brachialis may be palpated lateral to the lower portion of the biceps if the elbow is flexed and in the pronated position.[9] E asks S to bring the hand toward the face, flexing the elbow. E should observe for maintenance of forearm in supination (when testing for biceps) and that the wrist and fingers are relaxed or extended[9] (Fig. 6-14, *A*).

RESIST: E offers resistance at the distal end of the volar aspect of the forearm, pulling downward elbow extension[7,8] (Fig. 6-14, *B*).

Procedure for testing grades P, T, and 0

POSITION AND STABILIZE: S is lying supine with the shoulder abducted 90° and externally rotated. The elbow is extended and the forearm is supinated. (An alternative position is with S sitting upright and E sup-

porting the humerus in 90° abduction.) E stands at the head of the table on the side being tested. E stabilizes the humerus to prevent shoulder motion. The stabilizing hand can be used simultaneously for palpation.

PALPATE AND OBSERVE: Palpate as described earlier. E asks S to bring the hand toward the shoulder, flexing the elbow[7] while E watches for maintenance of forearm supination and relaxation of the fingers and wrist.[9]

GRADE: Grade strength according to standard definitions of muscle grades.

SUBSTITUTIONS: The brachioradialis will substitute for biceps, but the forearm will move to midposition during flexion of the elbow. Wrist and finger flexors may assist elbow flexion, which will be preceded by finger and wrist flexion.[7,9] The pronator teres may also assist. Forearm pronation during the movement may be evidence of this substitution.[9]

A 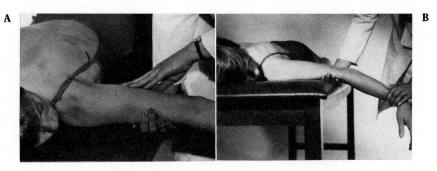 B

Fig. 6-15. Elbow extension. **A,** Palpate and observe. **B,** Resist.

Motion
Elbow extension

Muscles[7,8]	Innervation[7,8]
Anconeus	Radial nerve, C7-8
Triceps	Radial nerve, C7-8

Procedure for testing grades N to F

POSITION AND STABILIZE: S is lying prone with the humerus abducted 90° and in neutral rotation. The elbow is flexed 90°, and the forearm, which is perpendicular to the floor, is in neutral rotation. E stands next to S, just behind the arm to be tested.[6,8] E stabilizes the humerus by placing one hand for support under it, between S's arm and the table, to prevent shoulder motion and pressure of the arm against the table.[8]

PALPATE AND OBSERVE: E places fingers for palpation of the triceps over the middle of the posterior aspect of the humerus or the triceps tendon just proximal to the elbow joint on the dorsal surface of the arm.[7,9] E asks S to raise the hand up toward the ceiling, extending the elbow while E observes that the wrist and fingers remain relaxed (Fig. 6-15, *A*).

RESIST: E resists at the distal end of the forearm, pushing toward the floor or elbow flexion (Fig. 6-15, *B*).

Procedure for testing grades P, T, and 0

POSITION AND STABILIZE: S is lying supine with the humerus abducted 90° and in external rotation. The elbow is in full flexion, and the forearm is supinated. E is standing next to S just posterior to the arm to be tested.[7] E stabilizes the humerus by holding one hand over the middle or distal end of it to prevent shoulder motion.

PALPATE AND OBSERVE: E places fingers for palpation as described previously and asks S to move the hand away from the head, extending the elbow.

GRADE: Grade strength according to standard definitions of muscle grades.

SUBSTITUTIONS: Finger and wrist extensors may substitute for weak elbow extensors. In this instance, these movements will be seen first. When upright, gravity and eccentric contraction of the biceps will effect elbow extension from the flexed position. If the hand is fixed against a stationary object, the pectoralis major can be contracted toward adduction to effect locking of the elbow in extension.[8]

Motion
Forearm supination

Muscles[4,7,9]	Innervation[7]
Biceps	Musculocutaneous nerve, C5-6
Supinator	Radial nerve, C6

Procedure for testing grades N to F

POSITION AND STABILIZE: S is seated with the humerus adducted to the trunk, the elbow flexed to 90°, and the forearm in full pronation. E stands beside S on the side to be tested.[7] E stabilizes the humerus just proximal to the elbow to prevent shoulder motion.[7,8]

PALPATE AND OBSERVE: E places fingers for palpation over the supinator on the dorsolateral aspect of the forearm below the head of the radius. The muscle can best be felt when the radial muscle group (extensor carpi radialis and brachioradialis) is pushed up out of the way.[4] E may also palpate the biceps on the middle of the anterior surface of the humerus. E asks S to turn the hand palm up, supinating the forearm. Gravity may assist the movement after the 0° neutral position is passed (Fig. 6-16, *A*).

RESIST: E resists by grasping around the dorsal aspect of the distal forearm with the fingers and heel of the hand, turning the arm toward pronation (Fig. 6-16, *B*).

Procedure for testing grades P, T, and 0

POSITION AND STABILIZE: S is seated. The shoulder is flexed 90°, and the upper arm is resting on the supporting surface. The elbow is flexed 90°, and the forearm is in full pronation in a position perpendicular to the floor. E stands next to S on the side to be tested. E stabilizes the humerus just proximal to the elbow.

PALPATE AND OBSERVE: Palpate as described earlier. E asks S to turn the palm of the hand toward the face, supinating the forearm.

GRADE: Grade strength according to standard definitions of muscle grades.

SUBSTITUTIONS: With the elbow flexed, external rotation and horizontal adduction of the humerus will effect forearm supination. With the elbow extended, shoulder external rotation will place the forearm in supination. The brachioradialis can bring the forearm from full pronation to midposition. Wrist and thumb extensors assisted by gravity can initiate supination. E should observe for external rotation of the humerus, supination to midline only, and initiation of motion by wrist and thumb extension.[9]

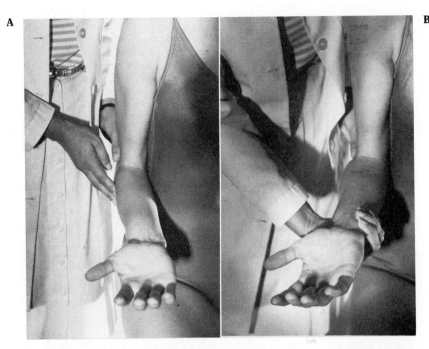

Fig. 6-16. Forearm supination. **A,** Palpate and observe. **B,** Resist.

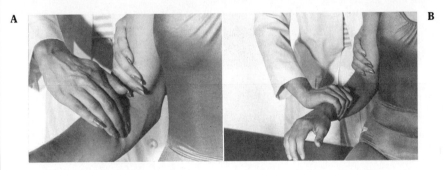

Fig. 6-17. Forearm pronation. **A,** Palpate and observe. **B,** Resist.

Motion

Forearm pronation

Muscles[4,9]	Innervation[7]
Pronator quadratus	Median nerve, C8, T1
Pronator teres	Median nerve, C6-7

Procedure for testing grades N to F

POSITION AND STABILIZE: S is seated with the humerus adducted to the trunk, the elbow flexed to 90°, and the forearm in full supination. E stands beside S on the side to be tested. E stabilizes the humerus just proximal to the elbow to prevent shoulder abduction.[7,8]

PALPATE AND OBSERVE: E places fingers for palpation of the pronator teres on the upper part of the volar surface of the forearm medial to the biceps tendon and diagonally from the medial condyle of the humerus to the lateral border of the radius.[7-9] E asks S to turn the hand palm down, pronating the forearm[7] (Fig. 6-17, *A*).

RESIST: E grasps the dorsal aspect of the distal forearm by using the fingers and heel of the hand and turns toward supination (Fig. 6-17, *B*).

Procedure for testing grades P, T, and 0

POSITION AND STABILIZE: S is seated. The shoulder is flexed 90°, the elbow is flexed 90°, and the forearm is in full supination. The upper arm is resting on the supporting surface, and the forearm is perpendicular to the floor. E stands next to S on the side to be tested.

PALPATE AND OBSERVE: Palpation is the same as previously described. E asks S to turn the palm of the hand away from the face, pronating the forearm.

GRADE: Grade strength according to standard definitions of muscle grades.

SUBSTITUTIONS: With the elbow flexed, internal rotation and abduction of the humerus will produce apparent forearm pronation.[7,9] With the elbow extended, internal rotation can place the forearm in a pronated position. The brachioradialis can bring the fully supinated forearm to midposition. Wrist flexion aided by gravity can effect pronation.[9]

Motion

Wrist extension with radial deviation

Muscles[7-9]	Innervation[9]
Extensor carpi radialis brevis	Radial nerve, C5-8
Extensor carpi radialis longus	Radial nerve, C5-8
Extensor carpi ulnaris	Radial nerve, C6-8

Procedure for testing grades N to F

POSITION AND STABILIZE: S is seated with the forearm resting on the supporting surface in pronation, the wrist at neutral, and the fingers and thumb relaxed. E sits opposite S[7,8] or next to S on the side to be tested. E stabilizes over the volar aspect of the mid to distal forearm[7,8] to prevent elbow and forearm motion.

PALPATE AND OBSERVE: E places fingers for palpation of the extensor carpi radialis longus and brevis tendons on the dorsal aspect of the wrist at the bases of the second and third metacarpals, respectively.[7,9] The tendon of the extensor carpi ulnaris may be palpated at the base of the fifth metacarpal, just distal to the head of the ulna[4,9] (Fig. 6-18, *A*). E asks S to bring the hand up from the supporting surface and move it medially (to the radial side) simultaneously, extending and radially deviating the wrist. The movement should be performed without finger extension, which could substitute for the wrist motion[7,9] (Fig. 6-18, *B*).

RESIST: E resists over the dorsum of the second and third metacarpals toward flexion and ulnar deviation[2] (Fig. 6-18, *C*).

Procedure for testing grades P, T, and 0

POSITION AND STABILIZE: S is positioned as described previously except that the forearm is resting in 45° of supination on its ulnar border. E stabilizes at the medial border of the forearm, supporting it slightly above the table surface.[6]

PALPATE AND OBSERVE: Palpation is the same as previously described. E asks S to bring the hand away from the body, extending the wrist and deviating the hand radially or maintaining midposition of the hand.

GRADE: Grade strength according to standard definitions of muscle grades.

SUBSTITUTIONS: These muscles can substitute for one another. In the absence of the extensor carpi radialis muscles, the extensor carpi ulnaris will extend the wrist in an ulnar direction. The combined extension and radial deviation will not be possible. The extensor digitorum communis and the extensor pollicis longus can initiate wrist extension, but finger or thumb extension will precede wrist extension.[9]

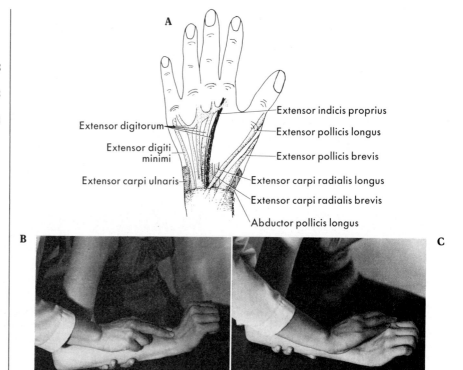

Fig. 6-18. **A,** Arrangement of extensor tendons at wrist. **B,** Wrist extension with radial deviation. Palpate and observe. **C,** Resist.

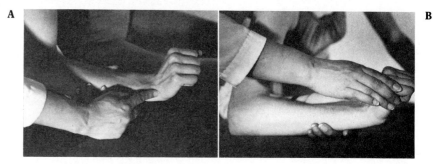

Fig. 6-19. Wrist extension with ulnar deviation. **A,** Palpate and observe. **B,** Resist.

Motion

Wrist extension with ulnar deviation

Muscles[7-9]	Innervation[8]
Extensor carpi radialis brevis	Radial nerve, C5-8
Extensor carpi radialis longus	Radial nerve, C5-8
Extensor carpi ulnaris	Radial nerve, C6-8

Procedure for testing grades N to F

POSITION AND STABILIZE: The position is the same as described for wrist extension with radial deviation.

PALPATE AND OBSERVE: Palpation is the same as for wrist extension with radial deviation. E asks S to bring the hand up from the supporting surface and move it laterally (to the ulnar side) simultaneously. E should observe that the movement is not preceded by thumb or finger extension[9] (Fig. 6-19, A).

RESIST: E resists over the dorsolateral aspect of the fifth metacarpal toward flexion and radial deviation[2] (Fig. 6-19, B).

Procedure for testing grades P, T, and 0

POSITION AND STABILIZE: S is positioned as described previously except that the forearm is in 45° pronation. E stabilizes S's arm at the volar aspect of the forearm, supporting it slightly above the supporting surface.[6]

PALPATE AND OBSERVE: Palpation is the same as described earlier. E asks S to bring the hand away from the body and move it ulnarly at the same time.

GRADE: Grade strength according to standard definitions of muscle grades.

SUBSTITUTIONS: In the absence of the extensor carpi ulnaris, the extensor carpi radialis longus and the extensor carpi radialis brevis can extend the wrist but will do so in a radial direction. The ulnar deviation component of the test motion will not be possible. Long finger and thumb extensors can initiate wrist extension, but the movement will be preceded by finger or thumb extension.[9]

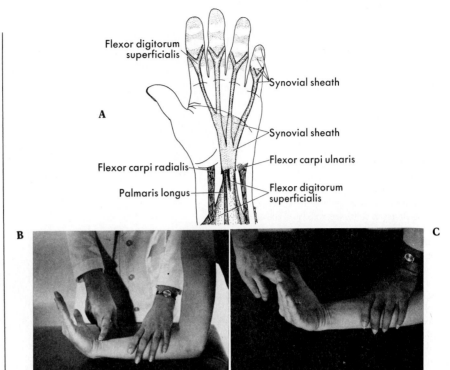

Fig. 6-20. **A**, Arrangement of flexor tendons at wrist. **B**, Wrist flexion with radial deviation. Palpate and observe. **C**, Resist.

Motion

Wrist flexion with radial deviation

Muscles[7]	Innervation[5,7,8]
Flexor carpi radialis	Median nerve, C6-8
Flexor carpi ulnaris	Ulnar nerve, C8, T1
Palmaris longus	Median nerve, C7-8, T1

Procedure for testing grades N to F

POSITION AND STABILIZE: S is seated with the forearm resting in nearly full supination on the supporting surface. The fingers and thumb should be relaxed. E is seated next to S on the side to be tested. E stabilizes the volar aspect of the midforearm to prevent elbow and forearm movements.[7,8]

PALPATE AND OBSERVE: E places fingers for palpation of muscle tendons. The flexor carpi radialis tendon can be palpated over the wrist at the base of the second metacarpal bone. The palmaris longus tendon is at the center of the wrist at the base of the third metacarpal and the flexor carpi ulnaris tendon can be palpated at the ulnar side of the volar aspect of the wrist at the base of the fifth metacarpal[4] (Fig. 6-20, A). E is shown palpating the flexor carpi radialis tendon. E asks S to bring the hand up from the supporting surface toward the face, deviating the hand toward the radial side simultaneously. E should observe that the fingers remain relaxed during the movement (Fig. 6-20, B).

RESIST: E resists in the palm at the radial side of the hand over the second and third metacarpals toward extension and ulnar deviation[7,8] (Fig. 6-20, C).

Procedure for testing grades P, T, and 0

POSITION AND STABILIZE: S is seated with the forearm in 45° pronation and the ulnar border of the hand resting on the supporting surface. E sits next to S on the side to be tested. E stabilizes at the medial border of the forearm to prevent elbow and forearm motion and to raise the hand slightly above the supporting surface.

PALPATE AND OBSERVE: Palpation is the same as described previously. E asks S to move the hand toward the body in a radial direction, flexing the wrist. E observes that S does not initiate the movement with finger flexion.

GRADE: Grade strength according to standard definitions of muscle grades.

SUBSTITUTIONS: The three wrist flexors can substitute for one another. If the flexor carpi radialis is weak or nonfunctioning in this test, the flexor carpi ulnaris will produce wrist flexion in an ulnar direction and the radial deviation will not be possible. The finger flexors can assist wrist flexion, but finger flexion will occur before the wrist is flexed. The abductor pollicis longus with the assistance of gravity can initiate wrist flexion.[9]

Motion
Wrist flexion with ulnar deviation

Muscles[7]	Innervation[5,7,8]
Flexor carpi radialis	Median nerve, C6-8
Flexor carpi ulnaris	Ulnar nerve, C8, T1
Palmaris longus	Median nerve, C7-8, T1

Procedure for testing grades N to F

POSITION AND STABILIZE: S is seated with the forearm resting in nearly full supination on the supporting surface. The fingers and thumb should be relaxed. E is seated opposite S or next to S on the side to be tested. E stabilizes the volar aspect of the middle of the forearm to prevent elbow and forearm movements.[7,8]

PALPATE AND OBSERVE: Palpation is the same as previously described for wrist flexion with radial deviation. E asks S to bring the hand up from the supporting surface, flexing the wrist, and simultaneously deviating it ulnarly (Fig. 6-21, *A*).

RESIST: E resists in the palm of the hand over the hypothenar eminence toward extension and radial deviation[8] (Fig. 6-21, *B*).

Procedure for testing grades P, T, and 0

POSITION AND STABILIZE: S is seated with the forearm resting in 45° of supination on the ulnar border of the arm and hand.[9] E sits opposite S or next to S on the side being tested. E should stabilize the forearm at the dorsomedial aspect to prevent elbow and forearm motion. S's arm can be supported slightly above the supporting surface.

PALPATE AND OBSERVE: Palpation is the same as described earlier. E asks S to bring the wrist toward the body, simultaneously flexing and deviating it ulnarly.

GRADE: Grade strength according to standard definitions of muscle grades.

SUBSTITUTIONS: The wrist flexors can substitute for one another. If the flexor carpi ulnaris is weak or absent, the flexor carpi radialis can produce wrist flexion in a radial direction and the ulnar deviation will not be possible. The finger flexors can also assist wrist flexion but the motion will be preceded by flexion of the fingers.[9]

Motion
Metacarpophalangeal (MP) flexion with interphalangeal (IP) extension

Muscles[1,4]	Innervation[7]
Dorsal interossei	Ulnar nerve, C8, T1
Palmar interossei	Ulnar nerve, C8, T1
Lumbricals 1 and 2	Median nerve, C6-7
Lumbricals 3 and 4	Ulnar nerve, C8, T1

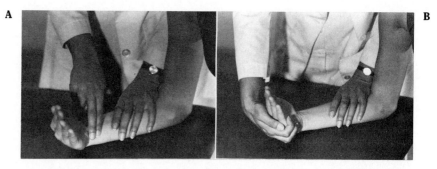

Fig. 6-21. Wrist flexion with ulnar deviation. **A,** Palpate and observe. **B,** Resist.

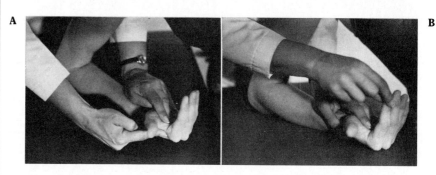

Fig. 6-22. MP flexion with IP extension. **A,** Palpate and observe. **B,** Resist.

Procedure for testing grades N to F

POSITION AND STABILIZE: S is seated with the forearm in supination and the dorsum of the hand resting on the supporting surface. The MP joints are extended and the IP joints are flexed. E sits next to S on the side being tested. E stabilizes S's palm to prevent wrist motion.

PALPATE AND OBSERVE: E places a finger for palpation of the first dorsal interosseous just medial to the distal aspect of the second metacarpal on the dorsum of the hand. The remainder of these muscles are not easily palpable because of their size and deep location in the hand.[9] E asks S to flex the MP joints and extend the IP joints simultaneously[8] (Fig. 6-22, *A*).

RESIST: E resists each finger separately by grasping the distal phalanx and pushing downward on the finger into the supporting surface toward MP extension and IP flexion. An alternative method is to apply pressure first against the dorsal surface of the middle and distal phalanges toward flexion, followed by application of pressure to the volar surface of the proximal phalanges toward extension[8] (Fig. 6-22, *B*).

Procedure for testing grades P, T, and 0

POSITION AND STABILIZE: S is seated with the forearm and wrist in midposition and resting on the ulnar border on the supporting surface. MP joints are extended and IP joints are flexed. E sits next to S on the

side being tested. E stabilizes the wrist and palm of the hand by holding at the dorsum of the hand to prevent wrist and forearm motion.

PALPATE AND OBSERVE: Palpation is the same as described previously. E asks S to flex the MP joints and extend the IP joints simultaneously.

GRADE: Grade strength according to standard definitions of muscle grades.

SUBSTITUTIONS: The flexor digitorum profundus and flexor digitorium superficialis may substitute for weak or absent lumbricals. If this is the case, MP flexion will be preceded by flexion of the distal and proximal IP joints.[9]

Motion
MP extension

Muscles[7-9]	Innervation[7]
Extensor digiti minimi	Radial nerve, C6-8
Extensor digitorum communis	
Extensor indicis proprius	

Procedure for testing grades N to F

POSITION AND STABILIZE: S is seated with the forearm pronated and the wrist in the neutral position. The MP and IP joints are flexed. E sits opposite S or next to S on the side to be tested. E stabilizes the wrist and metacarpals to prevent wrist motion by holding the hand slightly above the supporting surface.

PALPATE AND OBSERVE: E places fingers for palpation of the extensor digitorum tendons where they course over the dorsum of the hand. In some individuals, the extensor digiti minimi tendon can be palpated or visualized just lateral to the extensor digitorum tendon to the fifth finger. The extensor indicis proprius tendon can be palpated or visualized just medial to the extensor digitorum tendon to the first finger. E asks S to raise the fingers away from the supporting surface, extending the MP joints but maintaining the IP joints in flexion (Fig. 6-23, A).

RESIST: E resists each finger individually over the dorsal aspect of the proximal phalanx toward MP flexion[7,8] (Fig. 6-23, B).

Procedure for testing grades P, T, and 0

POSITION AND STABILIZE: Position and stabilization are the same as previously described except that S's forearm is in midposition and the hand and forearm are supported on the ulnar border.

PALPATE AND OBSERVE: Palpation is the same as described earlier. E asks S to move the fingers backward, extending the MP joints while keeping the IP joints flexed.

GRADE: Grade strength according to standard definitions of muscle grades.

SUBSTITUTIONS: With the wrist stabilized, no substitutions are possible. During functional movements, however, wrist flexion will produce incomplete finger extension through the tendon action of the finger extensors.[9]

Motion
PIP flexion, second through fifth fingers

Muscles[7,8]	Innervation[7,8]
Flexor digitorum superficialis	Median nerve, C7-8, T1

Procedure for testing grades N to F

POSITION AND STABILIZE: S is seated with the forearm in supination, the wrist at the neutral position, and the fingers extended. The hand and forearm are resting on the dorsal surface. E sits opposite S or next to S on the side being tested. E stabilizes the MP joint and proximal phalanx of the finger being tested.[7,8]

PALPATE AND OBSERVE: E uses the finger stabilizing the proximal phalanx for palpation of the flexor digitorium superficialis tendon on the volar surface of the proximal phalanx of the finger being tested. E's stabilizing finger may also palpate in this instance.[9] The tendon supplying the fourth finger may be palpated on the volar aspect of the wrist between the flexor carpi ulnaris and the palmaris longus tendons[4] if desired.

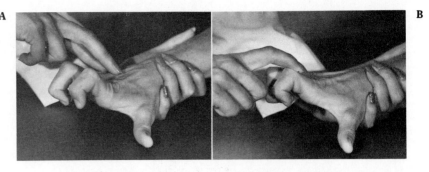

Fig. 6-23. MP extension. **A**, Palpate and observe. **B**, Resist.

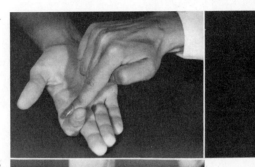

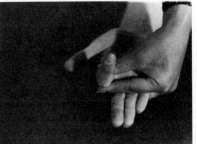

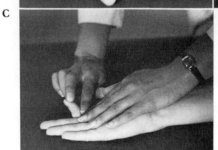

Fig. 6-24. PIP flexion. **A**, Palpate and observe. **B**, Position to assist with isolation of PIP joint flexion. **C**, Resist. Therapist checks for substitution by flexor digitorum profundus.

E asks S to flex the proximal interphalangeal (PIP) joint while maintaining the distal interphalangeal (DIP) joint in extension (Fig. 6-24, A). If isolating PIP flexion is difficult for S, E may hold all the fingers not being tested in MP hyperextension and PIP extension by pulling back over the IP joints. This maneuver inactivates the flexor digitorum profundus so that S cannot flex the distal joint[3]. Most individuals cannot perform isolated action of the PIP joint of the fifth finger[9] even with this assistance (Fig. 6-24, B).

RESIST: E resists with one finger at the volar aspect of the middle phalanx toward extension.[7,8] If E uses the index finger to apply resistance, the middle finger may be used to move the DIP joint back and forth to verify that the flexor digitorum profundus is not substituting (Fig. 6-24, C).

Procedure for testing grades P, T, and 0

POSITION AND STABILIZE: S is seated with the forearm in midposition and the wrist at the neutral position, resting on the ulnar border. E sits opposite S or next to S on the side to be tested. If stabilization during the motion is difficult in this position, the forearm may be returned to full supination, since the effect of gravity on the fingers is not significant.

PALPATE AND OBSERVE: Palpation and observation of movement is the same as described previously except that the movement is performed in a plane parallel to the floor.

GRADE: Grade strength according to standard definitions of muscle grades. If the test for grades P and below is done with the forearm in full supination, partial ROM against gravity may be graded P.[7]

SUBSTITUTIONS: The flexor digitorum profundus may substitute for the flexor digitorum superficialis if it has not been inactivated. DIP flexion will precede PIP flexion in this substitution. Tendon action of the flexor digitorum longus accompanies wrist extension and can produce an apparent flexion of the fingers through parital ROM.[9]

Motion

DIP flexion, second through fifth fingers

Muscles[7]	Innervation[7]
Flexor digitorum profundus	Median and ulnar nerves, C8, T1

Procedure for testing grades N to F

POSITION AND STABILIZE: S is seated with the forearm in supination, the wrist at the neutral position, and the fingers extended. E sits opposite S or next to S on the side being tested. E stabilizes the PIP joint and middle phalanx of the finger being tested to isolate flexor digitorum profundus action at the DIP joint.

PALPATE AND OBSERVE: E uses the finger stabilizing the middle phalanx to simultaneously palpate the flexor digitorum profundus tendon on the volar surface of the middle phalanx.[7,9] E asks S to bring the fingertip up away from the supporting surface, flexing the DIP joint (Fig. 6-25, *A*).

RESIST: E resists with one finger at the volar aspect of the distal phalanx toward extension[7,8] (Fig. 6-25, *B*).

Procedure for testing grades P, T, and 0

POSITION AND STABILIZE: S is seated with the forearm in midposition and the wrist at neutral position resting on the ulnar border. S may be positioned with the forearm supinated as previously described for PIP flexion for ease of handling and testing. Stabilization is the same as described previously.

PALPATE AND OBSERVE: Palpation is the same as described earlier. S is instructed to move the tip of the finger toward the body, flexing the DIP joint.

GRADE: Grade strength according to standard definitions of muscle grades except if the test for the grades P and below was done with the forearm in full supination, movement through partial ROM may be graded P.

SUBSTITUTIONS: No substitutions are possible during the testing procedure, since the flexor digitorum profundus is the only muscle that can act to flex the DIP joint when it is isolated. During normal hand function, however, wrist extension with tendon action of the finger flexors can produce parital flexion of the DIP joints.[9]

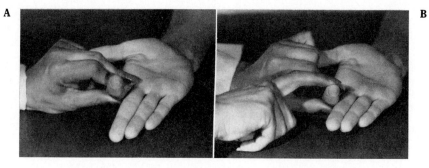

Fig. 6-25. DIP flexion. **A,** Palpate and observe. **B,** Resist.

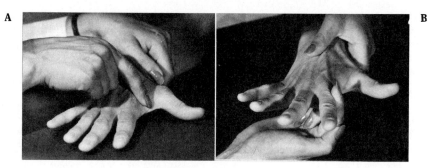

Fig. 6-26. Finger abduction. **A,** Palpate and observe. **B,** Resist.

Motion

Finger abduction

Muscles[7]	Innervation[7]
Abductor digiti minimi	Ulnar nerve, C8, T1
Dorsal interossei	Ulnar nerve, C8, T1

Procedure for testing grades N to F

POSITION AND STABILIZE: S is seated with the forearm pronated, wrist in neutral position, and fingers extended and adducted. E is seated opposite S or next to S on the side to be tested.[7] E stabilizes the wrist and metacarpals by holding S's hand slightly above the supporting surface.

PALPATE AND OBSERVE: E places fingers for palpation of the first dorsal interosseous on the lateral aspect of the second metacarpal or on the ulnar border of the fifth metacarpal to palpate the abductor digiti minimi.[7] The remaining interossei are not palpable. The test may be repeated twice if it is not possible to palpate both muscles simultaneously. E asks S to spread the fingers apart, abducting them at the MP joints (Fig. 6-26, *A*).

RESIST: E offers resistance to the first interosseous dorsalis by applying pressure on the radial side of the distal end of the proximal phalanx of the second finger in an ulnar direction (Fig. 6-26, *B*). Resistance to the second interosseous dorsalis is applied to the radial side of the distal end of the proximal phalanx of the middle finger in an ulnar direction. Resistance to the third interosseous dorsalis is applied to the ulnar side of the distal end of the proximal phalanx of the middle finger in a radial direction. Resistance to the fourth interosseous dorsalis is applied to the ulnar side of the distal end of the proximal phalanx of the ring finger in a radial direction. Resistance to the abductor digiti minimi is applied to the ulnar side of the distal end of the proximal phalanx of the little finger in a radial direction.[8] Resistance to the first dorsal interosseous only is seen in (Fig. 6-26, *B*.)

Procedure for testing grades P, T, and 0

The tests for these muscle grades are the same as described previously. Since the test motions were not performed against gravity, some judgment of the examiner must be used in grading. For example, full ROM in gravity-eliminated position with slight resistance may be graded F.

SUBSTITUTIONS: The extensor digitorum communis can assist weak or absent interossei dorsales but abduction will be accompanied by MP extension.[9]

Motion

Finger adduction

Muscles[7,8]	**Innervation[7]**
Palmar interossei 1, 2, and 3	Ulnar nerve, C8, T1

Procedure for testing grades N to F

POSITION AND STABILIZE: Positioning and stabilization is the same as described previously for finger abduction except that S's fingers are extended and abducted.

PALPATE AND OBSERVE: The palmar interossei are not readily palpable. E asks S to bring the first, fourth, and fifth fingers toward the middle finger until they are touching one another (Fig. 6-27, *A*).

RESIST: E grasps the first finger at the distal end of the proximal phalanx and pulls it in a radial direction. E similarly grasps the fourth and fifth fingers respectively and pulls them in an ulnar direction[8] (Fig. 6-27, *B*). These muscles are small and resistance will have to be modified to accommodate to the power of these small muscles.

Procedure for testing grades P, T, and O

The tests for these muscle grades are the same as described earlier. The examiner's judgment must be used in determining the degree of weakness. Achievement of full ROM with slight resistance may be graded F.

SUBSTITUTIONS: Flexor digitorum profundus and flexor digitorum superficialis can substitute for weak palmar interossei, but IP flexion will occur with finger adduction.[9]

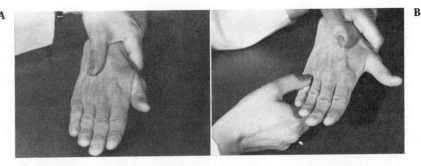

Fig. 6-27. Finger adduction. **A,** Therapist observes movement of fingers into adduction. Palpation of these muscles is not possible. **B,** Resist.

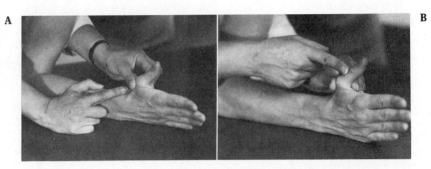

Fig. 6-28. Thumb MP extension. **A,** Palpate and observe. **B,** Resist.

Motion

Thumb MP extension

Muscles[7,8]	**Innervation[7,8]**
Extensor pollicis brevis	Radial nerve, C6-8

Procedure for testing grades N to F

POSITION AND STABILIZE: S is seated. The forearm is in midposition, the wrist is in neutral position, and the hand and forearm are resting on the ulnar border. The thumb is flexed into the palm at the MP joint and the IP is extended but relaxed. E sits opposite S or next to S on the side to be tested. E stabilizes the first metacarpal to isolate motion to the MP joint.

PALPATE AND OBSERVE: E places fingers for palpation of the extensor pollicis brevis tendon at the base of the first metacarpal on the dorsoradial aspect. It lays just medial to the abductor pollicis longus tendon on the radial side of the "anatomical snuff box,"[4] which is the hollow space created between the extensor pollicis longus and extensor pollicis brevis tendons when the thumb is fully extended and radially abducted. E asks S to extend the MP joint. The IP joint remains relaxed in extension (Fig. 6-28, *A*). It is difficult for many individuals to isolate this motion.

RESIST: E resists on the dorsal surface of the proximal phalanx toward MP flexion[7] (Fig. 6-28, *B*).

Procedure for testing grades P, T, and O

POSITION AND STABILIZE: Positioning and stabilization are the same as described previously except that the forearm is fully pronated and resting on the volar surface. E may stabilize the first metacarpal by holding the hand slightly above the supporting surface.

PALPATE AND OBSERVE: Palpation is the same as described earlier. MP extension is performed in a plane parallel to the supporting surface.

GRADE: Grade strength according to standard definitions of muscle grades.

SUBSTITUTIONS: The extensor pollicis longus may substitute for extensor pollicis brevis. IP extension will precede MP extension.[9]

Motion

Thumb IP extension

Muscles[7-9]	Innervation[7,8]
Extensor pollicis longus	Radial nerve, C6-8

Procedure for testing grades N to F

POSITION AND STABILIZE: S is seated. The forearm is in midposition, the wrist is in neutral position, and the hand and forearm are resting on the ulnar border. The MP joint of the thumb is extended or slightly flexed, and the IP joint is flexed fully into the palm. E sits opposite S or next to S on the side being tested. E stabilizes the first metacarpal and the proximal phalanx of the thumb to prevent carpometacarpal (CMC) and MP motion.

PALPATE AND OBSERVE: E places fingers for palpation of the extensor pollicis longus tendon on the dorsal surface of the hand medial to the extensor pollicis brevis tendon, between the head of the first metacarpal and the base of the second metacarpal[7] on the ulnar side of the anatomical snuff box.[4] E's hand can be positioned so that palpation and stabilization can be done simultaneously by placing the thumb over the extensor pollicis longus tendon on the dorsum of the first metacarpal. E asks S to bring the tip of the thumb up from the palm, extending the IP joint (Fig. 6-29, *A*).

RESIST: E resists on the dorsal surface of the distal phalanx down toward IP flexion (Fig. 6-29, *B*).

Procedure for testing grades P, T, and 0

POSITION AND STABILIZE: Positioning and stabilization are the same as previously described except that the forearm is fully pronated. E may stabilize S's hand so that it is held slightly above the supporting surface.

PALPATE AND OBSERVE: Palpation is the same as described previously. IP extension is performed in the plane of the palm, parallel to the supporting surface.

GRADE: Grade strength according to standard definitions of muscle grades.

SUBSTITUTIONS: A quick contraction followed by rapid release of the flexor pollicis longus will cause the IP joint to rebound into extension. IP flexion will precede IP extension.[9] Abductor pollicis brevis, flexor pollicis brevis, the oblique fibers of the adductor pollicis, and the first interosseous palmaris can extend the IP joint because of their insertions into the extensor expansion of the thumb.[8]

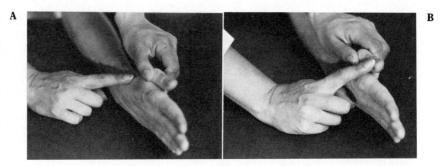

Fig. 6-29. Thumb IP extension. **A,** Palpate and observe. **B,** Resist.

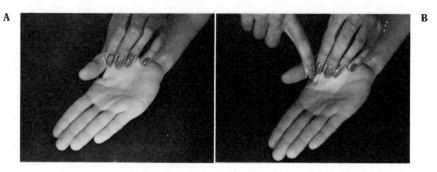

Fig. 6-30. Thumb MP flexion. **A,** Palpate and observe. **B,** Resist.

Motion

Thumb MP flexion

Muscles[7,8]	Innervation[7,8]
Flexor pollicis brevis	Median and ulnar nerves, C6-8, T1

Procedure for testing grades N to F

POSITION AND STABILIZE: S is seated with the forearm fully supinated, the wrist in the neutral position, and the thumb in extension and adduction. E is seated next to or opposite S.[7,8] E stabilizes the first metacarpal and the wrist to prevent CMC joint, wrist, or forearm movements.

PALPATE AND OBSERVE: E places fingers for palpation over the middle of the palmar surface of the thenar eminence,[7] just medial to the abductor pollicis brevis. The hand that is used to stabilize may also be used for palpation. E asks S to flex the MP joint while maintaining extension of the IP joint (Fig. 6-30, *A*). It may not be possible for some individuals to isolate flexion to the MP joint. In this instance, both MP and IP flexion may be tested together, considered a gross test for thumb flexion strength, and graded according to the examiner's judgment.

RESIST: E resists on the palmar surface of the first phalanx toward MP extension. When resistance is given, the IP joint may flex because the added effort to resist the pressure will recruit the assistance of the flexor pollicis longus muscle[8] (Fig. 6-30, *B*).

Procedure for testing grades P, T, and 0

POSITION AND STABILIZE: S is seated with the forearm in 45° supination, wrist in neutral position, and the thumb in extension and adduction. Stabilization is the same as described previously.

PALPATE AND OBSERVE: Palpation is the same as described earlier. E asks S to flex the MP joint so that the thumb moves over the palm of the hand.

GRADE: Grade strength according to standard definitions of muscle grades.

SUBSTITUTIONS: The flexor pollicis longus can substitute for flexor pollicis brevis. If this is the case, isolated MP flexion will not be possible and MP flexion will be preceded by IP flexion.[9]

Motion
Thumb IP flexion

Muscles[7-9]	Innervation[8]
Flexor pollicis longus	Median nerve, C7-8, T1

Procedure for testing grades N to F
POSITION AND STABILIZE: S is seated with the forearm fully supinated, the wrist in neutral position, and the thumb in extension and adduction. E is seated next to or opposite S. E stabilizes the first metacarpal and the proximal phalanx of the thumb in extension to ensure isolated movement of the IP joint.[8]

PALPATE AND OBSERVE: E places a finger for palpation of flexor pollicis longus tendon on the palmar surface of the proximal phalanx. In this instance the palpating finger may be the same one used for stabilization of the proximal phalanx. E asks S to flex the IP joint toward the palm[7] (Fig. 6-31, A).

RESIST: E resists with the index finger on the palmar surface of the distal phalanx toward IP extension (Fig. 6-31, B).

Procedure for testing grades P, T, and 0
POSITION AND STABILIZE: S is seated with the forearm supinated 45°, wrist in neutral position, and the thumb extended and adducted. Stabilization by E is the same as described earlier.

PALPATE AND OBSERVE: Palpation and observation are same as previously described.

GRADE: Grade strength according to standard definitions of muscle grades.

SUBSTITUTIONS: A quick contraction and release of the extensor pollicis longus may cause an apparent flexion of the IP joint. E should observe for IP extension preceding IP flexion.[9]

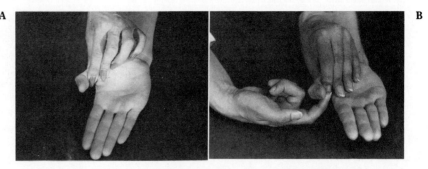

Fig. 6-31. Thumb IP flexion. **A,** Palpate and observe. **B,** Resist.

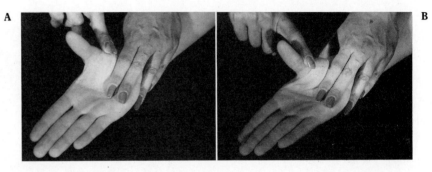

Fig. 6-32. Thumb palmar abduction. **A,** Palpate and observe. **B,** Resist.

Motion
Thumb palmar abduction

Muscles[8,9]	Innervation[8]
Abductor pollicis brevis	Median nerve, C6-8, T1

Procedure for testing grades N to F
POSITION AND STABILIZE: S is seated with the forearm in supination, the wrist in neutral position, the thumb extended and adducted, and the CMC joint rotated so that the thumb is resting in a plane perpendicular to the palm of the hand. E sits opposite S or next to S on the side to be tested.[8] E stabilizes the metacarpals and wrist by holding the volar aspect of the distal forearm, wrist, and palm.

PALPATE AND OBSERVE: E places fingers for palpation on the lateral aspect of the thenar eminence and lateral to the flexor pollicis brevis muscle.[7] E then asks S to raise the thumb away from the palm in a plane perpendicular to the palm[8] (Fig. 6-32, A).

RESIST: E resists at the lateral aspect of the proximal phalanx downward toward adduction[8] (Fig. 6-32, B).

Procedure for testing grades P, T, and 0
POSITION AND STABILIZE: S is positioned as described previously except that the forearm and hand are resting on the ulnar border. Stabilization is the same as described earlier.

PALPATE AND OBSERVE: Palpation is the same as previously described. E asks S to move the thumb away from the palm in a plane at right angles to the palm of the hand and parallel to the supporting surface.

GRADE: Grade strength according to standard definitions of muscle grades.

SUBSTITUTIONS: The abductor pollicis longus can substitute for the abductor pollicis brevis. However, abduction will take place more in the plane of the palm rather than perpendicular to it.[9]

Motion
Thumb radial abduction

Muscles[8]	Innervation[8]
Abductor pollicis longus	Radial nerve, C6-8

Procedure for testing grades N to F

POSITION AND STABILIZE: S is seated with the forearm in neutral rotation, the wrist in neutral position, and the thumb adducted and slightly flexed across the palm. The hand and forearm are resting on the ulnar border. E sits opposite S or next to S on the side being tested. E stabilizes the wrist and metacarpals of the fingers to prevent wrist and forearm motion. E may stabilize by supporting the ulnar border of the forearm and hand, holding S's hand slightly above the supporting surface.

PALPATE AND OBSERVE: E places fingers for palpation of the abductor pollicis longus tendon on the lateral aspect of the base of the first metacarpal. It is the tendon immediately lateral (radial) to the extensor pollicis brevis tendon.[4,7] E asks S to move the thumb out of the palm of the hand, abducting it in the plane of the palm (Fig. 6-33, *A*).

RESIST: E resists at the lateral aspect of the distal end of the first metacarpal toward adduction[8] (Fig. 6-33, *B*).

Procedure for testing grades P, T, and 0

POSITION AND STABILIZE: S is positioned as described previously except that the forearm is in full supination and the forearm and hand are resting in the dorsal surface. E stabilizes on the volar aspect of the wrist and palm of the hand.

PALPATE AND OBSERVE: Palpation is the same as previously described. E asks S to move the thumb out, away from the palm of the hand in the plane of the palm, and parallel to the supporting surface.

GRADE: Grade strength according to standard definitions of muscle grades.

SUBSTITUTIONS: The abductor pollicis brevis can substitute for the abductor pollicis longus. Abduction will not take place in the plane of the palm, however, but in a direction toward the ulnar side.[9]

Motion
Thumb adduction

Muscles[7,8]	Innervation[7,8]
Adductor pollicis	Ulnar nerve, C8, T1

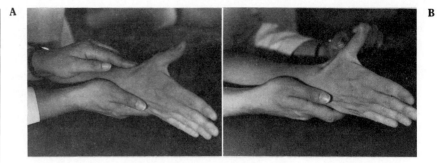

Fig. 6-33. Thumb radial abduction. **A,** Palpate and observe. **B,** Resist.

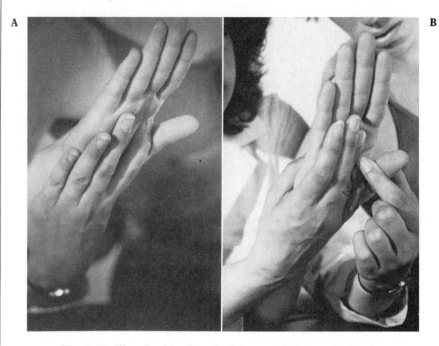

Fig. 6-34. Thumb adduction. **A,** Palpate and observe. **B,** Resist.

Procedure for testing grades N to F

POSITION AND STABILIZE: S is seated with the forearm pronated and the wrist in neutral position. The thumb is opposed and abducted. E is sitting opposite S or next to S on the side to be tested. E stabilizes the wrist and metacarpals and supports S's hand slightly above the supporting surface.[7]

PALPATE AND OBSERVE: E places fingers for palpation on the palmar side of the thumb web space.[9] E asks S to bring the thumb up to touch the palm[7] (Fig. 6-34, *A*). The palm is turned up in the figure to show the palpation point.

RESIST: E grasps the proximal phalanx of the thumb near the metacarpal head and pulls downward toward abduction (Fig. 6-34, *B*).

Procedure for testing grades P, T, and 0

POSITION AND STABILIZE: Positioning is the same as previously described except that the forearm is in midposition and the forearm and hand are resting on the ulnar border. E stabilizes the wrist and palm of the hand.

PALPATE AND OBSERVE: Palpation is the same as described previously. E asks S to bring the thumb in to touch the radial side of the palm of the hand or the second metacarpal bone.

GRADE: Grade strength according to standard definitions of muscle grades.

SUBSTITUTIONS: The flexor pollicis longus or extensor pollicis longus may assist weak or absent adductor pollicis. If one of these muscles substitutes, adduction will be accompanied by thumb flexion or extension preceding adduction.[7,9]

Motion
Opposition of the thumb to the fifth finger

Muscles[7,8]	Innervation[7,8]
Opponens digiti minimi	Ulnar nerve, C8, T1
Opponens pollicis	Median nerve, C6-8, T1

Procedure for testing grades N to F

POSITION AND STABILIZE: S is seated with forearm in full supination, wrist in neutral position, and thumb and fifth fingers extended and adducted. E sits opposite S or next to S on the side to be tested. E stabilizes the distal volar aspect of the forearm and wrist to prevent wrist and forearm motion.[8]

PALPATE AND OBSERVE: E places fingers for palpation of the opponens pollicis along the radial side of the shaft of the first metacarpal, lateral to the abductor pollicis brevis. The opponens digiti minimi cannot be easily palpated.[9] E asks S to bring the thumb out and across the palm to touch the pad of the distal phalanx of the thumb to the pad of the distal phalanx of the fifth finger (Fig. 6-35, *A*).

RESIST: E resists at the distal ends of the first and fifth metacarpals toward derotation of these bones and flattening of the palm of the hand[7] (Fig. 6-35, *B*).

Procedure for testing grades P, T, and 0

The same procedure described previously may be used for these grades if grading is modified to compensate for the movement of the parts against gravity. For example, movement through full ROM would be graded F and movement through partial ROM would be graded P.[7] An alternative would be to test opposition with the forearm perpendicular to the supporting surface resting on the elbow to effect opposition in a gravity-eliminated plane. Under these circumstances, the standard muscle grades would be assigned. The opponens pollicis and opponens digiti minimi should be graded separately according to resistance and ROM achieved by each component of opposition.

SUBSTITUTIONS: The abductor pollicis brevis will assist with opposition by flexing and medially rotating the CMC joint but the IP joint will extend. The flexor pollicis brevis will flex and medially rotate the CMC joint but the thumb will not move away from the palm of the hand. The flexor pollicis longus will flex and slightly rotate the CMC joint, but the thumb will not move away from the palm and the IP joint will flex strongly.[9]

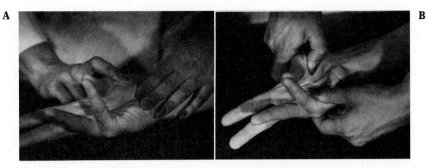

Fig. 6-35. Thumb opposition. **A,** Palpate and observe. **B,** Resist.

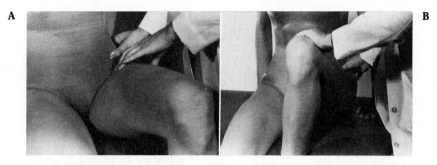

Fig. 6-36. Hip flexion. **A,** Palpate and observe. **B,** Resist.

Motion
Hip flexion

Muscles[4,7-9]	Innervation[4,7-9]
Iliacus	Femoral nerve, L2-3
Pectineus	Femoral nerve, L2-3
Psoas major	Lumbar plexus, L1-4
Rectus femoris	Femoral nerve, L2-4
Sartorius	Femoral nerve, L2-5, S1
Tensor fasciae latae	Superior gluteal nerve

Procedure for testing grades N to F

POSITION AND STABILIZE: S is seated with knees flexed over the edge of the table and feet above the floor. S may grasp the edge of the table with the hands or may fold the hands across the chest.[7,8] E stands next to S on the side being tested. E stabilizes the pelvis at the iliac crest on the side being tested to prevent pelvic tilt or trunk rotation.

PALPATE AND OBSERVE: E places fingers for palpation of the sartorius on the anterior surface of the thigh obliquely from superioanterior aspect to the inferior medial aspect. The psoas major and iliacus are difficult to palpate. The rectus femoris may be palpated on the middle- anterior aspect of the thigh just lateral to the sartorius.[4,9] E asks S to lift the leg up from the table, flexing the hip through the remainder of the ROM. E observes for internal rotation, external rotation, and abduction accompanying the flexion as signs of substitution or muscle imbalance in this muscle group (Fig. 6-36, *A*).

RESIST: E resists just proximal to the knee on the anterior surface of the thigh down toward the table into hip extension (Fig. 6-36, *B*).

Procedure for testing grades P, T, and 0

POSITION AND STABILIZE: S is lying on the side. E stands behind S, supporting the upper leg in neutral rotation and slight abduction with the knee extended.[7] The lower leg to be tested is extended at the hip and knee. The weight of the trunk may be adequate stabilization or E may stabilize the pelvis.

PALPATE AND OBSERVE: Palpation is the same as described previously. E asks S to bring the lower leg up toward the trunk, flexing the hip and knee.[7]

GRADE: Grade strength according to standard definitions of muscle grades.

SUBSTITUTIONS: The hip flexors can substitute for one another. If the iliacus and psoas major are weak or absent, hip flexion will be accompanied by other movements, such as abduction and external rotation (sartorius); abduction and internal rotation (tensor fasciae latae); and adduction (pectineus).[7,9] If the anterior abdominal muscles do not fix the pelvis to the trunk, the pelvis will flex on the thighs and the hip flexors may hold against resistance but not at maximal ROM.[8]

Motion
Hip extension

Muscles[7,8]	Innervation[7]
Gluteus maximus	Inferior gluteal nerve, L5, S1-2

Procedure for testing grades N to F

POSITION AND STABILIZE: S is lying prone with the hip in neutral position and the knee flexed about 90°. E stands next to S opposite the side to be tested.[8] E stabilizes the pelvis at the iliac crest on the side being tested to prevent extension of the lumbar spine. (The test may be performed with the knee extended to include action of the hamstring muscles if desired.[7])

PALPATE AND OBSERVE: E places fingers for palpation on the middle posterior surface of the buttock.[9] E asks S to lift the leg from the supporting surface, extending the hip while keeping the knee flexed to minimize action of the hamstring muscles on the hip joint (Fig. 6-37, *A*).

RESIST: E removes the palpating fingers and resists at the distal end of the posterior aspect of the thigh, downward toward flexion (Fig. 6-37, *B*).

Procedure for testing grades P, T, and 0

POSITION AND STABILIZE: S is lying on the side. E stands in front of S, supporting the upper leg in extension and slight abduction.[7] The lower leg to be tested is flexed at the hip and knee. E stabilizes the pelvis over the iliac crest to prevent trunk rotation, elevation of the pelvis, and extension of the lumbar spine.

PALPATE AND OBSERVE: Palpation is the same as described previously. E asks S to bring the lower leg backward, extending the hip, and maintaining flexion of the knee.

GRADE: Grade strength according to standard definitions of muscle grades.

SUBSTITUTIONS: Elevation of the pelvis and extension of the lumbar spine can produce some hip extension[7,9] In a supine position, gravity and eccentric contraction of the hip flexors can return the flexed hip to extension.[9]

Motion
Hip abduction

Muscles[7-9]	Innervation[7,8]
Gluteus medius	Superior gluteal nerve, L4-5, S1
Gluteus minimus	Superior gluteal nerve, L4-5, S1
Tensor fasciae latae	Superior gluteal nerve, L4-5, S1

Procedure for testing grades N to F

POSITION AND STABILIZE: S is lying on the side. The upper leg (to be tested) has the

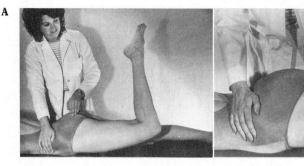

Fig. 6-37. Hip extension. **A,** Palpate and observe. **B,** Resist.

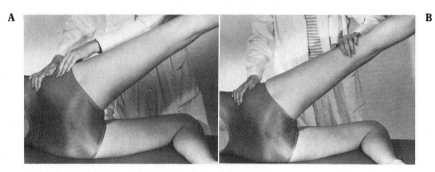

Fig. 6-38. Hip abduction. **A,** Palpate and observe. **B,** Resist.

knee extended and the hip slightly extended beyond the neutral position. The lower leg is flexed at the hip and knee to provide a wide base of support. E stands in front of S.[7,8] E stabilizes the pelvis over the iliac crest to prevent anterior or posterior tilt and elevation or depression of the pelvis.[8]

PALPATE AND OBSERVE: E places fingers for palpation of the gluteus medius on the lateral aspect of the ilium above the greater trochanter of the femur.[7] E asks S to lift the leg upward, abducting the hip (Fig. 6-38, *A*).

RESIST: E resists just proximal to the knee in a downward direction toward adduction (Fig. 6-38, *B*).

Procedure for testing grades P, T, and 0

POSITION AND STABILIZE: S is lying supine with both legs extended and in neutral rotation. E stands next to S opposite the side to be tested. E stabilizes the pelvis at the iliac crest on the side to be tested and the opposite limb at the lateral aspect of the calf.[7]

PALPATE AND OBSERVE: E may use the hand stabilizing over the pelvis to simultaneously palpate the gluteus medius by adjusting the position of the hand so that the fingers are touching the lateral aspect of the ilium above the greater trochanter as described previously. E asks S to move the free leg sideward, abducting the hip as far as possible and maintaining neutral rotation during this movement.

GRADE: Grade strength according to standard definitions of muscle grades.

SUBSTITUTIONS: Lateral muscles of the trunk may contract to bring the pelvis toward the thorax, affecting partial abduction at the hip.[7] If the hip is externally rotated, the hip flexors may assist in abduction.[9]

Motion
Hip adduction

Muscles[4,7-9]	Innervation[4,7,8]
Adductor brevis	Obturator nerve, L2-4
Adductor longus	Obturator nerve, L2-4
Adductor magnus	Obturator and sciatic nerves, L2-5, S1
Gracilis	Obturator nerve, L2-4
Pectineus	Femoral and obturator nerves, L2-4

Procedure for testing grades N to F

POSITION AND STABILIZE: S is lying on right side for test of right leg or on left side for test of left leg. The body is in a straight line with legs extended. E stands behind S. E supports S's upper leg in partial abduction while S holds on to the supporting surface for stability.[5,7,8]

PALPATE AND OBSERVE: E places fingers for palpation of any of the adductor muscles as follows: adductor magnus at the middle of the medial surface of the thigh; adductor longus at the medial aspect of the groin; and gracilis on the medial aspect of the posterior surface of the knee, just anterior to the semitendinosus tendon.[9] E asks S to raise the lower leg up from the supporting surface, keeping the knee extended. E observes that there is no rotation, flexion, or extension of the hip or pelvic tilting[8] (Fig. 6-39, A).

RESIST: E removes the palpating fingers and resists over the medial aspect of the leg just proximal to the knee downward toward abduction[7] (Fig. 6-39, B).

Procedure for testing grades P, T, and 0

POSITION AND STABILIZE: S is lying supine. The limb to be tested is abducted 45°. E stands next to S opposite the side to be tested. E stabilizes the pelvis at the iliac crest on the side to be tested and at the ankle of the opposite limb.[7]

PALPATE AND OBSERVE: Given the stabilization just described, palpation is not possible. It is suggested that E ask S to perform the test motion with the stabilization, then remove the hand stabilizing the opposite leg to use for palpation of one or more of the adductor muscles described earlier, and then ask S to repeat the test motion. Thus E can compare the accuracy of motion performed when not palpating with that performed while palpating to ensure that the muscles being tested are indeed the ones performing the motion. For the test motion E asks S to bring the leg being tested toward the opposite leg, adducting it to the midline.

GRADE: Grade strength according to standard definitions of muscle grades.

SUBSTITUTIONS: Hip flexors may substitute for adductors. S will internally rotate the hip and tilt the pelvis backward. The hamstring muscles may be used to substitute for adduction. S will externally rotate the hip and tip the pelvis forward.[7,9]

Motion
Hip external rotation

Muscles[7-9]	Innervation[7,8]
Gemellus inferior	Sacral plexus, L4-5, S1
Gemellus superior	Sacral plexus, L5, S1-2
Obturator internus	Sacral plexus, L5, S1-2
Obturator externus	Obturator nerve, L3-4
Piriformis	Sacral plexus, L5, S1-2
Quadratus femoris	Sacral plexus, L4-5, S1

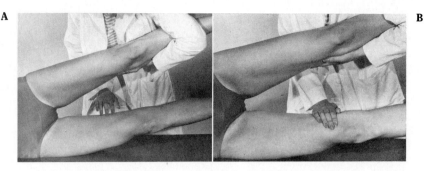

Fig. 6-39. Hip adduction. **A,** Palpate and observe. **B,** Resist.

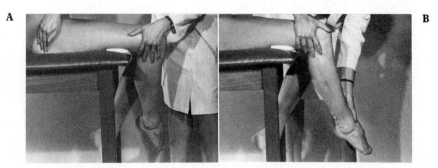

Fig. 6-40. Hip external rotation. **A,** Palpate and observe. **B,** Resist.

Procedure for testing grades N to F

POSITION AND STABILIZE: S is seated with knees flexed over the edge of the table. A small pad or folded towel is placed under the knee on the side to be tested. E stands in front of S toward the side to be tested. E places one hand on the lateral aspect of the knee on the side to be tested to prevent flexion or abduction of the hip. S may grasp the edge of the table to stabilize the trunk and pelvis.[7,8]

PALPATE AND OBSERVE: It is difficult or impossible to palpate these deep muscles. Action of the external rotators may be detected by deeply palpating posterior to the greater trochanter of the femur.[7] E places fingers for palpation and asks S to rotate the thigh outwardly by moving the foot medially (Fig. 6-40, A).

RESIST: E removes the palpating fingers, and with one hand stabilizing at the knee as described earlier, S resists with the other hand at the medial aspect of the ankle in a lateral direction toward internal rotation.[7,8,10] Resistance should be given carefully and gradually, since the use of the long lever arm can cause joint injury if sudden forceful resistance is given[7] (Fig. 6-40, B).

Procedure for testing grades P, T, and 0

POSITION AND STABILIZE: S is lying supine with hips and knees extended and hip to be tested internally rotated. E is standing next to S on the opposite side to be tested.[7] E stabilizes the pelvis on the side to be tested to prevent elevation or tilt of the pelvis.

PALPATE AND OBSERVE: Action of the external rotators may be detected by deeply palpating posterior to the greater trochanter of the femur.[7] E asks S to roll the thigh outward (laterally). Gravity may assist this motion once S has passed the neutral position. E may use one hand to palpate and the other to offer slight resistance during the second half of the movement to compensate for the assistance of gravity. If the ROM can be completed with slight resistance, a grade of P can be given.[7]

GRADE: Grade strength according to standard definitions of muscle grades for F to N muscles. Muscles are graded P if ROM in the gravity-eliminated position can be achieved against slight resistance during the last half of ROM. A grade of T can be assigned if contraction of external rotators can be detected by the deep palpation described earlier when the movement is attempted in the gravity-eliminated position.[7]

SUBSTITUTIONS: The gluteus maximus may substitute for the deep external rotators when the hip is in extension. The sartorius may substitute, but external rotation will be accompanied by hip abduction and knee flexion.[9]

Motion

Hip internal rotation

Muscles[4,7-9]	Innervation[7-9]
Gluteus medius	Superior gluteal nerve, L4-5, S1
Gluteus minimus	Superior gluteal nerve, L4-5, S1
Tensor fasciae latae	Superior gluteal nerve, L4-5, S1

Procedure for testing grades N to F

POSITION AND STABILIZE: S is seated on a table with the knees flexed over the edge. A small pad is placed under the knee on the side to be tested. E stands next to S on the side to be tested. E stabilizes the thigh at the medial aspect of the knee to prevent adduction of the hip. S may grasp the edge of the table to stabilize the pelvis and trunk.[7]

PALPATE AND OBSERVE: E places fingers for palpation of the gluteus medius between the iliac crest and the greater trochanter.[4] E asks S to rotate the thigh inwardly while moving the foot laterally. E should observe that S does not lift the pelvis on the side being tested[7] (Fig. 6-41, *A*).

RESIST: With one hand stabilizing at the medial aspect of the knee, E removes the palpating fingers and resists with that hand at the lateral aspect of the lower leg, pushing the leg medially and thus the thigh toward external rotation[7,8,10] (Fig. 6-41, *B*).

Procedure for testing grades P, T, and 0

POSITION AND STABILIZE: S is positioned supine with hips and knees extended. The hip to be tested is in external rotation. E stands opposite the side to be tested. E stabilizes the pelvis over the iliac crest on the side to be tested to prevent elevation or tilt of the pelvis.[7]

PALPATE AND OBSERVE: Palpation is the same as described previously. E asks S to rotate the thigh inwardly or medially. As in external rotation, gravity may assist the motion once the neutral position is passed but will not be as significant as in the test for external rotation.

GRADE: Grade strength according to standard definitions of muscle grades.

SUBSTITUTIONS: The tensor fasciae latae may substitute for the gluteus minimus, but the movement will be accompanied by some hip flexion. Trunk medial rotation may also effect some internal rotation of the hip.[9]

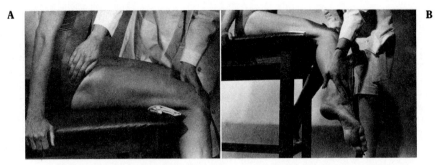

Fig. 6-41. Hip internal rotation. **A,** Palpate and observe. **B,** Resist.

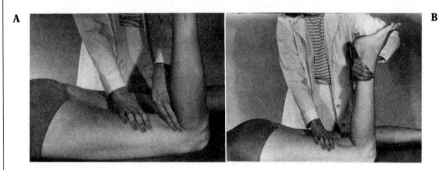

Fig. 6-42. Knee flexion. **A,** Palpate and observe. **B,** Resist.

Motion

Knee flexion

Muscles[4,7-9]	Innervation[4,7,8]
(Hamstrings)	
Biceps femoris	Sciatic nerve, L5, S1-3
Semimembranosis	Sciatic nerve, L4-5, S1-2
Semitendinosus	Sciatic nerve, L4-5, S1-2

Procedure for testing grades N to F

POSITION AND STABILIZE: S is lying prone with knees and hips in extension and neutral rotation.[5,7,8] E stands next to S opposite the side being tested toward the lower end of the supporting surface.[7] E firmly stabilizes the thigh over the posterior aspect above the tendinous insertion of the knee flexors to prevent hip motion.[8]

PALPATE AND OBSERVE: E places fingers on the lateral aspect of the posterior surface of the knee for palpation of the biceps femoris tendon as it nears its insertion on the head of the fibula or in the middle of the posterior surface of the knee for the semitendinosus tendon.[4,9] It is the most prominent tendon on the back of the knee.[4] E asks S to flex the knee slightly less than 90°[8] (Fig. 6-42, *A*).

RESIST: E resists by grasping S's leg over the posterior aspect of the ankle and pushing downward toward knee extension. Note that not as much resistance can be applied to knee flexion in this position as when tested with the hip flexed in a sitting position[8] (Fig. 6-42, *B*).

Procedure for testing grades P, T, and 0

POSITION AND STABILIZE: S is lying on the side with knees and hips extended and in neutral rotation. E stands next to S and supports the upper leg in slight abduction to allow testing of the lower leg. E stabilizes the thigh on the medial aspect.

PALPATE AND OBSERVE: E places fingers for palpation of the semitendinosus as described previously. This will allow simultaneous stabilization and palpation during the test motion. E asks S to flex the knee of the lower leg.

GRADE: Grade strength according to standard definitions of muscle grades.

SUBSTITUTIONS: The sartorius may substitute or assist the hamstrings, but hip flexion and external rotation will occur simultaneously.[7,9] The gracilis may substitute, causing hip adduction with knee flexion. The gastrocnemius may assist or substitute if strong plantar flexion of the ankle is allowed during knee flexion.[7]

Motion
Knee extension

Muscles[7]	Innervation[7]
Quadriceps femoris group	Femoral nerve, L2-4
Rectus femoris	
Vastus intermedius	
Vastus lateralis	
Vastus medialis	

Procedure for testing grades N to F
POSITION AND STABILIZE: S is sitting with knees flexed over the edge of the table and feet suspended off the floor. S may lean backward slightly to release tension on the hamstrings and grasp the edge of the table for stability.[7] E stands next to S on the side to be tested. E stablizes S's thigh by holding it firmly,[7,8] or E may place one hand under S's knee to cushion it from the edge of the table.[8]

PALPATE AND OBSERVE: E places fingers for palpation of any of the muscles in the quadriceps femoris group as follows: rectus femoris on the anterior aspect of the thigh; vastus medialis on the "anteromedial aspect of the lower third of the thigh;" and vastus lateralis on the "anterolateral aspect of the lower third of the thigh."[9] The vastus intermedius cannot be palpated.[9] E asks S to raise the foot toward the ceiling, extending the knee. Observe for hip movements as evidence of substitutions (Fig. 6-43, *A*).

RESIST: E resists on the anterior surface of the leg just above the ankle with downward pressure toward knee flexion.[7,8] S should not be allowed to "lock" the knee joint at the end of the ROM when full extension is achieved. Maintenance of a slight amount of knee flexion will prevent this. Resistance to a locked knee can cause joint injury[7] (Fig. 6-43, *B*).

Procedure for testing grades P, T, and 0
POSITION AND STABILIZE: S is lying on the side to be tested. The lower leg is positioned with the hip extended and the knee flexed 90°. E stands behind S. E supports the upper leg in slight abduction with one hand and with the other stabilizes the thigh of the leg to be tested on the anterior aspect.[7]

PALPATE AND OBSERVE: E palpates any of the muscles as previously described with the same hand used to stabilize S's thigh, then asks S to straighten the leg, thus extending the knee. Again, E should observe for hip movements.

GRADE: Grade strength according to standard definitions of muscle grades.

SUBSTITUTIONS: The tensor fasciae latae may assist or substitute for weak quadriceps. In this case hip internal rotation will accompany knee extension.[8,9]

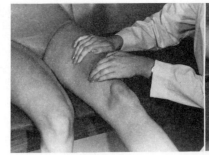
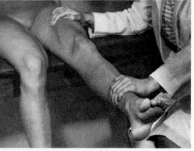

Fig. 6-43. Knee extension. **A**, Palpate and observe. **B**, Resist.

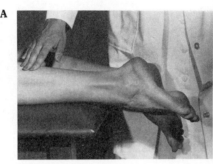
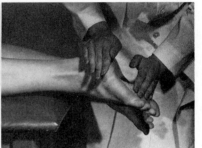

Fig. 6-44. Ankle plantar flexion. **A**, Palpate and observe. **B**, Resist.

Motion
Ankle plantar flexion

Muscles[4,7-9]	Innervation[8]
Gastrocnemius	Tibial nerve, S1-2
Plantaris	Tibial nerve, L4-5, S1
Soleus	Tibial nerve, L5, S1-2

Procedure for testing grades N to F
POSITION AND STABILIZE: S is lying prone with the hips and knees extended and the feet projecting beyond the edge of the table. E stands at the lower end of the table facing S's feet.[8] The weight of the leg is usually adequate stabilization.

PALPATE AND OBSERVE: E places fingers for palpation of the gastrocnemius on the posterior aspect of the calf of the leg or the soleus, slightly lateral to and beneath the lateral head of the gastrocnemius.[9] The achilles tendon above the calcaneus may also be palpated. E asks S to pull the heel upward, thus plantar flexing the ankle. E observes for flexion of the toes and forefoot before movement of the heel as evidence of substitutions[8,9] (Fig. 6-44, *A*).

RESIST: E applies resistance to the posterior aspect of the calcaneus as if pulling downward and the forefoot as if pushing forward.[7,8] If there is significant weakness, pressure to the calcaneus may be sufficient[8] (Fig. 6-44, *B*).

Procedure for testing grades P, T, and 0
POSITION AND STABILIZE: S is lying on the side to be tested. The hip and knee of the lower limb are extended and the ankle is in midposition. The upper limb may be flexed at the knee to keep it out of the way. E stands at the lower end of the table. E stabilizes the calf on the posterior aspect to prevent knee movements.[7]

PALPATE AND OBSERVE: E places fingers for palpation as previously described and asks S to pull the heel upward, pointing the toes down. E should observe for toe flexion, inversion, or eversion of the foot as evidence of substitutions.

GRADE: Grade strength according to standard definitions of muscle grades.

SUBSTITUTIONS: The flexor digitorum longus and flexor hallucis longus can substitute for plantar flexors, producing toe flexion and forefoot flexion with incomplete movement of the calcaneus. Substitution by the peroneus longus and peroneus brevis will cause foot eversion and substitution by the tibialis posterior will cause foot inversion. Substitution by all three will effect plantar flexion of the forefoot with limited movement of the calcaneus.[7,9]

Motion
Ankle dorsiflexion with inversion

Muscles[7,8]	Innervation[7,8]
Tibialis anterior	Peroneal nerve, L4-5, S1

Procedure for testing grades N to F

POSITION AND STABILIZE: S is seated with the legs flexed at the knees over the edge of the table. E sits in front of S, slightly to the side to be tested. S's heel can rest in E's lap.[7,8] E stabilizes S's leg just above the ankle to prevent any knee or hip motion.

PALPATE AND OBSERVE: E places fingers for palpation of the tibialis anterior tendon on the anterior medial aspect of the ankle.[7] Muscle fibers may be palpated on the anterior surface of the leg, just lateral to the tibia.[9] E asks S to pull the forefoot upward and inward, keeping the toes relaxed, thus dorsiflexing and inverting the foot. E should watch for extension of the great toe preceding the ankle motion as a sign of muscle substitution (Fig. 6-45, A).

RESIST: E resists on the medial dorsal aspect of the foot toward plantar flexion and eversion[7,8] (Fig. 6-45, B).

Procedure for testing grades P, T, and 0

POSITION AND STABILIZE: The same position and procedure just described may be used. To perform the test in the gravity-eliminated position and adhering to strict definitions of muscle grades, S should be lying on the side with the foot to be tested on the bottom and the knee slightly flexed. E or an assistant can support the upper leg in a position of slight hip abduction and knee flexion.

PALPATE AND OBSERVE: Observation and palpation are the same as described previously.

GRADE: If the against-gravity position is used in the procedure for grades P to 0, clinical judgment of the examiner must be used to determine muscle grades. Partial ROM against gravity can be graded P.[7] If the test is performed in the gravity-eliminated position for these grades, standard definitions of muscle grades may be used.

SUBSTITUTIONS: The peroneus tertius, a foot everter, can assist for foot dorsiflexion. However, dorsiflexion will be accompanied by foot eversion.[9] The extensor hallucis longus and extensor digitorum longus may also assist or substitute. Movement will be preceded by extension of the great toe or all of the toes.[7-9]

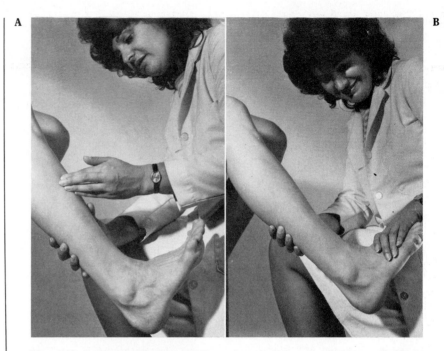

Fig. 6-45. Ankle dorsiflexion with inversion. **A,** Palpate and observe. **B,** Resist.

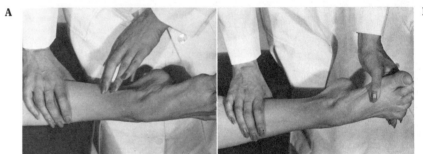

Fig. 6-46. Foot inversion. **A,** Palpate and observe. **B,** Resist.

Motion
Foot inversion

Muscles[7,8]	Innervation[7,8]
Tibialis posterior	Tibial nerve, L5, S1

Procedure for testing grades N to F

POSITION AND STABILIZE: S is lying on the side to be tested with the hip in neutral rotation, knee extended, and ankle in midposition. The upper leg may be flexed at the knee to keep it out of the way. E stands at the end of the table facing S's feet. E stabilizes the leg to be tested above the ankle joint on the dorsal surface of the calf, being careful not to put pressure on the tibialis posterior[7] to prevent knee or hip motion.

PALPATE AND OBSERVE: E places fingers for palpation of the tiabialis posterior tendon between the medial malleolus and navicular bone or above and just posterior to the medial malleolus. E asks S to move the foot upward (medially), inverting it (there normally will be some plantar flexion as well), and keeping the toes relaxed (Fig. 6-46, A).

RESIST: E resists on the medial border of the forefoot toward eversion[7] (Fig. 6-46, B).

Procedure for testing grades P, T, and 0

POSITION AND STABILIZE: S is lying supine with the hip extended and in neutral rotation, knee extended, and ankle in midposition. Stabilization is the same as described earlier.

PALPATE AND OBSERVE: Palpation is the same as described previously. E asks S to move the foot inward (medially), inverting it while keeping the toes relaxed.

GRADE: Grade strength according to standard definitions of muscle grades.

SUBSTITUTIONS: The flexor hallucis longus and flexor digitorum longus can substitute for the tibialis posterior. Movement will be accompanied by toe flexion or toes will flex when resistance is applied.[7-9] The tibialis anterior may assist in inversion if there is simultaneous dorsiflexion.[1,9]

Motion
Foot eversion

Muscles[7,8]	Innervation[7,8]
Peroneus brevis	Peroneal nerve,
Peroneus longus	L4-5, S1
Peroneus tertius	

Procedure for testing grades N to F

POSITION AND STABILIZE: S is lying on the side with the upper leg to be tested in hip extension and neutral rotation, knee extended, and ankle in midposition. The lower leg is flexed at the knee to keep it out of the way.[7,8] E stabilizes the leg above the ankle on its medial surface, supporting the foot slightly above the table surface.

PALPATE AND OBSERVE: E places fingers for palpation of the peroneus longus over the upper half of the lateral aspect of the calf just distal to the head of the fibula.[7,9] Its tendon can be palpated on the lateral aspect of the ankle, above and behind the lateral malleolus. The peroneus brevis tendon may be palpated on the lateral border of the foot proximal to the base of the fifth metatarsal.[7,9] Its muscle fibers can be found on the lower half of the lateral surface of the leg over the fibula.[7] E asks S to turn the sole of the foot outward, everting it. (NOTE: this movement is normally accompanied by some degree of plantar flexion.[8,9]) Observe for dorsiflexion or toe extension as evidence of substitutions (Fig. 6-47, *A*).

RESIST: E resists against the lateral border and the plantar surface of the foot toward inversion and dorsiflexion[8] (Fig. 6-47, *B*).

Procedure for testing grades P, T, and 0

POSITION AND STABILIZE: S is lying supine with hip extended and in neutral rotation, knee extended, and ankle in midposition. E stabilizes the leg from under the calf.

PALPATE AND OBSERVE: Palpation is the same as described earlier. E asks S to move the foot in a sideward or lateral direction, thus everting it.

GRADE: Grade strength according to standard definitions of muscle grades.

SUBSTITUTIONS: The peroneus tertius while everting the foot also dorsiflexes it. If it is substituting for the peroneus longus and peroneus brevis, dorsiflexion will accompany eversion. The extensor digitorum longus can also substitute for the peroneals, and toe extension will precede or accompany eversion.[9]

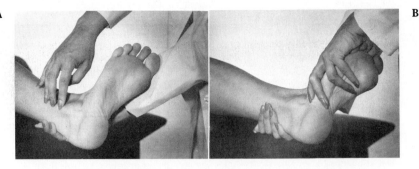

Fig. 6-47. Foot eversion. **A,** Palpate and observe. **B,** Resist.

FUNCTIONAL MUSCLE TESTING

It is not always necessary to perform a specific manual muscle test on a client referred for occupational therapy services. In some health care facilities the specific muscle testing is the responsibility of the physical therapy service. To avoid duplication of services, the occupational therapist may wish, then, to perform a quick functional muscle test to assess the strength and motion capabilities of the client. In dysfunctions where muscle weakness is not a primary or significant symptom, it may not be important to perform discrete muscle testing, but a general estimate of strength is desirable and adequate to plan treatment and measure progress. In still other instances a quick functional muscle test may be performed to identify areas of significant weakness that deserve more discrete testing. Thus the functional muscle test may serve as a screening tool.

The functional muscle test should be performed while the client is comfortably seated in a sturdy chair or wheelchair.

The client is asked to perform the test motion against gravity or in a gravity-eliminated position if the former is not feasible.

In all of the tests the subject is allowed to complete the test motion before the examiner applies resistance. The resistance is applied at the end of the ROM while the subject maintains the position and resists the force applied by the examiner. The therapist may make modifications in positioning to suit individual needs. As in the manual muscle tests, the examiner should stabilize proximal parts and attempt to rule out substitutions. It is assumed that the reader is familiar with joint motions, their prime movers, manual muscle testing, and muscle grades before performing this test.

REVIEW QUESTIONS

1. List three general classifications of physical dysfunction in which muscle weakness is a primary symptom.
2. Given F+ muscle strength and low endurance, in which kinds of activities can the client be expected to participate?
3. List at least three purposes for evaluating muscle strength.
4. Discuss five considerations and their implications in treatment planning that are based on the results of the muscle strength evaluation.
5. Define "endurance" and discuss its correlation with muscle strength.
6. How can muscle weakness be differentiated from joint limitation?
7. If there is joint limitation, can muscle strength be measured accurately? How is strength recorded when available ROM is less than normal?
8. What does the manual muscle test measure?
9. What does the manual muscle test *not* measure about motor function?
10. What are the criteria used to determine muscle grades?
11. In relation to the floor as a horizontal plane, describe or demonstrate what is meant by "with gravity assisting," "with gravity eliminated," "against gravity," and "against gravity and resistance."

12. List five factors that can influence the amount of resistance against which a muscle group can hold?
13. Define the muscle grades: N (5), G (4), F− (3−), F (3), P (2), P− (2−), T (1), and zero (0).
14. Define what is meant by "substitution."
15. How are substitutions most likely to be ruled out in the muscle testing procedure?
16. List the steps in the muscle testing procedure.
17. Is it always necessary to perform the manual muscle test to determine level of strength? If not, what alternative may be used to make a general assessment of strength? Generally describe the procedure.
18. Describe or demonstrate the muscle testing procedures for testing grades of normal to fair for the following muscle groups: scapula adduction, shoulder flexion, elbow extension, forearm pronation, wrist flexion, opposition, hip extension, knee flexion, and ankle dorsiflexion.

REFERENCES

1. Basmajian, J.F.: Muscles alive, ed. 4, Baltimore, 1978, Williams & Wilkins.
2. Bobath, B.: Adult hemiplegia: evaluation and treatment, ed. 2, London, 1978, William Heinemann Medical Books Ltd.
3. Brunnstrom, S.: Movement therapy in hemiplegia, New York, 1970, Harper & Row, Publishers, Inc.
4. Brunnstrom, S.: Clinical kinesiology, Philadelphia, 1972, F.A. Davis Co.
5. Chusid, J.: Correlative neuroanatomy and functional neurology, ed. 15, Los Altos, Calif., 1973, Lange Medical Publications.
6. Daniels, L., Williams, M., and Worthingham, C.: Muscle testing, Philadelphia, 1953, W.B. Saunders Co.
7. Daniels, L., and Worthingham, C.: Muscle testing, ed. 4, Philadelphia, 1980, W.B. Saunders Co.
8. Kendall, H., Kendall F., and Wadsworth, G.: Muscles: testing and function, ed. 2, Baltimore, 1971, Williams & Wilkins.
9. Killingsworth, A.: Basic physical disability procedures, Oakland, Calif., 1976, Cal-Syl Press.
10. Kottke, F., Stillwell, K., and Lehmann, J.: Krusen's handbook of physical medicine and rehabilitation, Philadelphia, 1982, W.B. Saunders Co.
11. Landen, B., and Amizich, A.: Functional muscle examination and gait analysis, J. Amer. Phys. Ther. Assoc. **43**:39, 1963.

CHAPTER 7

Evaluation of muscle tone and coordination

LORRAINE WILLIAMS PEDRETTI

MUSCLE TONE

Normal muscle tone is a continuous state of mild contraction of muscle. It is dependent on the integrity of peripheral and central nervous system (CNS) mechanisms and the properties of muscle, such as contractility, elasticity, ductility, and extensibility. A normal muscle at rest is not entirely atonic. It has a certain amount of resilience; when stretched passively, it offers a small amount of involuntary resistance. The maintenance of normal muscle tone is dependent on normal function of the cerebellum, motor cortex, basal ganglia, midbrain, vestibular system, spinal cord functions, and neuromuscular system.[4]

The normally functioning stretch reflex is essential in maintaining muscle tone. The stretch reflex can produce increased tension in certain muscle groups to provide a background of increased postural tone from which voluntary movement can proceed.[4] The stretch reflex is mediated by the muscle spindle, a sophisticated sensory receptor continuously reporting sensory information from muscles to the CNS. The muscle spindle has its own innervation. There are two types of motor innervation to the muscle spindle, gamma$_1$ and gamma$_2$. These are known as fusimotor neurons. The sensory innervation to the muscle spindle is from group Ia and group II fibers, which are sensitive to stretch of different regions of the muscle spindle. Stimulation of Ia fibers is the greatest driving force for firing lower motor neurons and causing muscle contraction or an increase of muscle tension. Fusimotor neurons can control the sensitivity or responsiveness of the Ia afferent fibers and are critical to the responsiveness of alpha motor fibers and the control of muscle tone.[7] For a more complete discussion of the anatomy of the muscle spindle and other proprioceptors that influence muscle tone, the reader is referred to Chapter 13.

Normal muscle tone

The estimation of muscle tone can only be made in relation to normal muscle tone. Although normal tone varies from one individual to another and is dependent on factors such as age, sex, and occupations, normal muscle tone is characterized by:

1. Effective cocontraction (stabilization) at proximal joints
2. Ability to move against gravity and resistance
3. Ability to maintain the position of the limb if it is placed passively by the examiner and then released[3,6]
4. Balanced tone between agonist and antagonist muscles
5. Ease of ability to shift from stability to mobility and vice versa as needed
6. Ability to use muscles in groups or selectively, if necessary[6]
7. Resilience or slight resistance in response to passive movement[4]

Flaccidity

Flaccidity is hypotonicity of msucle, that is, a decrease of normal muscle tone. Hypotonicity is usually the result of damage to the proprioceptive innervation of muscle,[10] a disruption of the reflex arc, or cerebellar disease and is seen temporarily in the "shock" phase after cerebral or spinal insult. It may also result from muscle disuse and prolonged immobilization.[2]

CHARACTERISTICS OF FLACCIDITY. Hypotonic muscles feel soft and flabby and offer less resistance to passive movement than does a normal muscle. Because of the laxity of the muscle, there may be an unusually wide range of motion (ROM) possible. If the flaccid limb is placed passively in a given position and then released, the subject cannot maintain the limb in the position. Rather, it is likely to drop heavily,[2] since the muscles are unable to resist gravity. Cocontraction (stability) of proximal joints is weak or absent.[6] Deep tendon reflexes are diminished or absent.[2,10]

OCCURRENCE OF FLACCIDITY. Flaccidity or hypotonicity of muscle occurs in primary muscle diseases, lower motor neuron disorders (such as peripheral neuropathies and polyneuritis), and cerebellar lesions and follows stroke or spinal cord injury during the shock phase. In these latter conditions the flaccidity usually gives way to increasing spasticity as the shock phase passes.

PURPOSES OF EVALUATION. The purposes for evaluating flaccidity are to (1) estimate muscle tone; (2) establish a baseline for reevaluation; (3) plan treatment, such as special splints and positioning, to prevent overstretching weak muscles; (4) select treatment methods for muscle strengthening; and (5) train in special methods or use of assistive devices to compensate for muscle weakness. If there is flaccidity, it is usually desirable to perform a manual muscle test to quantify the degree of flaccidity by grading strength and tone.

METHOD OF EVALUATION. Flaccidity is estimated by performing passive movements. The movements must be gentle. Without telling the subject what to expect, the therapist may take the subject's hand and gently move the fingers backward and then forward from tip to the wrist to produce slow undulating flexion and extension movements of fingers and wrist, thus estimating the tone in the flexors and extensors of the wrist and fingers. Similar movements can be performed at the larger joints of the upper and lower extremities with the examiner noting the degree of resistance to passive movement and any unusually wide ranges of motion.[2]

SCALE OF SEVERITY OF FLACCIDITY. The following scale is suggested in estimating the degree of flaccidity.

Mild flaccidity. Mild flaccidity is characterized by:

1. Decreased muscle tone; weak cocontraction of agonists and antagonist muscles in stabilizing joints

2. Ability of the limb to resist gravity briefly if placed in position and released[6]
3. Decreased muscle strength; functional motion still possible

Moderate to severe flaccidity. Moderate to severe flaccidity is characterized by:

1. Significantly decreased or absent muscle tone
2. No cocontraction possible
3. Limb drops immediately if placed against gravity and released[6]
4. Minimal or absent ability to move against gravity
5. Significant loss of strength; no functional motion possible

Spasticity

Upper motor neuron systems control fusimotor neurons to keep them inhibited. Damage to these upper motor neuron systems can cause a release or disinhibition of fusimotor neurons from central control. This results in their increased firing, which in turn causes the muscle spindle to become more sensitive and produces more firing of Ia afferent fibers. The final result is increased stimulation of the lower motor neurons with a resultant increased alpha motor activity called spasticity.[7]

CHARACTERISTICS OF SPASTICITY. Spasticity is characterized by hypertonic muscles, hyperactive deep tendon reflexes, clonus, and abnormal spinal reflexes.[12] The hypertonicity usually occurs in definite patterns of flexion or extension.[3,8,12] Typically the pattern of spasticity occurs in the antigravity muscles of the upper and lower extremities. In the upper extremity the flexor pattern usually dominates. It includes adduction (retraction) and depression of the scapula, internal rotation and adduction at the shoulder joint, elbow flexion with forearm pronation, wrist flexion, and finger flexion with adduction. In the lower extremity the antigravity muscles are the extensors, and the spastic pattern is elevation and retraction of the pelvis, external rotation and extension at the hip, and knee extension with inversion of the foot and plantar flexion at the ankle.[8]

In spasticity there is increased resistance to passive movement. After the initial resistance there may be a sudden relaxation of muscle known as the clasp-knife phenomenon.[4] This is thought to be a result of the function of the Ib sensory afferent fibers from the Golgi tendon organs (GTOs). The GTO is sensitive to both passive stretch and active contraction of the muscle. When applying passive stretch to a spastic muscle, the sudden relaxation or clasp-knife phenomenon is thought to be the result of the inhibition of the Ib fibers, preventing the firing of the overactive lower motor neurons so that the muscle will not be damaged because of the excessive resistance of the spastic muscle.[7]

OCCURRENCE OF SPASTICITY. Spasticity is commonly seen in upper motor neuron disorders, such as multiple sclerosis, cerebral palsy, spinal cord injury and disease, cerebrovascular accident, head injury, and brain tumors or infections. Any patient or client with an upper motor neuron disorder is a candidate for the routine evaluation of muscle tone.

FACTORS INFLUENCING SPASTICITY. The degree and patterns of spasticity are influenced by several factors. Spasticity is influenced by functions of the postural reflex mechanism, such as the righting and equilibrium reactions, and the presence of primitive postural reflexes, such as the tonic neck reflexes, tonic labyrinthine reflexes, and associated reactions. Therefore the position of the body and head in space and the head in relation to the body influence the degree and distribution of abnormal muscle tone.[3] Extrinsic factors that also have an influence on the degree of spasticity include the presence of contractures, anxiety, fear, environmental temperature extremes, painful physical conditions, and upsetting emotional experiences.[1] Conversely, relaxation, rest, good health, and satisfying life experiences tend to minimize the aversive influence of spasticity.[12]

Because of these internal and external influences, spasticity is changeable and fluctuating; it is not possible to measure it accurately and with certainty.[3,12] Bobath[3] proposes that a specific evaluation of spasticity is not necessary; rather, assessment of the distribution of abnormal tone should be

part of a comprehensive evaluation of the postural reflex mechanism. However, criteria have been suggested for estimating the severity of spasticity.[3,6] Using these criteria and being aware of spasticity's changing character and the factors that influence muscle tone, the therapist can estimate the degree and pattern of spasticity.

PURPOSES OF EVALUATION. The purposes of evaluating spasticity are, to (1) determine its presence, (2) estimate its severity, (3) observe the patterns in which it occurs, (4) establish a baseline against which to measure change, (5) determine its influence on performance of specific activities,[12] (6) select appropriate treatment approaches, (7) select appropriate treatment methods, and (8) structure internal and external environmental factors to minimize their effect on muscle tone.

METHOD OF EVALUATION. Spasticity is usually evaluated by estimating the degree of resistance to passive motion of a given muscle group or pattern of movement. The therapist should grasp the part gently but firmly and move it briskly through the desired motion or movement pattern. When spasticity is first developing (following the flaccid stage after stroke for example), it is necessary to move the part more quickly in an effort to detect mild stretch reflex activity, a sign of developing spasticity.

There are no standardized methods of evaluating muscle tone with absolute objectivity. When reporting the results of a spasticity evaluation, the occupational therapist should make note of the position in which the testing was done and any known internal and external environmental factors that may have influenced muscle tone. In addition, abnormal reflex influences on muscle tone should be observed and noted. Methods of testing reflexes are described in Chapter 8.

Bobath[3] assesses muscle tone as part of the evaluation of the postural reflex mechanism. This includes evaluation of righting reactions, equilibrium reactions, and automatic adaptation of muscles to changes in posture. The latter is tested by "placing" and provides an excellent means to detect resistance to passive movement and the failure of muscles to adapt quickly to postural change. The therapist moves the subject's body or limbs using specific movement patterns that should be learned or performed later in treatment. Normally muscle tone adapts quickly to changes in position. If the therapist's hands are removed, the limb does not fall, and there is no resistance to the movement as the limb is placed in the given position. Conversely, if spasticity is influencing the passive movement during placing, resistance is felt if the movement is in a direction opposite to the pattern of spasticity; uncontrolled assistance to the passive movement is felt if the movement is performed toward the pattern of spasticity. Bobath[3] provides an extensive evaluation with the specific movement patterns to be tested.

The effect of spasticity on performance of functional activities should be of particular concern to the occupational therapist. During activities, such as bed mobility, transfers, dressing, and toileting, the therapist should observe how and where spasticity interferes with righting and equilibrium reactions, protective reactions, weight shifting, weight bearing, position changing, movement speed, and coordination.

The use of the manual muscle test described in Chapter 6 is of no value in assessing spasticity, since the relative tone and "strength" of spastic muscles are influenced by the position of the head and body in space, failures in reciprocal innervation, abnormal cocontraction, and deficits in tactile and proprioceptive sensation. Therefore muscle tone and ability to hold against resistance are variable when there is spasticity.[3]

SCALE OF SEVERITY OF SPASTICITY. The following scale is suggested as a guide for estimating the degree of spasticity.

Mild spasticity. Mild spasticity is characterized by:

1. Mild or weak stretch reflexes evoked during passive movement and often not until late in the ROM
2. A slight decrease in balance of tone between agonist and antagonist muscles[6]

3. A mild increase of resistance to passive stretch[6]; yet possible for the therapist to move the part through the complete ROM with relative ease
4. A slight decrease in mobility; gross movements that are performed with fairly normal coordination[3,6]
5. A decreased ability to perform selective motion; fine movement that is impossible or performed clumsily[3]

Moderate spasticity. Moderate spasticity is characterized by:

1. Moderately strong stretch reflexes evoked during passive motion and often earlier in the range of movement than is seen in slight spasticity
2. A marked imbalance of tone between agonist and antagonist muscles[6]
3. Considerable resistance to passive stretch that is felt throughout the ROM; possible for the therapist to move the part through the complete ROM with some effort
4. Some gross movements that can be performed slowly and with much effort but with abnormal coordination.[3]

Severe spasticity. Severe spasticity is characterized by:

1. Strong stretch reflexes evoked during passive motion and often in the initial segment of the ROM
2. Marked resistance to passive movement[6]
3. Inability to complete the ROM passively because of the "strength" or severity of the spasticity
4. Presence of joint contractures[6] because severe spasticity makes effective ROM exercises nearly impossible and the spasticity may not respond well to techniques for relaxation
5. Severely decreased mobility and lack of any active movement[3,6]

Rigidity

Rigidity is an increase of muscle tone of agonistic and antagonistic muscles simultaneously. Both groups of muscles contract steadily, resulting in increased resistance to passive movement in any direction and throughout the ROM.[5,10] Rigidity is a sign of involvement of the extrapyramidal pathways in the circuitry of the basal ganglia, diencephalon, and brainstem.[5]

CHARACTERISTICS OF RIGIDITY. A feeling of constant resistance occurs throughout the ROM when the part is moved passively in any direction. This is called "plasticity" or lead pipe rigidity because of the similarity to the feeling of bending solder or a lead pipe. In rigidity the deep tendon reflexes are normal or only moderately increased.[5,10] Another type of rigidity in the cogwheel type in which there is a rhythmic "give" in the resistance throughout the ROM, much like the feeling of turning a cogwheel.[10] The clasp-knife phenomenon seen in spasticity is *not* characteristic of rigidity.

OCCURRENCE OF RIGIDITY. Rigidity occurs as a result of lesions of the extrapyramidal system, such as Parkinson's disease, some degenerative diseases, encephalitis, and tumors.[4] Cogwheel rigidity occurs in some types of parkinsonism and also after administration of high doses of reserpine or chlorpromazine and its derivatives. It can also occur after carbon monoxide poisoning.[2] Frequently there are lesions of both the pyramidal and extrapyramidal systems, and rigidity and spasticity of muscle may occur together.[5]

PURPOSES AND METHODS OF EVALUATION. The purposes and methods of evaluation are similar to those stated for spasticity. The degree of hypertonicity of muscle can be recorded using the same scale; however, the increased muscle tone will usually be noted in both agonist and antagonistic muscle groups. Whether there is lead pipe or cogwheel rigidity should be noted on the evaluation form.

Recording the results of an evaluation of muscle tone

Fig. 7-1 is a suggested form for recording the results of an evaluation of muscle tone. Using the definitions outline previously, the results are recorded as follows:

0—Moderate to severe hypotonicity (flaccidity)
1—Mild hypotonicity
2—Normal muscle tone
3—Mild hypertonicity (spasticity or rigidity)
4—Moderate hypertonicity
5—Severe hypertonicity

```
                    RECORDING ESTIMATED MUSCLE TONE


Name:_____ Age:_____

Diagnosis:_____

          _____



Directions to examiner:  The part should be moved passively and briskly
from the first position listed toward the second position listed.  Scores
of tonicity are recorded for the muscle group of the first motion listed
in each of the following tests so that if the scapula is moved from ad-
duction to abduction and moderate resistance is felt during the movement,
the hypertonicity resides in the adductors and a score of 4 should be
recorded.

Key:  D = Date of test
      R = Right side
      L = Left side
      P = Test position (P = Prone, S = Supine, ST = Sitting)

Scale of tonicity scores:
      0 = Moderate to severe hypotonicity
      1 = Mild hypotonicity
      2 = Normal muscle tone
      3 = Mild hypertonicity
      4 = Moderate hypertonicity
      5 = Severe hypertonicity
```

TRUNK

	D	R	P		D	L	P	REMARKS
Extension to lateral flexion								
Extension to flexion								
Flexion to extension								

UPPER EXTREMITY

	D	R	P		D	L	P	
Scapula								
Adduction to abduction								
Abduction to adduction								
Depression to elevation								
Shoulder								
Adduction to abduction (90°)								
Abduction to adduction								
Extension to flexion (90°)								
Flexion to extension								
Extension to hyperextension								
External rotation to internal rotation								
Internal rotation to external rotation								

Fig. 7-1. Form for recording estimated muscle tone.

	D	R	P	D	L	P	REMARKS
Elbow and forearm							
Extension to flexion							
Flexion to extension							
Supination to pronation							
Pronation to supination							
Wrist							
Extension to flexion							
Flexion to extension							
Fingers							
Extension to flexion							
Flexion to extension							
Thumb							
Extension to flexion							
Flexion to extension							
Upper extremity pattern							
Flexor pattern: Scapula depression and adduction, shoulder adduction, internal rotation, elbow flexion, forearm pronation, and wrist and finger flexion							
Extensor pattern: Scapula abduction, upward rotation, shoulder abduction, external rotation, elbow extension, forearm supination, and wrist and finger extension							
Other pattern: Describe							
Hip							
Extension to flexion							
Flexion to extension							
Adduction to abduction							
Abduction to adduction							
Internal rotation to external rotation							
External rotation to internal rotation							
Knee							
Extension to flexion							
Flexion to extension							
Ankle							
Dorsiflexion to plantar flexion							
Plantar flexion to dorsiflexion							
Inversion to eversion							
Eversion to inversion							
Toes							
Extension to flexion							
Flexion to extension							
Lower extremity pattern							
Extensor pattern: Elevation of pelvis, extension and external rotation of hip, knee extension, and inversion and plantar flexion at ankle							
Flexor pattern: Leveling of pelvis, flexion and internal rotation of hip, knee flexion, and eversion and dorsiflexion of ankle							
Other pattern: Describe							

REMARKS:

Fig. 7-1, cont'd. Form for recording estimated muscle tone.

Results of evaluation as a basis for treatment planning

An evaluation of muscle tone should suggest some directions of treatment for the therapist. If muscle tone is low, that is, if there is flaccidity, a manual muscle test to determine the exact degree of muscle weakness is indicated. If recovery of muscle function is expected, enabling exercise and therapeutic activities for improving strength may be selected for the treatment program. In addition, bed and chair positioning, splints, and other positioning devices, such as a wheelchair arm trough, may be necessary to protect weak muscles from overstretching and stronger antagonist muscles from becoming contracted. Strengthening exercise and activity must be directed toward the weaker muscle groups to effect a balance of strength and tone between agonist and anagonist muscles. Temporarily (or permanently if recovery of strength is not expected) the occupational therapist may have to assist the client in managing activities of daily living (ADL) in spite of mild to severe weakness. Some of the methods and devices for ADL described in Chapter 12 are useful for clients with muscle weakness.

If muscle tone is above normal, that is, hypertonic (rigid or spastic), treatment methods that use techniques of inhibition, such as the sensorimotor approaches described in Chapters 14 through 17 of this text, may be appropriate, depending on the disability, the severity and distribution of the hypertonicity, and concomitant problems. Application of cold is used to inhibit spasticity in some approaches. Since it can affect circulation, application of cold must be used cautiously (especially at proximal joints of the upper extremities) if there is cardiac involvement[8] or reduced blood supply to the brain. Inhibition of spasticity is necessary for maintaining joint ROM and for learning more normal movement patterns. If spastic agonist muscles can be inhibited, antagonist muscles may be facilitated and performance of movement

may be made possible, using one or another of the sensorimotor approaches to treatment. Spasticity reduction splints may be a part of treatment in some instances.[9,11,14]

Positioning and movement of parts in patterns opposite to spastic patterns is an important part of the neurodevelopmental treatment (Bobath) approach.[3] In this approach the reduction of spasticity is integrated with the development of a more normal postural reflex mechanism. Such positioning and movement is applied during ADL, crafts, games, and work activities for a total approach to treatment.

Whether spasticity is temporary or is persistent, severe, and unchangeable, the client must learn techniques to maintain ROM and to perform essential ADL under the circumstances of his or her motor function. Self-ROM techniques illustrated in Chapter 30 and one-handed dressing techniques described in Chapter 12 are examples of these.

COORDINATION

Coordination is the ability to produce accurate, controlled movement. Such movement is characterized by smoothness, rhythm, appropriate speed, refinement to the minimal number of muscle groups necessary to produce the desired movement, appropriate muscle tension, postural tone, and equilibrium for effective movement to occur.

To effect coordinated movement all of the elements of the neuromuscular mechanism must be intact. Coordinated movement is dependent on the contraction of the correct agonist muscles with simultaneous relaxation of the correct antagonist muscles together with the contraction of the joint fixator and synergist muscles. In addition, proprioception, body scheme, and the ability to accurately judge space and direct body parts through space with correct timing and to the desired target must be intact.[2]

Occurrence of incoordination

Coordination of muscle action is under the control of the cerebellum, and influenced by the extrapyramidal system. However, intact proprioception and knowledge of the body scheme and body-to-space relationships are essential

to the production of coordinated movement. Therefore many types of lesions can produce disturbances of coordination.[2] Disturbances of movement that are not caused by cerebellar lesions that can interfere with coordination include diseases and injuries of muscles and peripheral nerves, lesions of the posterior columns of the spinal cord, and lesions of the frontal and postcentral cerebral cortex. Paralysis of the limbs caused by a peripheral nervous system lesion prevents carrying out tests for coordination even though CNS mechanisms are intact.[10]

Signs of cerebellar dysfunction include the following[4]:

Ataxia: A reeling, wide-based, unsteady gait and a tendency to fall to the side of the lesion.

Adiadochokinesis: Inability to perform rapidly alternating movements, such as pronation and supination or elbow flexion and extension.

Dysmetria: Inability to estimate the ROM necessary to reach the target of the movement, such as when touching the finger to the nose or to an object on a table.

Dyssynergia: In effect a "decomposition of movement" in which voluntary movements are broken up into their component parts and appear jerky.

Tremor: An intention tremor that is associated with cerebellar disease, occurs during voluntary movement, is often intensified at the termination of the movement, and is often seen in multiple sclerosis.

Stewart-Holmes sign: Lack of a "check reflex" (the inability to quickly stop a motion to avoid striking something) so that, if the subject's arm is flexed against the resistance of the examiner and the resistance is released suddenly and unexpectedly, the subject's hand will hit his or her face or body.

Nystagmus: An involuntary movement of the eyeballs in an up and down, back and forth, or rotating direction.

Hypotonia: Decreased resistance to passive movement and floppiness of the limbs.

Dysarthria: Explosive or slurred speech caused by an incoordination of the speech mechanism.

Signs of extrapyramidal disease that produce incoordination include[4,10]:

Tremors: Resting tremors, such as the pill-rolling tremor seen in parkinsonism.

Choreiform movements: Irregular, purposeless, coarse, quick, jerky, and dysrhythmic movements of variable distribution that may also occur during sleep.

Athetoid movements: Continuous, slow, wormlike, arrythmic movements that primarily affect the distal portions of the extremities, occur in the same patterns in the same subject, and are not present during sleep.

Spasms: Involuntary contraction of large groups of muscles of the arm, leg, or neck.

Dystonia: Bizarre twisting movements of the trunk and proximal muscles of the extremities. Torsion spasms are included with spasmodic torticollis being the most common. Dystonic movements tend to involve large portions of the body and produce grotesque posturing with bizarre writhing movements.

Ballism: A rare symptom that is produced by continuous, gross, abrupt contractions of the axial and proximal musculature of the extremity, causes the limb to fly out suddenly, occurs on one side of the body (hemiballism), and is caused by lesions of the opposite subthalamic nucleus.

Clinical evaluation of coordination

Incoordination consists of errors in rate, range, direction, and force of movement. Therefore observation is an important element of the evaluation. The neurological examination for incoordination may include the nose-finger-nose test, the finger-nose test, the heel-knee test, the knee pat (pronation-supination) test, hand pat or foot pat tests, finger wiggling, and drawing a spiral.[2,10] Such tests can reveal dysmetria, dyssynergia, adiadochokinesis, tremors, and ataxia. Usually these examinations have been performed by the neurologist.

Occupational therapy evaluation of coordination

Since occupation is the hallmark of occupational therapy, the occupational therapist should seek to translate the clinical evaluation to a functional one. Selected activities and specific performance tests can reveal the effect of incoordination on function, the primary concern of the occupational therapist. The occupational therapist can observe for coordination difficulties during the ADL evaluation. The therapist can prepare simulated tasks that require coordinated muscle function, such as stationary bicycling, block stacking, stringing beads, writing, placing tiles, placing objects into containers, tossing and catching a bean bag, and playing a board game.[13] The therapist should observe for irregularity in the rate of movement, excessive ROM and force of movement, incorrect sequence of movement, and sudden corrective movements in an attempt to compensate for incoordination. Thus movement during the performance of various activities may appear irregular and jerky and overreach the mark.[10]

Several standardized tests of motor function and manual dexterity outlined by Smith[13] are available and can be used to evaluate coordination. Some of these include:

1. The Purdue Pegboard, available from Science Research Associates, Inc., 259 East Erie St., Chicago, Ill. 60611
2. Minnesota Rate of Manipulation Test, available from American Guidance Service, Inc., Publisher's Bldg., Circle Pines, Minn. 55014
3. Lincoln-Oseretsky Motor Development Scale, available from C.H. Stoelting Co., 424 N. Hohman Ave., Chicago, Ill. 60624
4. The Pennsylvania Bi-Manual Work Sample, available from Educational Test Bureau, American Guidance Service, Inc., Publisher's Bldg., Circle Pines, Minn. 55014
5. The Crawford Small Parts Dexterity Test, available from the Psychological Corporation, 304 East 45th St., New York, N.Y. 10017[13]

Results of evaluation as a basis for treatment planning

Admittedly, treatment of incoordination is difficult, and several approaches may be used. Incoordination arising from lesions of the pyramidal system may be improved using one or another of the sensorimotor approaches directed toward the normalization of muscle tone and the development of more normal movement patterns. Specific sensory input is used to change muscle tone and evoke adaptive motor responses. Activities graded on the basis of normal motor development may be helpful in attaining proximal stability and then mobility. Therapy directed toward the integration of primitive reflexes and the enhancement of higher cortical control mechanisms, such as the righting and equilibrium reactions, can help to improve coordination.

Some of the involuntary movements of cerebellar or extrapyramidal origin are difficult to manage or change. Pharmacological agents or surgical intervention may be employed by the physician in an effort to control tremors or other involuntary movements. Therapists have used weights on the extremities and proximal fixation in an effort to help the client gain an improvement in motor control. These are sometimes of some help but often not practical in day-to-day activities. Methods and devices to compensate for incoordination may be necessary to make ADL safer, more possible, and more satisfying. Some of these are described in Chapter 12.

REVIEW QUESTIONS

1. Define "muscle tone."
2. Describe the characteristics of "normal muscle tone."
3. Describe the characteristics of "hypotonicity" (flaccidity).
4. In which diagnoses does flaccidity usually occur?
5. Describe the characteristics of "spasticity."
6. In which diagnoses does spasticity usually occur?
7. How is rigidity unlike spasticity, and how is it like spasticity?
8. List five factors that can influence spasticity negatively?
9. Briefly describe the method for estimating muscle tone.
10. Which factors does the therapist need to keep in mind when estimating hypertonicity?
11. What is the special concern of the occupational therapist in assessing muscle tone?
12. Define "coordination."
13. List several factors on which normal coordination is dependent.
14. Which types of disabilities produce incoordination?
15. How is coordination evaluated?
16. What should the therapist observe when evaluating coordination using performance of ordinary activities?

REFERENCES

1. Anderson, T.P.: Rehabilitation of patients with completed stroke. In Kottke, F.J., Stillwell, G.K., and Lehmann, J.F.: Krusen's handbook of physical medicine and rehabilitation, Philadelphia, 1982, W.B. Saunders Co.
2. Bickerstaff, E.R.: Neurological examination in clinical practice, ed. 3, London, 1973, Blackwell Scientific Publications, Ltd.
3. Bobath, B.: Adult hemiplegia: evaluation and treatment, ed. 2, London, 1978, William Heinemann Medical Books, Ltd.
4. Chusid, J.G.: Correlative neuroanatomy and functional neurology, ed. 18, Los Altos, Calif., 1982, Lange Medical Publications.
5. De Myer, W.: Technique of the neurologic examination: a programmed text, ed. 2, New York, 1974, McGraw-Hill Book Co.
6. Farber, S.: Neurorehabilitation: a multisensory approach, Philadelphia, 1982, W.B. Saunders Co.
7. Felten, D.L., and Felten, S.Y.: A regional and systemic overview of functional neuroanatomy. In Farber, S.: Neurorehabilitation: a multisensory approach, Philadelphia, 1982, W.B. Saunders Co.
8. Johnstone, M.: Restoration of motor function in the stroke patient, ed. 2, New York, 1983, Churchill Livingstone, Inc.
9. King, T.I.: Plaster splinting as a means of reducing elbow flexor spasticity: a case study, Am. J. Occup. Ther. **36:**671, 1982.
10. Mayo Clinic and Mayo Clinic Foundation: Clinical examinations in neurology, ed. 5, Philadelphia, 1981, W.B. Saunders Co.
11. Mc Pherson, J.J., et al.: A comparison of dorsal and volar resting hand splints in the reduction of hypertonus, Am. J. Occup. Ther. **36:**664, 1982.
12. Okamoto, G.A.: Physical medicine and rehabilitation, Philadelphia, 1984, W.B. Saunders Co.
13. Smith, H.D.: Assessment and evaluation: specific evaluation procedures. In Hopkins, H.L., and Smith, H.D.: Willard and Spackman's occupational therapy, ed. 6, Philadelphia, 1983, J.B. Lippincott Co.
14. Snook, J.H.: Spasticity reduction splint, Am. J. Occup. Ther. **33:**648, 1979.

CHAPTER 8

Evaluation of reflexes and reactions

LORRAINE WILLIAMS PEDRETTI

Following central nervous system (CNS) injury or disease the nervous system may revert to an earlier level of development. Primitive reflexes may reappear, and equilibrium and protective reactions may be disturbed, limiting voluntary motor function and performance.

Fiorentino[5] has designed methods for testing the reflexes and reactions in children with CNS dysfunction. Many of these are appropriate for use with adults. Bobath[3] describes methods of evaluating muscle tone, abnormal motor patterns, voluntary movement, balance, and protective reactions of adults with hemiplegia. The reader is referred to these sources for a more detailed discussion of reflex maturation and evaluation.

SUMMARY OF REFLEXES AND REACTIONS
Spinal level

Reflexes mediated at the spinal level are the flexor withdrawal, extensor thrust, and crossed extension. These are normally present in the first 2 months of life.[5]

Brain stem level

Reflexes mediated at the brain stem level are static, postural reflexes that cause a change in muscle tone throughout the body. The changed tone is in response to a change of the position of the head in space or in relation to the body. The reflexes included are the asymmetrical tonic neck reflex (ATNR), symmetrical tonic neck reflex (STNR), and tonic labyrinthine reflex (TLR). Associated reactions and the positive and negative supporting reactions are also mediated at the brain stem level. These reflexes and reactions are present in the first 4 to 6 months of life.[5]

Midbrain level

Righting reactions are integrated at the midbrain level. They interact with one another to effect the normal head-to-body relationship in space and to each other. The righting reactions begin developing after birth and reach maximal effect at 10 to 12 months of age. As cortical control of voluntary movement increases, they are gradually inhibited and disappear by the end of the fifth year of life. Their effect on motor performance is to enable rolling over, sitting up, and assuming the quadrupedal position. Reactions included are the neck righting, body righting acting on the body, and labyrinthine righting and optical righting acting on the head.[5]

Cortical level

Cortical level reactions are the result of the efficient interaction of the cerebral cortex, basal ganglia, and cerebellum. The maturation of equilibrium reactions results in the ability to deal with bipedal motor skills. Equilibrium reactions occur when muscle tone is normalized and enable the adaptation to changes in the body's center of gravity. They begin to develop at 6 months of age and continue throughout life. Equilibrium and righting reactions that act to recover balance and maintain the normal position of the head in space should be possible in the prone, supine, quadrupedal, sitting, kneel-standing, squatting, and standing positions.[5]

Innate primary reactions[9]

Innate primary reactions are primitive movements present at birth that involve total patterns of flexion and extension. These include primary standing, reflex stepping, placing reactions of the upper and lower limbs, grasp reflex, sucking reflex, and rooting reflex. Primary standing is present from birth to 6 or 8 months of age.[9] Reflex stepping is normal in the first 4 to 8 weeks of life.[2] The placing reactions of the lower limbs are present in the first

month of life and those of the upper limbs are present for the first 6 months of life. The grasp, sucking, and rooting reflexes are present for the first 3 to 4 months of life.[9]

Automatic movement reactions

Automatic movement reactions are produced by changes of the position of the head in space. Included are the Moro reflex, Landau reflex, and protective extensor thrust. The Moro reflex is normal until 4 months of age. The Landau reflex is normally present from 6 months to 2½ years of age. The protective extensor thrust begins in the arms at about 6 months of age and is present throughout life.[5]

EVALUATION TECHNIQUES

The following are methods for evaluation of some of the reflexes and reactions just described. The methods may have to be adapted to accommodate to the size and physical abilities of the client being evaluated.

Spinal level
Extensor thrust[5]
POSITION: Supine lying, head in midposition, one leg extended and the other flexed
STIMULUS: Stimulation to sole of foot of flexed leg
NEGATIVE RESPONSE: Controlled maintenance of leg in flexion
POSITIVE RESPONSE: Uncontrolled extension of stimulated leg
NORMAL: Positive reaction up to 2 months of age
Flexor withdrawal[5]
POSITION: Supine lying, head in midposition, legs extended
STIMULUS: Stimulation to sole of foot
NEGATIVE RESPONSE: Maintained extension or voluntary withdrawal of stimulated leg
POSITIVE RESPONSE: Uncontrolled flexion of stimulated leg
NORMAL: Positive response up to 2 months of age

Brain stem level

Asymmetrical tonic neck reflex (ATNR)[2,5]

POSITION: Supine lying

STIMULUS: Rotation of head to either side

NEGATIVE RESPONSE: No reaction in limbs

POSITIVE RESPONSE: Extension of arm and leg on jaw side, flexion of arm and leg on skull side; response more pronounced in arms

NORMAL: Positive response up to 6 months of age; never obligatory, reflex response may not always occur, subject can move out of reflex position easily

Symmetrical tone neck reflex (STNR)[2,5,9]

POSITION: Quadruped

STIMULUS 1: Forward flexion of head

NEGATIVE RESPONSE: No change in muscle tone or position of limbs

POSITIVE RESPONSE: Increased flexor tone in arms and increased extensor tone in legs or flexion of arms and extension of legs

STIMULUS 2: Extension of head

NEGATIVE RESPONSE: No change in muscle tone or position of limbs

POSITIVE RESPONSE: Increased extensor tone in arms and increased flexor in legs or extension of arms and flexion of legs

NORMAL: Same as for ATNR

Tonic labyrinthine reflex (TLR)[2,5]

POSITION: Supine lying, head in midposition, limbs extended

STIMULUS 1: Supine position is stimulus

NEGATIVE RESPONSE: No increase in extensor tone of limbs when moved passively

POSITIVE RESPONSE: Increased overall extensor tone of neck, arms, and legs

POSITION: Prone lying, head in midposition, limbs extended

STIMULUS 2: Prone position in stimulus

NEGATIVE RESPONSE: No increase of flexor tone in neck, trunk, arms, or legs

POSITIVE RESPONSE: Increased overall flexor tone; inability to extend neck, back, or limbs, or adduct scapulae

NORMAL: Positive response up to 4 months of life, disappears by fifth month

Positive supporting reaction[2,5]

POSITION: Standing or holding subject in standing

STIMULUS: Pressure of soles against supporting surface; bounce subject several times on soles of feet

NEGATIVE RESPONSE: No increase in tone; legs flex voluntarily

POSITIVE RESPONSE: Legs develop supporting tone, become rigid, and support body weight for a short period

NORMAL: Positive reaction may occur normally from 3 to 8 months of age

Negative supporting reaction[2,5]

POSITION: Lift subject to standing

STIMULUS: Weight bearing

NEGATIVE RESPONSE: Loosening or relaxation of extension, progressing from proximal to distal musculature, which allows flexion for reciprocation

POSITIVE RESPONSE: Persistence of the positive supporting reaction; no release of extensor tone

NORMAL: Positive response should not persist beyond 8 months of age

Midbrain level

Neck righting[2,9]

POSITION: Supine lying, head in midposition, limbs extended

STIMULUS: Rotation of head to one side, actively or passively

NEGATIVE RESPONSE: Body does not rotate and follow rotation of head

POSITIVE RESPONSE: Body follows by turning in one piece, like a log, following in direction of head

NORMAL: Positive reaction up to 6 months of age; negative reaction should not persist beyond 1 month of age

Body righting reaction acting on the body[5,9]

POSITION: Supine lying, head in midposition, limbs extended

STIMULUS: Active or passive rotation of head

NEGATIVE RESPONSE: Body rotates in one piece, with a neck righting response

POSITIVE RESPONSE: Segmental rotation of trunk, first shoulders, then pelvis

NORMAL: Negative response—until 6 months of age; positive response—6 to 18 months of age

Labyrinthine righting reaction acting on the head[2,5,9]

POSITION: Prone, supine, or vertical positions in space; subject's vision is occluded

STIMULUS: Prone or supine positions are test stimuli or in vertical position body is tilted laterally

NEGATIVE RESPONSE: Head does not raise or right itself to normal face-vertical position

POSITIVE RESPONSE: Head tends to seek vertical position in space regardless of position of body and independent of vision

NORMAL: Positive response is present from 2 to 6 months of age throughout life

Optical righting reaction[5]

POSITION: Prone, supine, or vertical positions in space, with eyes open

Stimuli and responses are same as for labyrinthine righting reaction acting on head, described earlier

Cortical level

Equilibrium reaction[2,5,9]

POSITION: Supine lying, prone lying quadruped, sitting, kneel-standing, and standing

STIMULUS: Tipping or rocking subject or supporting surface, depending on position, sufficiently to disturb balance

NEGATIVE RESPONSES: Failure to make automatic movements to right head and body; no protective reactions

POSITIVE RESPONSES: Automatic movements to maintain balance, right head and body; protective reactions

NORMAL: Positive reactions in prone and supine begin at about 6 months of age; in quadruped position positive responses begin at about 8 months of age; in sitting at 10 to 12 months of age; in kneel-standing at about 15 months of age; and in standing from 15 to 18 months; these reactions remain throughout life

Innate primary reactions[9]

Reflex stepping[2,9]

POSITION: Supported in upright position with some weight bearing on feet

STIMULUS: Lean subject forward; contact and pressure of soles on supporting surface

RESPONSE: Rhythmic alternate stepping

NORMAL: First 4 to 8 weeks of life

Grasp reflex or tonic palmar reflex[6,9]

STIMULUS: Contact of object or pressure to palm of hand from ulnar side

RESPONSE: Flexing of fingers, grasping of stimulus object

NORMAL: Present at birth, diminishing by 4 or 5 months of age

Rooting reflex[2,9]

STIMULUS: Touching or stroking outward on corner of lips or on cheeks

RESPONSE: Tongue, lip, and head move to follow stimulus

NORMAL: From birth to 3 or 4 months of age

Sucking reflex[2,7]

STIMULUS: Stimulation to lips, gums, or front of tongue

RESPONSE: Sucking, swallowing motions

NORMAL: Present at birth, diminishing by 4 months of age[7]

Automatic movement reactions

Moro reflex[2,5,9]

POSITION: Semireclining or supine lying

STIMULUS: Dropping head backward from a semisitting position or a loud noise near the head

NEGATIVE RESPONSE: Minimal or absent movement of limbs

POSITIVE RESPONSE: Extension (or flexion) and abduction of arms and spreading of fingers

NORMAL: First 4 to 6 months of age

Landau reflex[5,9]

POSITION: Prone, suspended in space, supported under chest

STIMULUS: Passive or active neck extension

NEGATIVE RESPONSE: Spine and legs remain flexed

POSITIVE RESPONSE: Back and legs extend

NORMAL: Positive response begins about 4 to 6 months of age and disappears by 2 years of age[5,7]

Protective extension or parachute reactions[2,5]

POSITION: Suspended in prone position with arms extended overhead

STIMULUS: Move head suddenly toward the floor, holding subject at pelvis; for adults, where this position is not feasible, a sudden displacement of erect trunk will evoke protective extension, in the direction of the trunk movement, by arm or leg

NEGATIVE RESPONSE: Arms do not extend to protect head

POSITIVE RESPONSE: Protective extension of appropriate limb to protect head and attempt to recover balance

NORMAL: Begins in arms at about 6 months of age; develops first with forward responses, progresses to sideward, and then backward responses; is present throughout life

TREATMENT PLANNING

Primitive reflexes are essential to normal motor development. Responses to these reflexes prepare the individual for the progressive development of motor skills from rolling over to sitting, crawling, and standing, for example. In normal development the primitive spinal and brain stem reflexes gradually diminish and give way to the higher level righting and equilibrium reactions,[5] which are the foundations of normal motor function.[3] CNS lesions, such as a stroke or head injury, may cause primitive reflexes to be released from the normal inhibition exerted by higher centers of CNS control. In such instances the patient's motor performance may be dominated by primitive patterns of motor behavior that are on a reflexive level. The higher level of righting and equilibrium reactions and the normal adaptation of muscles to change in position are disturbed or absent, resulting in an abnormal postural reflex mechanism.[3,5]

A reflex assessment is necessary to determine the status of the primitive reflex integration and of the righting and equilibrium reactions. A delay in primitive reflex integration or a release of primitive reflexes will result in decreased segmentation of the trunk, decreased ability to perform isolated movement, decreased rotation in movement, decreased adaptation of muscles to postural change, decreased function of antigravity muscles, increased mass movement patterns (synergies), and increased dependence on stimuli from the environment for changes in posture.[4]

Formal assessment of reflexes should be accompanied by observation of the effect of reflexes on motor performance. For example, dysfunction in righting reactions can interfere with turning in bed and getting up. Dysfunction of equilibrium interferes with most functional skills and can be particularly noted during transfers, dressing, and ambulation activities. Other examples of abnormal postural reflexes and their effect on motor performance are outlined in Table 31-3.

To plan treatment effectively, the occupational therapist needs to know normal and abnormal reflexes and their effect on development and motor performance of the patient.[5] Knowledge of reflexes will also help the therapist understand their use or inhibition in the various sensorimotor approaches to treatment. The neurodevelopmental approach of Bobath (Chapter 16) and the sensory-integrative approach of Ayres[1] stress the importance of normal reflex activity, including muscle tone, for normal movement.[8] Both approaches employ techniques with the goal of inhibiting or integrating primitive reflexes while facilitating higher level righting and equilibrium reactions and more normal patterns of movement. The approach of Rood (Chapter 13) is based on the sequence of normal motor development and uses techniques for gradually increasing reflex maturation and normal motor skill development. The approach of Brunnstrom (Chapter 15) is based on the motor recovery process following a stroke, which is regarded as the recovery from an "evolution in reverse" that occurs as a result of a cerebral insult. In this approach primitive reflexes are sometimes used to evoke or reinforce desired movement patterns, since they are regarded as a normal part of the function of the recovering nervous system.

It is important to evaluate reflexes and reactions in adults with CNS disease to measure the level of CNS function; establish a baseline for recovery; inhibit or use the reflex activity as appropriate with the selected treatment approach; and determine the kind of positioning, motion, and sensory stimuli that could facilitate more mature motor responses.

REVIEW QUESTIONS

1. List the reflexes or reactions that are integrated at the spinal level, the brain stem level, the midbrain level, and the cortical level.
2. Name three automatic movement reactions and describe each.
3. Describe or demonstrate the procedures and give the norms for each of the following reflexes or reactions: extensor thrust, ATNR, TLR, neck righting, optical righting, and equilibrium reactions.
4. How is the sucking reflex different from the rooting reflex?
5. Describe Landau's reflex.
6. Why is it important for occupational therapists to understand and evaluate reflexes and reactions?
7. How can knowledge of reflex integration aid in selection of treatment methods?
8. Give four examples of how abnormal reflex activity interferes with normal movement.

REFERENCES

1. Ayres, A.J.: Sensory integration and learning disorders, Los Angeles, 1972, Western Psychological Services.
2. Banus, B.S., editor: The developmental therapist, Thorofare, N.J., 1971, Charles B. Slack, Inc.
3. Bobath, B.: Adult hemiplegia: evaluation and treatment, ed. 2, London, 1978, William Heinemann Medical Books Ltd.
4. Farber, S.: Neurorehabilitation: a multisensory approach, Philadelphia, 1982, W.B. Saunders Co.
5. Fiorentino, M.R.: Reflex testing methods for evaluating CNS development, Springfield, Ill., 1973, Charles C. Thomas, Publisher.
6. Peiper, A.: Cerebral function in infancy and childhood, New York, 1963, Consultants Bureau Enterprises.
7. Semans, S.: Developmental reactions, Stanford, Calif., 1968, Division of Physical Therapy, Stanford University. Mimeographed.
8. Tower, G.: Selected developmental reflexes and reactions: a literature search. In Hopkins, H.L., and Smith, H.D.: Willard and Spackman's occupational therapy, ed. 6, Philadelphia, 1983, J.B. Lippincott Co.
9. Trombly, C.A., and Scott, A.D.: Occupational therapy for physical dysfunction, Baltimore, 1977, Williams & Wilkins.

CHAPTER 9

Evaluation of sensation, perception, and cognition

LORRAINE WILLIAMS PEDRETTI

All persons with peripheral nervous system or central nervous system (CNS) disease or damage should be tested for sensory and perceptual dysfunction. Persons with thermal injuries are also candidates for sensory evaluation. Sensory receptors in the skin may have been destroyed, sensation may be disturbed following skin graft, or there may be peripheral nerve involvement in thermal injury. The sensory testing is usually not carried out until the postgrafting phase of rehabilitation, when there is good wound healing.

For clients with dysfunction of sensory receptors or peripheral neuropathy, tests of light touch, superficial pain, pressure, thermal sensitivity, position and motion sense (proprioception), and stereognosis should be applied. For those with CNS dysfunction, additional tests of body scheme, praxis, and visual perception should be applied. Examples of diagnoses that require sensory testing are thermal injuries (burns), peripheral nerve injuries and diseases, spinal cord injuries and diseases, brain injuries and diseases, and fractures and arthritis, when there is peripheral nerve involvement or to help determine if there is peripheral nerve involvement.

The purposes of performing sensory-perceptual evaluation are to determine the need for teaching precautions against injury or compensatory techniques such as visual guidance for movement and for initiating a program of sensory reeducation. Sensory loss may affect the client's use of splints and braces, since the client may be unaware of pressure points during use. Sensory loss may also affect controlled use of a dynamic splint, since the client's sensory feedback is faulty.

For these reasons the occupational therapist can use results of the sensory-perceptual evaluation to select appropriate treatment objectives and methods.

In addition, in some diagonoses sensory status and progress may provide valuable information that can indicate prognosis for recovery.[12]

TESTS FOR SENSATION

The following tests are based on evaluation tools of clinical neurology designed to test the sensation of adults with central or peripheral nervous system dysfunction.[4,11] It is important for the examiner to orient the subject to the test procedures and the rationale for administering the tests. The examiner should be sure the subject understands how to respond. The subject's vision can be occluded by shielding the parts to be tested from view. It is most desirable that the subject not be blindfolded or asked to keep the eyes closed.

A blindfold can be a source of sensory distraction and can be very anxiety provoking to subjects with sensory, perceptual, and balance disturbances. It is difficult for many individuals with CNS dysfunction to maintain eye closure because of apraxia and motor impersistence, in addition to the reasons just stated. Therefore to occlude vision it is preferable to use a folder or small screen under which the subject can place the hands and forearms.

Test for superficial pain[4,11,12]

PURPOSE: To make a gross evaluation of superficial pain sensitivity.

LIMITATIONS: Persons with receptive aphasia cannot be validly tested.

MATERIALS: A small curtain between two uprights or a manila folder to occlude subject's vision. A large safety pin or sharpened pencil.

CONDITIONS: A nondistracting environment where subject (S) is seated at a narrow table. Affected hand and forearm should rest comfortably on table. Examiner (E) sits opposite S on other side of table. If it is not possible to position S in this manner, the test may be administered while S is in bed or sitting in the wheelchair with arms resting on the lapboard.

METHOD: S's hand and forearm are hidden from S's view by placing them between uprights and under curtain or by E holding a manila folder over them. Affected hand and forearm are touched lightly at random locations, using sharp and dull stimuli in random order (Fig. 9-1). A few trial stimuli should be conducted with S watching to be sure that S understands test and knows how to respond. Test may be conducted entirely on an unaffected area first to establish a standard and determine that instructions are understood. If spasticity is a problem, E may support hand on dorsal surface and hold thumb in radial abduction and extension to secure relaxation for palmar testing. Each stimulus should be applied with same degree of pressure.

NOTES: Calloused or toughened areas (for example, palms) may be normally less sensitive than other areas. If S is fearful of a safety pin, a pencil or broken swab stick may be used.

RESPONSES: S should be asked to say "sharp" or "dull" in response to each stimulus. If S is aphasic or dysarthric, E should ask S to indicate a response by pointing to appropriate side of an open safety pin in S's view.

SCORING: E marks a plus at stimulus point on scoring chart for a correct response, a minus for an incorrect or unduly delayed response, and a zero for no response. Space for recording results of evaluation is presented in Fig. 9-2.

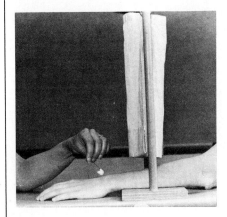

Fig. 9-1. Test for superficial pain sensitivity.

FORM FOR RECORDING SCORES ON
TESTS OF SENSATION

Department of Occupational Therapy

Name_____ Age_____ Sex_____

Diagnosis_____ Disability_____

Date_____

TEST FOR SUPERFICIAL PAIN	LEFT	RIGHT
Use a large safety pin and touch random locations with sharp and dull ends on anterior and posterior surfaces. Indicate on diagram: Intact: + Impaired: − Absent: 0	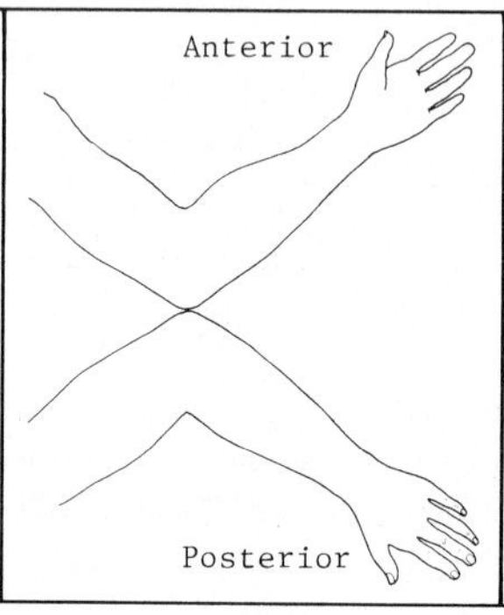 Anterior / Posterior	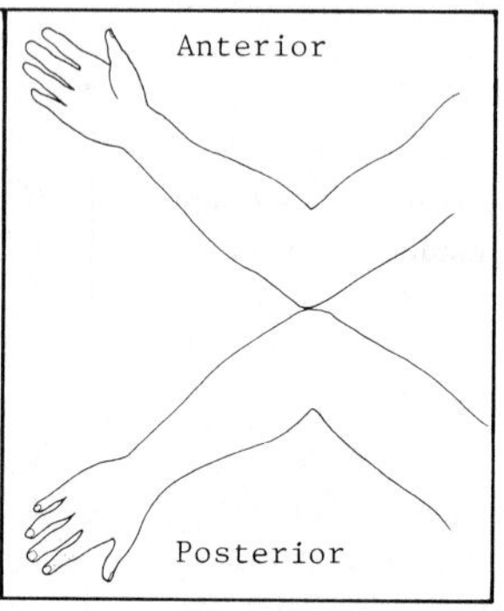 Anterior / Posterior

TEST FOR LIGHT TOUCH SENSITIVITY	LEFT	RIGHT
Use a cotton swab and touch random locations on anterior and posterior surfaces. Indicate on diagram: Intact: + Impaired: − Absent: 0	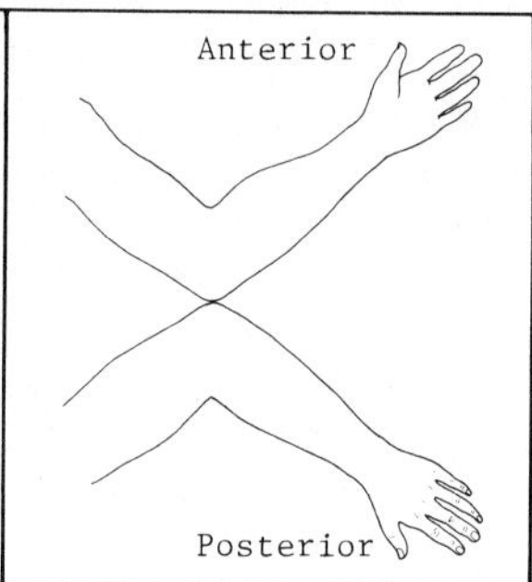 Anterior / Posterior	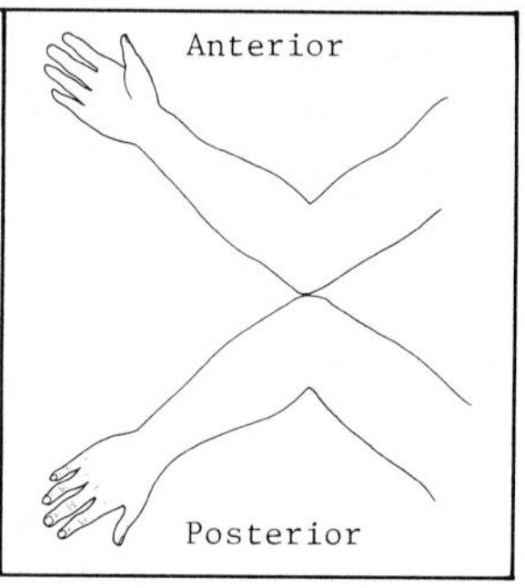 Anterior / Posterior

Fig. 9-2. Form for recording scores on test of sensation.

Test for light touch sensitivity[4,11,16]

PURPOSE: To determine S's ability to recognize and localize light touch stimuli.

LIMITATIONS: Patients with receptive aphasia cannot be validly tested.

MATERIALS: A small curtain between two uprights or a manila folder to occlude vision. A cotton swab.

CONDITIONS: A nondistracting environment where S is seated at a narrow table or as described previously for superficial pain if sitting at a table is not possible. Affected hand and forearm rest comfortably on table. E sits opposite S.

METHOD: S's hand and forearm are hidden from S's view by placing them under curtain or by E holding manila folder over them. Hand and forearm are touched lightly with a cotton swab at random locations. A few trial stimuli should be administered while S is watching to be sure S understands procedure and how to respond. Test may be administered on an uninvolved area first to establish a standard. If spasticity is a problem, E may support hand on dorsal surface and hold thumb in radial abduction and extension to secure relaxation of fingers for palmar testing (Fig. 9-3).

RESPONSES: After each stimulus, E asks if S was touched (recognition). S responds by nodding or saying "yes" or "no." Curtain or folder is removed after each stimulus, and S is asked to point to place where S was touched, using unaffected hand if possible. If this cannot be done, S is asked to describe location, and E should select locations that are easy to name (for example, over proximal interphalangeal joint).

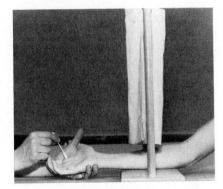

Fig. 9-3. Test of light touch sensitivity.

SCORING: On scoring chart E marks a plus for ability to recognize and localize touch stimuli, a minus for ability recognize only, and a zero for inability to recognize or localize a stimulus. Fig. 9-2 includes space for recording scores on test for touch sensitivity.

STANDARDS: Deviations of ⅗ to 1⅕ inches (1.5 to 3 cm) from the point of application of the stimulus are normal, depending on an area of hand or arm touched. Responses should be more accurate on hand than on forearm and more accurate on forearm than on upper arm.

Test for pressure sensitivity

Pressure sensitivity may be tested in exactly the same manner as described for light touch, except that E should press hard enough with the cotton swab to dent and blanch the skin. If light touch sensitivity is severely impaired or absent, pressure sensitivity may be intact and may provide important sensory feedback to compensate and enhance function.

Test for thermal sensitivity[4,7]

PURPOSE: To determine S's ability to discriminate between extremes of hot and cold and to detect variations in temperature at four levels.

LIMITATIONS: Persons with receptive aphasia cannot be validly tested.

MATERIALS: Four test tubes (¾-inch or 2 cm diameter) with stoppers.

CONDITIONS: A nondistracting environment where S is seated comfortably at a table with both hand and forearm resting on table, or alternatives described for previous tests.

METHOD:

Subtest I: Two test tubes are used, one filled with very cold water and one with very hot water. Ice water may be used for cold and hottest tap water tolerable to normal touch used for hot. Stoppers are placed in tubes. E touches sides of test tubes to skin surfaces to be tested in random order and at random locations, being sure to cover test area thoroughly (Fig. 9-4).

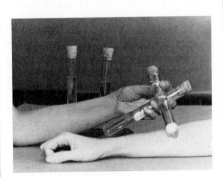

Fig. 9-4. Test for thermal sensitivity.

Subtest II: Four test tubes are used, one filled with very cold water, one with tepid water, one with warm water, and one with hot water. E should color code stoppers as follows: yellow—hot, green—warm, orange—tepid, and red—cold. Place stoppers in tubes. E asks S to touch or hold test tubes with affected hand(s) in random order. If S is unable to hold tubes, E may touch each one to S's palm and fingertips.

Subtest III: Using same four test tubes as in subtest II filled with water of like temperature, S is asked to hold each one with both hands simultaneously. If S is unable to hold tube with affected hand, E may hold tube to palmar surface of fingers of that hand while S touches tube with fingers of unaffected hand. S is asked to compare feeling of heat or cold in both hands, that is, does temperature feel same or different to affected and unaffected hands.

RESPONSES:

Subtest I: S responds "hot" or "cold" in response to each stimulus. If S is aphasic, E should work out an alternate nonverbal response before beginning tests.

Subtest II: S is asked to arrange test tubes on table from hottest to coldest in order from left to right. E checks correctness of order by color-coded stoppers and/or feeling tubes.

Subtest III: S is asked to tell whether sensation of warmth or cold is same to both hands or whether a given temperature is warmer or cooler to one hand or the other. This is an entirely subjective estimate and cognitive status of S may influence response.

SCORING (Fig. 9-5):

Subtest I: E marks a plus on form if temperature is correctly identified, and marks a zero if S cannot tell hot from cold. Subtests II and III are not administered if S cannot succeed at subtest I.

Subtest II: E marks appropriate blanks on form with a check and the appropriate letter to indicate S's responses.

Subtest III: E marks appropriate blanks on form with a check to indicate S's responses.

STANDARD: Normal adults should be able to complete all items on this test successfully.

```
TEST FOR THERMAL SENSITIVITY
    SUBTEST I.

        Test site (fill in location tested)              Score (+, 0)
                                          Dates
```

Use diagram to record scores on test of arms

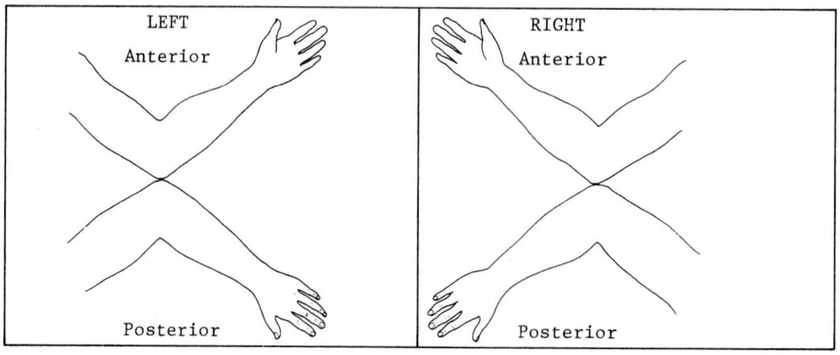

```
    SUBTEST II.                                     Date    Date    Date

        Arrange test tubes in correct order        _____   _____   _____
        Arrange test tubes in wrong order          _____   _____   _____

        Indicate arrangement of test tubes by filling in spaces below with
        H for hot, W for warm, T for tepid, and C for cold.

        Date: _____  _____  _____  _____  _____
              _____  _____  _____  _____  _____
              _____  _____  _____  _____  _____

    SUBTEST III.                                    Date    Date    Date

        Temperature feels the same to both hands    _____   _____   _____
        Temperature feels different to each hand    _____   _____   _____

          All feel warmer to affected hand          _____   _____   _____
          All feel cooler to affected hand          _____   _____   _____
          All feel warmer to unaffected hand        _____   _____   _____
          All feel cooler to unaffected hand        _____   _____   _____

          Hottest is intolerably hot to affected hand  _____  _____  _____
          Coldest is intolerably cold to affected hand _____  _____  _____
```

Fig. 9-5. Form for recording scores on test of thermal sensitivity.

Test for olfactory sensation

A loss of the sense of smell is known as anosmia. It may result from local chronic or acute inflammatory nasal disease or from intracranial lesions that may be the result of cerebral vascular accident, head injury, tumors, and infections.[4]

PURPOSE: To determine if the sense of smell is intact, impaired, or lost and whether the loss is unilateral or bilateral. E should note how anosmia interferes with function, for example, whether the client has an occupation where the sense of smell is critical to safety. In some disturbances where sense of smell is distorted and even pleasant odors are perceived as noxious (parosmia), the disturbance may interfere with the perception, enjoyment of food odors, and possibly eating.

LIMITATIONS: Persons with receptive aphasia cannot be validly tested. Persons with expressive aphasia who cannot communicate using symbols, such as pictures or words, to indicate responses cannot be validly tested. Test is quite subjective and E must rely on S's report.

MATERIALS: Five small opaque or dark-colored bottles containing essences, powders, or crystalline material of familiar odors. Coffee, almond, chocolate, lemon oil, and peppermint are some that are suitable.[4] Ammonia or other irritating chemical odors should *not* be used in a test of olfaction, since they stimulate all receptors of the mucous membranes and tend to be irritating.[7] If S cannot respond verbally, small cards with the word or a picture for each odor on them will be needed.

CONDITIONS: A nondistracting environment where no strong odors are present with S seated or semireclining.

METHOD: The cork of the bottle or a cotton swab moistened with essence is held under S's nostril; in the case of solid substances the container may be held under S's nostril. S is asked to compress one nostril or this may be done by E. S is then asked to take a breath to demonstrate that the remaining nostril is open. With vision occluded, if the substances could be recognized from their appearance, the cotton swab, cork, or bottle is then held under the open nostril, and S is asked to take two moderate sniffs. Each of the substances is tried with a short delay between them, and the nostrils are tested alternately using the same and different substances.[4,11]

RESPONSES: E asks S to (1) detect an odor, (2) identify the odor, (3) distinguish if the odors are the same or different to both nostrils.[4,11]

SCORING (Fig. 9-6): E marks a plus on the form if the odor is detected and correctly identified, a minus if an odor is detected, and a zero if no odor is detected. Whether or not the same odors are perceived as the same by both nostrils and whether S can differentiate between different odors presented to each nostril should be noted on the form.

STANDARD: Ability to detect and identify odors quickly, ability to detect odor without identification, and ability to detect and differentiate odors without identification may all be regarded as normal responses.[4] Distortion of the odor (parosmia) and inability to detect odors are regarded as dysfunction. If test responses are vague and variable, the results are unreliable, and it is best to postpone the test to a more favorable time.[4]

Test for gustatory sensation

Taste is subserved by the facial and glossopharyngeal nerve (cranial nerves VII and IX). Disturbances of taste may be caused by peripheral or CNS lesions.[11]

PURPOSE: Taste is not only basic to the enjoyment of food but is one of the sensory stimuli that triggers salivation and swallowing. Therefore taste sensation may be of concern to the occupational therapist as part of a comprehensive evaluation of oral-motor mechanisms and for planning feeding training programs.[14]

LIMITATIONS: The same limitations as were cited for the test of olfaction apply here. The most accurate method of administering the test requires that S keep the tongue extended. Therefore S must respond by pointing to a word or picture. In instances where S has speech but cannot recognize words or pictures, a verbal response should be allowed. If S is aphasic, E should observe for aversive responses to the sour and bitter stimuli.[14] The appreciation of taste depends on an intact sense of smell.[4]

MATERIALS: Sugar, salt, lemon or vinegar, and quinine in small containers to test the four basic tastes: sweet, salt, sour, and bitter. Cotton swabs.

CONDITIONS: A nondistracting environment where S is seated or semireclining. E should sit directly in front of S. S may close eyes, or S's vision should be occluded by a folder or blindfold if necessary. The oral cavity should be clean and free of residual food tastes.

METHOD: S is instructed to protrude the tongue and a small amount of the test substance on the tip of a wet cotton swab is applied to the appropriate place on the tongue: sweet—side/front of tongue, salt—all areas of tongue, sour—side/middle of tongue, and bitter—side/back of tongue.[14] If this is not effective, rubbing the substance along the side of the protruded tongue should be tried.[4,11]

RESPONSES: S is instructed to point to the response card before withdrawing the tongue and diffusing the taste to all areas of the tongue.[4,11]

SCORING (Fig. 9-6): E should record a plus if the taste is correctly identified and a minus if it cannot be identified.

STANDARD: Normal adults should be able to recognize all tastes accurately.

TESTS OF PERCEPTION
Test for proprioception[4,6,8,9,16]

PURPOSE: To evaluate S's senses of motion and position.

MATERIALS: Curtain on uprights shown on test for light touch sensitivity (Fig. 9-3) or a manila folder. For testing elbow and shoulder, if space and equipment permit, a curtained screen high and wide enough to conceal S's arm when held overhead or out in front when in a seated position. Curtain on screen should be full, continuous, and attached at top only. If such a screen is not available, a blindfold may be used that is as small and comfortable as possible.

CONDITIONS: Test should be conducted in privacy in a nondistracting environment. When fingers and wrist are being tested, S should be seated at a table with screen in front in a position to accommodate affected hand and forearm comfortably. E should sit opposite S on other side of screen in a position comfortable to accommodate S's hand for conducting test. When elbow and shoulder are being tested, S should be seated, and curtain screen placed at S's affected side. Curtain should be draped over the shoulder in such a manner that S is unable to see the affected arm. If screen is not available, blindfold should be used. If this position is not feasible, test may be conducted with S seated or reclining in bed or seated in a wheelchair.

RESPONSES: To determine appreciation of direction of movement S should be instructed to respond "up" (away from floor) and "down" (toward floor) or "out" (away from body) and "in" (toward body) as soon as he or she perceives direction of movement. Aphasic subjects may respond by pointing in appropriate direction. If there is one unaffected extremity, as in hemiplegia, S should be asked to imitate with unaffected extremity final position in which part rests after E has ceased movement to determine appreciation of position.

RECORDING SCORES OF OLFACTORY AND GUSTATORY SENSATION

Name: _____

Age: _____ Diagnosis: _____

Date: _____

Key: + = Can detect and identify odor
      - = Can detect odor, cannot identify odor
      O = Cannot detect or identify odor
      S = Can detect same odors, both nostrils
      D = Can detect different odors, both nostrils

OLFACTORY SENSATION   Left nostril   Right nostril   Comparisons

Dates						
Coffee						
Almond						
Chocolate						
Lemon						
Peppermint						

GUSTATORY SENSATION

Key: + = Identifies taste correctly
      - = Cannot identify taste

Dates			Remarks
Sweet			
Salt			
Sour			
Bitter			

Fig. 9-6. Form for recording scores of olfactory and gustatory sensation.

METHOD:

Test of fingers: Test positions are index finger flexion, middle finger extension, thumb extension, and little finger flexion. These should be presented in random order. No range should be carried to such an extreme as to elicit pain or a stretch reflex. S's hand and forearm should be placed under curtain, resting on dorsal surface. When testing a right hand, E should support S's hand with the left palm and hold thumb out of way with the left thumb if necessary. This position should induce relaxation of fingers if S has flexor spasticity. With the right hand E should grasp finger to be tested on each side at distal phalanx to avoid giving pressure cues with E's thumb and index finger. Finger being tested should be separated from others and should be kept from touching palm to avoid cues from contact. Position of E's hands is reversed when testing a left hand (Fig. 9-7).

Test of wrist: Test positions are wrist flexion and extension. The ranges should not be carried to such an extreme as to elicit tendon action or a stretch reflex. E's and S's hands are positioned as for testing fingers. However, E makes a somewhat firmer grasp at sides of S's hand, reducing contact between E's palm and back of S's hand.

Test of elbow and shoulder: Starting position for all motions is with S's arm at side, shoulder supported in 20° to 30° of abduction, elbow supported at 90° of flexion, and wrist stabilized at neutral. Test positions are elbow extension, shoulder flexion, shoulder internal rotation, and shoulder flexion-abduction (halfway between 90° of flexion and 90° of abduction). Test positions should be presented in random order. Ranges should not be carried to such an extreme as to elicit a stretch reflex or cause pain if there is joint tightness. S should be seated away from table. Curtained screen should be arranged at S's

test side as described or blindfold put in place. E should stand at S's test side and guide limb passively through test positions. When testing a right arm, E's right hand should be placed along ulnar border of S's hand and wrist, stabilizing wrist at neutral. E's left hand should be placed on dorsal surface of upper arm just proximal to elbow. Position is reversed when testing left arm. E may carry out all test positions for elbow and shoulder without changing position of hands (Fig. 9-8).

SCORING (Fig. 9-9):

Appreciation of direction of movement: E records plus if direction is correctly perceived or zero if direction is not perceived.

Appreciation of position: E records plus if correct response is given, minus if response is nearly correct, and zero if response is obviously incorrect or no response is given.

Remarks: On the recording form E comments on S's reactions, unusual statements, observations, and individual variations in test procedure adapted for specific dysfunctions.

Test for stereognosis[3,6,8,9,16]

PURPOSE: To evaluate S's ability to perceive tactile properties and identify common objects.

MATERIALS: Uprights with curtain described in test for light touch. Pencil, fountain pen, sunglasses, key, nail, large safety pin, metal teaspoon, quarter, and small leather coin purse.

CONDITIONS: Test should be conducted in privacy in a nondistracting environment. S should be seated at a table with curtain in front in a position that accommodates affected hand and forearm comfortably. E should sit opposite S. If S is unable to manipulate test objects because of motor weakness, E should assist S to manipulate them in as near normal a manner as possible.

METHOD: S's hand is under curtain, resting on dorsal surface on table. Objects are presented in random order. Manipulation

of objects is allowed and encouraged. Manipulation of objects may be assisted by E if S's hand is partially or completely paralyzed.

RESPONSES: S should be asked to name object or describe its properties if unable to name it. Aphasic patients may view a duplicate set of test objects after each trial and point to a choice.

SCORING: E marks plus if object is identified quickly and correctly and minus if there is a long delay before identification of object or if S can only describe properties (for example, size, texture, material, and shape) of object. E marks a zero if S cannot identify object or its properties (Fig. 9-9).

Test for body scheme*

PURPOSE: To evaluate S's ability to recognize and name individual fingers on self and E, identify body parts, differentiate between right and left, visualize body scheme, and recognize presence of disability.

MATERIALS: A lap board may be used for testing finger identification if S is in a wheelchair. Otherwise S may be seated at a table for finger identification test.

CONDITIONS: Test should be conducted in privacy in a nondistracting environment. S should be seated away from table to have a good view of self. E should sit on S's side at such an angle that S can see E clearly. If subject is hemiplegic, E should sit on unaffected side.

RESPONSES:

Finger identification: Names of fingers are to be clarified before test. They should be called thumb, index, middle, ring, and little fingers. S should be instructed to lift or point to appropriate finger as E names them.

Identification of body parts: S should be instructed to point to or raise appropriate parts of body as E names them. Correct part on either side of body is acceptable for full score.

Concept of right and left: S is to point to or raise appropriate parts of body as they are named. Part and side specified are essential for full score.

Visualization of body scheme and recognition of illness: S is to respond "yes" or "no" to a series of questions regarding body orientation and presence of illness. Aphasic subjects may nod "yes" or "no" in response.

*References 1, 2, 5, 9, 10, 16.

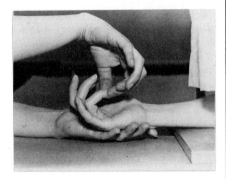

Fig. 9-7. Position sense test of fingers.

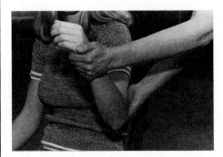

Fig. 9-8. Position and motion sense test of elbow and shoulder.

FORM FOR RECORDING TESTS OF PERCEPTION

Department of Occupational Therapy

Name_____ Age_____ Sex_____ Onset_____

Diagnosis/disability_____

Date_____

TEST OF PROPRIOCEPTION

	Shoulder flexion-abduction	Shoulder internal rotation	Shoulder flexion	Elbow extension	Wrist extension	Wrist flexion	Little finger flexion	Thumb extension	Middle finger extension	Index finger flexion
Appreciation of direction of movement										
Appreciation of position										

Remarks:

TEST OF STEREOGNOSIS

COMMON OBJECTS	+ – 0	DESCRIPTION
Pencil		
Fountain pen		
Sunglasses		
Key		
Nail		
Safety pin		
Teaspoon		
Quarter		
Leather coin purse		

Remarks:

Fig. 9-9. Form for recording scores on tests of stereognosis and proprioception.

TEST OF BODY SCHEME

FINGER IDENTIFICATION	+, 0	LOCATION NAMED, IF INCORRECT
Self: Thumb		
Ring		
Little		
Index		
Examiner: Thumb		
Index		
Ring		
Little		

IDENTIFICATION OF BODY PARTS	+, 0	LOCATION NAMED, IF INCORRECT
Hand		
Ear		
Cheek		
Knee		
Shoulder		
Mouth		

CONCEPT OF RIGHT AND LEFT	+, -, 0	LOCATION NAMED, IF INCORRECT
Right hand		
Left knee		
Right foot		
Left elbow		
Left ear		
Right shoulder		
Left thumb		
Right middle finger		

VISUALIZATION OF BODY SCHEME RECOGNITION OF ILLNESS	+, 0	SUBJECT'S COMMENTS
Feet at top of legs?		
Hand below elbow?		
Knee above hip?		
Are your weak, paralyzed?		
Arm and leg weak?		
Eyes above nose?		
One chin?		
Perfect health now?		
Right limbs as strong as left?		

Remarks:

Fig. 9-10. Form for recording scores on test of body scheme.

METHOD:

Finger identification: On himself S should be asked to identify thumb, ring, little, and index fingers, as E names them. On E, S should be asked to identify thumb, index, ring, and little fingers.

Identification of body parts: E should name hand, ear, cheek, knee, shoulder, and mouth, and S should point to or raise appropriate part.

Concept of right and left: E should name right hand, left knee, right foot, left elbow, left ear, right shoulder, left thumb, and right middle finger. S should lift or point to appropriate part and side.

Visualization of body scheme and recognition of illness: S should be instructed to respond with "yes" or "no" to following questions:

Are your feet at the tops of your legs?
Is your hand below your elbow?
Is your knee above your hip?
Are your (E names affected parts) weak, paralyzed?
Are your eyes above your nose?
Do you have one chin?
Are you now in perfect health?
Is your (right, left) leg as strong as (right, left)?
Is your mouth larger than your hand?

Questions may be modified to suit individual cases. Correct answers to questions regarding recognition of illness may vary from case to case.

SCORING (Fig. 9-10):

Finger identification: E records plus if correct identification is made and zero for incorrect identification. E also indicates incorrect locations named in response.

Identification of body parts: E records plus for correct identification and zero for incorrect identification.

Concept of right and left: E records plus for correct part and side, minus for correct part and wrong side or incorrect part and correct side, and zero for both incorrect part and side. E also specifies location of S's incorrect responses.

Visualization of body scheme and recognition of illness: E records plus for correct answers and zero for incorrect answers. E also records responses and comments S makes to questions.

DISCUSSION: Body scheme perception may also be evaluated by asking S to draw a picture of a man or woman, as appropriate, or assemble a human figure puzzle. These two tasks require several other perceptual and cognitive functions besides body scheme awareness. The examiner should be aware of this if the subject fails at these tasks. To validate responses on any of the methods the subject may be tested in all three ways.

Test for unilateral neglect[13]

Unilateral neglect is the inability to integrate and use perceptions from the left side of the body and the left side of space. An individual with unilateral neglect will ignore the left half of his or her body and may ignore objects on the left side of the environment. This phenomenon is common with left hemiplegia and may be present even if the visual fields are intact; it is compounded if accompanied by homonymous hemianopsia. In everyday activities the client bumps into things on the left side when walking or using a wheelchair, may neglect to shave the left side of the face, and may ignore food on the left half of the plate.[13]

Subtest I—ability to draw a house, clock, and flower[13]

PROCEDURE: S is given a separate sheet of paper for each drawing. S is asked to draw a house, draw a clock, and draw a flower in turn.

SCORING: Scoring is subjective based on observation of the form and content of the drawing. If the drawings include all of the parts in their proper places and in balanced proportion on right and left sides of the paper, there is probably not a unilateral neglect. Drawings that have missing parts on the left side, are thinner on the left, are skewed to the right, or done entirely on the right side of the paper are signs of unilateral neglect.

Subtest II—ability to copy a house, clock, and flower[13]

PROCEDURE: E provides a drawing of a house, clock, and flower (each separately) and provides S with clean paper. S is asked to copy each drawing in turn.

SCORING: Same as for Subtest I.

Subtest III—ability to recognize letters[13]

PROCEDURE: E types several lines of letters, double-spaced, and in random order across the top half of a sheet of typing paper. S is asked to look at each line from left to right and cross out all of the F's or any letter.

SCORING: Scoring is based on subjective observation. All occurrences of the requested letter crossed out from left to right of the page indicate that unilateral neglect may not be a problem. Letters missed on the left side of the page may be an indication of unilateral neglect.

TEST VALIDITY: Validity on tests for unilateral neglect may be improved by ruling out possible homonymous hemianopsia, constructional apraxia, poor vision, or inability to read letters of the alphabet.

Test of motor planning (praxis)

Ideational and ideomotor praxis include the ability to plan and copy demonstrated acts or carry out movements commonly associated with tools and implements (for example, comb or typewriter) or action words (for example, stir or kick). Constructional praxis is the ability to produce designs in two or three dimensions by copying, drawing, or constructing on command and spontaneously.[13] These skills are critical to success in rehabilitation programs, since much of the training in activities of daily living (ADL), exercises, activities, and work-related tasks involves carrying out demonstrated and verbal instructions, using tools and implements, and learning new movement patterns to perform old familiar tasks. The purpose of testing praxis is to determine the subject's capacity to plan and carry out the motor skills essential to progress. Other factors that can have a negative effect on the performance of these tasks are incoordination, unilateral neglect, homonymous hemianopsia, and impaired perception of visual-spatial relationships. Dysfunction in these subskills should be ruled out before testing.[13] The tests described are for quick clinical evaluation.

Tests of ideational and ideomotor apraxia

Subtest I—ability to copy demonstrated acts

PROCEDURE: E sits or stands opposite S. E performs random movements with arms and or legs (for example, strikes poses) and asks S to mimic or copy movements. Initially E should first use symmetrical postures, then asymmetrical, and then postures involving crossing midline. If S has one or more paralyzed limbs, E should not use mirror counterpart of that limb on self in demonstrations.

RESPONSES: Responses should be a mirror image of E's postures. Same procedure may be followed, using hand postures to evaluate fine motor planning, except that E sits next to S on unaffected side (if S is hemiplegic).

EVALUATION: Observe for speed and accuracy of responses.

Intact: S responds quickly and accurately to at least 90% of stimuli.

Impaired: S's responses are delayed or are less than 90% accurate.

Absent: S does not respond accurately to most of stimuli.

Subtest II—ability to perform movements associated with action words or tools

PROCEDURE: E hands S an implement used in daily life, (for example, comb or toothbrush) and asks S to show what to do with it or how to use it.

RESPONSES: S should actually perform or pantomime movements associated with implement.

EVALUATION: Any confusion or delays can be interpreted as some impairment. Inappropriate use of implement or complete inability to use it correctly can be interpreted as a significant dysfunction in praxis.

PROCEDURE: E asks s to pantomime movements that go with action verbs. Suggested test items are stir, rub, brush, comb, beat eggs, and typewrite.

RESPONSES AND EVALUATION: S should be able to carry these out quickly and accurately. Hesitation and delayed responses may be interpreted as impairment. Inaccurate or no response may be interpreted as a significant impairment of praxis.

Tests of constructional apraxia[13]

Subtest I—ability to copy forms (two dimensional)

PROCEDURE: S is provided with drawings of several geometric forms, such as a circle, square, triangle, diamond, and hexagon. These may be printed at the top of the test paper. S is asked to duplicate the drawing on the bottom half of the paper.

RESPONSES: (1) Drawings may be essentially correct with all of the lines in place and the arrangement of the drawing on the paper well-proportioned. (2) There may be lines omitted, rotations, or disproportions between parts of the drawing, but the form is still identifiable. (3) The drawing may be unrecognizable.

SCORING: Constructional praxis may be considered intact if most of the drawings are done as described in response 1, impaired if most are done as described in response 2, and absent if most are done as described in response 3.

Subtest II—ability to copy block bridges (three dimensional)[13]

PROCEDURE: E uses 1-inch cube blocks to build bridges for S to copy. E begins with a three-block bridge; if S is successful, E proceeds to a five-block bridge and so on to a seven block bridge. S is asked to copy each bridge with a separate set of blocks.

SCORING: Assessment of performance is by subjective observation of execution of the task. If S builds all of the bridges correctly within a reasonable amount of time, praxis may be considered intact. Difficulties in construction of the bridges may be a result of constructional apraxia, but incoordination, ideomotor apraxia, and visual-spatial deficits must be ruled out.[13]

Tests of visual form and space perception

Tests of visual form and space perception require constructional praxis. The second requires visual memory and number sequencing. Therefore poor performance could be partially or entirely a result of dysfunctions in these skills and not a result of visual form and space perception impairment. It is wise to test for praxis and visual memory before administering these tests. Also, performance on both tests could be affected by homonymous hemianopsia and neglect of the affected side.

Test of form perception and spatial relationships

MATERIALS: One set of parquetry blocks, pencil, and paper.

PROCEDURE: E sits next to S on unaffected side. E selects five pairs of blocks from set for self and for S (four squares, four triangles, two diamonds). E arranges block designs, first using two, then three, four, and five blocks and asks S to duplicate pattern *after* each set is presented. S may not construct patterns at same time that E is performing (Fig. 9-11).

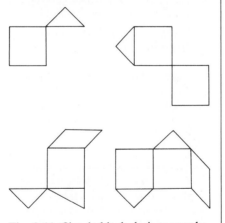

Fig. 9-11. Simple block designs may be used to assess form perception and spatial relationships.

EVALUATION: Evaluation of performance is based on E's experience and judgment. If form and space perception are intact, S will have no difficulty with this task and may be presented with increasingly complex visual-spatial patterns in same manner or may be challenged to copy block designs from paper patterns. Signs of dysfunction may be noted in (1) confusion between forms (for example, diamond and triangle), (2) reversals and inversions of patterns, (3) difficulty positioning block in relation to others (for example, uses a trial and error approach to setting a block down in pattern), (4) placing correct form in wrong position, and (5) omitting a form from pattern. If response is incorrect, E asks whether it look same as model. If response is "no," E challenges S to attempt to correct. Often S cannot make corrections but perceives pattern accurately.

Test of spatial relationships

MATERIALS: 8½ × 11-inch piece of plain paper and a pencil.

PROCEDURE: E draws a large circle on paper for S. E asks S to draw a clock face in circle, first arranging numbers, then placing hands at a designated hour.

EVALUATION: Again evaluation is based on E's experience and judgment. Signs of dysfunction may be noted in (1) tendency to space numbers incorrectly (for example, all squeezed together or spread out so they do not fit on clock face) and (2) tendency to be unable to place hands in correct positional relationships (Fig. 9-12).

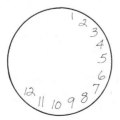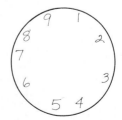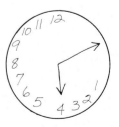

Fig. 9-12. Examples of responses that may be indicative of impaired perception of spatial relationships.

Test for homonymous hemianopsia (visual field defect)[11]

PROCEDURE: S is seated and asked to fix gaze on an object directly in front of him (6 to 10 feet or 1.8 to 3 m away). "Object" can be a volunteer or assistant who can observe that S maintains eye fixation. E stands at S's side and holds a pencil or small flashlight. E gradaully moves flashlight into S's peripheral visual field and asks S to say "now" or hold up his hand *as soon* as he sees flashlight. Flashlight should be held 10 to 15 inches (25 to 38 cm) from S's head. This should be repeated four to six times to determine accuracy of response (Fig. 9-13).

EVALUATION: Moving flashlight should be perceived at approximately 180° point on an imaginary circle around S's head at sides of eye. Responses may be recorded on a graph (Fig. 9-14).

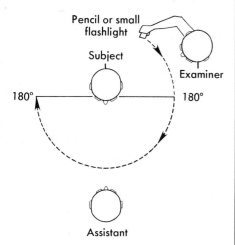

Fig. 9-13. Method of evaluating subject for homonymous hemianopsia (visual field defect).

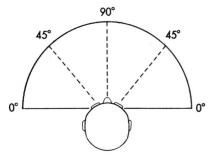

Fig. 9-14. Graph for recording visual field defect. On semicircle shade in number of degrees of estimated visual field defect.

COGNITIVE EVALUATION

Cognitive functions may be disturbed by head injury, stroke (cerebrovascular accident), or other diseases involving the brain. Subsequent to disease or injury impairments in functions such as judgment, memory, reasoning, problem solving, abstract thinking, concentration, sequencing, reading, computation, and generalization of learning may be evident. The therapist should observe for the following[15]:

1. Ability to follow simple or complex instructions
2. Ability to carry over learning from one day to the next
3. Ability to attend to the task at hand (attention and concentration)
4. Ability to follow several steps in a process
5. Ability to anticipate and understand cause and effect
6. Ability to solve problems
7. Ability to plan a sequence of steps to complete a task
8. Ability to interpret signs and symbols
9. Ability to read and perform computations for daily living

Some simple tests of mental functions are often used as part of the neurological examination, and the therapist may wish to use them before or in correlation with performance evaluation.

Memory[11]

Memory is actually an integrated process composed of at least three major steps. These are immediate retention of ongoing events, storage of new events and experiences, and recall of material in storage. Retention may be tested by asking S to repeat a given number of digits. E starts with two or three digits and progresses to seven digits. A normal seven-year-old child can repeat five digits, a ten-year-old can repeat six, and seven digits can be repeated by a fourteen-year-old. Retention may also be tested by asking S to repeat a three-part sentence, such as "I went to my room, ate lunch, and then came to therapy." If it is necessary to use a nonverbal response, S can be asked to carry out a three-step command.

Storage of recent events may be tested informally by asking what S ate at a recent meal, when the last therapy appointment took place, or who were S's recent visitors. S should also be questioned about orientation to time, place, and person.

Recall may be tested during an occupational therapy interview. Questions related to work and leisure histories, educational level, and family members are perfect material for testing recall.[11]

Calculations

Ability to perform calculations may be assessed in a variety of ways.[11] The method will need to be adapted for S's educational level and concomitant disorders, such as aphasia or agraphia. S may be asked to subtract 7 from 100 and then to continue to subtract 7 in succession. Completing simple mathematical problems in writing is another option. More advanced calculations, such as balancing a checkbook, may be used as well. If a nonverbal response is desired, S can be presented with several answers and asked to point to the correct one.[11]

The occupational therapist may evaluate ability to calculate during performance of daily living and therapeutic activities. Measuring foods, fabric, and project materials and calculating elapsed time for baking and cooking are functional applications of ability that E should evaluate.

Abstract thinking

Difficulty performing on an abstract level will result in vagueness and concreteness of responses.[11] To evaluate abstract thinking E may ask what the similarities are between various objects or persons, such as an apple and an orange, wood and coal, and a president and a king. S with difficulties in abstractions tends to be concrete in his or her answers, saying that the apple and orange are both round rather than that they are both fruits, for example. S may also be asked the meaning of simple proverbs, such as "a stitch in time saves nine," "a rolling stone gathers no moss," or "people in glass houses shouldn't throw stones." S with cerebral dysfunction is likely to interpret such sayings literally.[11]

In ordinary daily discourse such individuals often miss the abstract meanings of idiomatic speech that is a large part of American English. The therapist's instructions may be misunderstood, and attempts at subtle humor may be completely missed. S with difficulties in abstraction may not be able to abstract learning or performance from one situation to another or from one person to another. What is possible in the occupational therapy department cannot be done at home or in the hospital room, and what can be performed under the guidance of one therapist may be difficult or impossible when another is giving the instructions.

The occupational therapist should observe for cognitive deficits throughout the interaction with the client during evaluation and treatment procedures. The therapist should note apparent problems and describe in evaluation and progress reports behaviors that support the judgment. Methods for treatment of sensory, perceptual, and cognitive deficits are discussed in Chapters 30 and 31.

REVIEW QUESTIONS

1. Why is sensory and perceptual evaluation necessary and important to occupational therapy?
2. What types of disabilities should be routinely given sensory evaluation?
3. How is light touch sensitivity evaluated? Describe.
4. If the patient recognizes that he was touched but cannot localize the stimulus, what grade would be given on the test for light touch?
5. What are the alternatives for responses in the position sense test?
6. Why is it important to grasp the fingers and wrist laterally during the test for position sense?
7. What are some methods for occluding the patient's vision? What are the alternatives to blindfolding or asking the patient to keep his eyes closed?
8. Define "stereognosis," and describe how it can be evaluated.
9. Define "body scheme," and describe three ways it can be evaluated.
10. Define "motor planning."
11. Describe the clinical test for form perception and spatial relationships.
12. How can you evaluate for presence of a visual field defect?
13. Which odors are used in the olfaction test? Which types of odors should be avoided?
14. Give two examples of manifestations of deficits in abstract thinking during daily living activities.

REFERENCES

1. Ayres, A.J.: Development of the body scheme in children, Am. J. Occup. Ther. **15**:99, 1961.
2. Ayres, A.J.: Methods of evaluating perceptual-motor dysfunction, Proceedings of the Third International Congress, World Federation of Occupational Therapists, Philadelphia, 1962, University of Pennsylvania Printing Office.
3. Benton, A.L., and Schultz, L.M.: Observations of tactual form perception (stereognosis) in preschool children, J. Clin. Psychol. **5**:359, 1949.
4. Bickerstaff, E.R.: Neurological examination in clinical practice, ed. 3, London, 1973, Blackwell Scientific Publications, Ltd.
5. Critchley, M.: The parietal lobes, London, 1953, Edward Arnold and Co.
6. De Jong, R.: The neurologic examination, New York, 1958, Paul B. Hoeber, Inc.
7. De Myer, W.: Technique of the neurologic examination: a programmed text, ed. 2, New York, 1974, McGraw-Hill Book Co.
8. Head, H., et al.: Studies in neurology, London, 1920, Oxford University Press.
9. Kent, B.E.: Sensory testing of the upper limb of adult hemiplegics, master's thesis, Palo Alto, Calif., 1961, Stanford University.
10. MacDonald, J.C.: An investigation of body scheme in adults with cerebral vascular accidents, Am. J. Occup. Ther. **14**:99, 1960.
11. Mayo Clinic and Mayo Foundation: Clinical examinations in neurology, Philadelphia, 1981, W.B. Saunders Co.
12. Rancho Los Amigos Hospital: Procedures for gross sensory evaluation, Downey, Calif., Rancho Los Amigos Hospital. (Unpublished.)
13. Siev, E., and Frieshtat, B.: Perceptual dysfunction in the adult stroke patient: a manual for evaluation and treatment, Thorofare, N.J., 1976, Charles B. Slack, Inc.
14. Silverman, E.H., and Elfant, I.L.: Dysphagia: an evaluation and treatment program for the adult, Am. J. Occup. Ther. **33**:382, 1979.
15. Smith, H.D.: Assessment and evaluation: specific evaluation procedures. In Hopkins, H.L., and Smith, H.D.: Willard and Spackman's occupational therapy, ed. 6, Philadelphia, 1983, J.B. Lippincott Co.
16. Williams, L.A.: A suggested method for evaluating proprioception, stereognosis, and body scheme in adult patients with cerebral vascular accident for occupational therapists, master's project, San Jose, Calif., 1964, San Jose State College.

CHAPTER 10

Evaluation of performance skills

LORRAINE WILLIAMS PEDRETTI

The performance evaluation focuses on the client's abilities and limitations in performing activities of self-maintenance, work, and play-leisure. It is a primary purpose of occupational therapy to facilitate skill in performance of these essential tasks of living. It is important to help the client to create a balance in the quantity of activity in each of these three performance areas, which is healthy for him or her in terms of personality, skills, limitations, needs, values, and life-style.

For the therapist to assay the client's performance profile, the evaluation could begin with the charting of a daily or weekly schedule (see Chapter 4), an activities configuration,[1,10] an interest checklist,[5] or an occupational role history.[2,6] The activities configuration protocol can be used to gather data about the client's values, educational history, and work history, including current or recent work experience, past work experience, and vocational interests and plans. The interest checklist[5] can be used to determine degree of interest in five categories of activities: (1) manual skills, (2) physical sports, (3) social recreation, (4) activities of daily living (ADL), and (5) cultural and educational activities. The occupational role history is used to gather data about past and current occupational roles and the balance between work and leisure roles.[2] Although the interest checklist and the occupational role history were developed for a psychiatric population, they can be adapted for application to clients with a physical dysfunction. In the practice of occupational therapy for physical dysfunction, occupational performance can be overlooked if therapists focus on remedying specific performance components and fail to integrate these with the development of occupational role performance.

An interview and performance evaluation can yield a well-rounded picture of the client's occupational performance. Deficits and imbalances in occupational performance will be apparent. The performance evaluation is fundamental to the development of a comprehensive treatment plan, which deals with performance components that underlie those skills. The performance evaluations to be addressed in this chapter include ADL, home evaluation, driving evaluation, and prevocational and vocational evaluation.

ADL EVALUATION

Procedures for conducting the ADL evaluation are discussed in Chapter 12. The emphasis there is on evaluation of self-care tasks. Fig. 10-1 is a suggested form for recording results of self-care performance evaluation. There are a wide variety of such forms, although they are all somewhat similar. Many treatment facilities have developed their own forms. The practitioner must learn and use the system of recording used in the particular treatment facility.

Home management tasks are evaluated similarly to self-care tasks. The client should first be interviewed to elicit a description of the home and former and present home management responsibilities. Those tasks that the client will need to perform when returning home, as well as those that he or she would like to perform, should be ascertained during the interview. If there are communication disorders, aid of friends or family members may be enlisted to get the information needed. The client may also be questioned about his or her ability to perform each task on the activities list. However, the evaluation is much more meaningful if this is followed by a performance evaluation in the ADL kitchen or apartment of the treatment facility or in the client's home if possible.

The initial tasks should be simple one- or two-step procedures that are not hazardous, such as wiping a dish,

sponging off the table, or turning the water on and off. As the evaluation progresses, tasks graded in complexity and involving safety precautions should be performed, such as making a sandwich and a cup of coffee and vacuuming the carpet. It is assumed here that the therapist has already evaluated motor, sensory, perceptual, and cognitive skills. Consequently the therapist should select tasks and exercise safety precautions in keeping with the client's capabilities and limitations.

Traditionally, home management skills were thought to apply primarily to women clients. However, they are appropriate for men and sometimes for children and adolescents as well. In modern society men are more often living independently or sharing home management responsibilities with the partner. In some homes it will be necessary for a role reversal to occur after onset of a physical disability, and the woman partner may seek employment outside the home for the first time, while the disabled man remains at home. If he will be there alone, at the very least he needs to be able to prepare a simple meal, employ safety precautions, and get emergency aid if needed. The occupational therapist can evaluate potential for remaining at home alone through the activities of home management evaluation. Fig. 10-2 is a suggested form for recording results of the home management evaluation.

Text continued on p. 121.

OCCUPATIONAL THERAPY DEPARTMENT

ACTIVITIES OF DAILY LIVING EVALUATION

Name _____ Age _____ Diagnosis _____ Dom. _____

Mode of ambulation _____ Disability _____

Grading key: I = Independent   D = Dependent
             MiA = Minimal assistance   NA = Not applicable
             MoA = Moderate assistance   0 = Not evaluated
             MaA = Maximal assistance

TRANSFERS AND AMBULATION   BALANCE FOR FUNCTION

	Date	Independent	Assisted	Dependent
Tub or shower				
Toilet				
Wheelchair				
Bed and chair				
Ambulation				
Wheelchair management				
Car				

	Adequate	Inadequate
Sitting		
Standing		
Walking		

SUMMARY OF EVALUATION RESULTS

    Date

INTACT IMPAIRED   REMARKS
_____

INTACT	IMPAIRED		REMARKS
		SENSORY STATUS	
_____	_____	Touch	_____
_____	_____	Pain	_____
_____	_____	Temperature	_____
_____	_____	Position sense	_____
_____	_____	Olfaction	_____
_____	_____	Stereognosis	_____
_____	_____	Visual fields (hemianopsia)	_____
		PERCEPTUAL/CONCEPTUAL TESTS	
_____	_____	Follow directions	_____
_____	_____	Visual spatial (form)	_____
_____	_____	Visual spatial (block design)	_____
_____	_____	Make change	_____
_____	_____	Geometric figures (copy)	_____
_____	_____	Square, circle, triangle, diamond	_____
		Praxis	_____

Continued.

Fig. 10-1. ADL evaluation. (Adapted from Activities of Daily Living, evaluation form OT 461-1, Hartford, Conn., Sept. 1963, The Hartford Easter Seal Rehabilitation Center.)

```
                    Date
              INTACT   IMPAIRED                                    REMARKS

                                FUNCTIONAL RANGE OF MOTION
              _____ _____  Comb hair--two hands _____
              _____ _____  Feed self _____
              _____ _____  Button collar button _____
              _____ _____  Tie apron behind back _____
              _____ _____  Button back buttons _____
              _____ _____  Button cuffs _____
              _____ _____  Size zipper _____
              _____ _____  Tie shoes _____
              _____ _____  Stoop _____
                       _____  Reach shelf _____

              ADL SKILLS
```

EATING	Date					REMARKS
	Grade					
Butter bread						
Cut meat						
Eat with spoon						
Eat with fork						
Drink with straw						
Drink with glass						
Drink with cup						
Pour from pitcher						

UNDRESS	Date					REMARKS
	Grade					
Pants or shorts						
Girdle or garter belt						
Brassiere						
Slip or undershirt						
Dress						
Skirt						
Blouse or shirt						
Slacks or trousers						
Bandana or necktie						
Stockings						
Nightclothes						
Hair net						
Housecoat or bathrobe						
Jacket						
Belt and/or suspenders						
Hat						
Coat						
Sweater						
Mittens or gloves						
Glasses						
Brace						
Shoes						
Socks						
Overshoes						

Fig. 10-1, cont'd. ADL evaluation.

DRESS	Date					REMARKS
		Grade				
Pants or shorts						
Girdle or garter belt						
Brassiere						
Slip or undershirt						
Dress						
Skirt						
Blouse or shirt						
Slacks or trousers						
Bandana or necktie						
Stockings						
Nightclothes						
Hair net						
Housecoat or bathrobe						
Jacket						
Belt and/or suspenders						
Hat						
Coat						
Sweater						
Mittens or gloves						
Glasses						
Brace						
Shoes						
Socks						
Overshoes						

FASTENINGS	Date					REMARKS
		Grade				
Button						
Snap						
Zipper						
Hook and eye						
Garters						
Lace						
Untie shoes						
Velcro						

HYGIENE	Date					REMARKS
		Grade				
Blow nose						
Wash face, hands						
Wash extremities, back						
Brush teeth or dentures						
Brush or comb hair						
Set hair						
Shave or put on makeup						
Clean fingernails						
Trim fingernails, toenails						
Apply deodorant						
Shampoo hair						
Use toilet paper						
Use tampon or sanitary napkin						

Fig. 10-1, cont'd. ADL evaluation.

Continued.

COMMUNICATION	Date					REMARKS
	Grade					
Verbal						
Read						
Hold book						
Turn page						
Write						
Use telephone						
Type						

HAND ACTIVITIES	Date					REMARKS
	Grade					
Handle money						
Handle mail						
Use of scissors						
Open cans, bottles, jars						
Tie package						
Sew (baste)						
Sew button, hook and eye						
Polish shoes						
Sharpen pencil						
Seal and open letter						
Open box						

COMBINED PERFORMANCE ACTIVITIES	Date					REMARKS
	Grade					
Open-close refrigerator						
Open-close door						
Remove and replace object						
Carry objects during locomotion						
Pick up object from floor						
Remove, replace light bulb						
Plug in cord						

OPERATE	Date					REMARKS
	Grade					
Light switches						
Doorbell						
Door locks and handles						
Faucets						
Raise-lower window shades						
Raise-lower venetian blinds						
Raise-lower window						
Open-close drawer						
Hang up garment						

Fig. 10-1, cont'd. ADL evaluation.

OCCUPATIONAL THERAPY DEPARTMENT

ACTIVITIES OF HOME MANAGEMENT

Name_____ Date_____

Address_____

Age_____ Weight_____ Height_____ Role in family_____

Diagnosis_____ Disability_____

Mode of ambulation_____

Limitations or contraindications for activity_____

DESCRIPTION OF HOME
    1. Private house _____
          No. of tooms _____
          No. of floors_____
          Stairs   _____
          Elevators   _____

    2. Apartment house_____
          No. of rooms _____
          No. of floors_____
          Stairs   _____
          Elevators   _____

    3. Diagram of home layout (attach to completed form)

Will patient be required to perform the following activities? If not, who will perform?

    Meal preparation _____ _____
    Baking   _____ _____
    Serving   _____ _____
    Wash dishes   _____ _____
    Marketing   _____ _____
    Child care
      (under 4 years) _____ _____
    Washing   _____ _____
    Hanging clothes   _____ _____
    Ironing   _____ _____
    Cleaning   _____ _____
    Sewing   _____ _____
    Hobbies or
      special interest_____ _____

Does patient really like housework? Yes_____ No_____

Continued.

Fig. 10-2. Activities of home management. (Adapted from Occupational Therapy Department, University Hospital, Ohio State University, Columbus, Ohio.)

ACTIVITIES OF HOME MANAGEMENT

Sitting position: Chair_____ Stool_____ Wheelchair_____

Standing position: Braces_____ Crutches_____ Canes_____

Handedness: Dominant hand_____ Two hands_____ One hand only_____ Assistive_____

Grading key: I = Independent   MaA = Maximal assistance
                MiA = Minimal assistance   D = Dependent
                MoA = Moderate assistance   0 = Not evaluated

CLEANING ACTIVITIES	Date				REMARKS
	Grade				
Pick up object from floor					
Wipe up spills					
Make bed (daily)					
Use dust mop					
Shake dust mop					
Dust low surfaces					
Dust high surfaces					
Mop kitchen floor					
Sweep with broom					
Use dust pan and broom					
Use vacuum cleaner					
Use vacuum cleaner attachments					
Carry light cleaner tools					
Use carpet sweeper					
Clean bathtub					
Change sheets on bed					
Carry pail of water					

MEAL PREPARATION	Date				REMARKS
	Grade				
Turn off water					
Turn off gas or electric range					
Light gas with match					
Pour hot water from pan to cup					
Open packaged goods					
Carry pan from sink to range					
Use can opener					
Handle milk bottle					
Dispose of garbage					
Remove things from refrigerator					
Bend to low cupboards					
Reach to high cupboards					
Peel vegetables					
Cut up vegetables					
Handle sharp tools safely					
Break eggs					
Stir against resistance					
Measure flour					
Use eggbeater					

Fig. 10-2, cont'd. Activities of home management.

ACTIVITIES OF HOME MANAGEMENT—Cont'd

	Date	Grade				REMARKS
Use electric mixer						
Remove batter to pan						
Open oven door						
Carry pan to oven and put in						
Remove hot pan from oven to table						
Roll cookie dough or piecrust						

MEAL SERVICE

	Date	Grade				REMARKS
Set table for four						
Carry four glasses of water to table						
Carry hot casserole to table						
Clear table						
Scrape and stack dishes						
Wash dishes (light soil)						
Wipe silver						
Wash pots and pans						
Wipe up range and work areas						
Wring out dishcloth						

LAUNDRY

	Date	Grade				REMARKS
Wash lingerie (by hand)						
Wring out, squeeze dry						
Hang on rack to dry						
Sprinkle clothes						
Iron blouse or slip						
Fold blouse or slip						
Use washing machine						

SEWING

	Date	Grade				REMARKS
Thread needle and make knot						
Sew on buttons						
Mend rips						
Darn socks						
Use sewing machine						
Crochet						
Knit						
Embroider						
Cut with shears						

HEAVY HOUSEHOLD ACTIVITIES
WHO WILL DO THESE?

	Date				REMARKS
Wash household laundry					
Hang clothes					
Clean range					
Clean refrigerator					
Wax floors					
Marketing					
Turn mattresses					
Wash windows					
Put up curtains					

Continued.

Fig. 10-2, cont'd. Activities of home management.

ACTIVITIES OF HOME MANAGEMENT—Cont'd

                    Date   REMARKS

WORK HEIGHTS   SITTING/STANDING

Best height for   Wheelchair_____ Chair_____ Stool_____
   Ironing   _____
   Mixing   _____
   Dishwashing   _____
   General work   _____

Maximal depth of counter area (normal reach) _____

Maximal useful height above work surface _____

Maximal useful height without counter surface _____

Maximal reach below counter area _____

Best height for chair _____

Best height for stool with back support _____

SUGGESTIONS FOR HOME MODIFICATION
_____
_____
_____
_____
_____
_____
_____
_____
_____
_____
_____
_____
_____

Fig. 10-2, cont'd. Activities of home management.

HOME EVALUATION

When the discharge from the treatment facility is anticipated, a home evaluation should be carried out. The purpose of the home evaluation is to facilitate the client's maximal independence in the living environment. Ideally it should be performed by the physical and occupational therapists together on a visit to the client's home with the client and family members or housemates present. Budgetary and time factors may not allow two professional workers to go to the client's home, however. Therefore either the physical or occupational therapist should be able to perform the evaluation.

Before the visit the client and a family member should be interviewed to determine the client's and family's expectations and the roles the client will assume in the home and community. The cultural or family values regarding a disabled member may influence role expectations and whether or not independence will be encouraged. Willingness and financial ability to make modifications in the home can also be determined.[9]

Sufficient time should be scheduled for the home visit so that the client can demonstrate the required transfer and mobility skills. The therapist may also wish to ask the client to demonstrate selected self-care and home management tasks, which were learned at the treatment facility, in the home environment. The client should use the ambulation aids and any assistive devices that he or she is accustomed to during the evaluation. The therapist should bring a measuring device to determine, for example, width of doorways, height of stairs, and height of bed.

The therapist can begin by explaining the purposes and procedure of the home evaluation to the client and others present, if not done before the visit. The therapist can proceed to take the required measurements while surveying the general arrangement of rooms, furniture, and appliances. It may be helpful to sketch the size and arrangement of rooms for later reference and attach these to the home visit checklist (Fig. 10-3). Once this is completed, the client is involved in demonstrating his or her mobility and transfer skills as designated on the form and in demonstrating performance of essential self-care and home management tasks. The client's ability to use the entrance to the home and transfer to and from an automobile, if to be used, should be included in the home evaluation.

During the performance evaluation the therapist should be observing for safety factors, ease of mobility and performance, and limitations imposed by the environment. If the client requires assistance for transfers and other activities, the caretaker should be instructed in the methods that are appropriate.

At the end of the evaluation the therapist can make a list of problems. Additional safety equipment, assistive devices, home rearrangement, or alteration may be necessary to solve these. The most frequently needed changes are installation of a ramp or railings at the entrance to the home; removal of scatter rugs, extra furniture, and bric-a-brac; removal of door sills; addition of safety grab bars around the toilet and bathtub; rearrangement of furniture to accommodate a wheelchair; rearrangement of kitchen storage; and lowering of the clothes rod in the closet.[9]

When the home evaluation is completed, the therapist should write a report summarizing the information on the form and describing the client's performance in the home. The report should conclude with a summary of the problems the client is encountering and recommendations for their solution that would facilitate independence. Any equipment or alterations that are recommended should be specific in terms of size, building specifications, costs, and sources.

These recommendations are carefully reviewed with the client and his or her family. This is done with tact and diplomacy in a way that gives them options and freedom to refuse or consider alternative possibilities. Family finances may be a limiting factor in carrying out needed changes. The social worker may be involved in working out funding for needed equipment and alterations, and the client should be made aware of this service when cost is discussed.[9]

The therapist should include recommendations regarding the feasibility of the client's discharge to the home environment or remaining in or managing the home alone, if these apply.

If a home visit is not possible, much of the information can be gained by interviewing the client and family member following a trial home visit. The family member or caretaker may be instructed to complete the home visit checklist and provide photographs or sketches of the rooms and their arrangements. Problems encountered by the client during the trial home visit should be discussed and the necessary recommendations for their solution made, as described earlier.[9]

DRIVING EVALUATION

Adaptive driving has become possible for an increasing number of disabled persons. Special devices and adaptations to motor vehicles along with special training of the disabled driver have made it possible for some severely disabled persons to drive. There are evaluation programs that can be obtained through the state Department of Motor Vehicles and Licensing. Most large rehabilitation centers have driving evaluation programs.[7] Some have driving simulators for preroad testing.

The occupational therapist is usually not responsible for the actual driving evaluation. However, through various motor, sensory, perceptual, cognitive, and performance evaluations, pertinent information relevant to driving potential can be obtained and contributed by the occupational therapist. During evaluation and treatment of the client, the therapist is observing and assessing functions that subserve driving skills. These include reaction time; visual acuity; peripheral vision; color, figure-ground, spatial, vertical-horizontal perception; ocular movements; hearing; and involuntary movements. Cognitive and behavioral manifestations, such as attention, concentration, impatience, agitation, poor memory, confusion, problem-solving skills, safety awareness, and poor judgment can also be noted.[3,8]

Physical and performance skills that are necessary for driving can also be evaluated by the occupational therapist.

HOME VISIT CHECKLIST

Name _____ Therapist _____

Address _____ Date _____

Diagnosis _____ Disability _____

Type of home   Apartment _____ Floor, if apt. _____

                 Private home ____ No. of rooms _____ No. of floors _____

ENTRANCE TO HOME
1. Elevator _____ Stairs _____
2. Number of stairs _____
3. Height of stairs _____
4. Is there a handrail? _____ Left _____ Right _____ (facing house)
5. Are there other entrances that can be used? Describe _____
_____
_____
6. Is construction of a ramp feasible? _____
7. Is addition of a handrail feasible? _____
    Comments _____
_____
_____

BEDROOM
1. Width of doorway _____
2. Is there a doorsill? _____
3. Height of bed _____
4. Is bed suitable for attachment of   side rails? _____ trapeze bar? _____
5. Can furniture be arranged more conveniently? _____
6. Can patient reach closets? _____ bureaus? _____
7. Is there room for a wheelchair to maneuver? _____
8. Is there room for additional furniture (e.g., commode seat)? _____

BATHROOM
1. Width of doorway _____
2. Is there a doorsill? _____
3. Type of bathtub: roll rim _____ square rim _____ wide square rim _____
4. Can wheelchair get close to   sink? _____ toilet? _____ bathtub? _____
5. Is tub enclosed by   shower curtain? _____ sliding doors? _____
6. Is there a separate shower stall? _____
7. Is bathroom on same floor as   bedroom? _____ living room? _____ kitchen? _____
8. Is it feasible to install handrails on   bathtub? _____ walls? _____ toilet? _____
9. Additional comments _____
_____
_____
_____
_____

Fig. 10-3. Home visit checklist. (Adapted from The Hartford Easter Seal Rehabilitation Center, 1964, Hartford, Conn.)

KITCHEN
1. Width of doors _____
2. Is there a doorsill? _____
3. Is there room for movement of wheelchair? _____
4. Are cupboards within reach? _____
5. Can patient use kitchen utilities? _____ (range, sink, refrigerator)
6. Is rearrangement of furniture feasible? _____
7. Additional comments _____
    _____
    _____

OTHER ROOMS
1. Width of doors _____
2. Are there doorsills? _____
3. Are light switches in easy reach? _____
4. Would furniture rearrangement be feasible? _____
5. Is telephone conveniently located? _____
6. If needed, is there suitable space for installation of parallel bars? _____

FUNCTIONAL ACTIVITIES OF PATIENT
1. Can patient enter and leave home independently? _____
    If not, what assistance is needed? _____
2. Can the patient move about the home freely? _____
    If not, comment on limitations. _____
    _____
    _____

3. Which transfer activities is patient unable to perform independently?
    Bed to wheelchair _____
    Chair to bed _____
    Toilet _____
    Bathtub _____
    Shower _____
    Automobile _____
4. Self-care activities: Comment on performance and limitations imposed by home
    environment, if any. _____
    _____
    _____

5. Home management activities _____
    _____
    _____

PROBLEM LIST _____
_____
_____
_____
_____
_____

RECOMMENDATIONS FOR HOME MODIFICATION/SPECIAL EQUIPMENT _____
_____
_____
_____
_____
_____
_____
_____

Fig. 10-3, cont'd. Home visit checklist.

Muscle strength, joint range of motion, coordination, endurance, ability to use splints or other adapted devices, and transfer skills are some of these.[7,8]

Candidates for evaluation

The physician may play a primary role in facilitating the driving evaluation and certifying that the client is a candidate for driving. Okamoto[7] suggested the following criteria for selection of candidates:

1. The client wants to drive and is realistic about his or her limitations.
2. The client's condition is stable or improving.
3. The client is responsible and conscientious about taking medication. If there is a seizure disorder, drug compliance is excellent, and the client has been free of symptoms for at least 6 months.
4. The client has no history of drug or alcohol abuse.
5. The client has been well motivated to achieve maximal function and is competent in necessary ADL.
6. The client has adequate communication skills, visual-spatial perception, voluntary movement, and reasoning for safe driving.
7. The client is rational and demonstrates predictable behavior. Explosive, aggressive, hostile, paranoid, or suicidal behavior should not be present.
8. The client's family should be supportive and firm.

The driving evaluation

When data have been gathered and the client is thought to be a candidate for driving, a laboratory evaluation can be made. This may involve use of a stationary vehicle to determine transfer skills, basic ability to handle controls, and necessary adaptive equipment. A driving simulator, if available, can be used to assess the client's ability to handle hypothetical road situations. A driving inspector who specializes in evaluating diabled persons may next assess the client in a training car. The therapist can write or telephone the state Department of Motor Vehicles or local driving schools to ascertain the availability of such experts in a given region.[7]

Adaptive devices

Standard modifications or specially designed assistive devices and custom modifications may be necessary to enable driving. Power steering, power brakes, and automatic transmission may be adequate adaptations for the less severely disabled client. Hand controls will be required for the client who has significant lower extremity disability and for those with both lower and upper extremity disabilities. These hand controls may be push-pull, twist-push, or right angle–push types. The steering wheel may have a spinner or plain knob, latch, palm grip, tri-pin, driving ring, cuff, V-grip, or valve. Hooks or extensions may be used for brakes, turn signals, and gear selector. Pedals may be raised by attaching blocks or may need to be transferred to the opposite side. To facilitate transfers, sliding boards, bars, loops, straps, or floor boards are possible adaptive devices. For safe and comfortable seating, a cushion, safety belt, and chest harness may be used.[7] Special adaptations that are available for cars or vans include ramps and lifts for vans, car-top carriers for wheelchairs, and wheelchair locks that eliminate the necessity of transferring the individual to the seat of the van and allow him or her to drive from the wheelchair.[8] The van that is fitted with lifts, wheelchair locks, and force-amplifying control systems[3] has significantly increased the mobility of the severely disabled. The potential long-term benefits of such a van to the client must be evaluated against the high cost of the vehicle before it is obtained.[7]

The unsafe driver

The client may be eager to return to driving in spite of deficits, which may not be recognized or may be denied, that make driving hazardous.[8] The client may have a valid driver's license and commence driving against the advice of the physician and therapist. In such instances, Okamoto[7] suggests that the physician discuss the medical and legal implications with the client and the family; obtain a signed statement from the client or a family member that the discussion took place, risks were explained, and that driving is contraindicated; and for the patient who refuses to follow recommendations, a letter to

someone in the state Department of Motor Vehicles should be considered. The physician must use good judgment and should consult as needed with a lawyer or officer of the state medical association.

PREVOCATIONAL AND VOCATIONAL EVALUATION

Prevocational and vocational evaluation and training programs are specialized areas in occupational therapy. The ultimate goal of such programs is to estimate the client's vocational potential, measure basic skills necessary for work, and aid in setting appropriate vocational goals.

The occupational therapist is an appropriate evaluator of prevocational and vocational potential because of his or her personal skills and professional knowledge. The therapist is interested in working with people; has the ability to perceive, observe, and analyze performance and performance problems; has knowledge of dysfunctions; possesses teaching and motivating skills; can perform activity and task analyses; and knows or has the ability to learn a wide variety or work-related tasks and skills.[4]

Prevocational evaluation, usually performed by the occupational therapist, includes evaluation of physical assets and limitations; ADL performance, including transfer and transportation skills; perceptual and cognitive functions; and general educational abilities,[4] (for example, reading, computation, change making, and the recognition and interpretation of street signs and traffic signals).

Work evaluation assesses specific work skills using a real or simulated work situation.[4] Work habits and attitudes are also observed and evaluated. Work evaluation may be carried out by the occupational therapist following the prevocational assessment. However, work evaluation may also be performed by a vocational evaluator.

The prevocational or work evaluations may reveal the need to develop the necessary physical, performance, or psychosocial skills required of a worker. The occupational therapist may then engage the client in a work adjustment program. This has as its goals the development of physical capacities, such as transfer skills or speed of motion; psychosocial skills, such as ability to be supervised or get along with co-workers; and work habits, such as punctuality and perseverance at a task.

The vocational counselor coordinates the vocational evaluation. The vocational counselor gathers data from pertinent medical, psychological, social, educational, and vocational histories; examines environmental and cultural aspects of the client's situations[4] as they relate to employment; receives reports of prevocational and work evaluation; may counsel the client and administer specific aptitude or interest tests; and sets appropriate vocational goals with the client. The vocational counselor may assist the client in securing sheltered or competitive employment as a final outcome of the vocational evaluation program.

Role of the occupational therapist

The occupational therapist can function at all levels of evaluation, but his or her skills are most suitable for prevocational and work adjustment programs.

Before evaluation is started, the client should be at or near the individual maximal rehabilitation potential. The focus of the program will be different from that of the rehabilitation program because there is emphasis on

work speed, quality of products, concentration on task with minimal socialization, promptness, and perseverance. The occupational therapist evaluates physical resources (capacities, deficits), ADL, social behavior for work, emotional maturity, vocational development, general intellectual abilities, and performance of real or simulated jobs. Table 10-1 is a list of the skills and abilities that may be evaluated by the occupational therapist. A wide variety of forms have been devised to record the results of evaluation (Fig. 10-4).

A report of the findings of the prevocational and work evaluations should be prepared for the vocational counselor, who will use it to help the client select appropriate goals and determine the next step in the vocationally oriented program.

Methods of evaluation

A variety of methods can be used to evaluate work potential. Occupational therapists may use craft activities to assess such factors as use of tools, manual dexterity, work quality, computation, perceptual skills, and work speed. Work samples or simulated work stations may be used to evaluate specific work skills as well as work habits and attitudes. Commercial systems of evaluation are also available. Kester[4] lists and describes several such systems.

To develop work samples or work stations the vocational counselor or the occupational therapist may survey the community to determine the job market and types of industries and businesses that are supported there. Suitable jobs can be selected and analyzed for their performance requirements. Some employers may be willing to provide the necessary equipment and material for a work sample test or work station. Some possibilities are clerical jobs, assembly work, business machines operation, and garment construction. The *Dictionary of Occupational Titles* (DOT) is a helpful resource for job descriptions and requirements. It is published by the U.S. Department of Labor Employment and Training Administration and is available from the U.S. Government Printing Office.

More realistic work evaluation may be effected through assignment of the client to sheltered employment or a job within the health care facility or cooperating agency on a trial basis. Under these conditions the supervisor, who is someone other than the therapist or counselor, should be apprised of the client's skills and limitations, vocational goals, and specific aspects of performance that are to be observed and evaluated. The standards of evaluation should also be clear to the work supervisor, that is, is the client to perform at

---

Table 10-1
Skills and abilities for prevocational evaluation in occupational therapy

Physical resources-capacities	General abilities	Work behavior and attitudes	Work skills
Strength	Computational skills	Interpersonal skills, relationships	Dexterity
ROM	Reading skills	Reaction to supervision	Work speed
Sensation-perception-cognition	Mechanical aptitude	Cooperation with co-workers	Quality of work
Speech-hearing	Self-care independence	Interest	Use of tools and machines
Vision	Hygiene, appearance	Motivation	Ability to follow instructions
Ability and tolerance for	Transfer-transportation abilities	Concentration/perseverance at task	Verbal
Sitting		Emotional reactions	Written
Standing		Family concerns	Demonstrated
Walking		Child care	Designed
Running		Home management responsibilities affecting employment	Demonstrated aptitudes
Lifting-carrying			
Grasp-handling			
Pushing-pulling			
Climbing-crouching			
Presence of chronic pain			
Effect on performance			

PREVOCATIONAL EVALUATION

PATIENT PROGRESS REPORT*

Name_____ Address_____ Phone_____
Admission date_____ Schedule_____ Days per week_____ Hours per day_____
Type of transportation facility used _____ Driver's license_____
Diagnosis_____
Appliances used_____ Dominant hand_____
Period of evaluation: From _____ To _____
Jobs performed _____

OBSERVATIONS

PHYSICAL ASPECTS	WORK TIME (%)	SUP.	AV.	LTD.	POOR
Walking					
Standing					
Sitting					
Lifting (in lb)					
Carrying (in lb)					
Bending					
Climbing stairs					
Speech					
Hearing					
Vision					
Working speed					
Self-care					
Bimanual dexterity					
Finger dexterity Unaffected hand					
Finger dexterity Affected hand					

INTELLECTUAL ASPECTS					
Learning speed					
Retention					
Reading ability					
Work accuracy					
Arithmetical ability					
Judgment					
Problem solving					
Writing ability					

PERSONALITY ASPECTS					
Neatness					
Adaptability					
Regularity					
Punctuality					
Reliability					
Interest					
Initiative					
Ability to work independently					
Personal habits					
Interpersonal relations					
Conformance to rules					
Cooperativeness					
Perseverance					
Desire for employment					

COMMENTS: Include *brief* explanation pointing up any of above ratings checked.
Include brief summary of machines operated and jobs done.
Include any precautions to be observed with patient.

*NOTE: Rating terms, as used, are to be interpreted as being applicable to
performance in regular, competitive employment. Sup. = Superior,
AV. = Average, and Ltd. = Limited.

Fig. 10-4. Prevocational evaluation patient progress report. (Adapted from The Hartford
Easter Seal Rehabilitation Center, 1964, Hartford, Conn.)

minimal standards required for the job or will lesser performance be acceptable at this stage in rehabilitation?

Candidates for evaluation

Who is selected for prevocational evaluation? Generally employment should be a consideration for adolescents, young adults, and older adults who are involved in rehabilitation for physical dysfunction. This group will include those who have never worked, those who have worked and will be returning to the same or similar jobs, and those who have worked and must seek a change in occupation.

The candidate should have achieved or have the potential to achieve (1) adequate independence in self-care with or without attendant care, (2) adequate transportation to and from the work place with or without assistance, and (3) adequate physical performance and psychosocial skills to perform in a work setting. Inadequate vocational development may be a problem for some clients, especially those in the adolescent and young adult groups. With these individuals the prevocational program may need to include development of work habits, identification as a worker, and vocational exploration and choice making.

Alternatives to work

The result of the prevocational evaluation may be that the client is not a candidate for employment. Age, severity of the dysfunction, or serious psychosocial limitations can make the goal of employment unrealistic. What are the alternatives for such individuals?

Occupational therapists can play a primary role in helping to select alternatives and in actively developing or working in alternative programs. The occupational therapist should not overlook the client's leisure needs and should evaluate performance of potential avocational pursuits that can be done independently at home. This is an area that therapists have neglected and relegated to a lesser status in their professional work. Yet avocational pursuits are an integral part of each person's occupational performance and contribute to health and well-being.

The occupational therapist can facilitate support, maintenance, or activity

groups or day-care programs within the health care facility, if funding allows, or seek alternative community programs for the disabled. Examples of these are arthritis or stroke clubs that have been organized in many communities. Some disabled individuals are able to take part in senior citizen and adult education programs that are offered to all residents of a community.

It is necessary for the occupational therapist to explore the alternatives and evaluate the client for his or her ability to participate. It is often necessary for the occupational therapist, or a friend or family member whose help has been enlisted, to accompany the client to community programs the first few times to facilitate the client's adjustment and solve any problems that prohibit full participation.

The occupational therapist has an important role to play in prevocational evaluation. Together with the vocational counselor, social worker, and other pertinent members of the health care team, occupational therapy can facilitate the client's progress toward self-sufficiency through employment.

If employment goals are not a feasible outcome of the prevocational evaluation, occupational therapy can offer alternatives that can give meaning and satisfaction to the client's life.

REVIEW QUESTIONS

1. List the steps in the activities of home management evaluation.
2. What is the purpose of the home evaluation?
3. List the steps in the home evaluation.
4. Who should be involved in a comprehensive home evaluation?
5. What kinds of things are assessed in a home evaluation?
6. How does the therapist record and report results of the home evaluation and make the necessary recommendations?
7. Describe the role of the occupational therapist in the driving evaluation.
8. List eight criteria that can be used to select potential candidates for driving.
9. List six physical and performance skills that can help to determine driving potential.

10. Describe the differences between prevocational evaluation, work adjustment, and vocational evaluation.
11. What is the role of the occupational therapist in vocationally oriented programs?
12. List three criteria the client should meet before embarking on a vocational evaluation.
13. What are three methods that may be used to assess vocational potential?

REFERENCES

1. Cynkin, S.: Occupational therapy: toward health through activities, Boston, 1979, Little, Brown & Co.
2. Florey, L.L., and Michelman, S.M.: Occupational role history: a screening tool for psychiatric occupational therapy, Am. J. Occup. Ther. **36**:301, 1982.
3. Gurgold, G.D., and Harden, D.H.: Assessing the driving potential of the handicapped, Am. J. Occup. Ther. **32**:41, 1978.
4. Kester, D.L.: Prevocational and vocational assessment. In Hopkins, H.L., and Smith, H.D., editors: Willard and Spackman's occupational therapy, ed. 6, Philadelphia, 1983, J.B. Lippincott Co.
5. Matsusuyu, J.: The interest checklist, Am. J. Occup. Ther. **23**:323, 1969.
6. Moorhead, L.: The occupational history, Am. J. Occup. Ther. **23**:329, 1969.
7. Okamoto, G.A.: Physical medicine and rehabilitation, Philadelphia, 1984, W.B. Saunders Co.
8. Spencer, E.A.: Functional restoration: theory, principles and techniques. In Hopkins H.L., and Smith, H.D.: Willard and Spackman's occupational therapy, ed. 6, Philadelphia, 1983, J.B. Lippincott Co.
9. Trombly, C.A., and Scott, A.D.: Occupational therapy for physical dysfunction, Baltimore, 1977, Williams & Wilkins.
10. Watanabe, S.: Activities configuration, Regional institute on the evaluation process, Final Rep. RSA-123-T-68, New York, 1968, American Occupational Therapy Association.

PART 3

TREATMENT METHODS

CHAPTER 11

Therapeutic activities

LORRAINE WILLIAMS PEDRETTI

Therapeutic activities here are defined as arts, crafts, recreational, sports, leisure, self-care, home management, and work activities that may be used or adapted for use to meet one or more of the following therapeutic objectives: (1) to develop or maintain strength, endurance, work tolerance, range of motion (ROM), and coordination; (2) to practice and use voluntary, automatic movement in goal-directed tasks; (3) to provide for purposeful use of and general exercise to affected parts; (4) to explore vocational potential or train in work adjustment skills; (5) to improve sensation, perception, and cognition; and (6) to improve socialization skills and enhance emotional growth and development.

Early in the history of occupational therapy the psychological effects of the performance of purposeful activity were considered primary in the treatment of persons with physical dysfunction.[6] It was later recognized that physical benefits accrued from the performance of activity, and kinesiological considerations were also applied in the selection of appropriate therapeutic activities.

The uniqueness of occupational therapy lies in its emphasis on the extensive use of purposeful activity. This emphasis gives occupational therapy the theoretical foundation for its broad application to both psychosocial and physical dysfunction, as well as to health maintenance. In the context of occupational therapy purposeful activity is defined as "tasks or experiences in which the person actively participates" and that elicit coordination between physical, emotional, and cognitive systems.[3] During performance of purposeful activity, attention is directed to the task itself "rather than to the internal processes required for achievement of the task."[3] This definition reaffirms the concept that purposeful activity has an autonomous goal beyond the motor function required to perform the task.[1] For example, sawing wood may have the autonomous objective of securing parts for construction of a bookshelf, while the therapeutic objectives may be to strengthen shoulder and elbow musculature or to provide for release of aggression. Therefore purposeful motor function is the use of the neuromuscular system to accomplish the inherent or autonomous goal of the activity being performed. By this definition the conscious effort of the client performing the activity is focused on the ultimate objective of the movement and not on

the movement itself.[1] The client directs and is in control of the movement. As the client becomes absorbed in the performance of the activity, the affected parts are used more naturally and with less fatigue.[15] This notion is supported by neurophysiological experiments that have shown that concentration on motion has a detrimental effect on that motion and that muscles controlled by conscious attention and focused effort fatigue rapidly. Therefore it is neurologically more sound to focus attention on the activity and its autonomous goal than on the muscles or motions being used to accomplish the activity. The inherent goal of the activity may be so obvious that the unsophisticated observer may fail to see the more subtle therapeutic objectives. Likewise the client engaged in the activity may have difficulty comprehending its importance to his ultimate well-being.[1]

Traditionally occupational therapy has been associated with the use of arts and crafts as therapeutic modalities. Arts and crafts are still in use as treatment methods and constitute an effective and substantial portion of many occupational therapy programs. But occupational therapy is not restricted to the use of arts and crafts, and the scope of its treatment methods has changed and broadened considerably over the years. Other purposeful activities used in treatment programs include activities for daily living (for example, self-care, travel, communications, and home management activities). In prevocational programs simulated work activities or actual job samples are used to evaluate potential work skills of clients. Leisure or avocational activities may be used for exercising, physical conditioning, and establishing or maintaining the physical and psychosocial functions of the individual.

In addition to purposeful, goal-oriented activities therapists have become increasingly skillful in the use of therapeutic exercise and in sensorimotor approaches to treatment, both traditionally belonging to the field of physical therapy. These methods are used by some occupational therapists because they enable the development of the individual's ability to perform activities that will increase the level of independent functioning, a primary aim of occupational therapy. Occupational therapists also apply the principles of therapeutic exercise and of the sensorimotor approaches to treatment to activities for the greatest therapeutic benefit. The sensorimotor approaches are discussed in Chapters 13 through 17. Principles of therapeutic exercise are outlined in this chapter.

THERAPEUTIC EXERCISE

Therapeutic exercise is the prescription of bodily movement or muscle contraction to correct an impairment, improve musculoskeletal function, or maintain a state of well-being.[7,8] Many of its principles are applicable to therapeutic activity, and many occupational therapists use it in treatment programs. If used by occupational therapists, its purposes should be to prepare the client for performance of functional activities and to augment therapeutic activity and performance skills phases of the occupational therapy program.

General principles

After partial or complete denervation of muscle and during inactivity or disuse, muscle strength decreases. When strength is inadequate, substitution patterns or "trick movements"[16] are likely to develop. A substitution is the attempt to achieve a functional goal by using muscle groups and patterns of

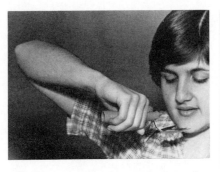

Fig. 11-1. Shoulder abduction is used to compensate for weak elbow flexion.

motion not ordinarily used because of loss or weakness of the muscles normally used to perform the movements.[16] An example is using shoulder abduction to achieve a hand-to-mouth movement if elbow flexors cannot perform against gravity (Fig. 11-1). When muscle loss is permanent, some substitution patterns may be desirable as a compensatory measure to improve performance of functional activities. However, many are not desirable, and it is often the aim of therapeutic exercise to prevent or correct substitution patterns.[16]

A muscle must contract to its maximal capacity to effect an increase in strength. Therefore strengthening exercises are not effective if the contraction is insufficient. Excess strengthening, on the other hand, may result in muscle fatigue, pain, and temporary reduction of strength.[9] If a muscle is overworked, it will fatigue and will not be able to contract. Selection of the type of exercise must suite the muscle grade and the client's fatigue tolerance level. Fatigue level varies from individual to individual, and the threshold for muscle fatigue decreases in pathological states.[9] Many clients may not be sensitive to fatigue or may push themselves beyond tolerance in the belief that this will hasten recovery. This means that the therapist must make a careful assessment of the client's muscle power and capacity for exercise. The therapist must also supervise the client closely and observe for signs of fatigue. These signs may be slowed performance, distractibility, perspiration, increase in rate of respiration, performance of exercise pattern through a decreased ROM, and inability to complete the prescribed number of repetitions.

Purposes

The general purposes of exercise are (1) to develop awareness of normal movement patterns and improve voluntary, automatic movement responses; (2) to develop strength and endurance in patterns of movement that are acceptable and necessary and will not produce deformity; (3) to improve coordination, regardless or strength; (4) to increase specific power of desired isolated muscles or muscle groups; (5) to aid in overcoming ROM deficits; (6) to increase strength of muscles that will power hand splints, mobile arm supports, and other devices; (7) to increase work tolerance and physical endurance through increased strength; and (8) to prevent or eliminate contractures developing as a result of imbalanced muscle power by strengthening the antagonistic muscles.[13]

Prerequisites for use

For therapeutic exercise to be effective the client must meet certain criteria. Therapeutic exercise is most effective in the treatment of orthopedic disorders, such as fractures and arthritis and lower motor neuron disorders that produce weakness and flaccidity. Examples of these are peripheral nerve injuries and diseases, poliomyelitis, GuillainBarré syndrome, infectious neuronitis, and spinal cord injuries and diseases.

Therapeutic exercise is contraindicated for clients who have poor general health or inflamed joints or who have had recent surgery.[12] As defined and described here, it cannot be used effectively with those who have spasticity and lack voluntary control of isolated motion or those who cannot control dyskinetic movement. These latter conditions are likely to occur in upper motor neuron disorders. It may not be useful where there is severely limited joint ROM as a result of well-established, permanent contractures.

The candidate for therapeutic exercise must be medically able to participate in the exercise regime, able to understand the directions for the exercise and its purposes, and interested and motivated to perform the exercise. The client must have available motor pathways, as demonstrated by muscle power on demonstrated muscle testing, and the potential for recovery or improvement of strength, ROM, coordination, or movement patterns, as the goal may be. It is important that some sensory feedback is available to the client. This means that sensation must be at least partially intact so that the client can perceive motion and position of the exercised part and have some sense of superficial and deep pain. Muscles and tendons must be intact, stable, and free to move. Joints must be able to move through an effective ROM for those types of exercise that use joint motion as part of the procedure. The client should be relatively free of pain during motion and should be able to perform isolated, coordinated movement. If there is any dyskinetic movement, the client shoud be able to control it so that the exercise procedure can be performed as prescribed.[12]

Precautions

Generally joints should be worked through pain-free ROM only.[8] Weak muscles should not be overstretched in the exercise procedure. Weak muscles that are overstretched will function less efficiently.[9] Excess fatigue of muscles should be avoided. Muscles around sites of recent surgery, such as tendon transplants, tendon grafts, skin grafts, and joint and bone reconstruction, should not be exercised until medical clearance has been obtained. Unless directed by the physician the therapist should not exercise inflamed joints with active or resistive techniques. Sometimes isometric contractions are advised to maintain muscle strength while not moving the inflamed joint.[11]

Types of muscle contraction used[5,9]

ISOMETRIC CONTRACTION. During an isometric contraction there is no joint motion, and the muscle length remains the same. A muscle and its antagonist may be contracted at any point in the ROM to stabilize a joint. This may be without resistance or against some outside resistance, such as the therapist's hand or a tabletop. An example of isometric exercise of triceps

against resistance is pressing against the tabletop with the ulnar border of the forearm while the elbow remains at 90°.

ISOTONIC OR CONCENTRIC CONTRACTION. During an isotonic contraction there is joint motion, and the muscle shortens. This may be done with or without resistance. Isotonic contractions may be performed in positions with gravity assisting or gravity eliminated or against gravity, according to the client's muscle grade and the goal of the exercise. An example of isotonic contraction of the biceps is lifting a fork to the mouth during eating. If a filled cup is lifted to the mouth, the biceps contracts against resistance.

ECCENTRIC CONTRACTION. When muscles contract eccentrically, the tension in the muscle increases or remains constant while the muscle lengthens. This may be done with or without resistance. An example of an eccentric contraction performed against no resistance is the slow lowering of the arm to the table. The biceps is contracting eccentrically in this instance. An example of eccentric contraction against resistance is the controlled return of a pail of sand lifted from the ground. Here, the bicep is contracting eccentrically to control the rate and coordination of the elbow extension in setting the pail on the ground.

Exercise classification

The type of exercise selected will depend on muscle grade, muscle endurance, joint mobility, diagnosis and physical condition, treatment goals, position of the client, and desirable plane of movement.

PASSIVE EXERCISE. The purpose of passive exercise is to maintain ROM, thereby preventing contractures and adhesions. It is used when absent or minimal muscle strength (grades O-T) precludes the active motion or when active exercise is contraindicated because of the client's physical condition. During the exercise procedure the joint or joints to be exercised are moved through their normal ranges manually by the therapist or client or mechanically by an external device, such as a pulley or counterbalance sling. The joint proximal to the joint being exercised should be stabilized during the exercise procedure[5] (Fig. 11-2).

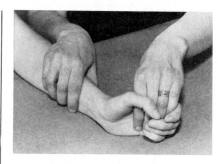

Fig. 11-2. Therapist is performing passive exercise of wrist.

PASSIVE STRETCH. The purpose of passive stretch or forced exercise is to increase ROM. Essentially this is passive exercise, as just described, with a gentle, firm push or pull at the end of the joint motion. If the client's muscle grades are adequate, the client can move the part actively through the available ROM, and the therapist can take it a little further thus forcing or stretching the soft structures around the joint.

The procedure requires a good understanding of joint anatomy and muscle function. It should be carried out cautiously under good medical supervision. Muscles to be stretched should be in a relaxed state.[9] The therapist should never force muscles when pain is present unless ordered by the physician to work through pain. Gentle, firm stretching held for a few seconds is more effective and less hazardous than quick, short stretching. The parts around the area being stretched should be stabilized and compensatory movements should be prevented. Incorrect stretching procedures can produce muscle tearing, joint fracture, and inflammatory edema.[8]

ACTIVE-ASSISTED EXERCISE. The goal of active-assisted exercise is to increase strength of trace to poor muscles while maintaining ROM as well. In active-assisted exercise the client moves the part actively through the range possible, and the remainder of the range is

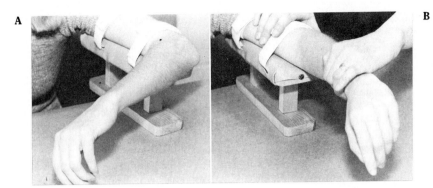

Fig. 11-3. A, Client extends elbow from full flexion toward extension in gravity-eliminated plane to degree possible actively. **B,** Therapist assists client to complete ROM.

completed by manual or mechanical assistance (Fig. 11-3). Mechanical assistance may be supplied by slings, pulleys, weights, springs, or elastic bands (Fig. 11-4). In the case of trace muscles the client merely contracts the muscle, and the therapist completes the entire ROM. This exercise is graded by decreasing the amount of assistance until the client can perform active exercises.[5,9]

ACTIVE EXERCISE. Active motion through the complete ROM with gravity eliminated or against gravity may be used for poor to fair muscles for the purpose of improving strength, with the added benefit of maintaining ROM as well. It may be used with higher muscle grades for the maintenance of strength and ROM when resistance is contraindicated. In this type of exercise the client moves the part through the complete ROM independently. If the exercise is performed in a gravity-eliminated plane, a powdered surface, skateboard, deltoid aid, or free-moving suspension sling may be used to reduce the resistance offered by friction. It is graded by adding resistance as strength improves.[5,9]

RESISTIVE EXERCISE. Resistive exercise is primarily for increasing strength of fair plus to normal muscles but may also be helpful for producing relaxation of the antagonistic muscles of the contracting muscles. This latter purpose can be useful if increased range is desired for stretching or relaxing spastic muscles.

The client performs muscle contraction against resistance and moves the part through the full ROM. The resistance applied should be the maximum that the muscle is capable of contracting against. Resistance may be applied manually or by weights, springs, elastic bands, sandbags, or special exercise devices. It is graded by progressively increasing the amount of resistance[5,9] (Fig. 11-5).

One specialized type of resistive exercise is the DeLorme method of progressive resistive exercise (PRE). PRE is based on the overload principle (increasing the load on the muscle) and the principle that muscles perform more efficiently if given a "warm-up" period. During the exercise procedure small loads are used initially. These are increased gradually after each set of 10 repetitions of the desired movement. The muscle is thus warmed up to prepare to exert its maximal power for the final 10 repetitions. The exercise procedure consists of three sets of 10 repetitions each, with resistance applied as follows: (1) First set, 10 repetitions at 50% of maximal resistance; (2) second set, 10 repetitions at 75% of maximal resistance; and (3) third set, 10 repetitions at maximal resistance. The client is instructed to inhale during the shortening contraction and exhale during the relaxation or eccentric contraction.[8]

An example of a PRE is a triceps extending the elbow against a 12-pound maximal resistance, performing 10 repetitions against 6 pounds of resistance, 10 repetitions against 9 pounds, and the final 10 repetitions against 12 pounds.

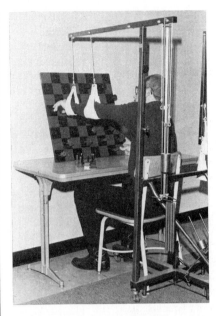

Fig. 11-4. Active-assisted exercise with deltoid aid assisting shoulder flexion in reaching activity.

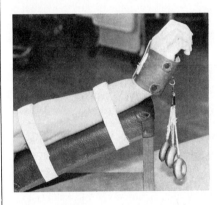

Fig. 11-5. Resistive exercise to wrist extensors, using forearm stabilizer and handcuff to compensate for inadequate grasp.

Maximal resistance, the amount of resistance the muscle can lift through the ROM 10 times, is determined by contracting the muscle and moving the part through the full ROM against progressively increasing loads for sets of 10 repetitions until the maximal load that can be lifted 10 times is reached.

At the beginning of the treatment program it is often difficult for the therapist to determine the maximal resistance that the client is capable of taking. This may be because (1) the client may not know how to exert maximal effort, (2) the client may be reluctant to exercise strenuously for fear of pain or reinjury, (3) the client may be unwilling or unable to endure discomfort, and (4) the client may have difficulty with timing of exercises.

Experience of the therapist and trial and error will aid in determining maximal resistance when this is difficult. The therapist should estimate the amount of resistance the client can take and then add or subtract resistance (for example, weight or tension) until the client can perform the sets of repetitions adequately.

The exercises should be performed once daily four or five times weekly and rest periods of 2 to 4 minutes should be allowed between each set of 10 repetitions. Modifications of the exercise procedure may be made to suit individual needs. Some possibilities are 10 repetitions at 25% of maximal resistance, 10 repetitions at 50%, 10 repetitions at 75%, and 10 repetitions at maximal resistance. Another possibility is 5 repetitions at 50% and 10 repetitions at maximal resistance. Still another possibility is to omit the second set of exercises. Adjustments in the first two sets of exercises may be made to suit the capacity of the individual.

Another approach is the "Oxford" technique, essentially a reverse of the DeLorme method. The exercise sequence begins with 100% resistance and decreases to 75% and then 50% on subsequent sets of 10 repetitions each.[8] The greatest gains may be made in the early weeks of the treatment program with smaller increases occurring at a slower pace in the subsequent weeks or months. During performance of the exercise the therapist should be aware of joint alignment of exercise device; proper fit and adjustment of device; ruling out substitute movements; and clear instructions of speed, ROM, and proper breathing.[7,13]

ISOMETRIC EXERCISE. In isometric exercises a muscle or group of muscles is actively contracted and relaxed without producing motion of the joint that it ordinarily mobilizes. The contractions may be performed against no outside resistance by asking the client to "set" the muscle, or resistance may be applied manually or by asking the client to hold against a wall, the edge of a table, or own hand.

The purpose of isometric exercise with no resistance is to maintain muscle strength when active motion is not possible. It may be used with any muscle grade above trace but is especially useful for clients in casts or with arthritis or burns when joint motion is not possible or is contraindicated.

The purpose of resistive isometric exercise is to increase muscle strength of fair plus to normal muscles when joint motion is not possible or not desirable. It is graded by increasing the amount of outside resistance or the degree of force the client holds against.

Isometric exercises should be performed for one exercise session per day 5 days a week. Maximal resistance should be applied for 5 to 6 seconds per contraction. A tension gauge should be used to accurately monitor the amount of resistance applied. It has been shown that daily single, brief isometric exercises are at least as effective and sometimes more effective than isotonic exercises for increasing strength. Isometric exercises also increase the endurance to a higher level than isotonic resistive exercises. However, brief isometric exercises performed at resting length are not always superior to isotonic exercises. There are many situations in which movement through complete ROM is a desirable aspect of the exercise program, for example, for increasing joint ROM, preventing contracture, and preparing for use of prosthetic devices. Isometric exercise has several specific applications, as in arthritis, when joint motion may be contraindicated, but muscle strength must be increased or maintained.[5,7,13]

COORDINATION EXERCISES.[7,8] It may be desirable to teach control of individual prime movers when they are so weak that they cannot be used normally. The purpose of the exercise is to improve muscle strength and muscle coordination into normal motor patterns. To achieve these ends the individual must learn precise control of the muscle. This is an essential step in the development of optimal coordination for persons with neuromuscular disease. To achieve these goals Kottke[7] described a procedure that he called *neuromuscular education*. To participate successfully in this type of exercise the client must be rational and be able to learn and follow instructions, cooperate, and concentrate on the muscular retraining. Before beginning the client should be comfortable and securely supported. The exercises should be carried out in a nondistracting environment. It is important that the client be alert, calm, and not tired. He should have good proprioception and an adequate pain-free arc of motion of the joint on which the muscle acts. Neuromuscular education can begin when there is at least 30° of pain-free motion.

The client's awareness of the desired motion and muscles that effect it is first increased by passive lengthening and relaxing of the muscle to stimulate the proprioceptive stretch reflex. This passive movement may be repeated several times. The client's awareness may be enhanced if the therapist also demonstrates the desired movement and if the movement is performed by the analogous unaffected part. The skin over the muscle belly and tendon insertion may be stimulated to enhance the effect of the stretch reflex. Stroking and tapping over the muscle belly may also be used to facilitate muscle action.[8]

The therapist should explain the location and function of the muscle, its origin and insertion, line of pull, and action on the joint. The therapist should then demonstrate the motion, and instruct the client to think of the pull of the muscle from insertion to origin. The skin over the muscle insertion can be stroked in the direction of the pull while the client concentrates on the sensation of the motion during the passive movement performed by the therapist.

The exercise sequence then begins with instructing the client to think about the motion while the therapist carries it out passively and strokes the skin over the insertion in the direction of the motion. The client then is instructed to assist by contracting the muscle while the therapist performs passive motion and stimulates the skin as before. Next the client moves the part through the ROM with assistance and cutaneous stimulation while the therapist emphasizes contraction of the prime mover only. Finally the client carries out the movement independently, using the prime mover.

Coordination exercises must be initiated against minimal resistance if activity is to be isolated to prime movers. If the muscle is very weak (trace to poor), the procedure may be carried out entirely in an active-assisted manner, so that the muscle contracts against no resistance and can function without activating synergists.

Progression from one step to the next depends on successful performance of the step without substitutions. Each step is carried out three to five times per training session for each muscle to be exercised, depending on the client's exercise tolerance.

Coordination is the combined activity of many muscles into smooth patterns and sequences of motion. Coordination is an automatic response monitored primarily through proprioceptive sensory feedback. To achieve a high degree of coordination proprioceptive mechanisms must be intact. Visual and tactile sensory feedback may be used to compensate or substitute for limited proprioception, but the coordination achieved will never be as great as when proprioception is intact.

The development of coordination depends on the repetitious performance of the desired precise patterns of motion to effect integration of the sensory stimuli and motor response. Initially the rate of performance may be slow. As a habit pathway is established, the activity can be performed with less effort and concentration and with increasing speed. A high degree of coordination

and speed does not develop until the pattern of motion becomes automatic and does not require the constant awareness of the performer. Coordination training should begin with simple movement patterns and progress to more complex patterns. Resistance should be minimal.[7,8]

Occupational therapists, often in conjunction with physical therapists, may initiate coordination training with neuromuscular education and progress to repetitious activities requiring desired coordinated movement patterns. Examples of exercise-like activities that demand repetitious patterns of nonresistive movement are placing small blocks, marbles, cones, paper cups, or pegs. These can later be translated to more purposeful activities, such as leather lacing, mosaic tile work, needlecrafts, or weaving.

If central nervous system impulses irradiate to muscles not involved in the movement pattern, incoordinated motion will result. Constant repetition of an incoordinated movement pattern will reinforce it, resulting in a persistent incoordination. Factors that increase incoordination are fear, poor balance, too much resistance, pain, fatigue, strong emotions, and prolonged inactivity.[7]

Summary

Several types of exercise have been described. These may be applied by the occupational therapist and may be used in conjunction with purposeful activity. They are more expertly applied by the physical therapist, who is extensively trained in their use. In many treatment facilities the physical therapist is responsible for the formal exercise program, and the occupational therapist helps the client to apply newly gained strength, range, and coordination in therapeutic activities and daily living skills. The respective therapists' roles may not be that sharply defined, with each sharing in exercise and activity aspects of the treatment program according to their skills, interests, and agreed-on division of labor.

PURPOSEFUL ACTIVITY
Theory of activity

Occupational therapy was founded on the concept that human beings have an "occupational nature,"[6] that is, it is natural for humans to be engaged in activity, and the process of being occupied contributes to the health and well-being of the organism.[1] Activity is valuable for the maintenance of health in the healthy individual and for the restoration of health after illness and disability. By engaging in relevant, meaningful, and purposeful activity an individual is able to effect changes in behavior and performance from dysfunctional toward more functional patterns. The occupational therapist acts as facilitator of the change process.[2] Therefore physical dysfunction can be ameliorated when the client participates in goal-directed activity.[1] The value of purposeful activity lies in the client's mental and physical involvement in an activity that provides the exercise needed to help develop purposeful use of the affected parts[15] and an opportunity to meet emotional, social, and personal gratification needs.[1]

Cynkin[2] in *Occupational Therapy: Toward Health Through Activities* maintains that occupational therapy deals with the activities of everyday life. The activities that form the pattern to one's life are taken for granted until some dysfunction occurs to disrupt the activities pattern. Occupational therapy was founded on the premise that performance of activities promotes physical and mental well-being. From this idea came the use of activities as therapeutic media for persons with mental or physical dysfunction. This implies that dysfunction can be modified, altered, or reversed toward function through engagement in activities.

Cynkin stated that

The uniqueness of occupational therapy rests with activities, in the belief (1) that activities are characteristic of and essential to human existence; (2) that culturally specific activities patterns can be detected and described by studying the manifest activities, values, and norms of different sociocultural groups; (3) that acceptable or unacceptable idiosyncratic variations can be found by studying the individual activities patterns of those groups; (4) that the individual leads a most satisfying way of life if able to carry out a set of activities approved by the group but also fulfilling personal needs and wants; (5) that such activity patterns can be equated with function; and (6) that activities themselves, systematically selected and combined in patterns tailored to each individual, are means for the development or restoration of function.*

Cynkin makes several assumptions about activities that relate to their nature, human nature, and change; these are summarized here. Activities fulfill many of an individual's needs and wants, and they are essential to physical and psychosocial growth and development and the achievement of mastery and competence. Activities are socioculturally regulated by the values and beliefs of the culture that defines acceptable behavior for groups of individuals in the culture. A society may be rigid or flexible in its interpretation of acceptable behaviors for various groups. In either case there is a point where deviations in behavior or activities patterns are deemed unacceptable. Changes in activities patterns can move or change from dysfunctional toward more functional. Individuals can change and desire change. Change takes place through motor, cognitive, and social learning.

Cynkin concludes from these assumptions that activities must be analyzed for "their inherent properties, socioculturally acquired characteristics, their meaning to individuals, and their potential as instruments of change."[2] A careful analysis by the occupational therapist is essential to use activities for therapeutic purposes. An analysis should yield information about the usefulness and application of purposeful activities as intervention strategies for physical dysfunction and health maintenance.

Principles of activity analysis

If activities are to be used as the core of occupational therapy, their usefulness as therapeutic modalities must be defined, analyzed, and classified.[2] Activities selected for therapeutic purposes should (1) be goal-directed, (2) have some significance and meaning to the client to meet individual needs in relation to social roles, (3) require the mental or physical participation of the client, (4) be designed to prevent or reverse dysfunction, (5) develop skills to enhance performance in life roles, (6) relate to the client's interests, (7) be adaptable, gradable, and age appropriate, and (8) be selected through knowledge and professional judgment of the occupational therapist in concert with the client.[4]

In the treatment of physical dysfunction if improvement of motor performance is the goal of the therapeutic activity, then an important aspect of the activity analysis is on muscles, joints, and motor patterns required to perform the activity. This is usually done by observation, palpation, joint measurement, and knowledge of kinesiology.

An activity should be analyzed under the specific circumstances that it is to be performed. Steps of the activity must be identified and broken down into the motions required to perform each step. ROM, degree of muscle strength, and type of muscle contraction to perform each step should be identified.

In developmental and upper motor neuron disorders activities also should be analyzed for their effect on the reinforcement, inhibition, or elicitation of primitive reflexes, equilibrium reactions, and normal and abnormal movement patterns. Stability or mobility requirements of the trunk, neck, and extremities should be analyzed. Required concentration and attention are also noted. Whether cortical or subcortical (automatic) control of movement is necessary should be determined. The sensory input and feedback provided by the activity should be observed for its potential effect on facilitation or inhibition of movement and performance. The client's cognitive functions, such as memory and ability to learn the activity process, and the value and meaning of the activity to the client must also be considered before selection of activity.[14]

Selecting appropriate and meaningful activities for the client should begin with obtaining and analyzing the individual's Activities Configuration Protocol. This model by Cynkin includes information about the client's values, educational history, work history, and vocational interests and plans. Additional information on social, community, and family roles would be helpful. This information may be obtained from interviews with the client and significant friends and family members. The reader is referred to the original source for the complete Activities Configuration Protocol.[2]

A carefully detailed account of the client's daily schedule can be very helpful in analyzing the client's activities pattern. The procedure for obtaining the daily schedule is described in Chapter 4.

Adaptation of activity

Activities may be adapted to suit the particular needs of the individual. If the required movement patterns or degree of resistance, for example, cannot be obtained when the activity is performed in the usual manner, simple adaptations or modifications may be made. These are usually accepted by the client if they are not complex and do not require motions that are strained and unnatural to the performance of the activity. The novice is cautioned that the value of the activity to the client may be diminished if it is designed to be performed in some contrived manner to achieve the desired movement patterns. Such methods require that the client focus on movements rather than on the process or end product.[14] This reduces satisfaction and defeats one of the primary purposes and benefits of purposeful activity described at the beginning of this chapter.

An example of a simple adaptation is positioning a large checkerboard in a vertical position to achieve the desired range of shoulder flexion while playing the game (Fig. 11-6). Positioning an object, such as a mosaic tile project, at increasing or decreasing distances from the client on the tabletop can affect the range needed to reach the materials. Handles may be extended to effect increased range, such as on a loom (Fig. 11-7).

Weights may be added to the client or to the equipment to increase the resistance required to perform the activity. A wrap sandbag with a Velcro fastener attached to the wrist could be used to increase resistance to arm movements during macrame or weav-

---

*From Cynkin, S.: Occupational therapy: toward health through activities, Boston, 1979, Little, Brown & Co.

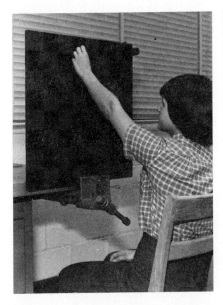

Fig. 11-6. Checkerboard is positioned vertically to increase ROM of shoulder flexion while playing game.

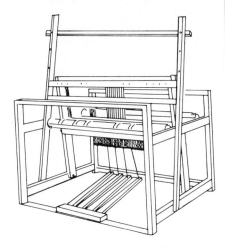

Fig. 11-7. Floor loom with adjustable vertically extended beater bar to require increasing ranges of shoulder flexion.

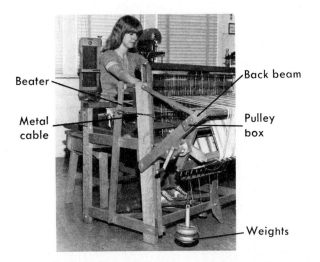

Fig. 11-8. Floor loom adapted with metal cable attached from beater through pulley on back beam from which weights are hung. Weights provide resistance to elbow flexors and shoulder extensors, as arranged.

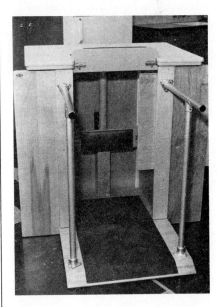

Fig. 11-9. Stand-up table with sliding door, padded knee support, and backrest.

ing. A pulley and weight system can be attached to the beater of the floor loom to increase resistance to the biceps or triceps, depending on whether the weight is attached to the back or the front of the loom (Fig. 11-8). Springs or elastic devices may be used to increase resistance on smaller pieces of equipment.[14]

Tool handles may be increased in size by using a larger dowel or padding the handle with foam rubber to accommodate limited ROM or facilitate grasp. Grasp mitts may be used when arm motion is desirable but grasp strength is inadequate to hold onto a tool or equipment handle. Adaptation of activity can be a challenge to the creativity and ingenuity of the occupational therapist. The therapist should remember that for the adaptations to be used effectively, the client must be able to use them in a good, comfortable position. The client must understand the need and purpose of the activity and the adaptations and be willing to perform the activity with the simple modifications. Peculiar and complicated adaptations that require frequent adjustment and modification should be avoided.[15]

Gradation of activity

Gradation of activity means that the activity should be appropriately paced and modified to demand the client's maximal capacities at any point in the client's progress or regress. There are many ways in which activities may be graded to suite the client's individual needs and the treatment objectives. Resistance may be increased by adding weights to the equipment or to the client, changing the texture of the materials, or changing to another more or less resistive activity. Endurance may be graded by moving from light to heavy work and increasing the length of the work period. Joint ROM may be graded by positioning materials to demand greater reach or excursion of joints or adapting equipment with lengthened handles. Standing and walking tolerance may be graded by increasing the length of time spent standing to work, perhaps at first in a stand-up table (Fig. 11-9), and increasing the time and distance spent in activities requiring walking. These may include home management and workshop activities.

Coordination and muscle control may be graded by decreasing amount of gross resistive movements and increasing fine controlled movements required in the purposeful activities. An example is progressing from sawing wood with a crosscut saw to using a coping saw to using a jewelers' saw to using chip-carving tools. Dexterity and speed of movement may be graded by practice, at increasing speeds, once movement patterns have been mastered through coordination training and neuromuscular education. Activities may also be graded for number of steps, complexity, problem solving, independent decision making, and social interaction requirements.

Selection of activity

In the treatment of physical dysfunction, activities are usually selected for their potential to improve physical performance skills and their potential psychosocial benefits. Activities selected for improvement of physical performance should provide desired exercise or purposeful use of affected parts. They should enable the client to transfer the motion, strength, and coordination gained to useful, normal daily activities.

If activities are to meet requirements for physical restoration, they must meet three basic criteria: (1) Activities should provide action rather than position of involved joints and muscles, that is, they should allow alternate contraction and relaxation of the muscles being exercised and allow the joints to course through their available ROM. (2) Activities should provide repetition of motion. This means that activities should allow for an indefinite but controllable number of repetitions of the desired movement patterns sufficient to be of benefit to the client. (3) Activities should allow for one or more kinds of gradation, such as for resistance, range, coordination, endurance, or complexity.[4,15]

The type of exercise that is needed must be considered. Active and resistive exercise are most often used in the performance of purposeful activity.[15] Requirements for passive and assistive exercise are less easily applied to purposeful activities, although not impossible.

Other important considerations in the selection of activity are (1) properties of the materials and equipment; (2) preparation and completion time; (3) complexity; (4) type of instruction and supervision required; (5) structure and controls in the activity; (6) learning requirements; (7) independence, decision making, and problem solving required; (8) social interaction potential; (9) communication skills required, and (10) potential gratification to the individual.

Prevocational activities must be selected for their ability to evaluate or develop work-related skills. Crafts, job samples, or work simulations may be selected for their similarities to skills required in the actual job. Physical skills required, work speed, concentration, ability to follow instructions and accept supervision, and work habits and attitudes may be assessed or developed through the use of such activities.[4]

The activity selected should have a reasonable goal or end product. Sanding wood or hammering numerous nails for no purpose other than to perform the associated movement patterns are poor activities[14] and might be replaced better by therapeutic exercise. These are examples of a tendency on the part of some occupational therapists to convert activities to exercise, an interesting phenomenon in light of the practice trends cited in Chapter 1.

An activity analysis model and a completed sample activity analysis follow, which offer the student or therapist a systematic approach to looking at activities for their therapeutic potential. This model includes the important factors that must be considered in the selection of activity that have been outlined.

Activity analysis model

A. **Activity or process under analysis:**

1. Describe the activity and its component steps.
2. Describe the necessary equipment and materials and positioning of the worker in relation to the equipment and materials.

B. **Criteria for use of the activity as an exercise.**
1. Action rather than position of muscles and joints.
   a. To which joints is movement localized?
   b. Which joints are in static or holding positions?
   c. Which muscle groups are used to perform the movements of the joints in motion? What types of muscle contraction are used?
   d. How much muscle strength is required to perform the activity/parts of activity (indicate muscle groups and estimated muscle grade needed for each)?
   e. Estimate amount of normal ROM that moving joints are coursing through. List and indicate minimal, moderate, and full.
2. Repetition of motion.
   a. Is the same movement/movement pattern performed repeatedly? Describe patterns.
   b. Is the number of repetitions controllable, that is, can the activity be stopped at any time without negating the goal of the activity or ruining the end product?
   c. Is the number of repetitions sufficient to effect the desired treatment goals?
3. Gradation.
   a. Is the activity gradable? How?
   b. How can the activity be graded if increased/decreased ROM is desired?
   c. How can the activity be graded if increased/decreased strength (resistance) is desired?
   d. How can the activity be graded if increased coordination (gross to fine movement patterns) is desired?
   e. What other types of gradation are possible?

C. **Sensory-perceptual-cognitive demands of the activity.**
  1. Sensory input from materials and performance.[10]
     a. Tactile
     b. Proprioceptive
     c. Vestibular
     d. Visual
     e. Olfactory
     f. Gustatory
     g. Pain
     h. Thermal
     i. Pressure
     j. Visceral
  2. Sensory integration processes.[10]
     a. Tactile-proprioceptive-vestibular functions.
        (1) Equilibrium and protective reactions: What are the sitting and standing balances required?
        (2) Postural and bilateral integration: Are postural adjustments and coordinated use of both body sides required?
        (3) Does the activity require tactile discrimination? Describe.
        (4) How essential is proprioceptive feedback to adequate performance?
        (5) Are the required motor planning skills simple or complex?
     b. Visual functions.
        (1) Does the activity require visual scanning? How much? Describe.
        (2) What types of differentiation and recognition are required?
           (a) Color
           (b) Size
           (c) Shape and form.
        (3) Does the activity require simple or complex perception of position in space and spatial relationships? Describe.
           (a) Fitting parts
           (b) Matching, fitting shapes or forms
           (c) Differentiating patterns
           (d) Observing, changing positions of parts
        (4) Is the figure-background perception required simple or complex? Describe.
        (5) Does the activity require gross or fine visual-motor coordination? Describe.
        (6) Does the activity require simple or complex sequencing or ordering of visual patterns (for example, arranging from top to bottom, left to right, or first to last)? Describe.
     c. Auditory functions.
        (1) Is hearing essential to the performance of the activity, that is, could activity be performed if one could not hear?
        (2) Is sound discrimination essential to adequately perform the activity? Why? Describe.
     d. Cognitive demands of the activity.
        (1) How critical is long-term memory (more than 2 days) to the performance of the activity?
        (2) How critical is short-term memory (1 hour to 2 days) to the performance of the activity?
        (3) Does the activity require the logical sequencing or ordering of steps or stages? Does the completion of one step depend on the anticipation of the next step and readiness for it?
        (4) Does the activity require analysis of problems and problem-solving skills (for example, recognizing errors, analyzing problems, determining solutions, and using the correct procedures to effect the solutions)?
        (5) Does the activity require the ability to do any of the following?
           (a) Read
           (b) Write
           (c) Speak
           (d) Comprehend oral instructions
           (e) Comprehend written instructions
           (f) Comprehend demonstrated instructions.
           (g) Comprehend diagrams
           (h) Learn another system of symbols
        (6) What level of concentration does the activity require?
        (7) Does the activity require generalization of learning from past experience or for future use?

D. **Safety factors.**
  1. Is there danger of cutting, piercing, or burning the skin?
  2. Is there danger of losing control of tools or machinery?

E. **Interpersonal aspects of the activity**[2]
  1. What is the number of people required or possible for participation?
  2. What is the nature of interpersonal transactions?
     a. Dependent
     b. Independent
     c. Cooperative
     d. Collaborative
     e. Competitive

F. **Sociocultural symbolism of the activity.**
  1. What does the activity symbolize in the culture?
  2. What does the activity symbolize in any specific subgroup within the culture?
  3. Does the activity connote sex role identification in the culture or to most individuals?

G. **Psychological-emotional responses to the activity.**
  1. What feelings does the activity evoke in the worker (for example, aggression, peace, or boredom)?
  2. Does the worker derive personal gratification from the performance of the activity?

H. **Therapeutic use of the activity.**
  1. List the autonomous or inherent objectives of the activity.
  2. List the possible therapeutic objectives.
     a. Physical
     b. Sensory integrative
     c. Psychosocial
     d. Vocational

SAMPLE ACTIVITY ANALYSIS

A. **Activity or process under analysis:** Pinch process in pinch pottery.
  1. A hole is made with the thumb in a ball of clay 3 to 4 inches in diameter (Fig. 11-10, A). The thumb and first two fingers then pinch around and around the hole from base to top of the ball or clay to gradually thin and spread the walls of the clay to

produce a small, round clay pot (Fig. 11-10, *B* and *C*).

2. The activity requires a ball of soft ceramic clay and a wooden table surface or a wooden work board on a metal or formica table. The table should be 30 to 32 inches high or a comfortable height for the worker when the worker is in an erect, sitting position at the table.

B. **Criteria for use of the activity as an exercise.**

1. Action rather than position of muscles and joints.

   a. Movement is localized to flexion and extension of the metacarpophalangeal (MP) and interphalangeal (IP) joints of digits one and two, opposition and abduction of the carpometacarpal joint of thumb, and flexion and extension of the MP and IP joints of the thumb.

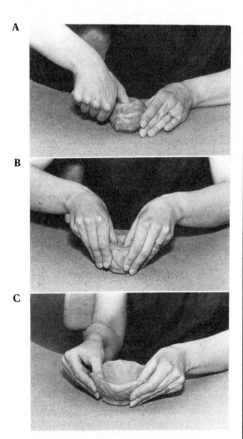

Fig. 11-10. A, Opening pinch pot with thumb. **B,** Walls of pot are gradually spread with pinching motion of fingers. **C,** Pinching continues in circular direction until desired size of pot is reached.

b. Static or holding positions are maintained at the wrist during the pinch process. However, the wrist makes many minor adjustments into radial and ulnar deviation and flexion and extension as the hand moves around and up and down the pot. The back and neck are stabilized. There is only slight movement at the shoulder and elbow to make adjustments in the position of the hand as it moves around the pot.

c. The opponens pollicis, flexors pollicis longus and brevis, and flexors digitorum profundis and superficialis are acting in concentric contraction. Palmar interossei are in isometric contraction to maintain adduction of the fingers. Lumbricales are acting concentrically to flex the MP joints and maintain extension of the IP joints of the fingers during the pinch process. The extensor digitorum communis, extensor indicis proprius, extensors pollicis longus and brevis, and abductor pollicis are in eccentric contraction, which accounts for their controlled lengthening during the pinch process and concentric contraction during the release from pinch.

d. The muscle strength required in the flexor groups and the opponens pollicis is at least fair plus, because the muscles must overcome the slight resistance of the clay. Poor strength is adequate for the extensors and thumb abductors, since they act to release the pinch, and there is no resistance to these motions. Muscle endurance must be adequate to repeat the movement pattern around the pot at least once before a rest is required.

e. Joints course through a minimal ROM. MP joints are in 60° to 90° of flexion, and IP joints are in nearly full extension during the pinch process.

2. Repetition of motion.

   a. The pinching motion with the thumb in opposition to the first two digits is repeated

until the pot has reached the desired height and thickness.

b. The number of repetitions is controllable, since the process may be stopped and the project damp-stored for future use at any time.

c. The number of repetitions is adequate for one or two treatment sessions. If more pinching activity is desirable, similar projects may be used.

3. Gradation. The activity cannot be graded for increasing ROM. It can be graded slightly for increasing strength by increasing the stiffness of the clay. It may also be graded for sitting tolerance by increasing the length of the work periods and for sitting balance by decreasing the amount of support for sitting.

C. **Sensory-perceptual-cognitive demands of the activity.**

1. Sensory input from materials and performance. There are tactile, proprioceptive, visual, slight olfactory, thermal, and pressure stimuli received from working with clay.

2. Sensory integration processes[10]

   a. Tactile-proprioceptive-vestibular functions.

      (1) The activity requires good sitting balance or trunk stabilization if balance is not adequate. Good head and neck control are required.

      (2) The activity requires the ability to make slight postural adjustments of trunk and proximal upper extremity joints and the use of both hands, one for supporting and moving the pot and the other for the pinching process.

      (3) Fine tactile discrimination is required to feel the texture, moisture content, and thickness of the clay. Visual functions may substitute to some extent.

      (4) Proprioceptive feedback is necessary for adequate performance to determine position of hand and fingers and degree of strength of pinch, so as not to progress too rapidly or break the clay by squeezing too hard.

(5) The motor planning skills required are relatively simple, since the same motor pattern and a familiar one already learned are repeated over and over. The motor pattern can be easily learned from visual or proprioceptive learning techniques.

b. Visual functions.
(1) The activity requires minimal visual scanning. Gaze is fixed on the object at the center of the work area.
(2) Differentiation and recognition.
  (a) The activity does not require color differentiation.
  (b) Size discrimination of the height and thickness of the walls is required. It can be obtained partially through tactile and proprioceptive feedback.
  (c) Shape and form perception through visual and tactile feedback is required to maintain the round shape of the pot.
(3) Requirements for position in space and spatial relationships are simple, since there is only one object and no fitting, matching of parts or shapes, or differentiating patterns.
(4) Figure-background perception required is simple, since there is only one object on a significantly contrasting background.
(5) The activity requires moderate to fine visual-motor coordination, since fine muscles are acting in a controlled manner in response to visual, tactile, and proprioceptive information.
(6) some simple visual sequencing is required to progress with the pinching in a circular manner and from bottom to top.

c. Auditory functions.
(1) Hearing is not essential to the performance of pinch pottery except to receive instructions. Demonstrated and written/illustrated instructions may be substituted.
(2) Sound discrimination is not required.

d. Cognitive demands of the activity.
(1) Long-term memory is not required.
(2) Short-term memory is essential if the project is to be completed in 2 to 3 days without reinstruction and continuous supervision.
(3) The activity requires sequencing of steps, and the completion of one step is necessary before the next can be started.
(4) The activity requires simple problem-solving skills for recognition of changes in shape and thickness of walls. Knowledge of the behavior of clay and its properties for analysis or of when to seek assistance to correct these problems is essential to the successful outcome of the end product.
(5) The activity requires the ability to comprehend oral or demonstrated instructions.
(6) The activity requires the ability to generalize from previous experience with pinch movements, soft materials, and round objects.

D. Safety factors.
1. There is no danger of cutting, piercing, or burning the skin.
2. There is no danger of losing control of tools or machinery, since none are used.

E. Interpersonal aspects of the activity.
1. The activity may be done alone or in a group of people performing the same or similar activities.
2. Interpersonal transactions may be independent if the worker is working alone or with others and needs little supervision and assistance; dependent if more assistance, supervision, prodding, or reassurance is required; and

competitive if all group members are making the same or similar objects, and there is a sense of competition, for example, for degree of attractiveness, use of the end product, speed of work, or admiration of supervisors.

F. Sociocultural symbolism of the activity.
1. The activity in American culture symbolizes the artistic or perhaps liberal or naturalistic groups of individuals in the society.
2. The activity is seen as a leisure rather than a work skill and may be associated with child's play by some individuals.
3. The activity may have a more feminine than a masculine identification to the older or more conservative segments of the society.

G. Psychological-emotional responses to the activity.
1. The soft, moist, pliable, and plastic properties of the clay may evoke peace and pleasure in many persons. Others may regard it as "messy" and dirty.
2. The potential for gratification is good, since the end product is easy to achieve, is creative, is as personal as the worker's own fingerprints, and is useful.

H. Therapeutic use of the activity.
1. The autonomous objectives of the activity are to derive pleasure and sense of worth from producing a creative object, produce a useful product, and interact with others with similar interests.
2. Therapeutic objectives.
  a. The physical objectives of the activity are to increase strength of opponens pollicis and flexor muscles of the fingers and thumb and improve coordination.
  b. The sensory-integrative objectives are to increase tactile, proprioceptive, and thermal sensory input to the hands and improve concentration and sequencing skills and form perception.
  c. The psychosocial objectives are to improve self-esteem and interaction skills, reduce anxiety, and provide an outlet for self-expression.
  d. There is little potential for vocationally related objectives in this activity.

REVIEW QUESTIONS

1. Define "therapeutic exercise."
2. What is meant by "substitution patterns"? Why do they occur?
3. What demand must be made on a muscle for its strength to increase?
4. What happens to a muscle that is fatigued?
5. List four signs of fatigue from excess exercise.
6. List at least four purposes of therapeutic exercise.
7. With which types of disabilities would you use therapeutic exercise? Which disabilities is it less useful for? Why?
8. To participate in a therapeutic exercise program the client must possess certain characteristics. List and discuss at least four of these requirements.
9. List four precautions or contraindications to therapeutic exercise, and explain why each can preclude the use of therapeutic exercise.
10. Define three types of muscle contraction, and given an example of how each occurs in daily activity.
11. What type of exercise should be used if muscle grades are fair plus to good? Why?
12. If a patient has joint pain and inflammation with good muscle strength, what type of exercise should be used? Why?
13. How is passive stretching different from passive exercise?
14. Describe the procedure and precautions for passive stretching.
15. When beginning PRE, how is the client's maximal resistance determined?
16. Describe the procedure for PRE to strengthen fair plus wrist extensors.
17. Describe the steps in coordination exercises.
18. List four objectives of therapeutic activities.
19. Name four classifications of activities that could be used for therapeutic objectives.
20. Discuss Cynkin's premises about activities in occupational therapy.
21. List at least five requirements that activities need to meet if they are to be used for therapeutic purposes.
22. How can activities be adapted to meet specific therapeutic objectives and allow for gradation of the therapeutic program?
23. list four ways in which activities may be graded.
24. What are the three criteria an activity must meet to be useful for exercise purposes?
25. Name and discuss at least five factors that should be considered in the selection of activities.
26. Can therapeutic activity and therapeutic exercise be used simultaneously in a treatment program? How and why?
27. Select one of the following activities, and complete an activity analysis according to the model provided.
    a. Sawing wood
    b. Pulling the beater on the floor loom
    c. Knitting
    d. Pulling leather lacing
    e. Rolling out dough
    f. Using a push broom

REFERENCES

1. Ayres, A.J.: Occupational therapy for motor disorders resulting from impairment of the central nervous system, Rehabil. Lit. **21**:302, 1960.
2. Cynkin, S.: Occupational therapy: toward health through activities, Boston, 1979, Little, Brown & Co.
3. Hinojosa, J., Sabari, J., and Rosenfeld, M.S.: Purposeful activities, Am. J. Occup. Ther. **37**:805, 1983.
4. Hopkins, H.L., Smith, H.D., and Tiffany, E.G.: The activity process. In Hopkins, H.L., and Smith, H.D., editors: Willard and Spackman's occupational therapy, ed. 5, Philadelphia, 1978, J.B. Lippincott Co.
5. Huddleston, O.L.: Therapeutic exercises, Philadelphia, 1961, F.A. Davis Co.
6. Kielhofner, G.: A heritage of activity: development of theory, Am. J. Occup. Ther. **36**:723, 1982.
7. Kottke, F.J.: Therapeutic exercise. In Krusen, F.H., Kottke, F.J., and Ellwood, P.M., editors: Handbook of physical medicine and rehabilitation, Philadelphia, 1965, W.B. Saunders Co.
8. Kottke, F.J.: Therapeutic exercise to maintain mobility. In Kottke, F.J., Stillwell, G.K., and Lehmann, J.F., editors: Krusen's handbook of physical medicine and rehabilitation, ed. 3, Philadelphia, 1982, W.B. Saunders Co.
9. Kraus, H.: Therapeutic exercise, Springfield, Ill., 1963, Charles C Thomas, Publisher.
10. Llorens, L.: Activity analysis for sensory integration (CPM) dysfunction, 1978. Mimeographed.
11. Melvin, J.L.: Rheumatic disease: occupational therapy and rehabilitation, ed. 2, Philadelphia, 1982, F.A. Davis Co.
12. Rancho Los Amigos Hospital: Muscle reeducation, Downey, Calif., 1963, Rancho Los Amigos Hospital. Mimeographed.
13. Rancho Los Amigos Hospital: Progressive resistive and static exercise: principles and techniques, Downey, Calif., Rancho Los Amigos Hospital. Mimeographed.
14. Trombly, C.A., and Scott, A.D.: Occupational therapy for physical dysfunction, Baltimore, 1977, Williams & Wilkins.
15. Willard, H.S., and Spackman, C.S., editors: Occupational therapy, ed. 4, Philadelphia, 1971, J.B. Lippincott Co.
16. Wynn-Parry, C.B.: Vicarious motions. In Basmajian, J.V., editor: Therapeutic exercise, ed. 3, Baltimore, 1978, Williams & Wilkins.

CHAPTER 12

Activities of daily living

LORRAINE WILLIAMS PEDRETTI

Activities of daily living (ADL) are tasks of self-maintenance, mobility, communication, and home management that enable an individual to achieve personal independence in his or her environment. Evaluation of and training in the performance of these important life tasks have long been important aspects of occupational therapy programs is virtually every type of health facility. Loss of ability to care for one's personal needs and manage the environment can result in loss of self-esteem, a deep sense of dependency, or even feelings of infantilism and can profoundly affect the role and function of the caretakers of the individual who has lost these performance skills.[10]

The role of occupational therapy in ADL, then, is to assess ADL performance skills, determine problems that interfere with independence, determine treatment objectives, and provide training or equipment to enhance the achievement of a higher level of independence. The occupational therapist may also be involved in ameliorating physical, cognitive, social, and emotional functions that are interfering with ADL performance. The need to learn new methods or use assistive devices to perform ADL may be temporary or permanent, depending on the particular dysfunction and the prognosis for recovery.

DEFINITION OF ADL

ADL include mobility, self-care, management of environmental hardware and devices, communication, and home management activities. These major classifications are further defined as follows: (1) mobility includes movement in bed, wheelchair mobility and transfers, indoor ambulation with special equipment, outdoor ambulation with special equipment, and management of public or private transportation; (2) self-care includes dressing, feeding, toileting, bathing, and grooming activities; (3) management of environmental hardware and devices includes the ability to use telephones, keys, faucets, light switches, windows, doors, scissors, and street control signals; (4) communication skills include the ability to write, operate a personal computer, read, type, or use the telephone, a tape recorder, or a special communications device; (5) home management activities include marketing, meal planning and preparation, cleaning, laundry, child care, and the ability to manage household appliances, such as vacuum cleaners, can openers, ranges, refrigerators, electric mixers, and hand-operated utensils.

FACTORS TO CONSIDER IN ADL EVALUATION AND TRAINING

Before commencing ADL performance evaluation and training the occupational therapist must assess performance components and consider several factors about the client and the individual environment. Physical resources, such as strength, range of motion (ROM), coordination, sensation, and balance, should be evaluated to determine potential skills and deficits in ADL performance and possible need for special equipment. Perceptual and cognitive functions should be evaluated to determine potential for learning ADL skills. General mobility in bed or wheelchair or ambulation should be assessed.

In addition to these relatively concrete and objective evaluations the occupational therapist should be familiar with the client's culture and its values and mores in relation to self-care, the sick role, family assistance, and independence. The values of the client and the client's peer group and culture should be important considerations in selecting objectives and initial activities in the ADL program. The balance of activities in the client's day, which demand time and energy, may influence how many ADL may be performed independently. The environment to which the client will return is an important consideration. Will the client return to live alone or with his or her family or a roommate? Will the client be going to a skilled nursing facility or to a board and care home permanently or temporarily? Will the patient be returning to work and community activities? The type and amount of assistance available in the home environment must be considered if the appropriate caretaker is to receive orientation and training in the appropriate supervision and assistance required. The finances available for assistant care, special equipment, and home modifications are important considerations. For example, a wheelchair-bound client who is wealthy may be willing and able to make major modifications in the home, such as installing an elevator, lowering kitchen counters, widening doorways, and replacing deep pile carpeting to accommodate a wheelchair life-style. A less well-off client may need the assistance of the occupational therapist in making less costly modifications, such as removing scatter rugs and door sills, installing a plywood ramp at the entrance, replacing the bathroom door with a curtain, and attaching a hand-held shower head to the bathtub faucet.

The ultimate goal of any ADL training program is for the client to achieve *his* or *her* maximal level of independence. It is important to note the "maximal level of independence" is defined differently for each client. For the client with mild muscle weakness in one arm caused by a peripheral neuropathy, complete independence in ADL may be the "maximal," whereas for the high-level quadriplegic feeding and oral hygiene activities with devices and assistance may be the maximal level of independence that can be expected. Therefore the potential for independence should be based on each client's unique personal needs, values, capabilities, limitations, and environmental resources.

Independence is a strong value in the American culture. It should not be pursued for its own sake on that basis or because it is a value of the rehabilitation personnel or family or friends of the client.

ADL EVALUATION
General procedure

When some data have been gathered about the client's physical, psychosocial, and environmental resources, the feasibility of ADL evaluation or training should be determined by the occupational therapist in concert with the client, supervising physician, and other members of the rehabilitation team. In some instances ADL should be delayed because of limitations of the client or in favor of more immediate treatment objectives that require the client's energy and participation.

Evaluation of ADL performance is often initiated with an interview, using an ADL checklist as a guide for questioning the client about individual capabilities and limitations. Several types of ADL checklists are available, but they cover similar categories and performance tasks. The ADL interview may serve as a screening device to determine the need for further assessment by observation of performance. This is determined by the therapist's professional judgment based on knowledge of the client, the dysfunction, and results of previous evaluations. A partial or complete performance evaluation is invaluable in assessing ADL performance. The phrase "one look is worth a thousand words" applies well here. The ADL interview alone, as a measure of performance, can be inaccurate, because the client may recall his or her performance before the onset of the dysfunction, may have some confusion or memory loss, and may overestimate or underestimate individual abilities, because he or she has had little opportunity to perform routine ADL since the onset of the physical dysfunction.

Ideally the occupational therapist should conduct the performance evaluation at the time and in the environment in which the activities to be evaluated usually take place. For example, a dressing evaluation could be arranged for early in the morning when the client usually is dressed by nursing personnel. Feeding evaluation should occur at regular meal hours. If this is not possible because of schedules, personnel, or environmental constraints in the treatment facility or client's home, the evaluation may be conducted during regular treatment sessions in the occupational therapy clinic under simulated conditions.

This is not as good, since it requires that the client perform or reperform routine self-maintenance tasks at irregular times in an artificial environment and can contribute to a lack of carryover for those clients who have difficulty generalizing learning.

The therapist should begin by selecting relatively simple and safe items from the ADL checklist for the client to perform and should progress to more difficult and complex items. The evaluation should not be completed all at once, since this would be fatiguing and somewhat artificial. Those items that would be unsafe or that very obviously cannot be performed should be omitted and the appropriate notation made on the evaluation form.

During the performance evaluation the therapist should observe the methods that the client is using or attempting to use to accomplish the task and try to determine causes of performance problems. Some of these might be weakness, spasticity, involuntary motion, perceptual deficits, or low endurance. If problems and their causes can be identified, the therapist has a good foundation for establishing training objectives, priorities, and methods and need for assistive devices. Other very important aspects of this evaluation that should not be overlooked are the client's need for respect and privacy and the ongoing interaction between the client and therapist. The client's feelings about having his or her body viewed and touched should be respected. Privacy should be maintained for toileting, grooming, and dressing tasks. The therapist with whom the client is most familiar and comfortable may be the most appropriate person to conduct the ADL evaluation and training. As the therapist interacts with the client during the performance of ADL, it may be possible to elicit the client's attitudes and feelings about the particular tasks; individual priorities in training; dependence and independence; and cultural, family, and personal values and customs about performance of daily living activities.

RECORDING RESULTS OF THE ADL EVALUATION. During the interview and performance evaluation the therapist makes the appropriate notations on the ADL checklists. These may include separate checklists for self-care, home management, mobility, and home environment evaluations. The information is then summarized succinctly for inclusion in the client's permanent records where interested professional co-workers can refer to it.

ADL TRAINING

If, after evaluation, it is determined that ADL training is to be initiated, it is important to establish appropriate short- and long-term objectives, based on the evaluation and on the client's priorities for independence. The following sequence of training for self-care activities is suggested: feeding, grooming, continence, transfer skills, toileting, undressing, dressing, and bathing. This sequence is based on the normal development of self-care independence in children.[15]

This sequence provides a good guide but may need to be modified to accommodate the specific dysfunction and the capabilities, limitations, and personal priorities of the client. One client was known to deem smoking a more important skill than feeding. Although the hand-to-mouth movement pattern in both activities is similar, and feeding was objectively estimated as a priority over smoking, the client was content to be fed by an assistant but became very involved in achieving smoking independence using mobile arm supports and assistive devices. Only after some independence was achieved here was feeding an acceptable activity.

The occupational therapist should estimate which ADL are possible and which are impossible for the client to achieve. The therapist should explore with the client the use of alternate methods of performing the activities and the use of any assistive devices that may be helpful. He or she should determine for which tasks the client will require assistance and how much should be given. It may not be possible to estimate these factors until the training program is underway.

The ADL training program may be graded by beginning with a few simple tasks and gradually increasing the number and complexity of tasks to be performed. Training should progress from dependent to assisted to supervised to independent, with or without assistive devices.[15] The rate at which grading can occur will depend on the client's recovery, endurance, skills, and motivation.

Methods of teaching ADL

The methods of teaching the client to perform daily living tasks must be tailored to suit each client's learning style and ability. The client who is alert and grasps instructions quickly may be able to perform an entire process after a brief demonstration and verbal instruction. Clients who may have perceptual problems, poor memory, and difficulty following instructions of any kind will require a more concrete, step-by-step approach, reducing the amount of assistance gradually as success is achieved. For such persons it is important to break the activity down into small steps and progress through them slowly, one at a time. Slow demonstration of the task or step in the same plane and in the same manner in which the client is expected to perform is very helpful. Verbal instructions to accompany the demonstration may or may not be helpful, depending on the client's receptive language skills and ability to process and integrate two modes of sensory information simultaneously.

Touching body parts to be moved, dressed, bathed, or positioned or passive movement of the part through the desired pattern to achieve a step or a task are helpful tactile and kinesthetic modes of instruction. These can be used to augment or substitute for demonstration and verbal instruction, again depending on the client's best avenues of learning. It is necessary to perform a step or complete task repetitiously to achieve skill, speed, or retention of learning. Tasks may be repeated several times during the same training session, if time and the client's physical and emotional tolerance allow, or they may be repeated on a daily basis until desired retention or level of skill is achieved. The process of "backward chaining" can be used in teaching ADL skills. In this method the therapist assists the client until the last step of the process is reached. The client then performs this step independently, which affords a sense of success and completion. When the last step is mastered, the therapist assists until the last two

steps are reached and the client then completes these two steps. The process continues with the therapist offering less and less assistance and the client performing successive steps of the task, from last to first, independently. This method is particularly useful in training patients with brain damage.[15]

Before beginning training in any ADL the therapist must make some preparations. The therapist should provide adequate space and arrange equipment, materials, or furniture for maximal convenience and safety. The therapist should be thoroughly familiar with the task to be performed and any special methods or assistive devices that will be used in its performance. The practitioner should be able to perform the task, as he or she expects the client to perform it, skillfully. After the preparation the activity is presented to the client, usually in one or more modes of demonstration and verbal instruction described earlier. The client then performs the activity either along with the therapist or immediately after being shown, with the amount of supervision and assistance required. Performance is modified and corrected as needed and the process is repeated to ensure learning. In the final phase of instruction when the client has mastered the task or several tasks, he or she is placed on his or her own to perform them independently. The therapist should follow up by checking on performance in progress and later arrange to check on adequacy of performance and carry-over of learning with nursing personnel, caretaker, or the supervising family members.[6]

Recording progress in ADL performance

The ADL checklists used to record performance on the initial evaluation usually have one or more spaces for recording changes in abilities and results of reevaluation during the training process. The sample checklist given later in this chapter is so designed and filled out. Progress is usually summarized for inclusion in the medical record. The progress report should summarize changes in the client's abilities and current level of independence and estimate the client's potential for further independence, attitude and motivation for

ADL training, and future goals for the ADL program.

When describing levels of independence occupational therapists often use terms like *moderate independence, maximal assistance,* and *minimal skill.* These quantitative terms have little meaning to the reader unless they are defined or supporting statements are used in progress summaries to give specific meaning for each. It also needs to be specified whether the level of independence refers to a single activity, a category of activities such as dressing, or all ADL. In designating levels of independence an agreed-on performance scale should be used to mark the ADL checklist. General categories and their definitions might be the following:

1. Independent. Can perform the activity or activities wihtout cueing, supervision, or assistance, with or without assistive devices, at normal or near normal speeds
2. Partially dependent. Can perform at least 50% of the activity or activities independently; may be considerably slower than normal performance, use assistive devices, and require some level of assistance
   a. Minimal assistance: Supervision, cueing, or less than 20% physical assistance
   b. Moderate assistance: Supervision, cueing, and 20% to 50% physical assistance
   c. Maximal assistance: Supervision, cueing, and 50% to 80% physical assistance
3. Dependent. Can perform only one or two steps of the activity or very few activities independently; may fatigue easily and perform very slowly; may require elaborate equipment and devices to perform basic skills such as feeding; needs more than 80% physical assistance

These definitions are broad and general. They can be modified to suit the program plan and approach of the particular treatment facility.

A sample case study, ADL and home management checklists, and summaries of an initial evaluation and progress report are included on pp. 144-150 (Figs. 12-1 and 12-2). The reader should keep in mind that the evaluation and progress summaries relate to the ADL portion of the treatment program only.

Text continued on p. 151.

Sample case study

J.V. is a 48-year-old married woman who suffered a cerebral thrombosis resulting in a CVA 6 months ago. She lives in a modest home with her husband and teenage daughter and was a full-time homemaker before the onset of her stroke. She was a cheerful and active woman who enjoyed cooking, baking, gardening, and visiting her neighbors and friends. The stroke resulted in the disturbance of cerebellar and brain stem functions. J.V. has a severe motor apraxia for speech, cannot close her mouth, drools, and walks with a broad-based ataxic gait. Since the onset of her disability J.V. has been very depressed, weeps frequently, is dependent for much of her self-care, and sits idly for long periods of time. She was referred to occupational therapy for evaluation and training in ADL, adjustment to disability, and development of drooling and swallowing control to facilitate feeding.

OCCUPATIONAL THERAPY DEPARTMENT

ACTIVITIES OF DAILY LIVING EVALUATION

Name __J. V.__ Age __48__ Diagnosis __CVA__ Dom. __Right__

Disability __Bilateral incoordination, ataxia, apraxia of mouth musculature__

Mode of ambulation __Independent__

> Grading key:
> I = Independent
> MiA = Minimal assistance
> MoA = Moderate assistance
> MaA = Maximal assistance
> D = Dependent
> NA = Not applicable
> 0 = Not evaluated

TRANSFERS AND AMBULATION

	Date	Independent	Assisted	Dependent
Tub or shower	8/1			D
Toilet	8/1		MiA	
Wheelchair	NA			
Bed and chair		I		
Ambulation			MiA	
Wheelchair management	NA			
Car			MiA	

BALANCE FOR FUNCTION

	Adequate	Inadequate
Sitting	I	
Standing	I	
Walking		MiA

Fig. 12-1. ADL evaluation. (Adapted from Activities of daily living evaluation form OT 461-1, Hartford, Conn., 1963, The Hartford Rehabilitation Center.)

Sample ADL progress report

J.V. has attended occupational therapy three times weekly for 3 weeks since the initial evaluation. Further evaluation of self-care skills revealed that J.V. is capable of some hygiene skills, except a tub bath, nail care, hair care, and makeup application. However, at home she remains almost entirely dependent on Mr. V. for self-care, whining, crying, and complaining of feeling weak.

Home management evaluation revealed considerable difficulty with most tasks except table setting, dusting, dish washing, and sweeping, which she can perform if given cues and supervision. Performance of more complex tasks is limited by psychomotor retardation, incoordination, distractibility, inability to sequence a process, and apraxia for fine hand activities. It was necessary to supervise J.V. closely and give step-by-step instructions while she performed household tasks. A few simple homemaking tasks were performed for several training sessions, but performance did not improve.

J.V. appears to be very depressed and lacks intrinsic motivation. It was suggested to her family that they offer less assistance for self-care, and involve her with them in household tasks that she can perform, under their supervision, if possible.

The occupational therapy program will continue with greater emphasis on achieving control of mouth musculature, a primary goal of J.V. ADL training will be delayed until J.V. is moving toward the achievement of this primary goal.

```
SUMMARY OF EVALUATION RESULTS

Date  8/1

Intact   Impaired                                          REMARKS

                    SENSORY STATUS

  X                 Touch_____
  X                 Pain_____
  X                 Temperature_____
           X        Position sense  More marked on left
           X        Olfaction_____
           X        Stereognosis    More marked on left
           X        Visual fields (hemianopsia)_____

                    PERCEPTUAL/CONCEPTUAL TESTS

  X                 Follow directions  Verbal
  X                 Visual spatial (form)_____
           X        Visual spatial (block design) Minimal impairment
  X                 Make change_____
           X        Geometric figures (copy) Some difficulty with triangle & diamond
                      square, circle, triangle, diamond_____
           X        Praxis  Mild apraxia evident on fine hand activities

                    FUNCTIONAL RANGE OF MOTION

  X                 Comb hair—two hands_____
  X                 Feed self_____
  X                 Button collar button_____
  X                 Tie apron behind back_____
  X                 Button back buttons_____
  X                 Button cuffs_____
  X                 Zip side zipper_____
           X        Tie shoes____ ⎤ Poor balance limits
           X        Stoop_____ ⎬ Reach and bending for these activities
           X        Reach shelf__ ⎦
```

Continued.

Fig. 12-1, cont'd. ADL evaluation.

ADL SKILLS

EATING	Date	8/1	8/25			REMARKS
		Grade				
Butter bread		I				
Cut meat		I				
Eat with spoon		I				
Eat with fork		I				
Drink with straw		D				Mouth apraxia
Drink with glass		D				prevents performance
Drink with cup		D				of these activities
Pour from pitcher		D				

UNDRESS	Date	8/1	8/25			REMARKS
Pants or shorts		I				Is physically
Girdle or garter belt		Mo A				capable of
Brassiere		Mi A				performing the
Slip or undershirt		I				activities as
Dress		I				indicated but
Skirt		I				Mr. V. reports
Blouse or shirt		I				that J.V. is
Slacks or trousers		I				dependent on him
Bandana or necktie		N A				for much assistance,
Stockings		Mo A				pleading fatigue,
Nightclothes		I				whining, and
Hair net		N A				crying for help
Housecoat/bathrobe		I				
Jacket		I				
Belt and/or suspenders		I				
Hat		I				
Coat		I				
Sweater		I				
Mittens or gloves		I				
Glasses		N A				
Brace		N A				
Shoes		Mo A				
Socks		Mo A				
Overshoes		Mo A				

DRESS	Date	8/1	8/25			REMARKS
Pants or shorts		Mi A				
Girdle or garter belt		Mo A				
Brassiere		Mo A				
Slip or undershirt		I				
Dress		I				
Skirt		I				
Blouse or shirt		I				
Slacks or trousers		I				
Bandana or necktie		N A				
Stockings		Mo A				
Nightclothes		I				
Hair net		N A				
Housecoat/bathrobe		I				
Jacket		I				
Belt and/or suspenders		I				
Hat		I				
Coat		I				
Sweater		I				
Mittens or gloves		I				
Glasses		N A				
Brace		N A				
Shoes		Mo A				
Socks		Mo A				
Overshoes		Mo A				

Fig. 12-1, cont'd. ADL evaluation.

FASTENINGS	Date	8/1	8/25			REMARKS
		Grade				
Button		I				
Snap		MoA				
Zipper		MiA				
Hook and eye		MaA				
Garters		D				
Lace		D				
Untie shoes		D				
Velcro		MiA				

HYGIENE	Date	8/1	8/25			REMARKS
Blow nose		O	I			
Wash face, hands		O	I			
Wash extremities, back		O	MaA			
Brush teeth or dentures		O	I			
Brush or comb hair		O	I			
Set hair		O	D			
Shave or put on makeup		O	MiA			
Clean fingernails		O	I, D			
Trim fingernails, toenails		O	D			
Apply deodorant		O	I			
Shampoo hair		O	D			
Use toilet paper		O	I			
Use tampon or sanitary napkin		O	NA			

COMMUNICATION	Date	8/1	8/25			REMARKS
Verbal		D				
Read		I				
Hold book		I				
Turn page		I				
Write		I				Writes name and few words
Use telephone		D				
Type		D				

HAND ACTIVITIES	Date	8/1	8/25			REMARKS
Handle money		O				
Handle mail		O				
Use of scissors		O				
Open cans, bottles, jars		O				
Tie package		O				
Sew (baste)		O				
Sew button, hook and eye		O				
Polish shoes		O				
Sharpen pencil		O				
Seal and open letter		O				
Open box		O				

COMBINED PERFORMANCE ACTIVITIES	Date	8/1	8/25			REMARKS
Open-close refrigerator		O	I			
Open-close door		O	I			
Remove and replace objects		O	I			
Carry objects during locomotion		O	D			
Pick up object from floor		O	D			
Remove, replace light bulb		O	D			
Plug in cord		O	O			

OPERATE	Date	8/1	8/25			REMARKS
		Grade				
Light switches		O	I			
Doorbell		O	I			
Door locks and handles		O	D			
Faucets		O	I			
Raise-lower window shades		O	D			
Raise-lower venetian blinds		O	D			
Raise-lower window		O	D			
Open-close drawer		O	I			
Hang up garment		O	I			

Fig. 12-1, cont'd. ADL evaluation.

OCCUPATIONAL THERAPY DEPARTMENT

ACTIVITIES OF HOME MANAGEMENT

Name _J. V._____ Date ___8/25_____

Address _Anytown, U.S.A._____

Age _48_____ Weight _135_____ Height _5'5"___ Role in family _Wife, mother____

Diagnosis _CVA_____ Disability _Bilateral ataxia, apraxia of mouth_

Mode of ambulation _Independent, no aids, mild ataxic gait_ _musculature_

Limitations or contraindications for activity_____
_____

DESCRIPTION OF HOME
1. Private house   _✓_
   No. of rooms   _6_ - kitchen, dining room, living room, 3 bedrooms
   No. of floors   _2_
   Stairs   _14_ - bedrooms on second floor
   Elevators   _0_

2. Apartment house   ____
   No. of rooms   ____
   No. of floors   ____
   Stairs   ____
   Elevators   ____

3. Diagram of home layout (attach to completed form)

Will patient be required to perform the following activities? If not, who will perform?
   Meal preparation _No_ _Daughter_____
   Baking   _No_ _Daughter (J.V. used to bake a lot)_____
   Serving   _Yes_ _____
   Wash dishes   _Yes_ _____
   Marketing   _No_ _Husband_____
   Child care   _No_ _____
     (under 4 years)
   Washing   _Yes_ _____
   Hanging clothes _NA_ _Has dryer_____
   Ironing   _No_ _Daughter_____
   Cleaning   _Yes_ _Light cleaning_____
   Sewing   _No_ _Does not sew_____
   Hobbies or   _Yes_ _Baking and gardening would be desirable activities_
     special interest   _____
Does patient really like housework? _No___
Sitting position: Chair _X__ Stool _X__ Wheelchair _NA____
Standing position: Braces _NA_ Crutches _NA_ Canes _NA_
Handedness: Dominant hand _Right_ Two hands _X_ One hand only____ Assistive____

Fig. 12-2. Activities of home management. (Adapted from Occupational Therapy Department, University Hospital, Ohio State University, Columbus, Ohio.)

Grading key: I = Independent
MiA = Minimal assistance
MoA = Moderate assistance
MaA = Maximal assistance
D = Dependent
0 = Not evaluated

CLEANING ACTIVITIES	Date	8/25				REMARKS
		Grade				
Pick up object from floor		D				
Wipe up spills		D				
Make bed (daily)		D				
Use dust mop		I				
Shake dust mop		D				
Dust low surfaces		I				
Dust high surfaces		D				
Mop kitchen floor		D				
Sweep with broom		I				
Use dust pan and broom		MiA				
Use vacuum cleaner		0				
Use vacuum cleaner attachments		D				
Carry light cleaning tools		I				
Use carpet sweeper		I				
Clean bathtub		D				
Change sheets on bed		D				
Carry pail of water		D				

MEAL PREPARATION	Date	8/25				REMARKS
Turn off water		I				
Turn off gas or electric range		I				
Light gas with match		D				
Pour hot water from pan to cup		D				
Open packaged goods		I				
Carry pan from sink to range		D				
Use can opener		D				
Handle milk bottle		I				
Dispose of garbage		D				
Remove things from refrigerator		D				
Bend to low cupboards		D				
Reach to high cupboards		D				
Peel vegetables		D				
Cut up vegetables		D				
Handle sharp tools safely		D				
Break eggs		D				
Stir against resistance		D				
Measure flour		D				
Use eggbeater		0				
Use electric mixer		D				
Remove batter to pan		D				
Open oven door		I				
Carry pan to oven and put in		D				
Remove hot pan from oven to table		0				
Roll cookie dough or piecrust		D				

Continued.

Fig. 12-2, cont'd. Activities of home management.

MEAL SERVICE	Date	8/25				REMARKS
Set table for four		I				
Carry four glasses of water to table		D				
Carry hot casserole to table		D				
Clear table		I				
Scrape and stack dishes		I				
Wash dishes (light soil)		I				
Wipe silver		I				
Wash pots and pans		MiA				
Wipe up range and work areas		MoA				
Wring out dishcloth		I				

LAUNDRY	Date	8/25				REMARKS
Wash lingerie (by hand)		D				
Wring out, squeeze dry		D				
Hang on rack to dry		I				
Sprinkle clothes		I				
Iron blouse or slip		D				
Fold blouse or slip						
Use washing machine						

SEWING	Date	8/25				REMARKS
Thread needle and make knot						
Sew on buttons						
Mend rip						
Darn socks						
Use sewing machine						
Crochet						
Knit						
Embroider						
Cut with shears						

HEAVY HOUSEHOLD ACTIVITIES. WHO WILL DO THESE?

	Date	8/25				REMARKS
Wash household laundry						
Hang clothes						
Clean range						
Clean refrigerator						
Wax floors						
Marketing						
Turn mattresses						
Wash windows						
Put up curtains						

WORK HEIGHTS

SITTING/STANDING

Wheelchair _____ Chair ___X___ Stool ___X___

Best height for
Ironing _17½" seated_
Mixing _26" on high stool at counter_
Dish washing _26" on high stool at counter_
General work _____

Maximal depth of counter area (normal reach) _25"_

Maximal useful height above work surface _33" if standing_

Maximal useful height without counter surface _68" if standing_

Maximal reach below counter area _20" if standing_

Best height for chair _17½"–can be used at adjustable ironing board_

Best height for stool with back support _24"–can be used at sink or food preparation counter_

SUGGESTIONS FOR HOME MODIFICATION

Remove scatter rugs in bedroom
Install guard rail on both sides of toilet
Install grab bars on wall next to bathtub
Place nonskid strips on bottom of bathtub

Fig. 12-2, cont'd. Activities of home management.

SPECIFIC ADL TECHNIQUES

In many instances specific techniques to solve specific ADL problems are not possible. Rather the occupational therapist may have to explore a variety of methods or assistive devices to reach a solution. It is sometimes necessary for the therapist to design a special device, method, splint, jig, or piece of equipment to make a particular activity possible for the client to perform. Many of the assistive devices available today through rehabilitation equipment companies were first conceived of and made by occupational therapists and clients. Many of the special methods used to perform specific activities also evolved through trial and error approaches of the therapists and their clients. Clients often have good suggestions for therapists, since they live with the limitation and are confronted regularly with the need to adapt the performance of daily tasks. The purpose of the following summary of techniques is to give the reader some general ideas about how to solve ADL problems for specific classifications of dysfunctions. The reader is referred to the references at the end of this section for more specific instruction in ADL methods.

Limited ROM[9,11,12,15]

The major problem for persons with limited joint ROM is to compensate for the lack of reach and joint excursion through such means as environmental adaptation and assistive devices. Some adaptations and devices are outlined here.

DRESSING ACTIVITIES. The following are general suggestions for facilitating dressing:

1. Use front-opening garments, one size larger than needed and made of fabrics that have some stretch.
2. Use dressing sticks (Fig. 12-3) with a garter on one end and neoprene-covered coat hook on the other for pushing and pulling garments off and on feet and legs. A pair of dowels with a cup hook on end of each can be used to pull socks on if a loop tape is sewn to the tops of the socks.
3. Use larger buttons or zippers with a loop on the pull tab.

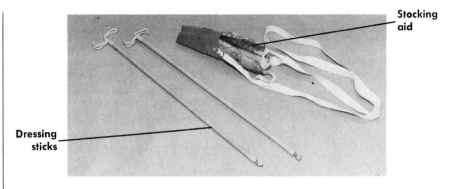

Fig. 12-3. Dressing sticks and stocking aid.

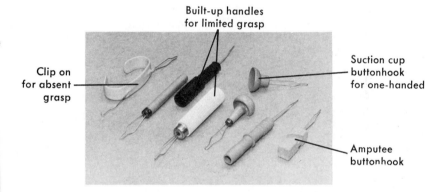

Fig. 12-4. Buttonhooks to accommodate limited or special types of grasp or amputation.

4. Replace buttons, snaps, hooks, and eyes with Velcro or zippers (for those clients who cannot manage traditional fastenings).
5. Eliminate the need to bend to tie shoelaces or use the finger joints in this fine activity by using elastic shoelaces or other adapted shoe fasteners.
6. Facilitate donning stockings without bending to the feet by using stocking aids made of garters attached to long webbing straps or buying those that are commercially available (Fig. 12-3).
7. Use one of several types of commercially available buttonhooks if finger ROM is very limited (Fig. 12-4).
8. Use scissor reachers for picking up socks and shoes, arranging clothes, removing clothes from hangers, and picking up objects on the floor (Fig. 12-5).

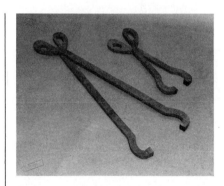

Fig. 12-5. Short and long scissor reachers.

FEEDING ACTIVITIES. The following are assistive devices that can facilitate feeding:

1. Built-up handles on eating utensils can accommodate limited grasp or prehension (Fig. 12-6).
2. Elongated or specially curved handles on spoons and forks may be needed to reach the mouth. A swivel spoon or spoon-fork combination can compensate for limited supination (Fig. 12-7).
3. Long plastic straws and straw clips on glasses or cups can be used if neck, elbow, or shoulder ROM limits hand-to-mouth motion or if grasp is inadequate to hold the cup or glass.
4. Universal cuffs or untensil holders can be used if grasp is very limited and even built-up handles do not work.
5. Plate guards or scoop dishes may be useful to prevent food from slipping off the plate.

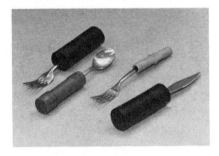

Fig. 12-6. Eating utensils with built-up handles.

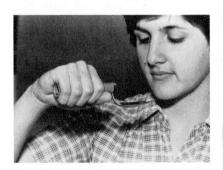

Fig. 12-7. Swivel spoon is used to compensate for limited supination.

HYGIENE AND GROOMING. Environmental adaptations that can facilitate bathing and grooming are as follows:

1. A hand-held shower head on flexible hose for bathing and shampooing hair can eliminate the need to stand in the shower and offers the user control of the direction of the spray. The handle can be built up or adapted for limited grasp.
2. A long-handled bath brush and sponge with a soap holder or long cloth scrubber can allow the user to reach legs, feet, and back. A wash mitt and soap on a rope can aid limited grasp (Fig. 12-8).
3. Long handles on comb, brush, toothbrush, lipstick, mascara brush, and safety or electric razor may be useful for limited hand-to-head or hand-to-face movements.
4. Spray deodorant, hair spray, and spray powder or perfume can "extend" the reach by the distance the material sprays. Special adaptations may be required by some individuals to operate the spray mechanism.
5. Electric toothbrushes and a Water-Pik may be easier to manage for oral hygiene than a standard toothbrush.
6. A short reacher can extend reach for using toilet paper.
7. Dressing sticks can be used to pull garments up after using the toilet. An alternative is the use of a long piece of elastic or webbing with garters on each end that can be hung around the neck and fastened to pants or panties, not allowing them to slip all the way to the floor during use of the toilet.

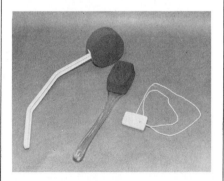

Fig. 12-8. Long-handled bath sponges and soap on a rope.

8. Safety rails can be used for bathtub transfers and safety mats or strips can be placed in the bathtub bottom to prevent slipping.
9. A bathtub seat, shower stool, or regular chair set in the bathtub or shower stall can eliminate the need to sit in the bathtub bottom or stand to shower and increases safety.

COMMUNICATION AND ENVIRONMENTAL HARDWARE. The following are examples of environmental adaptations that can facilitate communication:

1. Extended or built-up handles on faucets can accommodate limited grasp.
2. Telephones should be placed within easy reach. A clip-type receiver holder, extended receiver holder, or speakerphone may be necessary. A dialing stick or push-button phone are still other adaptations.
3. Built-up pens and pencils to accommodate limited grasp and prehension can be used. A wire stand pencil holder and several other commercially available or custom fabricated writing aids are possible (Fig. 12-9).
4. Electric typewriters or personal computers and book holders are aids that can facilitate communication for those with limited or painful joints.
5. Lever-type door knob extensions, car door openers, and adapted key holders can compensate for hand limitations.

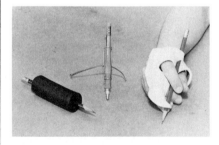

Fig. 12-9. Writing aids. **A,** Built-up pencil. **B,** Wire stand pencil holder. **C,** Thermoplastic custom-made writing device.

MOBILITY AND TRANSFER SKILLS. The individual who has limited ROM without significant muscle weakness may benefit from the following assistive devices:

1. A glider chair that is operated by the feet can facilitate transportation if there is limited hand and arm motion.
2. Platform crutches can prevent stress on hand or finger joints and accommodate limited grasp.
3. Enlarged grips on crutches or canes can accommodate limited grasp.
4. A raised toilet seat can be used if hip and knee motion is limited.
5. A walker with padded grips and forearm troughs can be used if there are marked hand, forearm, or elbow joint limitations.
6. A walker or crutch bags can facilitate the carrying of objects.

HOME MANAGEMENT ACTIVITIES.[8,12] Home management activities can be facilitated by a wide variety of environmental adaptations, assistive devices, energy conservation methods, and work simplification techniques. The principles of joint protection are essential for those with rheumatoid arthritis. These are discussed in Chapter 23. The following are suggestions to facilitate home management for individuals with limited ROM:

1. Store frequently used items on the fist shelves of cabinets just above and below counters or on counters where possible.
2. Use a high stool to work comfortably at counter height or attach a drop leaf table to the wall for planning and meal preparation area if a wheelchair is used.
3. Use a utility cart of comfortable height to transport several items at once.
4. Use reachers to get lightweight items (for example, cereal box) from high shelves.
5. Stabilize mixing bowls and dishes with nonslip mats.
6. Use lightweight utensils, such as plastic or aluminum bowls and aluminum pots.
7. Use electric can openers and electric mixers.

8. Use electric scissors.
9. Eliminate bending by using extended and flexible plastic handles on dust mops and brooms.
10. Facilitate sweeping by using dustpans and brushes with extended handles.
11. Eliminate bending by using wall ovens and counter top broilers.
12. Eliminate leaning and bending for ambulatory persons by using a top-loading automatic washer and elevated dryer. Wheelchair users can benefit from front-loading appliances.
13. Allow for sitting while ironing by using an adjustable ironing board.
14. Elevate the playpen and diaper table and use a Bathinette or plastic tub on the kitchen counter for bathing to reduce the amount of bending and reaching for the ambulatory mother during child care. The crib mattress can be raised, but this presents a safety factor when the child is more than a few months old.
15. Use larger and looser fitting garments with Velcro fastenings on children.

Problems of incoordination[1,9,15]

Incoordination in the form of tremors or ataxia or athetoid or choreiform movements can result from a variety of central nervous system (CNS) disorders, such as Parkinson's disease, multiple sclerosis, cerebral palsy, and head injuries. The major problems encountered in ADL performance are safety and adequate stability of gait, body parts, and objects to complete the tasks.

The degree of incoordinated movement may be influenced by fatigue, emotional factors, and fears. The client must be taught appropriate energy conservation and work simplification techniques along with appropriate work pacing and safety methods to avoid the fatigue and apprehension that could increase incoordination and affect performance.

DRESSING ACTIVITIES. Potential dressing difficulties can be reduced by using the following adaptations:

1. Front-opening garments that fit loosely can facilitate donning and removing garments.

2. Large buttons, Velcro, or zippers with loops on the tab can facilitate opening and closing fasteners. A buttonhook with a large, weighted handle may be helpful.
3. Elastic shoelaces, other adapted shoe closures, or slip-on shoes eliminate the need for bow tying.
4. Trousers with elastic tops for women or Velcro closures for men are easier to manage than those with hooks, buttons, and zippers.
5. Brassieres with front openings or Velcro replacements for the usual hook and eye may facilitate donning and removing this garment. A slip-over elastic-type brassiere or bra-slip may also eliminate the need to manage the brassiere fastenings. Regular brassieres may be fastened in front at waist level, then slipped around to the back and the arms put into the straps, which are then worked up over the shoulders.
6. Clip-on ties can be used by men who use a tie.
7. Dressing should be performed while sitting on or in bed or in a wheelchair or chair with arms to avoid balance problems.

FEEDING ACTIVITIES. For clients with problems of incoordination eating can be quite a challenge. Lack of control during eating is not only frustrating to the individual but can produce embarrassment and social rejection. Therefore it is important to make eating safe, pleasurable, and as neat as possible. The following are some suggestions for achieving this goal:

1. Use plate stabilizers, such as nonskid mats, suction bases, or even wet dish towels.
2. Use a plate guard or scoop dish to prevent pushing food off the plate. The plate guard can be carried away from home and clipped to any ordinary dinner plate (Fig. 12-10).
3. Prevent spills during the plate-to-mouth excursion by using weighted or swivel utensils to offer some stability. Weighted cuffs may be placed on the forearm to decrease involuntary movement (Fig. 12-11).

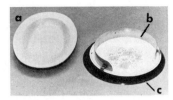

Fig. 12-10. A, Scoop dish. **B,** Plate with plate guard. **C,** Nonskid mat.

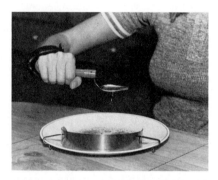

Fig. 12-11. Weighted wrist cuff and swivel utensil can sometimes compensate for incoordination or involuntary motion.

4. Use long plastic straws with a straw clip on a glass or cup with a weighted bottom to eliminate the need to carry the glass or cup to the mouth thus avoiding spills. Plastic cups with covers and spouts may be used for the same purpose.

5. Use a resistance or friction-type arm brace similar to a mobile arm support, which was shown to help control patterns of involuntary movement during feeding activities of adults with cerebral palsy and athetosis by Holser et al.[5] Such a brace may help many clients with severe incoordination achieve some degree of independence in feeding.

HYGIENE AND GROOMING. Stabilization and handling of toilet articles may be achieved by the following suggestions:

1. Articles such as shaver, lipstick, and toothbrush can be attached to a cord if frequent dropping is a problem. An electric toothbrush may be more easily managed than a regular one.

2. Weighted wrist cuffs may be helpful during the finer hygiene activities, such as applying makeup, shaving, or hair care.

3. An electric razor rather than a blade razor offers stability and safety.

4. A suction brush attached to the sink or counter can be used for nail or denture care (Fig. 12-12).

5. Soap should be on a rope and can be worn around the neck or hung over a bathtub or shower fixture during bath or shower to keep it in easy reach.

6. An emery board or small piece of wood with fine sandpaper glued to it can be fastened to the tabletop for filing nails.

7. Large size roll-on deodorants are preferable to sprays or creams.

8. Sanitary napkins that stick to undergarments may be easier to manage than those that require clipping to a sanitary belt or tampons.

9. A bath mitt with a pocket to hold the soap can be used for washing and eliminates the need for frequent soaping and rinsing and wringing a washcloth.

10. Nonskid mats should be used inside and outside the bathtub during bathing. Their suction bases should be securely fastened to the floor and bathtub before they are used. Safety grab bars should be installed on the wall next to the bathtub or fastened to the bathtub edge. A bathtub seat or shower chair provides more safety than standing while showering or transferring to

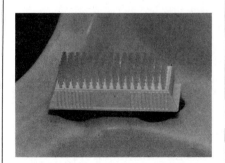

Fig. 12-12. Suction brush attached to bathroom sink.

bathtub bottom. Many incoordinated clients will require supervisory assistance during this hazardous activity. Sponge bathing while seated at a bathroom sink may substitute for bathing or showering several times a week.

COMMUNICATION AND ENVIRONMENTAL HARDWARE. The following adaptations can facilitate communication for clients who have incoordination:

1. Doorknobs may be more easily managed if adapted with lever-type handles or covered with rubber or friction tape.

2. Managing dials or push buttons may be facilitated by using weighted cuffs or by stabilizing arms against body or on tabletop to control involuntary movement. A telephone receiver holder may be helpful.

3. Writing may be managed by using a weighted, enlarged pencil or pen. An electric typewriter with a keyboard guard is a very helpful aid to communication.

4. Keys may be managed by placing them on an adapted key holder that is rigid and offers more leverage for turning the key. However, inserting the key in the keyhole may be very difficult unless the incoordination is relatively mild (Fig. 12-13).

5. Extended lever-type faucets are easier to manage than turn knobs or push-pull spigots. To prevent burns during bathing and kitchen activities cold water should be turned on first and hot water added gradually.

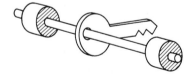

Fig. 12-13. Adapted key holder. Keys are slipped on small metal bar and rubber grommets or washers are slipped over ends to hold keys on. Similar adaptations are commercially available.

MOBILITY AND TRANSFERS.
Clients with problems of incoordination may use a variety of ambulation aids, depending on the type and severity of incoordination. In degenerative diseases it is sometimes necessary to help the client recognize the need for and accept ambulation aids. This may mean graduation from a cane to crutches to a walker and finally to a wheelchair for some persons. Clients with incoordination can improve stability and mobility by the following suggestions:

1. Instead of lifting objects, slide them on floors or counters.
2. Use suitable ambulation aids.
3. Use a utility cart, preferably a custom-made cart that is heavy and has some friction in the wheels.
4. Remove door sills, throw rugs, and shag carpeting.
5. Install banisters on indoor and outdoor staircases.
6. Substitute ramps for stairs wherever possible.

HOME MANAGEMENT ACTIVITIES.[8,9,15] It is important for the occupational therapist to make a careful assessment of homemaking activities performance to determine (1) which activities can be done safely, (2) which activities can be done safely if modified or adapted, and (3) which activities cannot be done adequately or safely and should be assigned to someone else. The major problems are stabilization of foods and equipment to prevent spilling and accidents and the safe handling of appliances, pots, pans, and household tools to prevent cuts, burns, bruises, electric shock, and falls. The following are suggestions for the facilitation of home management tasks:

1. Use a wheelchair and wheelchair lap board, even if ambulation is possible with devices. This will save energy and increase stability if balance and gait are unsteady.
2. If possible, use convenience and prepared foods to eliminate as many processes as possible, for example: peeling, chopping, slicing, and mixing.
3. Use easy-open containers or store foods in plastic containers once opened. A jar opener is also useful.

4. Use heavy utensils, mixing bowls, and pots and pans to increase stability.
5. Use nonskid mats on work surfaces.
6. Use electrical appliances such as crock pots, electric fry pans, and toaster-ovens, which are safer than using the range.
7. Use a blender and counter top mixer, which are safer than hand-held mixers and easier than mixing with a spoon or whisk.
8. If possible, adjust work heights of counters, sink, and range to minimize leaning, bending, reaching, and lifting, whether the client is standing or using a wheelchair.
9. Use long oven mitts, which are safer than potholders.
10. Use pots, pans, casserole dishes, and appliances with bilateral handles, which may be easier to manage than those with one handle.
11. Use a cutting board with stainless steel nails to stabilize meats and vegetables while cutting. When not in use the nails should be covered with a large cork. The bottom of the board should have suction cups or be covered with stair tread, or the board should be placed on a nonskid mat to prevent slippage when in use (Fig. 12-14).
12. Use heavy dinnerware, which may be easier to handle, since it offers stability and control to the distal part of the upper extremity. On the other hand, unbreakable dinnerware may be more practical if dropping and breakage are a problem.

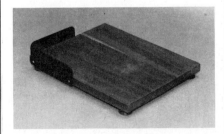

Fig. 12-14. Cutting board with stainless steel nails, suction cup feet, and corner for stabilizing bread is useful for clients with incoordination or who have one hand.

13. Cover the sink, utility cart, and counter tops with protective rubber mats or mesh matting.
14. Use a serrated knife, which is easier to control, for cutting and chopping.
15. Use a steamer basket or deep fry basket for preparing boiled foods to eliminate the need to carry and drain pots with hot liquids in them.
16. Turn foods during cooking and when serving foods with tongs, which may offer more control and stability than a fork, spatula, or serving spoon.[7]
17. Vacuum with a heavy upright cleaner, which may be easier for the ambulatory client. The wheelchair user may be able to manage a lightweight tank-type vacuum cleaner or electric broom.
18. Use dust mitts when dusting.
19. Eliminate fragile knickknacks, unstable lamps, and dainty doilies.
20. Eliminate ironing by using no-iron fabrics or a timed dryer or by assigning this task to other members of the household.
21. Use front-loading washers, a laundry cart on wheels, and premeasured detergents, bleaches, and fabric softeners.
22. Sit while working and use foam rubber bath aids, an infant bath seat, and a wide, padded dressing table with safety straps with Velcro fastening to offer enough stability for bathing, dressing, and diapering an infant. Child care may not be possible unless the incoordination is mild.
23. Use disposable diapers with tape fasteners, which are easier to manage than cloth diapers and pins.
24. Do not feed the infant with a spoon or fork unless the incoordination is very mild or does not affect the upper extremities. This task may need to be performed by another household member.
25. Provide clothing for the child that is large, loose, with Velcro fastenings, and made of nonslippery stretch fabrics.

Hemiplegia or use of only one upper extremity[1,8,9,15]

The suggestions for performing daily living skills apply to persons with hemiplegia, unilateral upper extremity amputations, and temporary disorders, such as fractures, burns, or peripheral neuropathy, which can result in the dysfuntion of one upper extremity.

The hemiplegic individual will require specialized methods of teaching, and many will have greater difficulty in learning and performing one-handed skills than persons with orthopedic or lower motor neuron dysfunction. This is because of involvement of the trunk and leg, as well as the arm, and therefore possible ambulation and balance difficulties. Also, sensory, perceptual, cognitive, and speech disorders may be present from a mild to severe degree. These affect the ability to learn and retain learning and performance. Finally, the presence of motor and ideational apraxia sometimes seen in this group of clients can have a profound effect on the client's potential for learning new motor skills or remembering old ones.

Therefore the client with normal perception and cognition and the use of one upper extremity may learn the techniques quicly and easily. The hemiplegic client needs to be evaluated for sensory, perceptual, and cognitive deficits to determine potential for ADL performance and to establish appropriate teaching methods, already described, to facilitate learning.

The major problems for the one-handed worker are reduction of work speed and dexterity, stabilization to substitute for the role normally assumed by the nondominant arm, and, for the hemiplegic, balance and precautions relative to sensory loss.

DRESSING ACTIVITIES. If balance is a problem, dressing should be done while seated in a locked wheelchair or sturdy armchair. Clothing should be within easy reach. Reaching tongs may be helpful for securing articles and assisting in some dressing activities. Assistive devices should be minimal for dressing and other ADL.

One-handed dressing techniques*
Dressing techniques for the hemiplegic that employ neurodevelopmental (Bobath) treatment principles are discussed in Chapter 16. The following one-handed dressing techniques can facilitate dressing for persons with use of one upper extremity.

Front-opening shirts may be managed by any one of three methods. The fist method can be used for jackets, robes, and front-opening dresses.

METHOD I
Donning shirt (Fig. 12-15)

1. Grasp shirt collar with normal hand and shake out twists (a).
2. Position shirt on lap with inside up and collar toward chest (b).
3. Position sleeve opening on affected side so it is as large as possible and close to affected hand, which is resting on lap (c).
4. Using normal hand place affected hand in sleeve opening and work sleeve over elbow by pulling on garment (d_1–d_2).
5. Put normal arm into its sleeve and raise up to slide or shake sleeve into position past elbow (e).
6. With normal hand gather shirt up middle of back from hem to collar and raise shirt over head (f).
7. Lean forward, duck head, and pass shirt over it (g).
8. With normal hand adjust shirt by leaning forward and working it down past both shoulders. Reach in back and pull shirt-tail down (h).
9. Line shirt fronts up for buttoning and begin with bottom button (i). Button sleeve cuff of affected arm. Sleeve cuff of unaffected arm may be prebuttoned if cuff opening is large or button may be sewn on with elastic thread or sewn on a small tab of elastic and fastened inside shirt cuff. A small button attached to crocheted loop of elastic thread is another alternative. Slip button on loop through button-hole in garment so that elastic loop is inside. Stretch elastic loop to fit around original cuff button. This simple device can be transferred to each garment and positioned before shirt is put on. Loop stretches to accommodate width of hand as it is pushed through end of sleeve.[14]

---

*Summarized from Activities of daily living for patients with incoordination, limited range of motion, paraplegia, quadriplegia, and hemiplegia, Cleveland, 1968, Highland View Hospital, Cuyahoga County Hospitals, Division of Occupational Therapy. Mimeographed, unpublished.

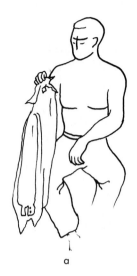

a

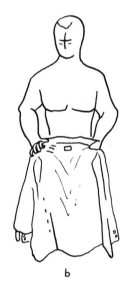

b

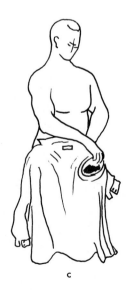

c

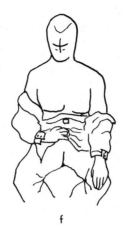

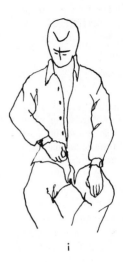

f

i

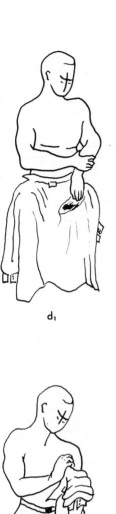

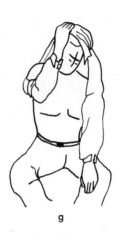

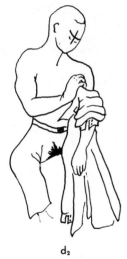

g

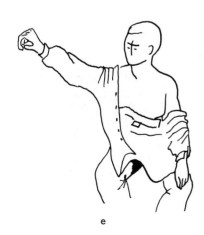

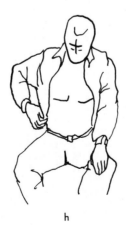

h

Fig. 12-15. Steps in donning shirt: method I. (Reproduced with permission of Mary S. Miller, Asst. Director of Occupational Therapy, Cuyahoga County Hospital, Cleveland, Ohio.)

Removing shirt
1. Unbutton shirt.
2. Lean forward.
3. With normal hand grasp collar or gather material up in back from collar to hem.
4. Lean forward, duck head, and pull shirt over head.
5. Remove sleeve from normal arm and then from affected arm.

METHOD II
Donning shirt
Method II may be used by clients who get shirt twisted or who have trouble sliding the sleeve down onto normal arm.

1. Position shirt as described in method I, steps 1 to 3.
2. With normal hand place involved hand into shirt sleeve opening and work sleeve onto hand, but do *not* pull up over elbow.
3. Put normal arm into sleeve and bring arm out to 180° of abduction. Tension of fabric from normal arm to wrist of affected arm will bring sleeve into position.
4. Lower arm and work sleeve on affected arm up over elbow.
5. Continue as in steps 6 through 9 of method I.

Removing shirt
1. Unbutton shirt.
2. With normal hand push shirt off shoulders, first on affected side, then on normal side.
3. Pull on cuff of normal side with normal hand.
4. Work sleeve off by alternately shrugging shoulder and pulling down on cuff.
5. Lean forward, bring shirt around back, and pull sleeve off affected arm.

METHOD III
Donning shirt (Fig 12-16)

1. Position shirt and work onto arm as described in method I, steps 1 to 4.
2. Pull sleeve on affected arm up to shoulder (a).
3. With normal hand grasp tip of collar that is on normal side, lean forward, and bring arm over and behind head to carry shirt around to normal side (b).
4. Put normal arm into sleeve opening, directing it up and out (c).
5. Adjust and button as described in method I, steps 8 and 9.

Removing shirt

The shirt may be removed using the same procedure described previously for method II.

Variation—donning pullover shirt
Pullover shirts can be managed by the following procedure:

1. Position shirt on lap, bottom toward chest and label facing down.
2. With normal hand roll up bottom edge of shirt back up to sleeve on affected side.
3. Position sleeve opening so it is as large as possible and use normal hand to place affected one into sleeve opening. Pull shirt up onto arm past elbow.
4. Insert normal arm into sleeve.
5. Adjust shirt on affected side up and on to shoulder.
6. Gather shirt back with normal hand, lean forward, duck head, and pass shirt over head.
7. Adjust shirt.

Variation—removing pullover shirt
Pullover shirts are removed by the following procedure:

1. Gather shirt up with normal hand, starting at top back.
2. Lean forward, duck head, and pull gathered back fabric over head.
3. Remove from normal arm and then affected arm.

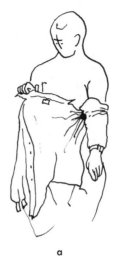

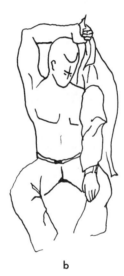

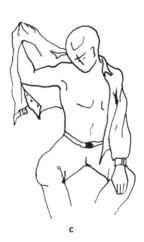

Fig. 12-16. Steps in donning shirt: method III. (Reproduced with permission of Mary S. Miller, Asst. Director of Occupational Therapy, Cuyahoga County Hospital, Cleveland, Ohio.)

Trousers may be managed by one of the following methods. These may be adapted for shorts and women's panties as well. It is recommended that trousers have a well-constructed button fly front opening. This may be easier to manage than a zipper. Velcro may be used to replace buttons or zippers. Trousers should be worn in a size slightly larger than worn previously and should have a wide opening at the ankles. They should be donned after the socks have been put on but before the shoes are put on.

METHOD I
Donning trousers (Fig. 12-17)

1. Sit in sturdy armchair or in locked wheelchair (a).
2. Position normal leg in front of midline of body with knee flexed to 90°. Using normal hand reach forward and grasp ankle of affected leg or sock around ankle (b_1). Lift affected leg over normal leg to crossed position (b_2).
3. Slip trousers onto affected leg up to position where foot is completely inside of trouser leg (c). Do *not* pull up above knee or difficulty will be encountered in inserting normal leg.
4. Uncross affected leg by grasping ankle or portion of sock around ankle (d).
5. Insert normal leg and work trousers up onto hips as far as possible $(e_1 - e_2)$. If wheelchair is used, place footrests in an up position.
6. If able to do so safely, stand and pull trousers over hips. To prevent trousers from dropping place affected hand in pocket or place one finger of affected hand into belt loop $f_1 - f_3$.
7. Sit down to button front (g). If standing balance is good, remain standing to pull up zipper or button (f_3).

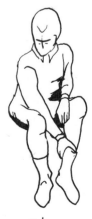

a, b₁

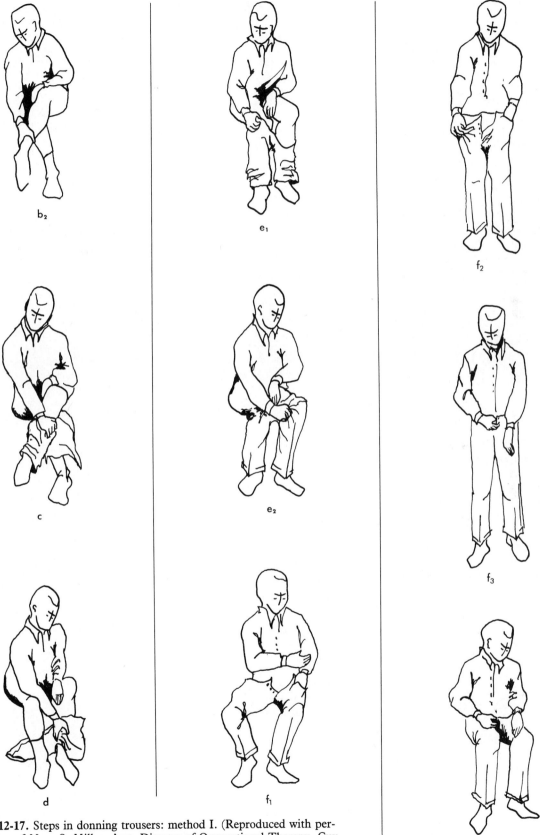

Fig. 12-17. Steps in donning trousers: method I. (Reproduced with permission of Mary S. Miller, Asst. Director of Occupational Therapy, Cuyahoga County Hospital, Cleveland, Ohio.)

Removing trousers

1. Unfasten trousers and work down on hips as far as possible while seated.
2. Stand, letting trousers drop past hips or work them down past hips.
3. Sit and cross affected leg over normal leg, remove trousers, and uncross leg.
4. Remove trousers from normal leg.

METHOD II

Donning trousers

Method II is used for clients who are in wheelchairs with brakes locked or are in sturdy straight armchairs that are positioned with back against wall and for clients who cannot stand independently.

1. Position trousers on legs as in method I, steps 1 through 5.
2. Footrests remain in down position. Elevate hips by leaning back against chair and pushing down with normal leg. As hips are raised, work trousers over hips with normal hand.
3. Lower hips back into chair and fasten trousers.

Removing trousers

1. Unfasten trousers and work down on hips as far as possible while sitting.
2. With footrests in *down* position lean back against chair, push down with normal leg to elevate hips, and with normal arm work trousers down past hips.
3. Proceed as in method I, steps 3 and 4.

METHOD III

Donning trousers

Method III is for clients who are in a recumbent position. It is more difficult to perform than those methods done sitting. If possible, bed should be raised to semireclining position for partial sitting.

1. Using normal hand, place affected leg in bent position and cross over normal leg, which may be partially bent to prevent affected leg from slipping.
2. Position trousers and work onto affected leg, first, up to the knee. Then uncross leg.
3. Insert normal leg, and work trousers up onto hips as far as possible.
4. With normal leg bent press down with foot and shoulder to elevate hips from bed and with normal arm pull trousers over hips or work trousers up over hips by rolling from side to side.
5. Fasten trousers.

Removing trousers

1. Hike hips as in putting trousers on in method III, step 4.
2. Work trousers down past hips, remove unaffected leg, and then remove affected leg.

Clothing items, such as brassieres, neckties, socks, stockings, and braces, may be difficult to manage with one hand. The following methods are recommended.

BRASSIERE

Donning

1. Tuck one end of brassiere into pants, girdle, or skirt waistband, and wrap other end around waist. Hook brassiere in front at waist level and slip fastener around to back (at waistline level).
2. Place affected arm through shoulder strap, and then place normal arm through other strap.
3. Work straps up over shoulders. Pull strap on affected side up over shoulder with normal arm. Put normal arm through its strap and work up over shoulder by directing arm up and out and pulling with hand.
4. Use normal hand to adjust breasts in brassiere cups.

NOTE: It is helpful if brassiere has elastic straps and is one size larger than usually worn. If there is some function in affected hand, a fabric loop may be sewn to back of brassiere near fastener. Affected thumb may be slipped through this to stabilize brassiere while normal hand fastens it. All elastic brassieres, prefastened or without fasteners, may be donned by adapting method I for shirts described previously.

Removing

1. Slip straps down off shoulders, normal side first.
2. Work straps down over arms and off hands.
3. Slip brassiere around to front with normal arm.
4. Unfasten and remove.

NECKTIE

Donning

Clip-on neckties are attractive and convenient. If conventional tie is used, the following method is recommended:

1. Place collar of shirt in up position and bring necktie around neck and adjust so that smaller end is at desired length when tie is completed.
2. Fasten small end to shirt front with tie clasp or spring clip clothespin.
3. Loop long end around short end (one complete loop) and bring up between V at neck. Then bring tip down through loop at front and adjust tie, using ring and little fingers to hold tie end and thumb and forefingers to slide knot up tightly.

Removing

Pull knot at front of neck until small end slips up enough for tie to be slipped over head. Tie may be hung up in this state and replaced by clipping it over head, around upturned collar, and knot tightened, as described in step 3 of donning necktie.

SOCKS OR STOCKINGS

Donning

1. Sit in straight armchair or in wheelchair with brakes locked.
2. With normal leg directly in front of midline of body cross affected leg over it.
3. Open top of stocking by inserting thumb and first two fingers near cuff and spreading fingers apart.
4. Work stocking onto foot before pulling over heel. Care should be taken to eliminate wrinkles.
5. Work stocking up over leg. Shift weight from side to side to adjust stocking around thigh.
6. Fasten stocking to garter. Velcro tabs may be substituted for garters.

NOTE: Stockings should be seamless and of soft, stretch-type fabric.

Removing

1. While sitting, unfasten garters.
2. Work socks or stockings down as far as possible with normal arm.
3. Cross affected leg over normal one as described in step 2 of donning socks or stockings.
4. Remove sock or stocking from affected leg. Dressing stick may be required by some clients to push sock or stocking off heel and off foot.
5. Lift normal leg to comfortable height or to seat level and remove sock or stocking from foot.

SHORT LEG BRACE

Donning (Fig. 12-18)

1. Sit in straight armchair or in wheelchair with brakes locked (a).
2. Bring normal leg to body midline. Cross hemiplegic leg over normal leg (b).
3. Pull tongue of shoe through laces and tuck under bottom part of lace, so that it does not push down into shoe as brace is donned (c).
4. Fold Velcro mesh flap back and hold back with calf band. With normal hand swing brace back and then forward so heel is between uprights. Swing shoe far enough forward so that toes can be inserted into shoe (d_1). Still holding onto upright bar of brace, turn shoe inward so that toes will go in at a slight angle, preventing catching toes at sides of shoe (d_2). Pull brace up onto leg as far as possible (e_1). If difficulty is encountered in getting brace up far enough on leg, raise affected leg by pulling up on crossbar, making foot easier to slip into shoe. Brace can now be held in position by pressure against crossbar between affected leg and normal leg, while shoehorn is inserted under heel in back (e_2). If there is difficulty in keeping brace on while inserting shoehorn, raise affected leg by pulling up

on crossbar to position where ankle of affected leg is resting against knee of normal leg, with uprights on each side (e₂).

6. By holding uprights, uncross affected leg and position at 90° angle to floor (f₁ – f₂). Shoehorn is now in position where heel is pressing on it. Alternately, direct pressure downward on the knee and move shoehorn back and forth, using normal hand, until foot slips into shoe (f₃ – f₅).

7. Fasten laces and straps. One of many methods of one-handed bow tying may be used. Elastic shoelaces or other commercially available shoe fasteners may be required if unable to tie shoes (g).

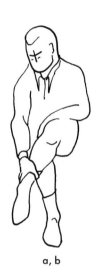

a, b

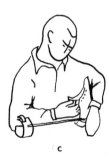

c

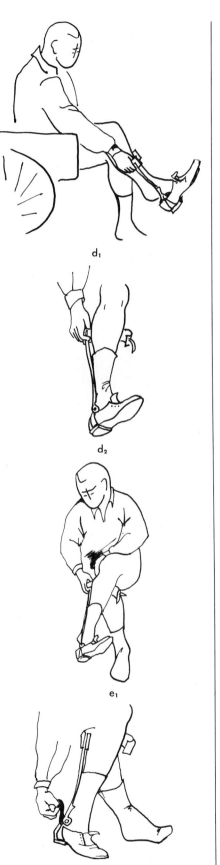

d₁

d₂

e₁

e₂

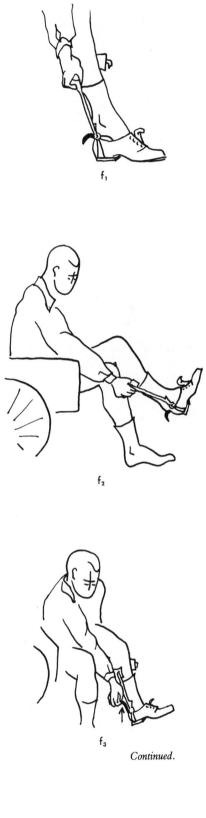

f₁

f₂

f₃

Continued.

Fig. 12-18. Steps in donning short leg brace. (Reproduced with permission of Mary S. Miller, Asst. Director of Occupational Therapy, Cuyahoga County Hospital, Cleveland, Ohio.)

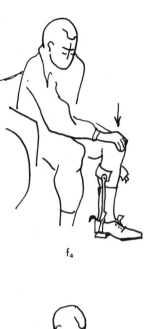

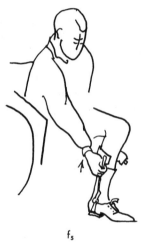

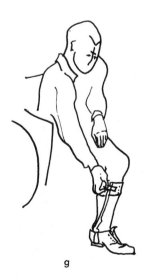

Fig. 12-18, cont'd. Steps in donning short leg brace.

Removing

Variation I

1. While seated as for donning, cross affected leg over normal leg.
2. Unfasten straps and laces with normal hand.
3. Push down on brace upright until shoe is off foot.

Variation II

1. Unfasten straps and laces.
2. Straighten affected leg by putting normal foot behind heel of shoe and pushing affected leg forward.
3. Push down on brace upright with hand and at same time push forward on heel of brace shoe with normal foot.

NOTE: Shoes may be donned by crossing legs, as described for stockings. Long-handled shoehorn may be helpful. Shoe tongue can have holes punched at top and shoelaces threaded through it to prevent tongue from being pushed into shoe when foot is forced in. Elastic shoelaces, buckles, or other adapted shoe closures are recommended for hemiplegic clients. Method for one-handed shoe tying is illustrated in Fig. 12-19 for those clients who prefer standard tie oxford.

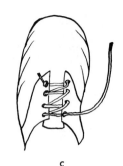

c

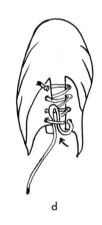

d

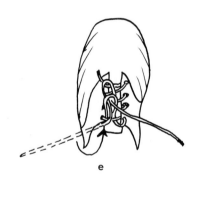

e

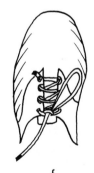

f

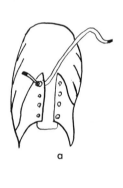

a

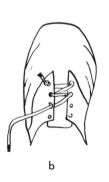

b

Fig. 12-19. One-hand shoe tying method. (Reproduced with permission of Mary S. Miller, Asst. Director of Occupational Therapy, Cuyahoga County Hospital, Cleveland, Ohio.)

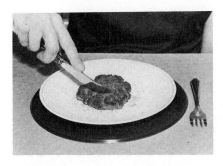

Fig. 12-20. Rocker knife for clients with one hand.

FEEDING ACTIVITIES. The only real problem encountered by the one-handed individual is managing a knife and fork simultaneously for meat cutting. This problem can be solved by the use of a rocker knife (Fig. 12-20) for cutting meat and other foods. It cuts with a rocking motion rather than a slicing back and forth action. The use of a rocking motion with a standard table knife or a sharp paring knife may be adequate to accomplish cutting tender meats and foods. If such a knife is used, the client is taught to hold the knife handle between the thumb and the third, fourth, and fifth fingers, and the index finger is extended along the top of the knife blade. The knife point is placed in the food in a vertical position, and then the blade is brought down to cut the food. The rocking motion, using wrist flexion and extension, is continued until the food is cut.

The occupational therapist should keep in mind that one-handed meat cutting involves learning a new motor pattern and may be difficult for clients with hemiplegia and apraxia.

HYGIENE AND GROOMING ACTIVITIES. With some assistive devices and the use of alternate methods hygiene and grooming activities can be accomplished by those with use of one hand or use of one side of the body. The following are suggestions for achieving hygiene and grooming with one hand:

1. Use an electric razor rather than a safety razor.

2. Use a bathtub seat or chair in the shower stall, wash mitt, long-handled bath sponge, safety rails on the bathtub or wall, soap on a rope or suction soap holder (Little Octopus), and suction brush for fingernail care.

3. Sponge bathe while sitting at the lavatory, using the wash mitt, suction brush, and suction soap holder. The uninvolved forearm and hand may be washed by placing a soaped washcloth on the thigh and rubbing the hand and forearm on the cloth.

4. Care for fingernails as described previously for clients with incoordination.

5. Use spray deodorants rather than creams or roll-ons, since they can be more easily applied to the uninvolved underarm.

6. Use a suction denture brush for care of dentures. The suction fingernail brush may also serve this purpose.

COMMUNICATION AND ENVIRONMENTAL HARDWARE. The following are suggestions to facilitate writing, reading, and using the telephone:

1. The primary problem in writing is stabilization of the paper or tablet. This can be overcome by using a clip board or paper weight or by taping the paper to the writing surface. In some instances the affected arm may be positioned on the tabletop to stabilize the paper passively.

2. If dominance must be shifted to the nondominant extremity, writing practice may be necessary to improve speed and coordination. One-handed writing and typing instruction manuals are available.

3. Book holders may be used to stabilize a book while reading or holding copy for typing and writing practice.

4. The telephone is managed by lifting the receiver to listen for the dial tone, setting it down, dialing or pressing the buttons, then lifting the receiver to the ear. To write while using the telephone a telephone receiver holder that is on a stand or that rests on the shoulder must be used.

MOBILITY AND TRANSFERS. Specific transfer techniques for clients with hemiplegia are described in Chapter 18.

HOME MANAGEMENT ACTIVITIES.[8] A wide variety of assistive devices is available to facilitate home management activities. Whether the client is disabled by the loss of function of one arm and hand, as in amputation or peripheral neuropathy, or whether both arm and leg are affected along with possible visual, perceptual, and cognitive dysfunctions, as in hemiplegia, will determine how many home management activities can realistically be performed, which methods can be used, and how many assistive devices can be managed. The reader is referred to the references listed at the end of this chapter for details of home management with one hand. The following are some suggestions for one-handed homemakers:

1. Stabilization of items is a major problem for the one-handed homemaker. Stabilize foods for cutting and peeling by using a board with two stainless steel or alumium nails in it. A raised corner on the board stabilizes bread while making sandwiches or spreading butter. Suction cups or a rubber mat under the board will keep it from slipping. Rubber stair tread may be glued to the bottom of the board.

2. Use sponge cloths, Dycem pads, wet dishcloths, or suction devices to keep pots, bowls, and dishes from turning or sliding during food preparation.

3. To open a jar, stabilize it between the knees or in a partially opened drawer while leanng against it or use a Zim jar opener (Fig. 12-21).

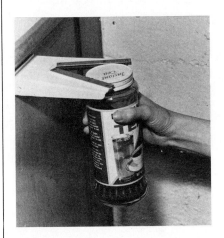

Fig. 12-21. Zim jar opener.

4. Open boxes, sealed paper, and plastic bags by stabilizing between the knees or in a drawer, as just described, and cutting open with a household shears.

5. Open an egg by holding it firmly in the palm of the hand, hitting it in the center against the edge of the bowl, and then using the thumb and index finger to push the top half of the shell up and the ring and little finger to push the lower half down. Separate whites from yolks by using an egg separator or a funnel.

6. Eliminate the need to stabilize the standard grater by using a grater with suction feet.

7. Stabilize pots on counter or range for mixing or stirring by using a pan holder with suction feet (Fig. 12-22).

8. Eliminate the need to use hand-cranked or electric can openers requiring two hands by using a one-handed electric can opener.

9. Use a utility cart to carry items from one place to another. One that is weighted or constructed of wood may be used as a minimal support during ambulation for some clients.

10. Transfer clothes to and from the washer or dryer by using a clothes carrier on wheels.

11. Use electrical appliances, such as a lightweight electrical hand mixer, blender, and food processor, which can be managed with one hand and save time and energy. Safety factors and judgment need to be evaluated carefully when electrical appliances are considered.

12. Floor care becomes a greater problem if ambulation and balance, as well as one arm, are affected. For those clients with involvement of one arm only, a standard dust mop, carpet sweeper, or upright vacuum cleaner should present no problem. A self-wringing mop may be used if the mop handle is stabilized under the arm and the wringing lever operated with the normal arm. Clients with balance and ambulation problems may manage some floor care from a sitting position. Dust mopping or using a carpet sweeper may be possible if gait and balance are fairly good without the aid of a cane.

These are just a few of the possibilities to solve home management problems for one-handed individuals. The occupational therapist must evaluate each client to determine how the dysfunction affects performance of homemaking activities. One-handed techniques take more time and may be difficult for some clients to master. Activities should be paced to accommodate the client's physical endurance and tolerance for one-handed performance and use of special devices. Work simplification and energy conservation techniques should be employed.

New techniques and devices should be introduced on a graded basis as the client masters one technique and device and then another. Family members need to be oriented to the client's skills, special methods used, and work schedule. The therapist with the family and client may facilitate the planning of homemaking responsibilities to be shared by other family members and the supervision of the client, if that is needed.

If special equipment and assistive devices are needed for ADL, it is advisable to acquire these through the health agency, if possible. The therapist can then train the client in their use and demonstrate to a family member before sending these items home.

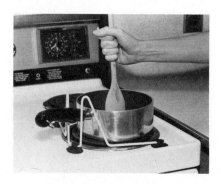

Fig. 12-22. Pan stabilizer.

ADL for wheelchair-bound individuals with good to normal arm function (paraplegia)

Clients who are confined to a wheelchair need to find ways to perform ADL from a seated position, transport objects, and adapt in an environment designed for standing and walking. Given normal upper extremity function, the wheelchair ambulator can probably perform independently.

DRESSING ACTIVITIES.* It is recommended that wheelchair-bound clients put on clothing in this order: stockings, undergarments, braces (if worn), trousers or slacks, shoes, shirt, or dress.

TROUSERS
Donning

Trousers and slacks are easier to fasten if they button or zip in front. If braces are worn, zippers in side seams may be helpful. Wide bottom slacks of stretch fabric are recommended. Procedure for putting on trousers, shorts, slacks, and underwear is as follows:

1. Use side rails or trapeze to help pull self up to sitting position.
2. Sit on bed and reach forward to feet or sit on bed and pull knees into flexed position.
3. Holding top of trousers flip pants down to feet.
4. Work pant legs over feet and pull up to hips. Crossing ankles may help get pants on over heels.
5. In semireclining position roll from hip to hip and pull up garment.
6. Reaching tongs may be helpful to pull garment up or position garment on feet.

Removing

Remove pants or underwear by reversing procedure for donning. Dressing sticks may be helpful to push pants off feet.

SOCKS OR STOCKINGS
Donning

1. Apply socks or stockings while seated on bed.
2. Pull one leg into flexion with one hand.
3. Use other hand to slip sock or stocking over foot and pull it on.

---

*Summarized from Activities of daily living for patients with incoordination, limited range of motion, paraplegia, quadriplegia, and hemiplegia, Cleveland, 1968, Highland View Hospital, Cuyahoga County Hospitals, Division of Occupational Therapy. Mimeographed, unpublished.

NOTE: Soft stretch socks or stockings are recommended. Panty hose that are slightly large may be useful. Elastic garters or stockings with elastic tops should be avoided. Dressing sticks or a stocking device may be helpful to some clients.

Removing

Remove socks or stockings by flexing leg as described for donning, pushing sock or stocking down over heel. Dressing sticks may be needed to push sock or stocking off heel and toe and to retrieve it.

SLIPS AND SKIRTS

Donning

1. To apply slips and skirts sit on bed, slip garment over head, and let it drop to waist.
2. In semireclining position, roll from hip to hip and pull garment down over hips and thighs.

NOTE: Slips and skirts slightly larger than usually worn are recommended. A-line, wraparound, and full skirts are easier to manage and look better on a person seated in a wheelchair than narrow skirts.

Removing

1. In sitting or semireclining position unfasten garment.
2. Roll from hip to hip, pulling garment up to waist level.
3. Pull garment off over head.

SHIRTS

Donning

Shirts, pajama jackets, robes, and dresses opening completely down front may be put on while client is seated in wheelchair. If it is necessary to dress while in bed, following procedure can be used:

1. Balance body by putting palms of hands on mattress on either side of body. If balance is poor, assistance may be needed or bed backrest may be elevated. (If backrest cannot be elevated, one or two pillows may be used to support back.) With backrest elevated both hands are available.
2. If difficulty is encountered in usual methods of applying garment, open garment on lap with collar toward chest. Put arms into sleeves and pull up over elbows. Then hold on to shirttail or back of dress, pull garment over head, adjust and button.

NOTE: Fabrics should be wrinkle-resistant, smooth, and durable. Roomy sleeves and backs and full skirts are more suitable styles than closely fitted garments.

Removing

1. Sitting in wheelchair or bed, open fastening.
2. Remove garment in usual manner.
3. If this is not feasible, grasp collar with one hand while balancing with other hand. Gather material up from collar to hem.
4. Lean forward, duck head, and pull shirt over head.
5. Remove sleeve from supporting arm and then from working arm.

SHOES

Donning

Shoes may be applied by one of the following variations.

Variation I

1. In sitting position on bed pull one knee at a time into flexed position with hands.
2. While supporting leg in flexed position with one hand, use free hand to put on shoe.

Variation II

1. Sit on edge of bed or in wheelchair for back support.
2. Bend one knee up to flexed position, supporting leg with arm, and with free hand slip shoe on.

Variation III

1. Sit on edge of bed or in wheelchair for back support.
2. Cross one leg over other and slip shoe on.
3. Put foot on footrest and push down on knee to push foot into shoe.

Removing

1. Flex or cross leg as described for appropriate variation.
2. For variations I and II remove shoe with one hand while supporting flexed leg with other hand.
3. For variation III remove shoe from crossed leg with one hand while maintaining balance with other hand, if necessary.

FEEDING ACTIVITIES. Eating activities should present no special problem for the wheelchair-bound individual with good to normal arm function. Wheelchairs with desk arms and swing-away footrest are recommended so that it is possible to sit close to the table.

HYGIENE AND GROOMING. Face and oral hygiene and arm and upper body care should present no problem. Reachers may be helpful to secure towels, washcloths, makeup, deodorant, and shaving supplies from storage areas, if necessary. Tub baths or showers require some special equipment.

Transfer techniques for toilet and bathtub will be discussed in Chapter 18. The following are suggestions for facilitating bathing activities:

1. Use a hand-held shower head and keep a finger over the spray to determine sudden temperature changes in water.
2. Use long-handled bath brushes with soap insert for ease in reaching all parts of the body.
3. Use soap bars attached to a cord around the neck.
4. For sponge bath in wheelchair cover the chair with a sheet of plastic.
5. Use shower chairs or bathtub seats.
6. Increase safety during transfers by installing grab bars on wall near bathtub or shower and on bathtub.
7. Fit bathtub or shower bottom with nonskid mat or adhesive material.

COMMUNICATION AND ENVIRONMENTAL HARDWARE. With the exception of reaching difficulties in some situations, use of the telephone should present no problem. Short-handled reachers may be used to grasp the receiver from the cradle. Dialing could be accomplished with a short, rubber-tipped, ¼-inch dowel stick. Use of writing implements, typewriter, tape recorder, and personal computer should be easily possible for these clients.

Managing doors may present some difficulties. If the door opens toward the person, opening it can be managed by the following procedure:

1. If doorknob is on right, approach door from right, and turn doorknob with left hand.
2. Open door as far as possible and move wheelchair close enough so it helps keep door open.
3. Holding door open with left hand turn wheelchair with right hand and wheel through door.
4. Start closing door when halfway through.

If the door is very heavy and opens out or away from the person, the following procedure is recommended:

1. Back up to door so knob can be turned with right hand.
2. Open door and back through so big wheels keep it open.
3. Also use left elbow to keep door open.
4. Wheel backward with right hand.[3]

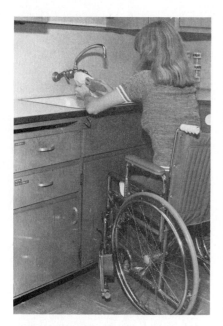

Fig. 12-23. Wheelchair footrests are swung away to allow closer access to sink.

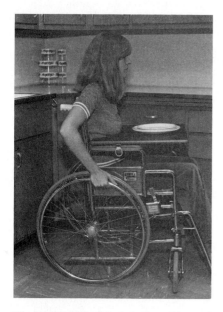

Fig. 12-24. Wheelchair lapboard is used to transport items.

MOBILITY AND TRANFERS. Specific transfer techniques will be discussed in Chapter 18.

HOME MANAGEMENT ACTIVITIES.[8] When performing homemaking activities from a wheelchair, the major problems are work heights, adequate space for maneuverability, access to storage areas, and transfer of supplies, equipment, and materials from place to place. If funds are available for kitchen remodeling, reducing counters and range to a comfortable height for wheelchair use is recommended. However, such extensive adaptation is often not feasible. Suggestions for home management are as follows:

1. Remove cabinet doors to eliminate the need to maneuver around them for opening and closing. Frequently used items should be stored toward the front of easy-to-reach cabinets above and below the counter surfaces.
2. If entrance and inside doors are not wide enough, use a wheelchair narrower or make doors slightly wider by removing strips along the door jambs.
3. A wheelchair cushion can increase the user's height so that standard counters may be used.
4. Use detachable desk arms and swing-away detachable footrests to allow the wheelchair user to get as close as possible to counters and tables and also to stand at counters, if that is possible (Fig. 12-23).
5. Transport items safely and easily by using a wheelchair lapboard. The lapboard may also serve as a work surface for preparing food and drying dishes. It also protects the lap from injury from hot pans and prevents utensils falling into the lap (Fig. 12-24).
6. Fasten a drop leaf–type board to a bare wall or slide-out board under a counter to give the wheelchair homemaker one work surface that is a comfortable height in a kitchen that is otherwise standard.
7. Fit cabinets with custom- or ready-made lazy Susan devices to eliminate need to reach to rear space (Fig. 12-25).
8. Ranges should ideally be at a lower level. If this is not possible, place the controls at the front of the

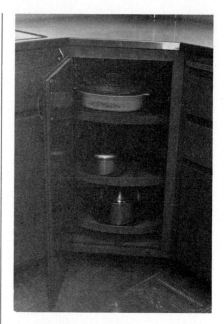

Fig. 12-25. Lazy Susan–type kitchen storage cabinet.

range, and hang a mirror angled at the proper degree over the range so that the homemaker can see contents of pots.
9. Substitute small electric cooking units for the range if it is not safely manageable.
10. Use front-loading washers and dryers.
11. Vacuum carpets with a carpet sweeper or tanktype cleaner that rolls easily and is lightweight or self-propelled. A retractable cord may be helpful to prevent tangling of cord in wheels.

ADL for the wheelchair-bound individual with upper extremity weakness (quadriplegia)

In general, persons with muscle function from spinal cord levels C7 and C8 can follow the methods just described for paraplegia. Individuals with muscle function from C6 can be relatively independent with adaptations and assistive devices, whereas those with muscle function from C4 and C5 will require a considerable amount of special equipment and assistance. Clients with muscle function from C6 may benefit from the use of a wrist-driven flexor hinge splint. Externally powered splints and arm braces or mobile arm supports are recommended for C3, C4, and C5 levels of muscle function.[1]

DRESSING ACTIVITIES[2,13]

Criteria. Dressing training can be commenced when the spine is stable.[2,13] Minimal criteria for upper extremity dressing are (1) fair to good muscle strength in deltoids, upper and middle trapezii, shoulder rotators, rhomboids, biceps, supinators, and radial wrist extensors; (2) ROM of 0° to 90° in shoulder flexion and abduction, 0° to 80° in shoulder internal rotation, 0° to 30° in external rotation, and 15° to 140° in elbow flexion; (3) sitting balance in bed or wheelchair, which may be achieved with the assistance of bed rails or wheelchair safety belt; and (4) finger prehension achieved with adequate tenodesis grasp or wrist-hand orthosis (formerly the flexor-hinge splint). Additional criteria for dressing the lower extremities are (1) fair to good muscle strength in pectoralis major and minor, serratus anterior, and rhomboid major and minor; (2) ROM of 0° to 120° in knee flexion and 0° to 110° in hip flexion; (3) body control for transfer from bed to wheelchair with minimal assistance; (4) ability to roll from side to side, balance in side lying, or turning from supine position to prone position and back; and (5) vital capacity of 50% or better.[13]

Contraindications. Dressing is contraindicated if any of the following factors are present: (1) unstable spine at site of injury, (2) pressure sores or tendency for skin breakdown during rolling, scooting, and when transferring, (3) uncontrollable muscle spasms in legs, and (4) less than 50% vital capacity.[2,13]

Sequence of dressing. The recommended sequence for training to dress is put on underwear and trousers while still in bed, then transfer to a wheelchair and put on shirts, socks, and shoes.[13] Some clients may wish to put the socks on before the trousers, since they may help the feet to slip through the trouser legs more easily.

Expected proficiency. Total dressing, which includes both upper and lower extremity dressing skills, can be achieved by clients with spinal cord lesions at C7 and below. Total dressing can be achieved by clients with lesions at C6 but lower extremity dressing may be difficult or impracticable in terms of time and energy for these clients. Upper extremity dressing can be achieved by clients with lesions at C5 to C6 with some exceptions. It will be difficult or impossible for these clients to don a brassiere, tuck a shirt or blouse into a waistband, and fasten buttons. Factors such as age, physical proportions, coordination, concomitant medical problems, and motivation will affect the degree of proficiency in dressing skills that can be achieved by any client.[2]

Types of clothing. Clothing should be loose and have front openings. Trousers need to be a size larger than usually worn to accommodate the urine collection device or leg braces if worn. Wraparound skirts and rubber pants are helpful for women clients. The fastenings that are easiest to manage are zippers and Velcro closures. Since the quadriplegic client often uses the thumb as a hook to manage clothing, loops attached to zipper pulls, undershorts, and even the back of the shoes can be helpful. Belt loops on trousers will be used for pulling and should be reinforced. Brassieres should have stretch straps and no boning in them. Front-opening styles can be adapted by fastening loops and adding Velcro closures; back-opening styles can have loops added at each side of the fastening. Shoes can be one-half to one size larger than normally worn to accommodate edema and spasticity and to avoid pressure sores. Shoe fastenings can be adapted with Velcro, elastic shoe laces, large buckles, or flip-back tongue closure. Loose woolen or cotton socks without elastic cuffs should be used initially. As skill is gained, nylon socks, which tend to stick to the skin, may be possible. If neckties are used, the clip-on type or a regular tie that has been preknotted and can be slipped over the head may be manageable for some clients.[2,13]

The following dressing techniques can facilitate dressing for persons with upper extremity weakness.

TROUSERS AND UNDERSHORTS
Donning

1. Sit on bed with bed rails up. Trousers are positioned at foot of bed with trouser legs over end of bed and front side up.[13]
2. Sit up and lift one knee at a time by hooking right hand under right knee to pull leg into flexion, then put trousers over right foot. Return right leg to extension or semiextended position while repeating procedure with left hand and left knee.[2] If unable to maintain leg in flexion by holding with one arm or through advantageous use of spasticity, dressing band may be used. This is a piece of elasticized webbing that has been sewn into a figure eight pattern, with one small loop and one large loop. Small loop is hooked around foot and large loop is anchored over knee. Band is measured for individual client so that its length is appropriate to maintain desired amount of knee flexion. Once the trousers are in place, knee loop is pushed off knee and dressing band is removed from foot with dressing stick.[4]
3. Work trousers up legs using patting and sliding motions with palms of hands.
4. While still sitting with pants to mid-calf height, insert dressing stick in front belt loop. Dressing stick is gripped by slipping its loop over wrist. Pull on dressing stick while extending trunk, returning to supine position. Return to sitting position and repeat this procedure, pulling on dressing sticks and maneuvering trousers up to thigh level.[13] If balance is adequate, an alternative is for client to remain sitting and lean on left elbow and pull trousers over right buttock, then reverse process for other side. Another alternative is for client to remain in supine position and roll to one side; throw opposite arm behind back; hook thumb in waistband, belt loop, or pocket; and pull trousers up over hips. These maneuvers can be repeated as often as necessary to get trousers over buttocks.[2]
5. Using palms of hands in pushing and smoothing motions, straighten the trouser legs.
6. In supine position, trouser placket is fastened by hooking thumb in loop on zipper pull, patting Velcro closed, or using hand splints and button hooks if there are buttons.[2,13]

Removing

1. Lying supine in bed with bed rails up, unfasten belt and placket fasteners.
2. Placing thumbs in belt loops, waist band, or pockets, work trousers past hips by stabilizing arms in shoulder extension and scooting body toward head of bed.

3. Use arms as described in step 2 and roll from side to side to get trousers past buttocks.
4. Coming to sitting position and alternately pulling legs into flexion as described previously, push trousers down legs.[13]
5. Trousers can be pushed off over feet with dressing stick or by hooking thumbs in waistband.

CARDIGANS OR PULLOVER GARMENTS

Cardigan and pullover garments include blouses, vests, sweaters, skirts, and front-opening dresses.[2,13] Procedure for putting on these garments is as follows:

Donning

1. Garment is positioned across thighs with back facing up and neck toward knees.
2. Place both arms under back of garment and in armholes.
3. Sleeves are then pushed up onto arms past elbows.
4. Using a wrist extension grip, hook thumbs under garment back and gather material up from neck to hem.
5. To pass garment over head, adduct and externally rotate shoulders and flex elbows while flexing head forward.
6. When garment is over head, relax shoulders and wrists, and remove hands from back of garment. Most of material will be gathered up at neck, across shoulders, and under arms.
7. To work garment down over body, shrug shoulders, lean forward, and use elbow flexion and wrist extension. Wheelchair arms may be used for balance if necessary. Additional maneuvers to accomplish task are to hook wrists into sleeves and pull material free from underarms or lean forward, reach back, and slide hand against material to aid in pulling garment down.
8. Garment can be buttoned from bottom to top with aid of button hook and wrist-hand orthosis if hand function is inadequate.

Removing

1. Sit in wheelchair and wear wrist-hand orthosis. Unfasten buttons (if any) while wearing splints and using button hook. When this is accomplished, splints are removed for remaining steps.
2. For pullover garments, hook thumb in back of neckline, extend wrist, and pull garment over head while turning head toward side of raised arm. Balance can be maintained by resting against opposite wheelchair armrest or pushing on thigh with extended arm.

3. For cardigan garments, hook thumb in opposite armhole and push sleeve down arm. Elevation and depression of shoulders with trunk rotation can be used to get garment to slip down arms as far as possible.
4. One cuff can be held with opposite thumb while elbow is flexed to pull arm out of sleeve.

BRASSIERE (Back opening)[2,13]
Donning

1. Place brassiere across lap with straps toward knees and inside facing up.
2. Using a right-to-left procedure, hold end of brassiere closest to right side with hand or reacher and pass brassiere around back from right to left. Lean against brassiere at back to hold it in place, while hooking thumb of left hand in a loop that has been attached near brassiere fastener. Right thumb is hooked in a similar loop on right side and brassiere is fastened in front at waist level.
3. Hook right thumb in edge of brassiere and using wrist extension, elbow flexion, shoulder adduction, and internal rotation, brassiere is rotated around body so that front of brassiere is in front of body.
4. While leaning on one forearm, hook opposite thumb in front end of strap and pull strap over shoulder, then repeat procedure on other side.

Removing

1. Hook thumb under opposite brassiere strap, and push down over shoulder while elevating shoulder.
2. Pull arm out of strap, and repeat procedure for other arm.
3. Push brassiere down to waist level, and turn around as described previously to bring fasteners to front.
4. Unfasten brassiere.

SOCKS
Donning

1. Sit in wheelchair or on bed if balance is adequate in cross-legged position with one ankle crossed over opposite knee.
2. Pull sock over foot with wrist extension grip and patting movements with palm of hand.[2,13]
3. If trunk balance is inadequate and cross-legged position cannot be maintained, foot can be propped on stool, chair, or open drawer while opposite arm is around upright of wheelchair for balance. Wheelchair safety belt or leaning against wheelchair armrest on one side are alternatives to maintain balance.
4. Stocking aid or sock cone (see Fig. 12-3) may be used to assist in donning socks while in this position. Sock cone is powdered and sock is applied to it by using

thumbs and palms of hands to smooth sock out on cone. Inside of cone is powdered to reduce friction against cone.
5. Cord loops of sock cone are placed around the wrist or thumb and cone is thrown beyond foot.
6. Cone is maneuvered over toes by pulling cords using elbow flexion. Insert foot as far as possible into cone.
7. To remove cone from sock after foot has been inserted, move heel forward off wheelchair footrest using wrist extension of hand not operating sock cone behind knee and continue pulling cords of cone until it is removed and sock is in place on foot. Sock is smoothed using palms with patting and stroking motion.[13]

Removing

1. While sitting in wheelchair or lying in bed, use dressing stick or long-handled shoe horn to push sock down over heel. Legs should be crossed if possible.
2. Dressing stick with cuphook on end can be used to pull sock off toes.[3]

SHOES
Donning

1. Position that is used for donning socks can be used for putting on shoes.
2. Use extended-handle dressing aid and insert it into tongue of shoe, then place shoe opening over toes. Dressing aid is removed from shoe, and shoe is dangling on toes.
3. Using palm of hand on sole of shoe, pull shoe toward heel of foot. One hand is used to stabilize leg while other is pushing against sole of shoe to work shoe onto foot. Thenar eminence and sides of hand are used for this pushing motion.
4. With feet flat on floor or on wheelchair footrest and knees flexed 90°, place a long-handled shoe horn in heel of shoe and press down on flexed knee.
5. Fasten shoes.[13]

Removing

1. Sitting in wheelchair with legs crossed as described previously, unfasten shoes.
2. Shoe horn or dressing stick is used to push on heel counter of shoe, dislodging it from heel, then shoe will drop or can be pushed to floor with dressing stick.[13]

FEEDING ACTIVITIES.[1] Eating may be assisted by a variety of devices, again depending on the level of muscle function. Levels C5 and above require mobile arm supports or externally powered splints and braces. A wrist splint and universal cuff may be used together if a wrist-hand orthosis (flexor hinge splint) is not used. The universal cuff holds the eating utensil, and the splint

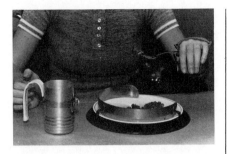

Fig. 12-26. Feeding with aid of universal cuff, plate guard, nonskid mat, and clip-type cup holder to compensate for absent grasp.

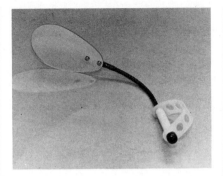

Fig. 12-27. Skin inspection mirror.

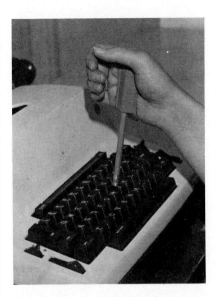

Fig. 12-28. Typing with aid of universal cuff and typing stick.

stabilizes the wrist. A nonskid mat and a plate with plate guard may provide adequate stability of the plate for pushing and picking up food (Fig. 12-26). The spoon-plate is an option for independent feeding for patients with high spinal cord injuries. It is a portable device that can be adjusted in height to the level of the patient's mouth. The plate is fabricated of a high temperature thermoplastic, such as Kydex. The plate is formed over a mold that has a rim bowled to the approximate depth and length of a spoon. The patient rotates the device with mouth and neck control. Food is removed from the rim of the plate with the mouth. Successful use of the device depends on adequate oral control, head and trunk control, and motivation. The reader is referred to the original source for information on fabricating or obtaining this device.[16]

A regular or swivel spoon-fork combination can be used when there is minimal muscle function (C4 to C5). A long plastic straw with a straw clip to stabilize it in the cup or glass eliminates the need for picking up these drinking vessels. A bilateral or unilateral clip-type holder on a glass or cup makes it possible for many individuals with hand and arm weakness to manage liquids without a straw.

Built-up utensils may be useful for those with some functional grasp or tenodesis grasp. Cutting food may be managed with a quad quip knife if arm strength is adequate to manage the device.

HYGIENE AND GROOMING.[1] General suggestions to facilitate hygiene and grooming are as follows:

1. Use a shower or bathtub seat and transfer board for transfers.
2. Extend reach by using long-handled bath sponges with loop handle or built-up handle.
3. Eliminate need to grasp washcloth by using bath mitts.
4. Hold comb and toothbrush with a universal cuff.
5. Use a clip-type holder for electric razor.
6. Suppository inserters for quadriplegics who can manage bowel care independently with this aid can be used.
7. Use skin inspection mirror with long stem and looped handle for independent skin inspection (Fig. 12-27).

Devices selected and methods must be adapted to the degree of weakness for each individual client.

COMMUNICATION AND ENVIRONMENTAL HARDWARE. The following are suggestions for facilitating communication:

1. Turn pages with an electric page turner, mouth stick, or head wand if hand and arm function are inadequate.
2. Insert pen, pencil, typing stick, or paintbrush in a universal cuff that has been positioned with the opening on the ulnar side of the palm (Fig. 12-28) for typing, writing, operating a tape recorder, and painting.
3. Dial the telephone with the universal cuff and a pencil positioned with eraser down or with mouth stick or

head wand if hand and arm function are absent. The receiver may need to be stationed in a telephone arm and positioned for listening. Special adaptations are available to substitute the need to replace the receiver in the cradle.
4. Use electric typewriters, which are easier to use than standard ones, or personal computers.
5. Built-up pencils and pens or special pencil holders are needed for clients with hand weakness.
6. Sophisticated electronic communications devices operated by mouth, suck and blow, and head control are available for clients with no upper extremity function.[15]
7. Two mouthsticks and a cassette tape holder allow C3, C4, or C5 quadriplegic patients to operate a tape recorder or radio independently. The first mouthstick, a rod about 19.7 inches (50 cm) long with a friction tip, is used to depress the operating buttons and adjust the volume and selector dials of the radio. The second mouthstick is a metal rod that separates into two prongs at its end. These prongs are 4 inches (10.1 cm) apart and the mouthstick is used to place the cassettes from the cassette

holder to the tape recorder and remove the cassettes from the recorder. The cassette tape stand has eight levels and is designed to hold eight tapes. It is a vertical stand made of metal and tilted backward to a 70° angle. The reader is referred to the original source for specifications on construction of these devices.[7]

MOBILITY AND TRANSFERS. Wheelchair transfer techniques for the individual with quadriplegia will be described in Chapter 18. Mobility will depend on degree of weakness. Electric wheelchairs operated by hand or mouth controls have greatly increased the mobility of persons with severe upper and lower extremity weakness. Vans fitted with wheelchair lifts and stabilizing devices have made it possible for such clients to be transported thus to pursue community, vocational, educational, and avocational activities with an assistant.

Adaptations for hand controls have made it possible for many clients with function of at least C6 level to drive independently.

HOME MANAGEMENT ACTIVITIES. Many individuals with upper extremity weakness who are bound to wheelchair ambulation will be dependent or partially dependent for homemaking activities. Clients with muscle function of C6 or better may be independent for light homemaking with appropriate devices, adaptations, and safety awareness. Many of the suggestions for wheelchair maneuverability and environmental adaptation outlined for the paraplegic apply here as well. In addition, the client with upper extremity weakness will need to use lightweight equipment and special devices. The *Mealtime Manual for People With Disabilty and the Aging* compiled by Judith Lannefeld Klinger[8] is an excellent resource for many specific suggestions that apply to the homemaker with weak upper extremities.

REVIEW QUESTIONS

1. Define "activities of daily living" (ADL) and list four classifications of tasks that may be considered in ADL.
2. What is the role of occupational therapy in restoring ADL independence?
3. List at least three activities that would be considered self-care skills, three mobility skills, three communication skills, and three home management skills.
4. List three factors that the occupational therapist must consider before commencing ADL performance evaluation and training. Describe how each could limit or effect ADL performance.
5. What is the ultimate goal of the ADL training program?
6. Discuss the concept of maximal independence, as defined in the text.
7. List the general steps in the procedure for ADL evaluation.
8. Describe how the occupational therapist can use the ADL checklist.
9. How does the occupational therapist, with the client, select ADL training objectives after the ADL evaluation?
10. Describe three approaches to teaching ADL skills to a client with perception or memory deficits.
11. List the important factors to include in an ADL progress report.
12. Define three general levels of independence, as defined in the text.
13. Demonstrate the use of at least three assistive devices mentioned in the text.
14. Teach another individual how to don a shirt, using one hand.
15. Teach another individual how to don and remove trousers, as if hemiplegic.
16. Teach another individual how to don and remove trousers, as if the legs were paralyzed.

REFERENCES

1. Activities of daily living for patients with incoordination, limited range of motion, paraplegia, quadriplegia, and hemiplegia, Cleveland, 1968, Highland View Hospital, Cuyahoga County Hospitals, Division of Occupational Therapy. Mimeographed, unpublished.
2. Bromley, I.: Tetraplegia and paraplegia: a guide for physiotherapists, ed. 2, London, 1981, Churchill Livingstone.
3. Buchwald, E.: Physical rehabilitation for daily living, New York, 1952, McGraw-Hill, Inc.
4. Easton, L.W., and Horan, A.L.: Dressing band, Am. J. Occup. Ther. **33**:656, 1979.
5. Holser, P., Jones, M., and Ilanit, T.: A study of the upper extremity control brace, Am. J. Occup. Ther. **16**:170, 1962.
6. Hopkins, H.L., Smith, H.D., and Tiffany, E.G.: Therapeutic application of activity. In Hopkins, H.L., and Smith, H.D., editors: Willard and Spackman's occupational therapy, ed. 6, Philadelphia, 1983, J.B. Lippincott Co.
7. Kelly, S.N.: Adaptations for independent use of cassette tape recorder/radio by high-level quadriplegic patients, Am. J. Occup. Ther. **37**:766, 1983.
8. Klinger, J.L.: Mealtime manual for people with disabilities and the aging, Camden, N.J., 1978, Campbell Soup Co.
9. Malick, M.H., and Almasy, B.S.: Activities of daily living and homemaking. In Hopkins, H.L., and Smith, H.D., editors: Willard and Spackman's occupational therapy, ed. 6, Philadelphia, 1983, J.B. Lippincott Co.
10. Malick, M.H., and Almasy, B.S.: Assessment and evaluation: life work tasks. In Hopkins, H.L., and Smith, H.D., editors: Willard and Spackman's occupational therapy, ed. 6, Philadelphia, 1983, J.B. Lippincott Co.
11. Melvin, J.L.: Rheumatic disease: occupational therapy and rehabilitation, Philadelphia, 1977, F.A. Davis Co.
12. The Professional Manual Subcommittee of the Educational Committee, Allied Health Professional Section of the Arthritis Foundation: Arthritis manual for allied health professionals, New York, 1973, The Arthritis Foundation.
13. Runge, M.: Self-dressing techniques for patients with spinal cord injury, Am. J. Occup. Ther. **21**:367, 1967.
14. Sokaler, R.: A buttoning aid, Am. J. Occup. Ther. **35**:737, 1981.
15. Trombly, C.A., editor: Occupational therapy for physical dysfunction, Baltimore, 1983, Williams & Wilkins.
16. Wykoff, E., and Mitani, M.: The spoon plate: a self-feeding device, Am. J. Occup. Ther. **36**:333, 1982.

CHAPTER 13

Neurophysiology of sensorimotor approaches to treatment

GUY L. McCORMACK

Occupational therapy is an ever-expanding field. To treat patients who have neurological dysfunctions the therapist should have an operational understanding of neurophysiology. With this knowledge the therapist can help patients achieve the ability to perform purposeful activities and understand why certain motor disturbances exist. This chapter will review the basic neurophysiological rationale for the therapeutic approaches that are described in subsequent chapters.

DIVISIONS OF THE NERVOUS SYSTEM

The nervous system is often subdivided into the peripheral, autonomic, and central nervous systems.

Peripheral nervous system

The peripheral nervous system begins in the skin and in the special sense organs. It carries information along 31 pairs of spinal nerves, related ganglia, and 12 pairs of cranial nerves.[20,41] The receptors in the skin possess the ability to discharge when stimulated by certain kinds of mechanical energy. The receptors (end organs) in the skin transmit sensory impulses along specific fibers. These nerve fibers vary greatly in their diameter, degree of myelination, and conduction velocity.[42] Generally speaking, the greater the diameter of the fiber and the thicker the myelin sheath, the faster the rate of conduction.[14] There is no universal method of classification of the nerve fibers. Two classifications of nerve fibers are presently in use. One is an electrophysiological classification based on the speed of conduction of sensory and motor fibers. This classification uses an alphabetical system consisting of three groups: A, B, and C. The A and B fibers are thicker in diameter and myelinated, whereas C fibers are thin and unmyelinated.[20] The A fibers are further divided into subgroups called alpha, beta, gamma,

and delta. The A fibers contain two motor components: alpha fibers, which supply skeletal (extrafusal) muscle, and gamma fibers, which innervate muscle spindle (intrafusal) muscle.

The second classification pertains only to sensory fibers and uses Roman numerals to designate fiber size and fiber origin. This includes group Ia for the primary ending of the muscle spin-

dle; group Ib for the Golgi tendon organs; group II for secondary sensory ending from muscle spindles; group III for touch, pressure, pain, and temperature receptors; and group IV for nonspecific unmyelinated pain and temperature fibers. Table 13-1 summarizes the two classifications and differentiates the major modalities. Table 13-2 compares proprioception with pain and temperature.

Table 13-1
Nerve fiber classification

Letter	Roman numeral	Functional component	Fiber diameter (μm)*
A alpha	Group I		12-22
	Ia	Primary muscle spindle ending (stretch)	
	Ib	Golgi tendon organ (contraction)	
A beta	Group II	Secondary sensory ending from muscle spindle (maintained stretch)	6-13
		Encapsulated endings	
		Cutaneous afferents from skin and joints (joint position-pressure)	
A gamma		Motor to muscle spindle (static-dynamic)	—
B		Motor—branch of alpha motor neuron	—
		Preganglionic autonomic efferents	
A delta	Group III	Bare nerve endings, cutaneous mechanoreceptors; cold and nociceptors	1-6
C fibers	Group IV	Unmyelinated, nonspecific sensory reception; cold, warm, and nociceptors	1-1.5

*Micron millimeters.

Table 13-2
Comparison of proprioception with pain and temperature

Proprioception		Pain and temperature	
A alpha (I)	**A alpha (III)**	**A delta (III)**	**C (IV)**
Muscle stretch			
Muscle contraction	Muscle stretch		
	Position sense		
	Vibration		
	Velocity detection		
	Pressure		
		Cold	Cold
		Light touch	Touch
		Pain	Pain
			Warmth

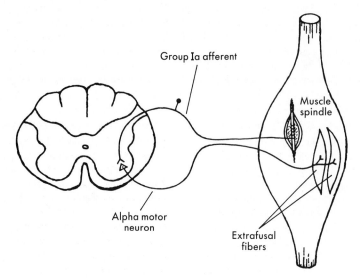

Fig. 13-1. Monosynaptic stretch reflex (reflex arc).

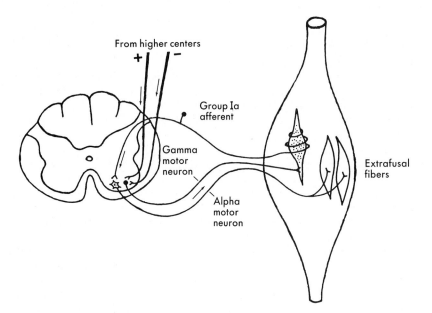

Fig. 13-2. Gamma loop (added gamma neuron to reflex arc).

Once the sensory impulse reaches the spinal cord, it may cross to the opposite side, ascend the spinal cord, or connect directly with a motor neuron. This transfer of coded information from one neuron to another represents a synaptic transmission. When the sensory neuron synapses directly with a motor neuron in the spinal cord and carries that impulse back out to activate a muscle, it is called a monosynaptic reflex arc[26] (Fig. 13-1). This reflex arc is a basic neuronal circuit that causes stereotyped reactions to stimuli from the environment. To remain intact the reflex arc must have a complete receptor unit, sensory fiber, synapse within the spinal cord, motor neuron, and viable myoneural connection.[11] If any of these components are destroyed, the reflex arc is abolished. Reflex arcs enable the nervous system to react to stimuli that may be potentially harmful without exerting conscious effort. Thus touching the cornea of the eye results in a blink, touching a hot object results in a withdrawal reflex, or foreign objects in the windpipe cause coughing. The reflex arc is used to examine the integrity of the nervous system or to elicit crude components of movement.[21]

Alpha motor neurons are the largest of the anterior horn cells. They can be stimulated through the reflex arc by the Ia primary afferents and group II secondary afferents of the muscle spindles.[47] Alpha motor neurons are also influenced by higher centers and by fibers from the corticospinal, raphe spinal, reticulospinal, and lateral vestibulospinal tracts.[51] Anytime a motor act is elicited, be it voluntary or reflexive, the impulse must travel to the muscle by way of an alpha motor neuron. Because the alpha motor neuron is the last remaining connection between the spinal cord and extrafusal muscle, it is called the "final common pathway."[13] If the cell body or axon of the alpha motor neuron is destroyed, the reflex arc is abolished, and the muscle will become hypotonic. This would constitute a lower motor neuron dysfunction, and efforts to activate that muscle through sensory stimulation would be nonproductive unless some regeneration had occurred.

The gamma loop or the fusimotor system plays a very important role in sensorimotor treatment techniques.

Gamma motor neurons innervate the intrafusal muscle fibers within the muscle spindles of skeletal muscle.[2,42] The intrafusal muscle fibers align themselves parallel to the extrafusal (skeletal) fibers. Any change in the length of the muscle will also modify the length of the intrafusal fibers. The motor fibers supplying the intrafusal muscles are smaller than the thinly myelinated gamma fibers. Their cell bodies are found in the anterior horn of the spinal cord along with the alpha motor neuron.[36,44]

The static gamma motor neurons terminate primarily on the nuclear chain fibers but also branch to nuclear bag fibers. The static gamma motor neurons are regulated by nuclei in the cerebellum, reticular system, basal ganglia, and vestibular system. The static gamma motor neurons are involved during a maintained shortening or contraction of muscle.[47]

The principle function of the gamma motor neuron is to adjust the length of the intrafusal fibers during contraction of the muscle, which enables the muscle spindle to automatically reinforce the power of contraction.[42]

Gamma and alpha motor neurons work in a collaborative fashion. The gamma loop (Fig. 13-2) is described as a servoassistance mechanism that aids in the production and control of movement. This collaborative effort between alpha and gamma motor neurons is known as coactivation.[44] The anatomical and sensory aspects of the muscle spindle are discussed in the forthcoming section on receptors.

Autonomic nervous system

The autonomic nervous system regulates glands, smooth muscles, and cardiac muscles. This system functions predominantly at the subconscious level but is integrated with other body activities and influenced by events in the environment.[10] Functionally, the autonomic nervous system consists of two branches, the sympathetic and parasympathetic systems.

SYMPATHETIC NERVOUS SYSTEM. The sympathetic nervous system expends energy and is known to be a catabolic system. The cell bodies of the preganglionic sympathetic neurons exit the spinal cord at levels T1 to L2

(thorax-lumbar outflow) and enter the paravertebral ganglion chain that runs adjacent to either side of the spinal column.[14,17] The sympathetic chain extends from the top to the bottom of the spinal column so impulses can travel up or down the chain for considerable distances. To activate glands or internal organs the sympathetic impulse must travel through a two-neuron chain. The preganglionic neurons arise from the intermediate gray column of the spinal cord. The postganglionic neuron is located in the paravertebral ganglia and innervates the smooth muscles of all the organs. Each spinal nerve receives a branch from the sympathetic trunk ganglia that are distributed to the blood vessels, erector pili muscles of hair, and secretory organs of the skin throughout the distribution of the nerve.[44] The viscera of the pelvic and abdominal cavities are innervated by sympathetic branches of the splanchnic nerves.[9] The sympathetic nervous system liberates neurotransmitters that are norepinephrine-like substances classified as adrenergic.[20]

The nervous system is stimulated when the individual experiences strong emotions, such as fear and rage, and by exposure to cold or pain. This stimulation produces a generalized physiological response, allowing the adrenal glands to liberate substances into the bloodstream that reinforce the effects of sympathetic neurons. As a result, the blood vessels in the skin and digestive systems constrict, whereas the blood vessels in the cardiac and skeletal muscles dilate. The bronchioles of the lungs and pupils of the eyes also dilate. Heart rate and force of contraction increase. The sweat, lacrimal, and salivary glands increase secretions. Last, the spleen may release extra red blood cells into the bloodstream in case of blood loss. In summary, the major function of the sympathetic nervous system is to mobilize the body during stress or emergency situations.

PARASYMPATHETIC NERVOUS SYSTEM. In contrast, the parasympathetic nervous system conserves energy and is known to be an anabolic system.[22] The preganglionic cell bodies arise from the craniosacral regions of the central nervous system. The cranial portion consists of cranial nerves III,

VII, IX, and X. Cranial nerve X (vagus nerve) supplies the organs of the thorax. The sacral portion arises from spinal segments S2, S3, and S4. The sacral division communicates with pelvic splanchnic nerves and supplies muscular walls of the colon, rectum, and urinary and reproductive tracts. The postganglionic terminals of the parasympathetic system liberate acetylcholine and are classified as cholinergic.[22,30]

The parasympathetic system can act simultaneously with the sympathetic system during the fight or flight situation. During exaggerated fear the sacral segment may produce involuntary emptying of the bladder and rectum. In contrast to the sympathetic response the parasympathetic system acts to dilate blood vessels in the skin and digestive tract, constrict bronchial tubes, contract the pupils of the eyes, and increase motility of the gastrointestinal tract. During sexual arousal the parasympathetic system controls penile and clitoral erection, and the sympathetic branch mediates ejaculation.[17]

Much is yet to be learned about the autonomic nervous system. For instance, there appears to be complex synaptic connections joining skin efferents and visceral afferents with the autonomic neurons. Thus sensory stimulation to some areas of the skin can influence the action of certain internal organs. Several reflex arcs have been identified, but the interneuronal pathways have not been clearly delineated.[44,48]

In recent years it has been found that the autonomic nervous system can be manipulated through facilitory and inhibitory techniques. Gellhorn[19] has described anatomical and physiological factors contributing to states of stress and relaxation on a continuum. The fight or flight state combines increased sympathetic activity, arousal of the cortex, and increased muscle tone. Gellhorn termed this the ergotropic response. The other end of the continuum is a state that combines increased parasympathetic activity, cortical relaxation, and decreased muscle tone. This state has been termed the trophotropic end of the continuum.

In the process of using facilitory or inhibitory activities the therapist should determine where the patient's capabilities fall along this ergotropic-trophotropic continuum. If the goal is to reduce spasticity, the patient should be toward the trophotropic (parasympathetic) end. However, if the goal is to promote learning or increase tonicity in muscles, the activities should be stimulating and compatible with the ergotropic (sympathetic) response.

Central nervous system

THE SPINAL CORD. The central nervous system (CNS) consists of the spinal cord, brainstem, cerebellum, subcortical nuclei, and the cerebral cortex.[17,30] The spinal cord is phylogenetically old and less complex than other structures in the CNS. The spinal cord is less than an inch (2.54 cm) in diameter with enlargements in the lower cervical and in the lower lumbar regions to accommodate the outflow to the extremities. The spinal cord begins at the foramen magnum and extends caudally to vertebrae level L1 or L2.[42,52] The spinal cord is subdivided into segments. The spinal segments do not align opposite the corresponding vertebrae because the cord is about 9⅘ inches (25 cm) shorter. There are 31 pairs of spinal nerves: 8 cervical, 12 thoracic, 5 lumbar, 5 sacral, and 1 coccygeal. Each spinal nerve has dorsal and ventral roots that form the sensory and motor components. All the sensory (afferent), somatic, and visceral fibers enter the spinal cord by way of the dorsal roots. All motor fibers (efferent) exit the spinal cord via the ventral roots. In a transverse section the spinal cord appears to have a butterfly-shaped area of gray substance surrounded by white matter. The white matter is composed of longitudinal ascending and descending fiber tract systems. The cell bodies of the efferent fibers are located in the gray matter. The gray matter can be further subdivided into 10 laminae, each extending the length of the cord. The white matter of the spinal cord is divided into three pairs of funiculi (anterior, lateral, and dorsal).[41,47] Some generalizations may be made about the sensory and motor tracts of the spinal cord. In respect to the motor tracts the older phylogenetic systems are located in the anterior and anterolateral quadrants of the cord. Efferent impulses are transmitted along these tracts to be excitatory to extensor motor neurons and inhibitory to flexor motor neurons. The anterolateral quadrant of the spinal cord contains the phylogenetically newer motor systems. These neurons tend to be excitatory to flexors and inhibitory to extensors.[51] A similar relationship exists in the sensory tracts. The anterolateral tracts (spinothalamic) are phylogenetically old and mediate pain, temperature, and touch along small diameter fibers. This is felt to be a primitive protective system. Conversely, the dorsal columns of the spinal cord (lemniscal system) represent a newer sensory system conveying discriminative sensory information from the skin and deep structures to the cerebral cortex. This system is rapidly conducting because the fibers are large and well myelinated and undergo few synapses en route to the cortex.[3,51]

BRAINSTEM. The brainstem has been regarded by Ayres[3] as the center of sensory integration. That is, all perceptual processes basic to learning are dependent on sensory integration at the brainstem level. The brainstem consists of the medulla oblongata, pons, midbrain, and thalamus.[45] The brainstem contains the 12 cranial nerves, reticular system, major nuclei, and ascending and descending tract systems. The lowest portion of the brainstem, the medulla, contains nuclei for five cranial nerves, the reticular formation, the vestibular system, and the respiratory and cardiac functions. All the major ascending and descending tracts pass through the medulla.[22] The pons is a large mass that lies above the medulla. The pons plays an important role as a relay station between the cerebellum and the cerebral cortex. The pons contains four cranial nerves, pontine nuclei, and major fiber tracts.[7,20] The midbrain is a relatively short section of the brainstem but contains several important structures. Some of these structures are the corpora quadrigemina (superioinferior colliculi), red nucleus, substantia nigra, crura cerebri, and cranial nerves III and IV.[20,41] Two major motor tracts arising from the midbrain are the rubrospinal and tectospinal tracts. A lesion to the midbrain region results in strong extensor tone or rigidity.[11]

The cerebellum is located in the posterior cranial fossa. It is attached to the pons, medulla, and midbrain by the cerebellar peduncles. The cerebellum is divided into three lobes. The flocculonodular lobe (archicerebellum) located in the posterioinferior region communicates with the vestibular system. The anterior lobe (paleocerebellum) receives proprioceptive information via the spinocerebellar tracts; the posterior lobe (neocerebellum) is located between the other two lobes and communicates with the motor cortex.[1,14,26]

THALAMUS. The thalamus is a complex structure that makes up the rostral portion of the brainstem. With the exception of the olfactory system all sensory information passes through the thalamus en route to the cortex.[51] For this reason the thalamus has been regarded as a sensory relay station. In the past it was believed that the thalamus participated in the realization of crude sensation.[30] However, recent evidence suggests that the thalamus participates in refining or consolidating sensory information before it reaches the cortex.[45] The thalamus may also play a role in emotion and behavior through its connections with the limbic system.[1] Cerebrovascular accidents may cause destruction to parts of the thalamus resulting in the so-called thalamus syndrome. This condition can cause exaggerated pain or unpleasant sensations to nonnoxious stimuli.[11]

HYPOTHALAMUS. The hypothalamus lies inferior to the thalamus and forms the ventral floor of the third ventricle. There is evidence that the hypothalamus exerts a direct or indirect influence on every function of the body.[42] The hypothalamus has widespread connections with the autonomic and endocrine systems. The hypothalamus contributes to the control of cardiovascular and respiratory functions, body temperature, food intake, reproductive behavior, and emotions.[40,44]

LIMBIC SYSTEM. The limbic system, sometimes called the visceral brain, is a collection of interconnected structures contributing to emotional responsiveness and affective behavior.[15] The principle structures of the limbic system are the cingulate gyrus, septal area, insula, parahippocampal gyrus, amygdala, and hippocampal formation.[1,20] Although the limbic system is not directly related to motor systems, its emotional and behavior components affect autonomic and somatic responses. Moore[37] has expounded on the importance of the limbic system in rehabilitation techniques. This system governs feeding, fighting, and reproductive behaviors. It is also responsible for short-term memory.

BASAL GANGLIA. The major structure of the basal ganglia are the caudate nucleus, putamen, and globus pallidus. The basal ganglia may also be functionally related to the amygdaloid nucleus, claustrum, subthalamic nucleus, and substantia nigra.[1,14] The basal ganglia receive much input from the cerebral cortex and transmit it into many circuits and feedback loops. Attempts to delineate the functions of the basal ganglia have credited it with the refinement of complex movement, automatic movement patterns, associated movements, and regulation of postural tone in antigravity muscles.[11,17]

CEREBRAL CORTEX. The cortex makes up the outermost region of the cerebrum. It has been attributed to intellectual functions, memory storage, language, consciousness, perception, and complex motor activities.[14] The cortex is composed of six layers of densely packed neuron cell bodies. The cortex has been anatomically divided into four lobes and 52 distinct areas, based on types of cell groupings.[42] Clinically, some of the most significant areas would include the primary motor strip (area 4) supplementary motor area (area 6), prefrontal cortex (areas 9 through 12), Broca's area (areas 44 and 45), Wernicke's area (area 22), sensory strip (areas 1, 2, and 3), and supramarginal gyrus (area 40). Lesions to the areas just mentioned result in profound sensory or motor dysfunction.[10,13]

BASIS FOR RATIONALE OF THE SENSORIMOTOR APPROACHES TO TREATMENT

The neuron

The neuron is unique among all cells in the body because of its ability to transmit coded information for long distances. The neuron varies in form and structure, depending on its role in the transport of information. Each neuron has a cell body containing a nucleus, dendrites that receive stimuli, an axon that conducts impulses away from the cell body, and axon terminals.[7] To convey information the neuron must have two properties, conductivity of electrical impulses and neurotransmission of a chemical substance.[15,26] These two properties are briefly described in the following.

The neuron has an excitable membrane that is activated by the difference between the interior of the cell and the fluid surrounding it. If there is an ionic balance existing between the cytoplasm of the neuron and the extracellular fluid, the cell is in a state of resting potential (expressed in voltage as -70 mV).[40] This balance is achieved by the permeability of the cell membrane to sodium (Na^+) and potassium (K^+) ions. The interior of the nerve cell contains high concentrations of potassium and low concentrations of sodium and chloride (Cl^-), whereas the extracellular fluid contains low potassium and high concentrations of sodium and chloride. When a neuron membrane is excited by an outside stimulus, changes in potential occur along the cell membrane.[44] If the stimulus is strong enough, the cell reaches its threshold and discharges an *action potential* (nerve impulse). The impulse then travels along the axon with a constant rate of electrical energy until it reaches the terminal ending. A *graded potential* is a small change in resting potential and the membrane voltage. It is not sufficient to discharge impulses along the axon but is carried by dendrites and cell bodies.[44] Under some circumstances, several weak stimuli (subthreshold) may impinge on the neuron (spatial summation) to cause an action potential to develop. This phenomenon is called summation.[15] This is a very important concept in therapy because it means neurons can be stimulated to action potential by increasing

the sensory input. If, for example, a traumatic lesion has destroyed neuronal circuits that normally stimulate a group of neurons to discharge, alternative pathways can be developed by consistent sensory stimulation. Bach-y-Rita[4] has used the analogy of the telephone line to describe this process. If a phone line were damaged between two cities on the east and west coasts, messages could be rerouted through less direct lines. The new network would be slower and as efficient but would nevertheless transmit messages that would improve over time. Neurons have the ability to adapt and change the direction of impulses through axon collaterals.[43] Synaptic transmissions get stronger and more efficient with use.[40]

NEUROTRANSMISSION. Neurotransmission represents the chemical aspect of interneuronal communication. It occurs between the presynaptic and postsynaptic membranes of two nerve cells. Normally there is a space or cleft between two communicating neurons called a synapse. A synapse can occur between the dendrite, axon, or cell body of a receiving neuron. The transmission of information is propagated by a release of a chemical substance (neurotransmitter) that is capable of either producing or preventing electrical changes in the postsynaptic neuronal membrane.[41] If the neurotransmitter traverses the synapse and causes an action potential in the subsequent neuron, it is facilitory. However, if the neurotransmitter causes a hypopolarization of the postsynaptic cell membrane, it is called inhibitory.[47] Synaptic junctions between neurons vary considerably throughout the nervous system. The average motor neuron may have about 6000 axon collateral synapses. Thus each neuron is capable of receiving several thousand messages from different sources. Generally speaking, sensory neurons conduct impulses in only one direction, away from the area where the stimulus originated.[7] The intensity of the stimulus may determine the action potential, yet the distance the impulse travels is dependent on the properties of the cell receiving the communication.[20] Impulses can travel along several different circuits. Some neurons have many collateral branches that synapse with many neurons and form a *divergent circuit* to several regions of the nervous system. On the other hand, a single neuron may receive synaptic messages from several other neurons. This process is called *convergence*.[44] In this case the neuron must process both the excitatory and inhibitory impulses converging on it and decide to fire or inhibit the transmission. When the excitatory synapses predominate, action potentials are discharged and facilitation has occurred. Another facilitory circuit is called positive feedback or *reverberating excitation*. Hypothetically, this occurs in a circuit where neurons further down the chain feed back excitation to the preceding neurons. Reverberating excitation occurs through axon collaterals and forms a continuous feedback loop, causing the neuron to discharge for a long time.[45] Reverberating circuits have been associated with short-term memory or arousal states generated within the reticular system.[26] It is postulated that cutaneous stimulation (icing or brushing) may also initiate reverberating excitation.[29]

Neurons may also transmit through inhibitory circuits, which automatically suppress too much excitation. Typical inhibitory circuits include reciprocal inhibition through interneurons (Renshaw cells) or by groups of inhibitory neurons occupying parallel positions to excitatory neurons (surrounded inhibition).[44] Within the CNS there are regions where inhibitory circuits play a greater role in suppressing excitatory impulses.[14] These neuronal circuits help to smooth out or prevent unwanted actions during movement. When the CNS is damaged, there is an imbalance between the excitatory and inhibitory circuits.[43] Consequently, patients may exhibit degrees of paralysis, alterations of reflex patterns, or changes in muscle tone.[21] When the inhibitory circuits are damaged, their dampening effects on excitatory neurons are "released." This phenomenon is called *disinhibition*. Clinically, it may be seen as spasticity, rigidity, tremors, or athetosis.

Guyton[26] has described another phenomenon called *rebound*, which is related to fatigue of spinal level reflexes. Rebound occurs immediately after a reflex response has been evoked. Following the reflex response there is a period of fatigue and the same reflex becomes more difficult to elicit. Strangely enough, reflexes of the antagonist muscles can be elicited more briskly. This is a manifestation of reciprocal innervation and is a contributing factor to rhythmical movements. The term *rebound* has also been used to describe generalized reciprocal responses to prolonged use of thermal stimuli. For instance, if a patient stays in a heated therapeutic swimming pool too long, his biological thermoregulatory system (posterior hypothalamus) may work as a thermostat and increase the activitiy in the parasympathetic nervous system, causing a state of relaxation. An hour later the autonomic nervous sytem can generate a sympathetic response, and the patient may become agitated and excitable and have an increase in muscle tone. The therapist must weigh the value of certain sensorimotor techniques with respect to long-term or short-term gains. Some inhibitory techniques, if used too long, can trigger a reciprocal sympathetic response. It should also be noted that high-intensity cutaneous stimulation can cause similar rebound phenomenon.

Myelination

Myelin is a spirally deposited, fatlike substance that wraps around the axons of rapidly conducting nerve fibers.[7] It is produced by Schwann and oligodendroglial cells. The myelin sheath is important to the function of the nervous system because it increases the velocity of the impulses up to 100 times.[11] Myelination begins relatively late in development—not until the end of the third fetal month. Many of the tracts in the nervous system myelinate at different times. The vestibulospinal tract, tectospinal tract, and reflex arc begin myelination by the end of the fifth month.[15] The corticospinal tracts, which are responsible for voluntary skilled movements, continue myelination into the second year. Some areas of the reticular formation and the cerebellum continue to myelinate into early adulthood. The

association fibers of the cortex may continue to myelinate throughout life.

Most myelinated nerve fibers exist predominately in the cranial and spinal nerves. Therefore unmyelinated fibers are more abundant in the autonomic nervous system.[52] There is some evidence to suggest that sensory stimulation during the developmental years may improve the myelination process.[48]

Dendritic growth

Dendrites are the small branches (spines) projecting from the cell body of a neuron. Dendrites form synaptic connections with other neurons. Greenough[25] has conducted definitive animal studies to demonstrate the importance of environmental stimuli on the developing brain. The studies have shown that sensory stimulation promotes dendritic growth. It is postulated that the proliferation of dendrites contributes to intelligence and adaptive behavior in humans.[40]

Neuroplasticity

Recent neuroscientific studies have demonstrated that the CNS has some capacity to adapt or recover from traumatic injury.[4,43] The ability of neurons to adapt depends on (1) activation of latent neurons that may have been previously suppressed, (2) the ability of neurons adjacent to the lesion to sprout collateral axons that form new synapses, and (3) changes in neurotransmitter sensitivity. For example, denervated muscles can develop increased sensitivity to neurotransmitters through anatomical, physiological, or biochemical changes. This phenomenon may be part of an adaptive process to compensate for loss of innervation.[4,48]

To compensate for a lesion the damaged nervous system must be "forced" into recovery. Studies have shown that when the damaged system is forced into action it recovers to a greater extent. For instance, animals with lesions and hemiparetic extremities have shown better recovery when the uninvolved limbs are restrained and the affected limbs are forced into use.[4]

Peripheral control hypothesis versus the central control mechanism

Many of the sensorimotor theorists follow the assumption that the nervous system is stimulated and altered solely by stimuli that arise from the peripheral environment. There is much scientific evidence to support this premise, but there is also accumulating evidence to show the nervous system has built-in internal control mechanisms.[40] These central control mechanisms may be compared with "printed circuits" or genetic programs for repetitive movements. For example, the so-called subcortical movements may be manifestations of innate movements passed down through evolutionary development. Animal studies and clinical observations on humans have shown that movements can be initiated both internally and externally. The central control hypothesis may have implications for rehabilitation techniques in the near future.

SOMATOSENSORY SYSTEM

The term *somatosensory* can be defined as the body's awareness of external stimuli. The body contains many types of sensory receptors that keep us informed about changes in our immediate environment. These end organs can be viewed therapeutically as "portals" through which stimuli can be systematically programmed into the nervous system. Although the information on sensory receptors is incomplete, it is important for the occupational therapist to have a basic understanding of the characteristics these receptors possess.

For the purposes of sensorimotor therapy, sensory receptors (end organs) are classified into five categories in this discussion: (1) interoceptors, (2) exteroceptors, (3) proprioceptors, (4) kinesioceptors, and (5) meridian points.

Interoceptors

Interoceptors monitor events within the body and are located within the walls of the respiratory, cardiovascular, gastrointestinal, and genitourinary systems.[52] Interoceptors can detect a variety of stimuli, such as distention of a cavity wall, or monitor pH levels in the bloodstream. Many interoceptors are activated during therapeutic activities. The *carotid sinus* is a baroreceptor located in the walls of the carotid artery.[24] It is stimulated by blood pressure changes and linked to the parasympathetic nervous system. In therapy it is brought into action during inversion techniques.[15] Anytime the head approaches a position below the level of the shoulders, the increase in blood pressure distends the carotid sinus and fires impulses along the glossopharyngeal nerve (CN IX) to cardiovascular inhibitory centers of the vagus nerve, which in turn slows heart rate and reduces blood pressure. This is a negative feedback system that must be used with caution. Clinicians have used the carotid sinus to reduce hypertension and to produce a state of generalized inhibition.[11,15,51]

The *mucous membranes* of the oral cavity provide another area where interoceptors are used for therapeutic intervention. The mucous membranes contain receptors that are stimulated by several modalities, such as temperature, touch, stretch, and taste. Stimulation to this area will discharge impulses to the brainstem via the sensory components of the trigeminal nerve (CN V), facial nerve (CN VII), glossopharyngeal nerve (CN IX), and vagus nerve.[10] Occupational therapists use oral stimulation primarily for functional activities of daily living that are related to feeding.

Therapists have used cutaneous stimulation and vibration to affect the interoceptors in the wall of the bladder or detrusor muscle to facilitate or inhibit the micturition reflex. Stimulation has been applied dermatomally or to the skin directly over the bladder.[15] These techniques should not be used without proper understanding of neurophysiology or supervision by a physician.

The use of temperature input is another way interoceptors are used in sensorimotor techniques. Neutral warmth and icing techniques not only influence cutaneous receptors but act on thermoregulatory centers in the spinal cord, brainstem, and hypothalamus.[45,47] Temperature input has been used primarily to reduce hypertonicity in skeletal muscles or for symptomatic pain. However, it should be stressed that external changes in skin temperature can also affect the circulatory, endocrine, and autonomic nervous systems, which produce internal physiological responses.

Exteroceptors

Exteroceptors are found immediately under the skin, in the external mucous membranes, or in special sense organs.[42,52] These receptors respond to stimuli that arise outside of the body. Exteroceptors vary tremendously in their structure, function, and reaction to mechanical stimuli. Following is a brief summary of the primary cutaneous exteroceptors.

FREE NERVE ENDINGS. The subcutaneous tissues are richly innervated by free nerve endings. These are unencapsulated receptors with projecting, unmyelinated branches for sensory detection. Free nerve endings are widely distributed in the skin and viscera. They are thought to be nonspecific receptors for pain, crude touch, and temperature.[1] The free nerve endings associated with pain outnumber all other receptors along the midline axis of the body.[40] Free nerve endings transmit impulses by way of unmyelinated "C" nerve fibers.[48] In general the free nerve endings involved with touch are rapidly adapting. Those that are associated with dull pain perception are slowly adapting.[40] For therapeutic purposes free nerve endings are activated with thermal or brushing techniques and elicit primitive protective responses. Stimulation to free nerve endings can also cause states of arousal.[29] It is believed that free nerve endings, along with other receptors, can synapse with gamma motor neurons and bias the muscle spindle.

HAIR END ORGANS. Hair end organs are actually a type of free nerve ending that wraps around the base of a hair follicle.[42] These receptor organs are activated by the bending or displacement of hair. They are rapidly adapting and transmit impulses predominately along A delta-size (group III) fibers.[40] In therapy hair receptors are stimulated during light touch or stroking of the skin. Although they are rapidly adapting, hair end organs discharge into neuron pools that reach the reticular system and probably bias the muscle spindle through the fusimotor system.

MEISSNER'S CORPUSCLES. Meissner's corpuscles are elongated, encapsulated end organs found just beneath the epidermis in hairless (glabrous) skin. They are particularly abundant in the skin of the fingertips, tip of the tongue, lips, and pads of the feet.[51] Histological studies show that these receptors maintain a close relationship with the skin. The corpuscles are primarily rapidly adapting receptors that transmit along the thicker A beta (group II) fibers. Meissner's corpuscles are largely responsible for fine tactile discrimination. They are very important in digital exploration and sensory substitution skills, such as reading braille. These receptors transmit discriminatory messages to the somatosensory cortex by way of the dorsal columns of the spinal cord.[42,51]

PACINIAN CORPUSCLES. Pacinian corpuscles are the largest encapsulated receptors. They are almost as widely distributed as free nerve endings and are located in the deep layers of the skin, in viscera, mesenteries, ligaments, and near blood vessels.[40] Pacinian corpuscles are probably the most rapidly adapting receptors in the body.[42] They respond to deep pressure but are amazingly sensitive to slight indentations in the skin.[48] Pacinian corpuscles also discharge with a steady train of impulses when exposed to vibration. Therefore with vibratory stimuli the pacinian corpuscle is a slowly adapting receptor. Although the Pacinian corpuscle fires when vibrated, it has not been demonstrated to play a role in the tonic vibration reflex.[23,51]

The pacinian corpuscle has some interesting therapeutic features. It discharges along fast-conducting A beta (group II) fibers to the dorsal columns of the spinal cord. Stimulation to a single corpuscle in the skin can excite an area of the postcentral gyrus of the cortex.[11] Research has shown that the pacinian corpuscle can suppress pain perception at the cutaneous level.[36,40] It may

also contribute to the inhibition of muscles when pressure is applied over tendinous insertions.[15] Furthermore, the pacinian corpuscle may play a role in the desensitization of hypersensitive skin in children who exhibit tactile defensiveness.[3] It is interesting to note that the sole of the foot contains an abundance of these receptors. Thus the sole of the foot might be an excellent target area when using vibratory stimuli for sensory stimulation. The stimulation should be done with low frequency vibration and light pressure so that the positive supporting reaction is not elicited.

MERKEL'S TACTILE DISKS. Merkel's tactile disks are nonencapsulated receptors found in the deepest layer of the epidermis in hairless skin. These receptors are located most commonly on the volar surface of the fingers, lips, and external genitalia. Merkel's tactile disks are slowly adapting touch-pressure receptors. They transmit along A beta (group II) myelinated fibers.[40,51] These receptors are very sensitive to slow movements across the skin's surface. They have been related to the sense of tickle and pleasurable touch sensations.[48]

Proprioceptors

Proprioceptors monitor the awareness of position, posture, movement, and equilibrium. These receptors are found in muscles, tendons, and joints. The process of proprioception can be conscious or subconscious. Conscious proprioceptors will be covered under kinesioceptors (joint receptors). Subconscious proprioception pertains to information received from muscle spindles, Golgi tendon organs, and the vestibular apparatus. Subconscious proprioception derived from Golgi tendon organs and muscle spindles transmits to the cerebellum. The vestibular apparatus may have connections to the cerebral cortex.[51]

GOLGI TENDON ORGANS. Golgi tendon organs (GTO) are spindle-shaped receptors found in the musculotendinous region of the proximal and distal insertions.[7] In the past the GTO was believed to be a high-threshold protective receptor designed to inform the nervous system when muscle tension was reaching damaging proportions. New evidence has shown the

GTO has a greater sensitivity to muscle contraction.[36,39] Therefore it more specifically monitors the tendon tension produced by muscle contraction rather than by muscle tension produced by stretch. In addition, GTO appears to complement the action of the muscle spindle. For example, during isometric contraction of the biceps brachii, tendon tension will be developed, and the GTO will discharge (action potential). In contrast, the muscle spindle will remain relatively silent because muscle length has not changed. If the same muscle (biceps brachii) is completely relaxed and passively stretched (elbow extended), the muscle spindle would fire, and the GTO would remain relatively silent because little tension is put on the tendon. Therefore the GTO and muscle spindle work collaboratively to inform the nervous system about the muscle length and tension.[42]

The GTO transmits along A alpha (Ib) afferent fibers. It is a slowly adapting receptor that discharges at a rate nearly proportional to the tension of muscle contraction.[36] With respect to spinal reflexes the GTO is associated with autogenic inhibition.[26] In other words, it can cause inhibition of the primary muscle that is contracting against resistance. This occurs because the Ib fiber synapses with inhibitory interneurons in the spinal cord that cause inhibition of the anterior horn cells that innervate the contracting muscle. Clinically, this is seen as a sudden lengthening reaction.[13,21] This phemonenon is commonly seen in patients with spasticity and is called the clasp-knife reflex.[14] According to Moore,[39] other joint receptors may also contribute to this phenomenon.

MUSCLE SPINDLES. Muscle spindles are complex, encapsulated receptors that lie deep within skeletal muscle. Their principal function is to monitor changes in length of a muscle and the rate at which the length changes.[42]

Anatomically, the muscle spindle (Fig. 13-3) is a slender, encapsulated structure that houses four to six bundles of specialized muscle fibers called intrafusal muscles. There are two main types of intrafusal fibers, nuclear chain and nuclear bag fibers.[2] Nuclear bag fibers have an enlarged, noncontractile

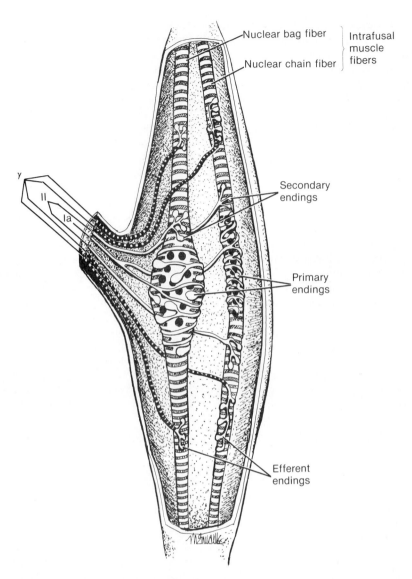

Fig. 13-3. Muscle spindle (sensory and motor attachments). (From Nolte, J.: The human brain: an introduction to its functional anatomy, St. Louis, 1981, The C.V. Mosby Co.)

Labels on figure:
Nuclear bag fiber
Nuclear chain fiber
Intrafusal muscle fibers
Secondary endings
Primary endings
Efferent endings

has a low threshold and is selectively sensitive to the onset of muscle stretch. Some authors have subdivided the Ia primary afferent into phasic and tonic functions.[29] Therefore anytime the muscle is put through a quick stretch within normal range, it will fire the Ia phasic component. The Ia tonic component is believed to originate around the nuclear chain fiber. Therefore the Ia tonic component is less sensitive to quick stretch but fires when the stretch is maintained in the submaximal range.[2,36,46]

A second afferent fiber wraps around the nuclear bag and nuclear chain adjacent to the equatorial region (predominately on the nuclear chain fibers). This fiber was originally called the flower-spray ending because of its appearance. It is now called the secondary ending or group II fiber. The function of the secondary endings is not fully understood.[26] Classically, secondary endings are less sensitive to the onset of stretch but fire during maintained stretch, especially when the muscle is elongated to its maximal range.[2,20,42] The function of the secondary ending is controversial. However, in classic theory maintained stretch will fire the secondary endings and produce facilitation of the flexor and inhibition of the extensor regardless of which muscle receives the stretch.[29] The problem with this principle is determining which muscles are the physiological flexors and which are the anatomical flexors. For example, by definition a physiological extensor serves to elongate an extremity. Subsequently, if an individual assumes the quadruped position with the palms of the hands flat on the floor and "flexes" the wrist, the forelimbs are elongated; physiologically, this would represent extension. Kottke[31] has suggested that the secondary endings feed into multisynaptic pathways to cause flexion or exension synergies. Thus, if the extensors are stimulated, the secondary endings in extensors will cause extensor synergies. If the flexors are stimulated, the secondary endings in flexors cause flexor synergies.

The primary spinal level reflex associated with the muscle spindle is reciprocal innervation. This is a basic stretch

central region containing many nuclei and tapered, contractile (plate) endings. The nuclear chain fibers are smaller and contain a single row of nuclei in the equatorial region. As mentioned earlier, the muscle spindle receives motor innervation from gamma motor neurons.[4] The intrafusal fibers do not contribute to extrafusal muscle strength or joint movement but regulate the tension in the muscle spindle.[35] Hence, as the extrafusal fibers contract, the intrafusal fibers contract concurrently to maintain some tension in the equatorial region and restore its sensitivity. In summary,

the gamma motor neurons regulate the tension of the intrafusal fibers so their sensitivity remains constant as the extrafusal fibers change their length.[2,36,46]

The muscle spindle also contains two types of sensory endings. The first type is called the Ia primary fiber (annulospiral ending), which bifurcates within the spindle and wraps around the equatorial regions of both the nuclear bag and nuclear chain. Because of this spiral arrangement, the Ia primary afferent is stretched like a spring when the equatorial region of the intrafusal muscle elongates. The Ia primary ending reflex where one muscle group is facilitated and the opposing muscles are inhibited.[44] For example, when the biceps is stretched, it is facilitated, and the antagonist muscle (the triceps) is inhibited. This relationship is called reciprocal inhibition.[26,51] Therapists have used the reflex functions of the muscle spindle in a number of ways. Because the Ia primary ending has a low threshold, it can be fired by quick stretch, vibration, tapping over the muscle belly, or any action that causes elongation of the extrafusal fibers.[15] The results will usually be the same. The muscle receiving the stimulus will be facilitated and the antagonist inhibited. The properties of the muscle spindle have been described in isolation. Yet in reality anytime a muscle is stretched or contracted, a multitude of skin and receptors are firing concurrently.

VESTIBULAR APPARATUS. The vestibular apparatus is classified as a proprioceptive organ.[14] It consists of three semicircular canals attached to a vestibule, which is further subdivided into the saccule and utricle. The semicircular canal system is the kinetic labyrinth. This system is sensitive to head movement and rotatory acceleration or deceleration.[40,42] The vestibule (utricle and saccule) is regarded as the static labyrinth. This system is sensitive to head position and linear acceleration or deceleration.[45] The vestibular system acts as a complex relay center that influences many systems of the body. Thus vestibular stimulation has a profound influence on the development of the nervous system.[3] However, as a proprioceptive organ, the vestibular system serves (1) to stabilize the position of the head in space, (2) to stabilize the position of the eyes in space during head movements, (3) to regulate posture and movement through tonic and phasic reflexes, and (4) to exert a powerful influence over the antigravity muscles of neck, trunk, and limbs.[40] The receptor organs in the semicircular canals are the crista ampullaris. In the vestibule, the receptor organ is called the macula or otolith. The vestibular apparatus sends impulses to four nuclei in the upper medulla and disperses to centers throughout the nervous system.

The descending tracts consist of the lateral and medial vestibulospinal tracts. Ascending fibers travel in the medial longitudinal fasciculus to extraocular muscles and other centers. Still other fibers connect with cranial nerves, the autonomic nervous system, and the cerebellum.[11,26,31] An understanding of the vestibular apparatus allows the therapist to alter muscle tone, elicit reactions in selected muscle groups, or enhance facilitory or inhibitory states.[15]

Kinesioceptors

Kinesioceptors are joint receptors that represent the conscious division of proprioception because they transmit to the cerebral cortex. Anatomically, joint receptors are located in joint capsules, ligaments, and tendons. These include Ruffini's end organs, Golgi-Mazzoni corpuscles, Vator-Pacini corpuscles, Golgi-type endings, and free nerve endings.

RUFFINI'S END ORGANS. Ruffini's end organs are exclusively joint receptors found only in fibrous joint capsules.[51] These receptors respond vigorously at the beginning of joint movement, but their discharge rate declines as the joint reaches a different position. These receptors also fire when touch pressure is applied over the surface of the joint.[56]

GOLGI-MAZZONI CORPUSCLES. Golgi-Mazzoni corpuscles take on a similar appearance to pacinian corpuscles. They are small, encapsulated receptors found in joint capsules and tendon surfaces.[51,52] It is interesting to note that the Golgi-Mazzoni receptors are abundant in the connective tissues of the hands. These are rapidly adapting receptors that detect rapid joint movements.[42] They also discharge under deep pressure or vibratory stimuli.[36]

VATER-PACINI CORPUSCLES. Vater-Pacini corpuscles are found in joint capsules and ligaments. They discharge at a greater rate as the joint reaches its maximal range of motion.[36] These receptors may serve a protective function to inform the cortex when the joint has reached its end position of range.

GOLGI-TYPE ENDINGS. Golgi-type endings are another variation of the Golgi tendon organ found mostly in the joint ligaments. These receptors seem to monitor the rate of joint movement.

They are slowly adapting and discharge most rapidly when joint movement is initiated.[10,51]

As previously mentioned, free nerve endings are widely distributed throughout all the soft tissues of the body. It would appear that these receptors support the joint receptors by providing a crude awareness of joint movement. Free nerve endings would also mediate touch, pain, and temperature sensations in the joint region.[52]

The major function of joint receptors is to inform the nervous system about joint position, velocity of movement, and perhaps the direction of movement. At this time there is no evidence to prove that joint receptors contribute to the force of muscle contraction.[42] From this brief summary it appears that joint receptors supply the conscious awareness of joint position and joint movement. As a group, joint receptors provide another means of sensory input. The therapist should incorporate activities that stress the conscious awareness of joint movements as part of the sensorimotor repertoire.

Meridian points (acupoints)

The meridians provide a unique system for cutaneous stimulation that is not yet fully understood.[50] In Eastern philosophy the meridians are described as channels and form a complex network of flowing energy throughout the body. In Chinese tradition there are 12 to 14 meridians, each corresponding to major organs or to other functions. In Eastern medicine illness is described in terms of imbalances or obstruction of the energy that travels through the meridians. Techniques, such as acupressure, acupuncture, or forms of massage, are purported to release the energy from its trapped locations. In the past the concept of using meridian points in therapy seemed improbable. However, there is mounting research evidence to support the fact that some form of energy exists in specific regions of the skin.[27,48] Many studies have linked the meridian points to the release of endorphins (enkephalins)[50] and the autonomic nervous system.[8,9]

The Eastern techniques of cutaneous stimulation have been used for over 2000 years. Therapists should keep an open mind in looking at new theories to develop new techniques as information becomes available.

TRACT SYSTEM

Sensorimotor techniques are aimed at stimulating specific receptors and tract systems. From a sensory stimulation standpoint there are four tract systems through which sensory input travels.[10,40]

Sensory tracts

SPINOTHALAMIC. The first system is called protopathic because it is phylogenetically old and serves a protective function.[3] Anatomically, this system constitutes the anterior and lateral spinothalamic tracts. The spinothalamic system contains fibers of the A delta (group III) and C fibers (group IV). This is a slowly conducting system because most of its fibers are unmyelinated and small in diameter.[41] This system mediates pain, temperature, crude touch, and visceral pain. The first order neuron of this system enters the lateral portion of the dorsal horn of the spinal cord, synapses with interneurons, crosses to the opposite side of the cord, and ascends in an anterolateral spinothalamic tract. An important feature of this system is that it gives off numerous collaterals to the reticular-activating system.[3,45,51] The second order neuron continues its ascent to nonspecific nuclei of the thalamus. From there the third order neuron terminates with many areas of the cerebral cortex. In summary the spinothalamic system serves a protective function that is excitatory to the cortex because of its many collaterals in the reticular formation.

LEMNISCAL. The second system is phylogenetically advanced and is called epicritic because it has a high degree of specificity. Anatomically, this sensory tract system makes up the dorsal columns of the spinal cord and is called the lemniscal system.[11] The lemniscal system contains fibers from the A alpha (group I) and A beta (group II) classifications. Since this system contains well-myelinated, thick fibers with few collaterals, it is a fast conducting system.

The lemniscal system carries impulses from the discriminative receptors (Meissner's corpuscles, pacinian corpuscles, and Ruffini's end organs). Therefore this system mediates stereognosis, 2-point discrimination, pressure, vibration, and other senses of fine recognition. The lemniscal system is well defined. The first order neuron enters the medial portion of the dorsal root and ascends in the dorsal columns of the cord on the same side it enters. This system gives off few collaterals to the reticular formation and synapses on the ventrobasal nuclei of the thalamus. The third order neuron terminates in areas 3, 1, and 2 of the somatosensory cortex.[3,45,51] To summarize, the lemniscal system has a high degree of specificity and carries discriminative information.

PROPRIOCEPTIVE. The proprioceptive tracts make up the third sensory pathway. Proprioception refers to the conscious or unconscious awareness of body position and movement of bodily segments. The proprioceptive pathways are of particular interest to the occupational therapist because they regulate movements toward purposeful activities.

Conscious proprioception is regulated by the lemniscal (dorsal column) system. This pathway begins in joint receptors and ends in the parietal lobe of the cerebral cortex where conscious awareness takes place. Conscious proprioception enables the cortex to refine our voluntary movements for skillful activities.[13,17]

Unconscious proprioception is mediated by the spinocerebellar tracts. This pathway begins in the afferents of the muscle spindle and Golgi tendon organ and terminates in the cerebellum. Unconscious proprioception is concerned with muscle tension, muscle length, and speed of movement. The spinocerebellar tracts do not ascend to the cortex.[51] However, the cerebellum serves as a feedback mechanism for the motor cortex so it can modify or correct voluntary movements as they are being initiated.

TRIGEMINAL. The trigeminal nerve (CN V) makes up the fourth and last division of the sensory tract systems. The trigeminal nerve is unique in many ways. It is responsible for direct transmission of tactile, proprioceptive, pain

and temperature sensation in the skin of the facial region. The posterior of the head and neck is supplied by C2, C3, and C4 of the cervical spinal roots.[10,45,52] Therefore the trigeminal nerve transmits information directly to sensory nuclei that are connected to the reticular formation, cerebellum, and cerebral cortex. The sensory end organs and afferent fibers are separated into ophthalmic, maxillary, and mandibular divisions.

The trigeminal nerve is one of the earliest sensory roots to myelinate and respond to touch stimulation. Stimulation to the perioral area evokes a protective avoiding reaction at 7 ½ fetal weeks. The discriminative receptors begin their development and differentiation at about the fourth fetal month.[11] Because of the nerve's early ontogenetic development, some sensorimotor therapists begin cutaneous stimulation to the trigeminal nerve.

The motor branch of the trigeminal nerve supplies the muscles of mastication, tensor tympani muscle of the ear, and tensor veli palatini muscle of the soft palate.[14,30]

DERMATOMES

With the exception of the facial region the skin of the body receives its sensory innervation in a segmental fashion by nerve roots of the spinal cord. The area of skin supplied by a single dorsal root and its ganglion constitutes a dermatome.[39] The dermatomes are arranged on the surface of the body in a sequence corresponding to the related spinal cord segments. Cutaneously, the highest dermatomal level represents the posterior of the head, whereas the lowest is in the anal region.[10] Fig. 13-4 shows the segmental arrangement of dermatomes from the neck down to the anal region. There is much overlap in the segmental borders of the dermatomes, particularly in the trunk. It is important for the occupational therapist to have a fundamental understanding of dermatomal segments. The dermatomes are the skin areas that delineate the sensory regions of the skin. Each sensory dermatome that feeds into the spinal cord has a motor component for the respective segment. What is more,

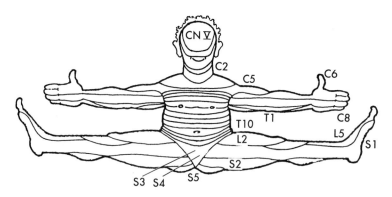

Fig. 13-4. Dermatomes (segmental levels). (From Clark, R.G.: Clinical neuroanatomy and neurophysiology, ed. 5, Philadelphia, 1975, F.A. Davis Co.)

all areas of the skin are not alike. For example, the facial area and the volar surface of the hands contain a greater number of discriminative receptors, whereas the central axis of the trunk contains more protective (protopathic) and autonomic afferents.

In many cases cutaneous stimulation is applied dermatomally in an effort to activate selected muscle groups.[25] Dermatomes are also important in evaluating the integrity of peripheral nerves and the spinal cord segments.

CUTANEOUS REFLEX

An important concept in sensory stimulation is the existence of the cutaneous fusimotor reflex. This reflex was first demonstrated on polio patients by Kenny and later substantiated by Hagbarth.[27,31] In essence, studies have found that stimulation to certain areas of the skin can influence the specific muscles of the body. The cutaneous reflex is not a simple monosynaptic reflex arc. Instead, it is a polysynaptic system that entails cutaneous afferents, gamma motor neurons, and Ia afferents of the muscle spindle. Any stimulation to a dermatome will discharge cutaneous receptors that synapse with gamma motor neurons at the same spinal segment in the ventral horn of the spinal cord. The gamma motor neurons will cause intrafusal fibers to contract. This causes the Ia afferents to discharge, which in turn sends impulses back into the spinal cord where they synapse with alpha motor neurons. If the stimulus is strong

enough to cause the alpha motor neuron to discharge, a reflexive contraction or increase in tone occurs in the muscle innervated at that segmental level. The activity of the cutaneous receptors and the gamma system is proportional to the intensity of the stimuli.[27,29] However, it should be emphasized that the cutaneous stimulus should be applied to the dermatome that corresponds to the muscles to be activated. This technique seems to work best on the dermatomes that overlie the muscles to be activated. In patients with spinal cord injury or with CNS lesions the response may be exaggerated. This occurs because the supraspinal centers are detached or the excitatory neurons are disinhibited.[4,21]

HIERARCHICAL ORGANIZATION OF POSTURE AND MOVEMENT

Research on animal preparations and observations of human subjects with regional lesions suggest that neuromuscular function is based on reflex activity.[1,11] The evolution of the nervous system has allowed the more advanced reflexes to become superimposed on the more primitive. Therefore it is postulated that pathological reflexes are manifestations of primitive reflexes that are normally supressed by supraspinal centers. This concept is now being challenged by proponents of the central control hypothesis, but it still provides a useful model for the therapists who use sensorimotor approaches. The concept is helpful in understanding the hierarchical organization of posture and motor control for testing and treatment. Table 13-3 summarizes and serves as a

reference. The following is a brief summary of the segmental centers for motor control.*

Spinal level

The spinal level regulates the more primitive, stereotypical movements. These are principally stretch reflexes arising from muscles. Because these reflexes are generated from muscles, they are often called myotatic reflexes. Spinal reflexes are "phasic" in that they occur rapidly and extinguish very fast. These reflexes are believed to be primitive responses to potentially harmful stimuli. Therefore a painful stimulus or quick stretch produces spinal level responses. The spinal level reflexes include (1) flexor withdrawal, (2) crossed extension, (3) extensor thrust, (4) positive supporting reaction, (5) negative supporting reaction, and (6) cutaneous-fusimotor reflexes. These reflexes are fairly predictable when elicited in infants or individuals with CNS lesions. They abide by the principles of reciprocal innervation and autogenic inhibition. They are evoked by primary and secondary endings in muscle spindles, Golgi tendon organs, and nonspecific cutaneous receptors.

Lower brainstem

The lower brainstem includes the nuclei in the medulla and the facilitory portion of the reticular formation. These centers have long-lasting effects on posture and therefore are called "tonic" reflexes. For example, the nuclei for the vestibular system are constantly discharging into motor neuron pools to sustain head and body alignment. The static labyrinthine reflex arises from the vestibule (utricle and saccule) and discharges during changes in head position and linear acceleration. The kinetic labyrinth includes the three semicircular canals and responds to head movement and rotatory motions. These reflexes regulate muscle tone (especially extensors) and balance reactions. The tonic neck reflexes are also exerting tonic influences on limbs and postural muscles in response to stretch imposed on the neck muscles. The tonic lumbar reflex arises from joint and muscle proprioceptors in the lum-

---

* References 1, 10, 11, 13, 20, 21, 26, 31, 47, 51.

Table 13-3
Hierarchical organization of postural reflexes

Level	Reflex	Stimulus	Receptor	Motor response	Pathlogical sign
Cerebral cortex (basal ganglia and cerebellum)	Optical righting	Visual cues	Eyes	Righting of head	Decorticate rigidity Spasticity Babinski's sign Hoffmann's sign Clasp-knife reflex
	Placing reaction Hopping reaction	Surface contact	Various * proprioceptors	Weight bearing on palmar sole when placed on hard surface	
Upper brainstem (midbrain and diencephalon)	Labyrinthine righting	Tilt body	Vestibular apparatus	Face vertical and mouth horizontal	
	Neck righting	Stretch of neck muscles	Muscle spindles	Rights body in respect to neck	Romberg's sign Tremor
	Body on head righting	Pressure on side of body	Exteroceptors	Rights head in respect to gravity	Decerebrate rigidity
	Body on body reaction	Rotation of head or thorax	Exteroceptors	Rights head or thorax	
	Tonic lumbar reflex	Lateral flexion or rotation of trunk	Joint and muscle proprioceptors	Reciprocal movements of limbs, trunk, and pelvis for gait pattern	Ataxia Asynergies, weakness
Lower brainstem (medulla and reticular formation)	Tonic labyrinthine reflex (kinetic and static)	Head inversion (gravity)	Vestibular apparatus	Increased extensor tone	"Vestibular shoot"
	Tonic neck reflex	Rotation, flexion or extension of neck	Joint receptors Neck proprioceptors	Alterations in extensor or flexor tone of the limbs	Asynergistic movements; tonic changes in muscle tone
Spinal cord (reflex arc)	Flexor withdrawal	Nociceptive	Exteroceptive	Withdrawal of stimulated extremity	
	Crossed extension	Nociceptive	Exteroceptive	Flexion of stimulated limb and extension-abduction of contralateral limb	
	Extensor thrust	Nociceptive	Exteroceptive	Extension-abduction of contralateral limb	
	Positive supporting reaction	Contact with sole or palm	Proprioceptors and distal flexors	Leg extended to support body	Marie-Foix reflex
	Negative supporting reaction	Stretch	Proprioceptors in extensors	Release of positive supporting reaction	Flexion reflex and clonus
	Cutaneous-fusimotor reflex	Cutaneous stimuli	Exteroceptors and spindle afferents	Prolonged increase in muscle tone at segmental level	Hyperreflexia Hypertonia Romberg's sign Degrees of paralysis

*Pacinian corpuscles, Ruffini end organs, Golgi-Mazzoni muscle spindles, and several exteroceptors.

bar segments. This reflex is divided into symmetrical and asymmetrical components. The symmetrical response occurs when the trunk is ventroflexed, causing flexion of all four extremities, and dorsiflexed, causing extension of all four extremities. The asymmetrical response is stimulated by rotation or lateral flexion of the trunk. Trunk rotation to one side results in flexion of the ipsilateral upper extremity and extension of the lower extremity. Simultaneously the contralateral upper extremity extends and the lower extremity flexes. These opposite effects contribute to the normal reciprocal movements of the limbs during gait pattern. Lateral flexion of the trunk results in ipsilateral upper extremity flexion and lower extremity extension. The contralateral response produces extension of the upper extremity and flexion of the lower. Lower brainstem reflexes include (1) tonic labyrinthine reflexes (static or kinetic), (2) tonic neck reflexes (asymmetrical or symmetrical), and (3) tonic lumbar reflexes. These reflexes arise from the proprioceptors in the neck muscles and trunk and the receptor organs in the vestibular apparatus.

Upper brainstem

The upper brainstem includes the midbrain and the diencephalon (hypothalamus and thalamus). This level includes "tonically" induced reflexes for more refined postural adjustments. Because these reflexes assist with the maintenance of the upright position, they are "righting" or "displacement reactions."[13]

The upper brainstem includes (1) labyrinthine righting reactions, (2) neck righting, (3) body-and-head righting, and (4) body-on-body righting.

Central control centers

The integrated circuits between cerebral cortex, basal ganglia, and cerebellum supply an added dimension to posture and movement. Voluminous research has been done to single out the functions of these structures. They seem to work as feedback circuits to refine higher level motor functions. In general, skilled voluntary movement

arises from the cerebral cortex. Descending impulses send collaterals to both the basal ganglia and the cerebellum. The basal ganglia are credited with the regulation of the more rhythmical automatic movement patterns.[14] The cerebellum tends to monitor the rate, range, force, and direction of movement. Therefore once the voluntary movement has been initiated by the cortex, the subcortical structures refine and feed back information during the motor act.[1] Some reflexes or reactions associated with the cerebral cortex are (1) optical righting reflexes, (2) placing reactions, and (3) hopping reactions.

SPECIAL SENSE MECHANISMS
Olfactory

The special senses are often alluded to in sensorimotor techniques, but specific procedures are limited at this time. The following discussion will outline some of the salient features of the special sense organs and how they might be used in therapy.

The physiological components of the olfactory system are not well understood. There are many theories about how smell is transduced into neuronal messages, but the scientific facts are somewhat limited. Basically olfaction is a chemical process.[30] The receptors for smell are located in specialized epithelium in the roof of the nasal cavity. The olfactory epithelium contains three types of cells and small glands that secrete mucous substances for dissolving odorous materials. The receptor cells contain fine hairlike cilia, which are the most exposed nerve endings in the entire body. The olfactory epithelium is estimated to contain 100 million receptor cells, yet it only occupies an area the size of a dime.[17,26] The afferent fibers from these cells converge with the second order neurons in a ratio of 1000:1.[1]

The receptor cells for olfaction respond to a variety of stimuli. Some sources indicate that humans can distinguish between 2000 to 4000 different odors.[34] However, each of these odors may generate different impulses from the olfactory receptors and pass directly to many regions of the brain. The principal regions are the temporal lobe of the cortex (area 28), structures in the

limbic system, and subcortical nuclei and autonomic nuclei of the hypothalamus.[17,40] Furthermore, olfaction is the only sensory modality that bypasses the thalamus en route to the cortex.[24] So if the thalamus is damaged, olfactory stimulation can still reach certain portions of the CNS.

When using olfactory stimuli, the therapist should keep in mind that the receptors for smell adapt rather quickly. As many as 50% will cease firing after the first few seconds of stimulation.[26] Therefore the strength of the odor has to be increased by about 30% to reactivate the adapted receptors. To allow for adaptation the therapist can use three vials of the same scent, each one containing a concentration 30% greater than the first. The therapist should start with a diluted scent first, then a solution of 60%, and last a solution of full strength. This process will increase the time the therapist can use a given scent for olfactory stimulation. Consequently, some noxious chemicals, such as ammonia and vinegar, cause irritation of the mucous linings in the nasal cavity. As a result, it causes more activity in the trigeminal nerve rather than the olfactory. These odors are more useful for stimulating avoidance reactions or facial expressions.

Gustatory

Gustation or taste is also a chemical process. However, the act of eating is a multisensory experience that uses somatosensory receptors as well. The taste receptors are located in the tongue, soft palate, and upper regions of the throat.[40] The tongue contains three different types of taste buds that occupy specific locations. Basically there are four primary taste sensations: sweet, sour, salty, and bitter. Many flavors are combinations of the four taste sensations.[44] However, action potentials show the base of the tongue responds best to bitter, the outer edges to sour and salty, and the tip to sweet.[30]

The taste receptors transmit along the fibers of four cranial nerves: the glossopharyngeal (IX), trigeminal (V), facial (VII), and vagus (X). These cranial nerves transmit to nuclei in the brainstem, reticular formation, spinal and cranial reflex centers, thalamus, and regions of the parietal lobe of the cortex.[40,41]

Before beginning gustatory stimulation the therapist should evaluate swallowing and the gag reflexes to see if the glossopharyngeal (IX) and vagus (X) nerves are intact. Gustatory discrimination is similar to olfaction in that it adapts readily and requires about a 30% change in concentration to distinguish differences.[25,44] Also before a substance can be tasted, it must be somewhat water soluble. Therefore the therapist can use one of each primary flavor mixed in distilled water so the concentrations can be graded from weak to strong. Again the first solution should contain a 1:3 ratio, that is, one part flavor and three parts distilled water. Three vials can be mixed for each taste stimulus. The second vial can contain a solution 30% stronger than the first, and the last can be full strength. These solutions can be applied to the tongue with an eye dropper so they contact specific portions of the tongue. For example, the sweet flavor can be made with low calorie sweeteners and distilled water. In this case the drops would be applied to the tip of the tongue. The sour taste can be made with vinegar and distilled water and applied to the middle sides of the tongue. Salt flavor can be made with table salt or sodium flouride and applied to the anterior edges of the tongue.[9,40] Because bitter tastes are detected in lower concentrations and can trigger avoidance reactions, they should be used last. In addition, sour and bitter tastes may also elicit "taste reflexes" that stimulate the parotid and submaxillary glands to secrete saliva. This is a natural way of promoting swallowing, but it may dilute the taste stimuli.

Auditory

The auditory system enables the perception of events that are taking place at a distance. This is a sophisticated sense that transduces sound waves into mechanical energy and ultimately neuronal impulses. The receptor cells for audition are housed in the cochlea in a structure called Corti's organ.[10,40] This structure contains hair cells similar in appearance to the cells in the vestibular system. The impulses from the receptor cells pass along nerve fibers of the spiral ganglion through the nerve root of cranial nerve VIII to special nuclei in the superior portion of the medulla. Second order neurons project to the contralateral side of the brainstem or ascend ipsilaterally to the olivary and accessory nuclei. Still other collaterals synapse on neurons in the reticular system or ascend by way of the lateral lemniscus to the inferior colliculus. Third order neurons ascend to the medial geniculate body and then to the auditory cortex (Brodmann's area 41).[26]

The auditory system has its own set of reflexes that are related to protective behavior. It connects to the reticular formation and then evokes responses in the autonomic nervous system. In the midbrain the inferior colliculi feed into the tectospinal tract. This system is activated by sudden sounds, such as a car backfiring. Such a sound would transmit auditory input to centers believed to trigger reflexive movements of the head, neck, and upper extremities. The auditory system may be used with moderation in therapy. This does not imply that the therapist should use sudden sound stimuli to evoke reflex responses. However, it does imply that auditory stimuli feed into motor neuron pools that influence postural reflexes. It may also imply that the auditory stimuli going to the reticular formation can produce excitatory or inhibitory states, depending on the nature of the sound. For example, a novel sound stimulus tends to be excitatory. A constant sound stimulus, such as the waves of the ocean or city traffic, is suppressed by the reticular system. Soft melodic music is said to be restful, whereas "hard rock" music would have an excitatory effect. Some therapists use the sound of their voice as an inhibitory or excitatory stimulus. If the activity is designed to promote movement, the therapist should use simple, one-word commands, such as "reach," "pull," "stop," or "look." On the other hand, if the activity is designed to be inhibitory, the therapist should speak to the patient in a soft monotone. This is particularly helpful for elderly patients who have difficulty hearing sounds of high-pitched frequencies.[9]

Visual

The visual system is one of the most relied-on senses for orientation in space. Vision is a remarkable biochemical process that transduces light stimuli into neuronal impulses. Basically light is an electromagnetic energy that passes through the lens of the eye to be casted on the retina. The retina is actually an extension of the brain. It is composed of specialized receptor cells (rods and cones) and photopigments that absorb the light stimulus. This causes an action potential, and impulses are conducted along visual pathways.[1,7] The visual pathway projects posteriorly to form the fiber tracts of cranial nerve II where it becomes the optic nerve. The visual pathway can be very confusing because the retina of each eye contains fibers from the nasal portion that cross at the optic chiasm. The fibers arising from the temporal portions of each retina do not cross at the optic chiasm but continue uninterrupted to the lateral geniculate bodies of the thalamus. From this juncture the fibers proceed posteriorly until they terminate on the occipital lobes of the cortex. The visual cortex is composed of Brodmann's area 17, which is the visual receptive area. Areas 18 and 19 are believed to be involved with visual reflexes and visual perception. Area 8 in the frontal lobe is associated with voluntary eye movements.[14]

The visual system mediates a number of protective and postural reflexes. For example, connections to the superior colliculus mediate reflexes for quick localization of potentially harmful stimuli. Connections to cranial nerves III, IV, VI and the vestibular apparatus provide a stabilizing influence on the eyes during head rotation. Other visual reflexes may include the light reflex, visual fixation, convergence, accommodation, pupillary constriction, blinking, and ciliospinal reflex.[1,10] Much evidence suggests that the visual motor system is linked to chains of motor neurons that modulate posture and movement.[40] In essence the extraocular muscles direct the eyes toward a stimulus in the periphery. If the eyes are turned laterally to converge on the object in the visual field, the head will rotate in an effort to center the eyes. Rotation of the neck sets off a volley of postural responses (tonic neck and righting reactions) that attempt to realign the trunk with the neck. Therefore the eyes lead, the head follows, and the trunk and limbs adjust accordingly.

NEW FRONTIERS IN THERAPY

Although the nervous system is composed of many subdivisions, it functions as an integrated whole. Since the therapist cannot see the internal functions of the CNS, examination must be done through clinical observation. Sometimes the nervous system gives subtle clues about what is going on inside. The occupational therapist must be a skilled observer to interpret subtle signs, such as body language, behaviors, and motor deficits, that the patient exhibits.

Neurolinguistic programming

A new approach to understanding the process of human communications offers some hints for understanding how an individual perceives sensory input. This approach is called neurolinguistic programming.[6,32] Although neurolinguistic programming is in its infancy, it offers some interesting ways to observe and communicate with patients. As the name implies, the nervous system is programmed to process information similar to a computer. Studies have shown that people process incoming information by channelling it through a dominant sensory modality. In our culture most people are biased to one of the three sensory-based categories: kinesthetic, visual, or auditory. Because the occupational therapist engages the patient in purposeful activities, it is important to ascertain which sensory modality the patient prefers to use. To do this, neurolinguistic programming provides some helpful hints. During the time the therapist is interviewing or evaluating the patient, some simple observations can be made. These findings may not be absolute but are true for many individuals. First, the observer should focus on the patient's oculomotor system or the movement of the eyes. Interestingly, the direction in which a person is looking is in correlation with the individual's thinking process. For example, when a person is speaking and the eyes are turned upward or defocused straight ahead, that person is most likely visualizing what is being described. If the patient looks upward frequently, it could mean the patient is a visual learner. Therefore functional activities may be more successful for this patient if introduced more visually or graphically. The therapist may reinforce this visualization process by looking upward and posing hypothetical questions. Many times the patient will follow the lead and answer the questions by looking upward to imagine the situation.

The person who is oriented to processing information auditorily usually oscillates the eyes from side to side. If the person is engaged in internal speech or talks to self while performing a task, the eyes usually turn in the direction of the nondominant hand. The auditory individual will prefer sounds or words for learning. Thus the therapist may present functional activities more verbally and discriptively.

The kinesthetic person tends to be oriented towards emotions or physical action. The most common eye pattern is to look down towards the dominant hand while experiencing sensations or emotions. This patient may profit from activities that are more physically oriented.

Hand gestures and breathing patterns may also reveal auditory, visual, or kinesthetic tendencies. People have been known to point toward or touch the sense organ that is associated with their thinking process. The auditory person gestures toward his ear; the visual gestures in the direction of the eyes; and the kinesthetic may point toward the heart, an organ equated with emotions. Kinesthetic persons exhibit deep abdominal respirations. Shallow thoracic breathing has been linked with visual perception, and even breathing with prolonged expiration is associated with auditory perception.

Touch communication

Touch is another important aspect of interpersonal communication. It has been shown that touch is a form of primal communication, perhaps more powerful than the spoken word alone.

Montagu[37] has emphasized the importance of touch from an anthropological standpoint. More recently, Krieger[33,34] has demonstrated how the "laying on of hands" produces measurable physiological benefits. "Therapeutic touch," as it is called, is a process by which the therapist assesses or in a sense treats certain conditions by placing the hands within proximity of the patient. It is postulated that some form of energy is transmitted from the therapist to the patient.[33] The ancient practice of laying on of hands is not unique to occupational therapy. However, research is showing that touch or cutaneous stimulation may have many more implications than previously imagined. Some evidence suggests that touch changes the relationship of positive and negative ions, which in turn regulates "wellbeing" or "wellness."

Endorphins

The recent discovery of endorphins and enkephalins may also bring credence to therapeutic activities. Recent research has shown that various types of cutaneous stimulation can release these opiate-like substances in the midbrain, limbic system, pituitary gland, and other structures of the nervous system. Endorphins and enkephalins have been found to block pain transmission and to alter emotions, moods, and intestinal motility.[8,9,20,42] How these substances actually work is a matter of speculation at present, but it is likely that cutaneous and proprioceptive stimulation and certain activities may indeed release endorphins. The occupational therapist should stay abreast of new developments in the neurosciences. Because what seems to be speculation today may become new paradigms for therapeutic intervention tomorrow.

REVIEW QUESTIONS

1. What are the two classifications of nerve fibers?
2. What is the primary function of gamma loop (fusimotor neuron)?
3. Differentiate between the functions of the sympathetic and the parasympathetic branches of the autonomic nervous system.
4. Why is the brainstem so important to sensorimotor integration?
5. Describe the two properties a neuron must possess to convey information.
6. Explain the terms *reverberating, excitation,* and *disinhibited.*
7. Describe the factors contributing to the rebound phenomenon.
8. List three factors associated with neuroplasticity.
9. Discuss how interoceptors are used in sensorimotor techniques.
10. Describe some of the therapeutic features associated with the pacinian corpuscle.
11. Contrast the basic functions of the Golgi tendon organ with the muscle spindle.
12. Describe the functions of the Ia afferent and secondary endings of the muscle spindle.
13. Describe the anatomical components of the static and kinetic labyrinthine systems.
14. List four functions of the vestibular system.
15. What are the functions of joint receptors?
16. Differentiate between the spinothalamic and the lemniscal tract systems.
17. Why is the trigeminal nerve considered to be an individual sensory tract system?
18. Describe how dermatomes relate to spinal cord segments and the topographic arrangement on the skin.
19. Describe the "cutaneous reflex" and its significance in sensorimotor therapy.
20. List the reflexes associated with each level of the nervous system.
21. Describe how the olfactory system can be used in sensorimotor therapy.
22. Discuss how gustation can be used in sensorimotor therapy.
23. How can auditory stimuli be used in sensorimotor therapy?
24. How can visual stimuli be used in sensorimotor therapy?
25. Describe how neurolinguistic programming can be used in occupational therapy.

REFERENCES

1. Afifi, A., and Bergman, R.: Basic neuroscience, Baltimore, 1980, Urban & Schwarzenberg, Inc.
2. Appelberg, B., Beson, P., and LaPorte, Y.: Effects of dynamic and static fusimotor gamma fibers on the responses of primary and secondary endings, J. Physiol. (Lond.) **177:**29, 1965.
3. Ayres, J.: The development of sensory integrative theory and practice, Dubuque, Iowa, 1974, Kendall/Hunt Publishing Co.
4. Bach-y-Rita, P., (editor): Recovery of function: theoretical considerations for brain injury rehabilitation, Baltimore, 1980, University Park Press.
5. Balian, R., and Riggs, H.: Myelination of the brain in the newborn, Philadelphia, 1969, J.B. Lippincott Co.
6. Bandler, R., and Grinder, J.: The structure of magic, Palo Alto, Calif., 1975, Science & Behavior Books.
7. Barr, M.: The human nervous system, ed. 2, New York, 1974, Harper & Row, Publishers, Inc.
8. Basbaum, A., Clanton, C., and Fields, H.: Opiate and stimulus produced analgesia: functional anatomy of a medullospinal pathway, Proc. Natl. Acad. Sci. U.S.A. **73:**4685, 1976.
9. Basbaum, A., and Fields, H.: Endogenous pain conrol mechanisms: review and hypothesis, Ann. Neurol. **4:**451, 1978.
10. Basmajian, J.: Primary anatomy, ed. 7, Baltimore, 1976, The Williams & Wilkins Co.
11. Brown, D.: Neurosciences for allied health therapies, St. Louis, 1980, The C.V. Mosby Co.
12. Brudny, J., et al.: Helping hemiparetics to help themselves: sensory feedback therapy, JAMA **241:**814, 1979.
13. Chusid, J.: Correlative neuroanatomy and functional neurology, ed. 18, Los Altos, Calif., 1982, Lange Medical Publications.
14. Clark, R.: Clinical neuroanatomy and neurophysiology, ed. 5, Philadelphia, 1975, F.A. Davis Co.
15. Farber, S.: Neurorehabilitation: a multisensory approach, Philadelphia, 1982, W.B. Saunders Co.
16. Feigenson, J.S.: Stroke rehabilitation: effectiveness, benefits and cost: some practical considerations, (editorial), Stroke **10:**1, 1979.
17. Gardner, E.: Fundamentals of neurology, ed. 6, Philadelphia, 1975, W.B. Saunders Co.
18. Gartland, J.: Fundamentals of orthopaedics, ed. 3, Philadelphia, 1979, W.B. Saunders Co.
19. Gellhorn, E.: Principles of autonomic-somatic integration, Minneapolis, 1967, University of Minnesota Press.
20. Gilman, S., and Winans, S.: Manter and Gatz's essentials of clinical neuroanatomy and neurophysiology, ed. 6, Philadelphia, 1982, F.A. Davis Co.
21. Gilroy, J., and Meyer, J.S.: Medical neurology, ed. 3, New York, 1979, Macmillan Publishing Co., Inc.
22. Golberg, S.: Clinical neuroanatomy made ridiculously simple, Miami, 1979, Medical Master, Inc.
23. Goodwin, G.M., McCloskey, D.I., and Matthews, P.: The contribution of muscle afferents to kinesthesia shown by vibration illusions of movement and by the effects of paralyzing joint afferents, Brain **95:**705, 1972.
24. Goss, C.M.: Gray's anatomy, ed. 28, Philadelphia, 1970, Lea & Febiger.
25. Greenough, W.: Experimental modification of the developing brain, Am. Sci. **63:**30, 1975.
26. Guyton, A.: Structure and function of the nervous system, Philadelphia, 1972, W.B. Saunders Co.
27. Hagbarth, K.E.: Excitatory and inhibitory skin areas for flexor and extensor motoneurons, Acta. Physiol. Scand. **26:**1, 1952.
28. Hughes, J.: Isolation of an endogenous compound from the brain with pharmacological properties similar to morphine, Brain Res. **88:**295, 1975.
29. Huss, J.: Sensorimotor treatment approaches. In Hopkins, H.L., and Smith, H.D., editors: Willard and Spackman's occupational therapy, ed. 4, Philadelphia, 1971, J.B. Lippincott Co.
30. Jacob, S., and Francone, C.: Structure and function in man, Philadelphia, 1974, W.B. Saunders Co.
31. Kottke, F., Stillwell, K. and Lehmann, J.: Krusen's handbook of physical medicine and rehabilitation, ed. 3, Philadelphia, 1982, W.B. Saunders Co.
32. Knowles, R.: Through neuro-linguistic programming, Am. J. Nurs. **83:**1010, 1983.

33. Krieger, D.; Healng by the laying-on of hands as a facilitator of bioenergetic change: the response of invivo human hemoglobin, Int. J. Psychoenergetic Systems **1**:121, 1976.

34. Krieger, D.: Therapeutic touch: searching for evidence of physiological change, Am. J. Nurs. **79**:660, 1979.

35. Matthews, P.B.C.: Mammalian muscle receptors and their central actions, London, 1973, Edward Arnold (Publishers), Ltd.

36. McCloskey, D.I.: Kinesthetic sensibility, Physiol. Rev. **58**:763, 1978.

37. Montagu, A.: Touching: the human significance of the skin, ed. 2, San Francisco, 1978, Harper & Row, Publishers, Inc.

38. Moore, J.: A new look at the nervous system in relation to rehabilitation techniques, Am. J. Occup. Ther. **22**:6, 1965.

39. Moore, J.: The Golgi tendon organ and the muscle spindle, Am. J. Occup. Ther. **28**:7, 1974.

40. Mountcastle, V.B.: Medical physiology, ed. 14, St. Louis, 1980, The C.V. Mosby Co.

41. Noback, C.: The human nervous system, basic principles of neurophysiology, ed. 2, New York, 1975, McGraw-Hill, Book Co.

42. Nolte, J.: The human brain: an introduction to its functional anatomy, St. Louis, 1981, The C.V. Mosby Co.

43. Rosner, B.S.: Recovery of function and localization of function in historical perspective. In Stein, D.G., Rosen, J.J., Butlers, N., editors: Plasticity and recovery of function in the central nervous system, New York, 1974, Academic Press, Inc.

44. Schmidt, R.: Sensory physiology, New York, 1977, Springer-Verlag New York, Inc.

45. Schmidt, R.: Fundamentals of neurophysiology, New York, 1978, Springer-Verlag New York, Inc.

46. Scholz, J., and Campbell, S.: Muscle spindles and the regulation of movement, Phys. Ther. **60**:1416, 1980.

47. Selkurt, E.E.: Basic physiology for the health sciences, ed. 2, Boston, 1982, Little, Brown & Co.

48. Vallbo, A., Hagbarth, H., and Torebjard, H.: Somatosensory, proprioception sympathetic activity in human peripheral nerves, Physiol. Rev. **59**:919, 1979.

49. Vierck, C.J.: Alterations of spatio-tactile discrimination after lesions of primate spinal cord, Brain Res. **58**:69, 1973.

50. Wensel, L.: Acupuncture in medical practice, Reston, Va., 1980, Reston Publishing Co., Inc.

51. Werner, J.K.: Neuroscience a clinical perspective, Philadelphia, 1980, W.B. Saunders Co.

52. Williams, P., and Warwick, R.: Functional neuroanatomy of man, ed. 35, Philadelphia, 1975, W.B. Saunders Co.

CHAPTER 14

The Rood approach to the treatment of neuromuscular dysfunction

GUY L. McCORMACK

Margaret S. Rood was trained and registered in both occupatioal and physical therapy. Her theory originated in the 1940s and has continued to undergo revisions to the present day.[46] Since Rood did not write extensively, she seemed to prefer clinical teaching to disseminate her ideas. Most of the literature that describes the Rood approach is based on interpretations by accomplished therapists. It is postulated that Rood may have been ahead of her time. She integrated neurophysiological and developmental literature with clinical observations. At times her level of understanding was beyond the comprehension of the average clinician. Many knowledgeable therapists, such as Shereen Farber, Jean Ayres, Joy Huss, Margot Heininger, and Shirley Randolph, have been greatly influenced by Rood's work. The purpose of this chapter is to summarize and clarify the major tenets of Rood's theory.

Rood's basic hypothesis may be paraphrased as: appropriate sensory stimulation can elicit specific motor responses. Rood combined controlled sensory stimulation with ontogenetic sequences of motor behavior to achieve a purposeful muscular response.[36] Thus muscle action can be "activated, facilitated and inhibited through the sensory system."[52]

GOALS

The goals of Rood's theory are summarized in the following discussion.

Normalize muscle tone

Patients with neurological dysfunction may have muscle tone ranging from hypertonic to hypotonic. Controlled muscle tone is a prerequisite to movement. Normal muscle tone flows smoothly and is constantly changing during a motor act. For example, to turn on the ignition of a car, one has to

have fairly good eye-hand coordination, postural control of the trunk muscles, coinnervation of the proximal arm muscles, forearm pronation and supination, and moderately fine prehension and dexterity in the hands. Subsequently, the demands placed on the various muscle groups are different. Rood recognized this when she categorized muscles into heavy work and light work groups. Rood also believed that a voluntary motor act is based on inherent reflexes and by modification of those reflexes at higher centers.[52] Therefore Rood began therapy by eliciting motor responses on a reflex level and incorporating developmental patterns to augment the motor response. The heavy work muscles are activated before the light work muscles except in the case of feeding and speech muscles.[51]

Treatment begins at the developmental level of functioning

The patient is evaluated developmentally and treated in a sequential manner. The patient does not proceed to the next level of sensorimotor development until some measure of voluntary (supraspinal) control is achieved. This principle follows the cephalo-caudal rule. Treatment begins from the head and proceeds downward segment by segment to the sacral area. The flexors are stimulated first, the extensors second, the adductors third, and the abductors last.[57]

Movement is directed toward a purposeful goal

Rood realized that the patient's motivation plays an important role in the rehabilitation. The patient must first accept the activitiy as a meaningful event. Secondly, the patient must develop a subcortical program in his or her central nervous system (CNS) to perform a

motor act in a coordinated manner. Neurologically, the pyramidal system (corticospinal) is used to control reflex activity and to perform isolated voluntary acts.[38] However, the coordination of the agonist muscle, antagonist muscle, and synergies is a function of the extrapyramidal system. Complex motor patterns rely on subcortical centers for modification and correction so that the cortex can concentrate on the purpose of the act.

Repetition is necessary for the training of muscular responses

The importance of repetition to achieve coordination has been emphasized by Kottke.[38,39] Thousands of repetitions are required to formulate *engrams*. Engrams are interneuronal circuits involving specific neurons and muscles to perform a pattern of motor activity. Repetition, however, can be monotonous. Therefore activities that incorporate similar motor patterns add purpose and value to the exercise.

PRINCIPLES OF TREATMENT

In a journal acticle in 1956[51] Rood suggested four principles in the treatment of neuromuscular dysfunction. Following is an interpretation of those principles.

Tonic neck and labyrinthine reflexes can assist or retard the effects of sensory stimulation

The tonic neck receptors lay in the neck region and respond to changes in the relationship of the head to the neck. The tonic neck reflexes (TNR) are divided into the symmetrical and asymmetrical.[32,35] According to Rood, the TNRs have a modifying influence on extensor tone, especially the "postural part." Fukuda[24] studied postural reflexes in humans and offered the following summary. Dorsiflexion of the neck extends the upper extremities and flexes the lower extremities. Ventral flexion of the neck flexes the upper extremities and extends the lower extremities. Torsion or rotation of the neck toward one shoulder produces an increase in the extensor tone of the upper and lower extremities on the face side of that shoulder.

The labyrinthine receptors lay in the ampullae of the semicircular canals and in the vestibule.[13] These receptors are affected by the "position of the head in relation to gravity." Rood's description of labyrinthine influences on posture is somewhat unclear.

The following is a composite summary from several authors and is illustrated in Fig. 14-1 for clarification. In the normal upright bipedal stance (180°) (Fig. 14-1, *A*) TNR and tonic labyrinthine reflexes (TLR) cause slight flexion of the elbow joint and extension of the lower limbs.[48] As the face moves clockwise to the quadruped position

(Fig. 14-1, *B*), the TNR and TLR are neutralized.[48] In this position the vertebral column is almost horizontal, eliminating gravitational pressure on the intervertebral joints, and the face is looking downward, which reduces the activity of the TLR. In addition, weight bearing is evenly distributed between the upper and lower extremities. If the subject assumes the prone position (Fig. 14-1, *C*) in the horizontal plane (−90°), the static TLR diminishes while the TNRs prevail.[31,37] If the subject assumes a position in which the head is lower than the shoulders (Fig. 14-1, *D*), extensor tone increases in selected muscles (extensor carpi ulnaris, extensor carpi radialis, and soleus).[58] A position of total inversion (Fig. 14-1, *E*) would elicit righting reactions,[38] whereas a supine position with the head below the horizontal plane (Fig. 14-1, *F* and *G*) constitutes a combined TNR and TLR.[37] A client in the supine-semireclining position (Fig. 14-1, *H*) at

60° above horizontal is in a position that maximizes the static TLR.[39] This position causes abduction, flexion, and external rotation of the arms and increased extensor tone in the trunk and lower extremities. Hellenbrant[32] and his associates reported that this supine head-up position (45° to 60° above horizontal) suppresses the TNR. Rood[51] suggested that if the subject is lying on the side with the ear toward the earth's surface, "the arm and leg of the down side will exhibit extensor tone while the up side will be predominated by flexor tone."

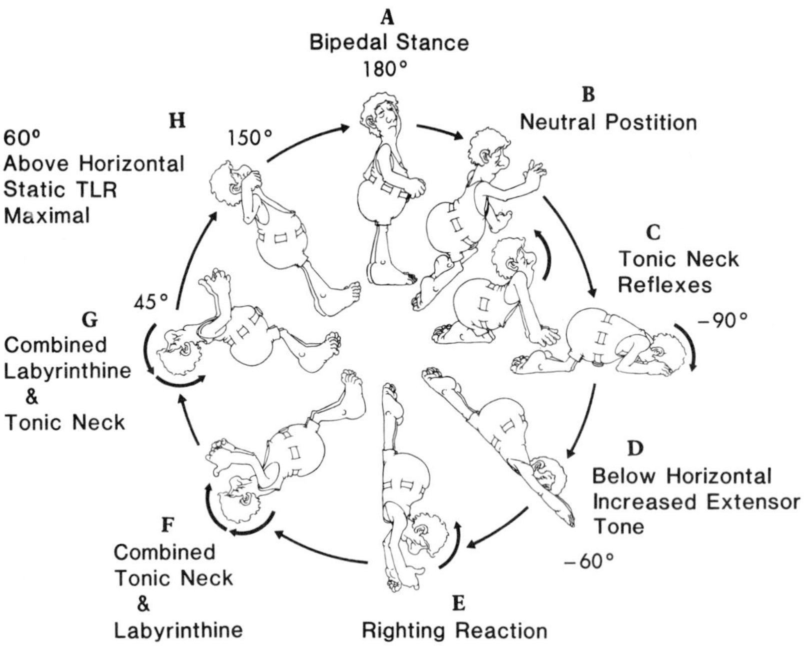

Stimulation of specific receptors can produce three major reactions

The three major reactions that can be produced by stimulation of specific receptors are protective responses, alterations in homeostasis, and adaptive responses aimed toward learning. In 1970 Rood presented four rules of sensory input to clarify the procedure.[31] The first rule is "A fast brief stimulus produces a large synchronous motor output. This type of stimulus is used to confirm that the reflex arc is intact." The second rule states "A fast repetitive sensory input produces a maintained response." A stimulus, such as fast brushing with a battery-operated brush, activates nonspecific receptors that transmit impulses along the C fibers. According to Rood, this stimulus feeds into the fusimotor system that can drive the alpha motor neuron of the muscle. The third rule states "A maintained sensory input produces a maintained response." The force of gravity is an example of a maintained sensory input.[34] Gravity is an ever present force that has a constant effect on the sensory system. Whether standing, sitting, or lying, the exteroceptors of the skin are in contact with a surface, thus discharging impulses into the nervous system. The fourth rule is "Slow, rhythmical, repetitive sensory input deactivates body and mind." Any constant low-frequency stimuli, such as slow rocking in an easy chair, soft music, or even firm pressure to the upper lip, abdomen, soles of the feet, or palms of the hands, activates the parasympathetic system, causing a generalized calming effect.[21]

Fig. 14-1. Composite summary: tonic labyrinthine reflexes. **A,** Bipedal stance. **B,** Neutral position. **C,** Tonic neck reflexes (TNR). **D,** Below horizontal increased extensor tone. **E,** Righting reaction. **F,** Combined TNR and TLR. **G,** Combined TLR and TNR. **H,** Sixty degrees above horizontal static TLR maximum.

Table 14-1

Characteristics of stabilizer and mobilizer muscles

Characteristics	Stabilizers	Mobilizers
Function	Heavy work (holding patterns and maintainance of posture)	Light work (repetitive or rhythmical patterns of distal musculature and skilled movement)
Anatomy	Deep, close to bone and medial axis of body; fan shaped with broad attachments	More superficial and lateral to midline axis; fusiform shaped, tendinous distal attachment
Fibers	Red fibers (aerobic); run obliquely	White fibers (anaerobic), more energy; run parallel to long axis of muscle
Joints	Cross one major joint (uniarthrodial)	Cross two or more joints (multiarthrodial)
Specific muscles	Deep tonic extensors of neck and trunk, scapular adductors (rhomboid major and minor), downward rotators	Two joint extensors (longhead of the triceps brachii, gastrocnemius, flexors, and adductors)
Innervation	More reflexive (tonic) under extrapyramidal, vestibulospinal, reticulospinal, and medial motor system	More voluntary or willed under lateral corticospinal and rubrospinal tracts
Activating stimuli	High threshold exteroceptors and proprioceptors (for example, inverted position, joint [approximation] compression of more than body weight)	Low threshold exteroceptive, light stretch, light moving, touch, quick stretch, and traction
Exercise	Isometric resistance	Isometric or isotonic resistance
Testing	Inversion, joint compression of more than body weight	Quick stretch and light moving touch
Muscle innervation	Greater number of II and fewer Golgi tendon organs	Greater number of Ia afferents

Modified from Farber, S.: Sensorimotor evaluation and treatment procedures for allied health personnel, Indianapolis, 1974, Indiana University and Purdue University at Indianapolis Medical Center; Rood, M.: Occupational therapy in the treatment of the cerebral palsied, Phys. Ther. Rev. **32:**220, 1952; Stockmeyer, S: An interpretation of the approach of Rood to the treatment of neuromuscular dysfunction, NUSTEP proceedings, Am. J. Phys. Med. **46:**900, 1967.

Muscles have different duties

Some muscles predominate as stabilizers, whereas other muscles undertake the duties of mobilization. According to Rood, both groups can be activated as needed through sensory stimulation. Table 14-1 is a summary of the characteristics of the stabilizer and mobilizer muscles.

Heavy work muscles should be integrated before light work muscles

The principle of integrating heavy work muscles before light work muscles primarily refers to the use of the upper extremities. For example, fine fingertip manipulation is not functional if the proximal muscles are not strong enough to lift or stabilize the position of the arm.

SEQUENCE OF MOTOR DEVELOPMENT

Rood proposed four sequential phases of motor control.[4,52,57]

Reciprocal inhibition (innervation)

Reciprocal inhibition is an early mobility pattern that subserves a protective function. It is a phasic (quick) type of movement that requires contraction of the agonist muscle as the antagonist muscle relaxes. This basic movement pattern is primarily a reflex governed by spinal and supraspinal centers.

Cocontraction (coinnervation)

Cocontraction provides stability and is considered to be a tonic (static) pattern. This provides the ability to hold a position or an object for a longer duration. Cocontraction is defined as simultaneous contraction of the agonist muscle and antagonist muscle with the antagonist supreme.[21]

Heavy work

Heavy work is described by Stockmeyer[57] as "mobility superimposed on stability." In this pattern the proximal muscles contract and move while the distal segment is fixed. A good example is creeping. In the quadruped position the distal segments, wrist, and ankles are in a fixed position. The proximal joints, such as the neck and thorax, are stable while the shoulder and hip girdles are free to move.

Skill

Skill is the highest level of motor control and combines the effort of mobility and stability.[50] To execute a skilled pattern, the proximal segment is stabilized while the distal segment moves freely. The art of oil painting typifies this pattern as the artist stands back from the canvas, holds his or her arm at full length, and manipulates the brush freely in the hand.

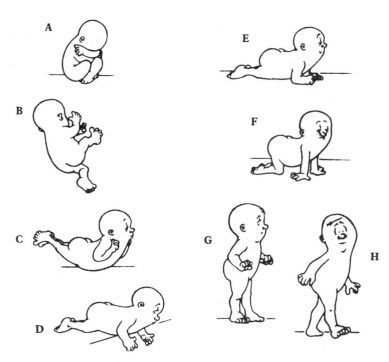

Fig. 14-2. Ontogenetic motor patterns. **A,** Supine withdrawal. **B,** Roll over toward side lying. **C,** Pivot prone. **D,** Neck cocontraction. **E,** Prone on elbows. **F,** Quadruped pattern. **G,** Static standing. **H,** Walking.

ONTOGENETIC MOTOR PATTERNS

The sequence of motor development described previously occurs as the patient is put through the skeletal function sequence that Rood called ontogenetic motor patterns.[57] The eight ontogenetic motor patterns are briefly described and related to their neurological benefits and are illustrated in Fig. 14-2.

Supine withdrawal (supine flexion)

Supine withdrawal is a total flexion response toward the vertebral level of T10.[52] This is a protective position because the flexion of the neck and the crossing of the arms and legs protects the anterior surface of the body. This is a mobility posture requiring reciprocal innervation. Yet is also requires heavy work of the proximal muscles and trunk.[57] Therapeutically, supine withdrawal aids in the integration of the TLR. Rood recommended this pattern for patients who do not have reciprocal flexion pattern and for patients dominated by extensor tone[57] (Fig. 14-2, *A*).

Roll over (toward side lying)

When rolling over, the arm and leg flex on the same side of the body. This is a mobility pattern for the extremities and activates the lateral trunk musculature.[57] This pattern is encouraged for patients who are dominated by tonic reflex patterns in the supine position. The rolling action also stimulates the semicircular canals which in turn activate the neck and extraocular muscles (Fig. 14-2, *B*).

Pivot prone (prone extension)

The pivot-prone position demands a full range of extension of the neck, shoulders, trunk, and lower extremities. This pattern has been called both a mobility and stability pattern. This position is difficult to assume and hold. Therefore it plays an important role in preparation for stability of the extensor muscles in the upright position.[52] The pivot-prone position has been associated with the labyrinthine righting reaction of the head. The ability to maintain the position indicates integration of the symmetrical TNRs and the TLRs (Fig. 14-2, *C*).

Neck cocontraction (coinnervation)

Neck cocontraction is the first real stability pattern. In keeping with the cervicocaudal rule and cervicorostral rule, cocontraction of the neck precedes cocontraction of the trunk and extremities. As the head bobs up and down, the extensors and rotators are stretched. This action is said to activate both flexors and deep tonic extensors of the neck.[51] However, it is important to make sure the neck flexors are well established before the prone position is assumed. To raise the head against gravity, the patient needs to have good cocontraction of the flexors and extensors of the neck.[22] Neurologically, this pattern elicits the tonic labyrinthine righting reaction when the face is perpendicular to the floor. As the head flexes, it stretches the proprioceptors in the neck and upper trapezius, causing them to contract against the forces of gravity (Fig. 14-2, *D*).

On elbows (prone on elbows)

Following cocontraction of the neck and prone extension, weight bearing on the elbows is the next pattern to achieve. Bearing weight on the elbows stretches the upper trunk musculature to influence stability of the scapular and glenohumeral regions. This position gives the patient better visibility of the environment and an opportunity to shift weight from side to side. It is also inhibitory to the symmetrical TNR[5] (Fig. 14-2, *E*).

All fours (quadruped position)

The quadruped position follows stability of the neck and shoulders. The lower trunk and lower extremities are brought into a cocontraction pattern. Initially the position is static and the abdomen may sag at the T10 level, causing stretching of the trunk and limb girdles. This stretching develops cocontraction of the trunk flexors and extensors.[31] Eventually weight shifting forward, backward, side to side, and diagonally provides a mobility superimposed on the stability phase. The weight shifting may be preparatory to equilibrium responses (Fig. 14-2, *F*).

Static standing

Assuming the upright bipedal position, static standing is thought to be a skill of the upper trunk because it frees the upper extremities for prehension and manipulation.[57] At first, weight is equally distributed on both legs and then weight shifting begins. This position brings in higher level integration, such as righting reactions and equilibrium reactions (Fig. 14-2, *G*).

Walking

The gait pattern unites skill, mobility, and stability. According to Murray,[44] normal locomotion entails the ability to support the body weight, maintain balance, and execute the stepping motion. Walking includes a stance phase, push off, swing, heel strike, and stride length.[57] Walking is a sophisticated process requiring coordinated movement patterns of various parts of the body (Fig. 14-2, *H*).

SPECIFIC FACILITATION TECHNIQUES USED IN TREATMENT
Cutaneous facilitation

Cutaneous facilitation can be used to stimulate the exteroceptors of the skin.[3,60] The exteroceptors are those end organs located immediately under the skin in subcutaneous tissues or in external mucous membranes.[61] Exteroceptors respond to stimuli arising from the external environment. In general, the exteroceptive system subserves protective withdrawal responses and produces states of alertness and rapid movements of the limbs.[7,12,19] The principle sensory modalities transmitted by the exteroceptive system are pain, temperature, and touch.[27] These modalities are transmitted to the spinal cord along A delta (Group III) and C fibers (Group IV), which are thin, have little or no myelination, and are slow conducters.[21] Nondiscriminative exteroceptive impulses travel to higher centers of the CNS by way of the spinothalamic and spinoreticular tracts. The more discriminative exteroceptive stimuli, vibration, stereognosis, and fine touch (conscious proprioception), ascend along the lemniscal (dorsal) columns.[4,19] Exterocep-

tive stimuli, such as icing and brushing, should be used judiciously because they have a profound effect on the reticular activating system and the autonomic nervous system.[31] Specific techniques of cutaneous facilitation are described later.

LIGHT MOVING TOUCH. Touch is important for normal growth and development.[42] Light touch stimuli send input to limbic structures and have been shown to increase corticosteroid levels in the bloodstream.[54] Corticosteroids aid in increasing resistance against disease, tissue repair, and fluid and electrolyte balance.[3] Rood used a light moving touch or stroking of the skin to activate the superficial mobilizing muscles. These muscles are classified as the light work group that perform skilled tasks.[52,57] Neurologically, the light stroke stimulus activates low threshold hair end organs and free nerve endings. The stimuli send impulses along A delta size sensory fibers, which synapse with the fusimotor system. As a result, light moving touch causes reciprocal innervation, which is clinically seen as a phasic withdrawal response.[45] Light moving touch is applied with the fingertip, camel hair brush, or cotton Q-tip. Originally, the frequency of the touch stimulus was done "two times per second and at least ten times, and then repeated three to five times."[51] The formula now suggested is to apply three to five strokes and allow 30 seconds to elapse between strokes.[21,31] The 30-second rest period is important because it prevents a presynaptic inhibitory response called primary afferent depolarization. This is a synaptic mechanism that prevents overstimulation.[22,53] Light moving touch is applied to the facial region after firm pressure is maintained on the upper lip.[22] This causes a generalized inhibitory response before the light moving stimulus is applied to the perioral region. The first area stimulated is the area from the nose to the chin (perioral midline). The stimulus may have to be applied several times before a response is elicited. In infants the response may cause a flexion pattern of the upper and perhaps the lower extremities.[22] A similar type of stimulus is to apply light stroking from the corner of the lip to the cheek (perioral lateral). This stimulus activates superficial

musculature of the neck and the head tilts laterally toward the side of the stimulus. In adults a unilateal flexion pattern can be facilitated by applying a light moving touch to the navel region or dermatome T10.[22] The stimulus is applied several times in a midline to lateral direction. Light moving touch can also be applied to the dorsal web spaces of the fingers and toes to elicit a withdrawal pattern of the extremities. More rapid results may be obtained[51,52] if light moving touch is applied to the palm of the hands or sole of the feet because it facilitates a "tickle withdrawal response" of greater magnitude.

FAST BRUSHING. In 1964 Rood introduced a battery-operated brush to stimulate the C fibers, which send many collaterals to the reticular activating system.[59] The stimulation to this system was reported to have its maximal effect 30 minutes after stimulation.[51] Therefore fast brushing was used before all other forms of stimulation because of its prolonged latency effect. Spicer and Matyas[55] compared brushing and icing as therapeutic modalities. They found brushing to be a better stimulus than icing but the greatest effect occurs during the time the stimulation is applied. Neurologically, fast brushing is a nonspecific, high-intensity stimulus that increases the fusimotor activity of selected muscles. The key to fast brushing is to apply it over the dermatomes of the same segment that supplies the muscle that is to be facilitated.[25,31] Fig. 14-3 shows the anterior and posterior distribution of the dermatomes. Table 14-2 shows the spinal segment, the location of the dermatome, the muscles facilitated at the spinal level, and the primary function. The stimulus is applied for three to five seconds and repeated after 30 seconds have elapsed.[52] Fast brushing can be applied adjacent to the vertebral column over the posterior primary rami to facilitate the deep tonic muscles of the back[57] (Figs. 14-4 and 14-5). Heininger and Randolph[31] have suggested that the inverted position is more effective for this purpose. The anterior primary rami can also be brushed to tonically facilitate

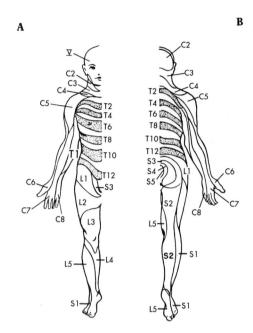

Fig. 14-3. A and B, Dermatomes.

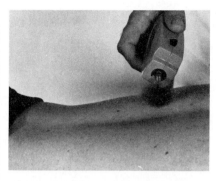

Fig. 14-4. Fast brushing to deep proximal muscles.

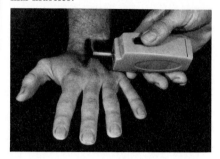

Fig. 14-5. Fast brushing to web spaces of fingers.

Table 14-2
Dermatomes

Spinal segment	Dermatome location	Muscles facilitated	Function
CN V	Anterior facial region	Mastication	Ingestion
CI 3	Neck region	Sternocleidomastoid, upper trapezius	Head control
C4	Upper shoulder region	Trapezius (diaphragm)	Head control
C5	Lateral aspect of shoulder	Deltoid, biceps, rhomboid major and minor	Elbow flexion
C6	Thumb and radial forearm	Extensor carpi radialis, biceps	Shoulder abduction wrist extension
C7	Middle finger	Triceps, extensors of wrist and fingers	Wrist flexion, finger extension
C8	Little finger, ulnar forearm	Flexor of wrist and fingers	C8 finger flexion
T1	Axilla and proximal medial arm	Hand intrinsics	Abduction and adduction of fingers
T2-12	Thorax	Intercostals	Respiration
L1-2	Inside of thigh	Cremasteric reflex, accessory muscles	Elevation of scrotum
T4,T6	Nipple line	Intercostals	Respiration
T7-11	Midchest region Lower rib	Abdominal wall, abdominal muscles	T5-7 "superficial" abdominal reflex
T10	Umbilicus	Psoas, iliacus	Leg flexion
L2	Proximal anterior thigh	Iliopsoas, adductors of thigh	Reflex voiding
L3-4	Anterior knee	Quadriceps, tibialis anterior, detrusor urinae	Hip flexion, extensors of knee, abductors of thigh
L5	Great toe	Lateral hamstrings	Flexion at knee, toe extension
L5-S1	Foot region	Gastrocnemius, soleus, extensor digitorum longus	Flexor withdrawal, urinary retention
S2	Narrow band of posterior thigh	Small muscles of foot (flexor digitorum, flexor hallucis)	Bladder retention

the superficial muscles. Again the stimulus is applied to the dermatomal segment (T2 to T12) that corresponds to specific muscle groups.[51] Brushing appears to work best on isolated muscle groups where the dermatome lays over the muscle to be facilitated.[36]

Fast brushing is contraindicated for certain areas of the skin. The outer ring of the trigeminal nerve where C2 dermatome begins has a tremendous overlap of free nerve endings. This area also has an extensive input to the reticular system. The pinna of the ear also has an abundant nerve supply. It receives sensory fibers from the trigeminal, facial, and vagus cranial nerves as well as the auricular and occipital nerves that surface from C2 and C3 spinal segments.[26,27] Dermatomal skin areas L1 and L2 connect with sympathetic fibers in the spinal cord and innervate the detrussor urinae. Fast brushing to this area can cause voiding. Stimulation to dermatomes S2 to S4 can improve bladder retention in incontinent patients.[52] This technique appears to work as an overflow mechanism similar to the referred pain phenomenon. The smooth muscle of the bladder responds to a stretch reflex controlled by the proprioceptors in its wall.[27] Fast brushing over dermatome S2 to S4 sends impulses to the proprioceptors of the sphincter muscle, thereby causing involuntary constriction of the sphincter muscles.[27]

ICING. Ice is an extreme in thermal facilitation. Ice has been used for facilitation of muscle activity and autonomic nervous system responses.[51] Unfortunately, icing is a powerful stimulus and the results are not predictable. Rood has described three uses for icing.[51,52] First, A icing or quick icing is used for patients with hypotonia and in a state of relaxation. A icing probably activates the more myelinated A delta fibers, causing a reflex withdrawal response in the superficial muscles.[57] The ice is applied to the skin in three quick swipes and the water blotted with a terry cloth towel between each swipe (Fig. 14-6). To elicit a withdrawal response of the limbs, the ice is applied to the dorsal web spaces or the palms and soles of the hands and feet[52] (Fig. 14-7). Second, C icing is a high-intensity nociceptive stimulus that affects the nonspecific C fibers.[52] This type of icing is used to

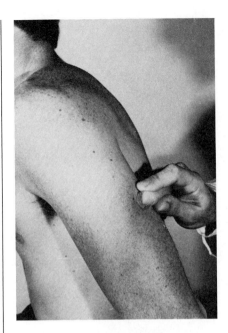

Fig. 14-6. "A" icing.

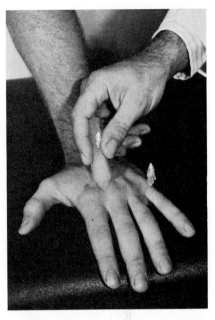

Fig. 14-7. Icing to dorsal web spaces of fingers.

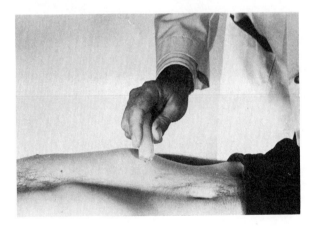

Fig. 14-8. "C" icing.

facilitate maintained postural responses. The ice cube is pressed to the skin of a dermatome serving the same spinal segment of the target muscles to be stimulated. The excess water is wiped away and the response may take as long as 30 minutes because it must travel through spinal circuits and the reticular activating system.[52] Third, autonomic icing is a stimulus affecting the sympathetic nervous system and probably influences glandular output of the thyroid and adrenal glands[51] (Fig. 14-8). This is an area that needs more research. Rood has described the use of ice to promote

the reciprocal pattern between the diaphragm and the abdominal muscles.[51] Ice is administered to the upper right quadrant of the abdomen (T7 through T9) along the angle of the lower rib. The stimulus is applied briefly two or three times from midline to the lateral direction. The melted water should be blotted instead of stroked.[51] This technique has been reported to increase breathing patterns, voice production, and general vitality.[51]

Ice chips have been used inside of the mouth to stimulate the mucosa, to facilitate closure of the mouth, and to aid swallowing.[36] Ice can be used rather safely on the inner walls of the cheeks and the posterior of the tongue because there are fewer free nerve endings in this area.[16] In some patients ice applied to the lips can cause opening of the mouth.

Icing should be used more selectively than fast brushing. Aside from the mucosa of the mouth, ice should never be applied above the neck to the trigeminal nerve distribution or to the pinna of the ear. Furthermore, ice should not be applied along the midline axis of the body. The midline axis contains a greater concentration of free nerve endings and a greater capacity to feed into the sympathetic outflow of the autonomic nervous system.[16] In patients with spinal cord injury at the level of C4, C5, icing along midline may be in autonomic dysreflexia, which can bring on seizures, palpitations of the heart, and vasoconstriction. In general, the exteroceptive stimulation can be unpredictable. It is a divergent system that recruits other neurons and can cause discharge long after the stimulus is applied.[29] In the 1970s Rood began to abandon the use of exteroceptive stimuli and endorsed the use of proprioceptive input.[31]

Proprioceptive facilitory techniques

Proprioceptive stimulation refers to the facilitation of muscle spindles, Golgi tendon organs, joint receptors, and the vestibular apparatus.[41,60] In general, proprioceptive stimulation gives the therapist more control over the motor response. Proprioceptors adapt more slowly than exteroceptors and can produce sustained postural patterns.[12] There is little or no recruitment in the proprioceptive system. Therefore the motor response lasts as long as the stimulus is applied.[20,53]

HEAVY JOINT COMPRESSION. Heavy joint compression is defined as joint compression greater than body weight applied through the longitudinal axis of the bone.[4] The amount of force is more than that of the normal body weight above the supporting joint[22] (Fig. 14-9). Heavy joint compression is used to facilitate cocontraction at the joint undergoing compression. This can

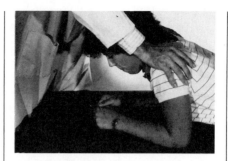

Fig. 14-9. Heavy joint compression.

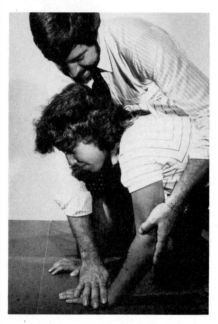

Fig. 14-10. Joint compression to elbow with stretch to wrist extensors in quadruped position.

be combined with developmental patterns, such as prone on elbows, quadruped (Fig. 14-10), sitting, and standing positions. The joint compression may be done manually by the therapist or done with weighted wrist cuffs or sandbags. Clinically, joint compression seems to be most effective when applied through the longitudinal axis of long bones such as the humerus (glenohumeral joint) and the femur (acetabulum).

STRETCH. Stretch is a physiological stimulus used to activate the proprioceptors in selected muscles of the body.[52] Quick stretch employs the principles of reciprocal innervation. The muscle undergoing stretch is facilitated through the Ia afferent of the muscle

spindle and by alpha motor neurons. Quick stretch is applied by holding the proximal bony prominences of the limb to be stretched while the distal joint is moved in one direction. For example, the elbow joint is secured while the forearm is pushed into flexion to stretch the triceps. The response is immediate and short-lived. Quick stretch is used on light work muscle groups, such as physiological flexors and adductors.[57]

INTRINSIC STRETCH. Intrinsic stretch pertains to Rood's use of the intrinsic muscles to promote stability of the scapulohumeral region.[57] For example, in the on-elbows position, shoulder stability can be enhanced if the patient engages in an activity requiring a resistive grasp. Resistance is a form of stretching because it increases fusimotor activity of the muscle spindle. Another variation of this principle can be used in the quadruped position if the patient bears more weight on the ulnar side of his or her hand.[57] Therapists have used cones, float trowels, and horizontal bars angled downward toward the lateral side of the forearm to distribute more weight on the ulnar side of the hands.[22,57]

SECONDARY ENDING STRETCH. Rood has combined resistance and maintained stretch to facilitate ontogenetic skeletal patterns. For instance, to promote the supine withdrawal pattern, the patient is placed supine on a mat with the knees flexed and feet flat on the supporting surface. A small book is placed under the head and a folded towel under the lumbosacral regions. The book and towel put the deep extensor muscles on full stretch. In principle, anytime a muscle is put on full stretch, it fires the secondary endings, which is always facilitory to the flexors and inhibitory to the extensors regardless of which muscle is being stretched.[31,57] Rood called this procedure "driving the flexors through the extensors." To reinforce the reciprocal action of this maneuver, the patient is offered resistance to the flexors, adductors, and internal rotators of the shoulders by compressing a device, such as a bicycle pump.

STRETCH PRESSURE. Stretch pressure affects both the exteroceptors and the Ia afferents of the muscle spindle. The stimulus is applied by placing the pads of the thumbs and index and middle fingers on the skin over a superficial muscle. Firm downward pressure and stretching motion is achieved as the thumb moves away from the fingers.[21,22] The degree of pressure and stretch should be sufficient to cause deformation of the skin and stretch the underlying muscle fibers. The stimulus should not exceed three seconds. This technique can be applied dermatomally or directly over the muscle belly. Since this stimulus is offensive to some patients, a lubricant can be used to reduce the friction on the skin.

RESISTANCE. Rood used heavy resistance to stimulate both primary and secondary endings of the muscle spindle.[52] Resistance is used in an isotonic fashion in developmental patterns to influence the stabilizer muscles. According to Stockmeyer,[57] resistance to contraction of muscles in the shortened range facilitates muscle spindle afferents in the deeper, tonic postural muscles. Fast brushing was used over the stabilizers about 30 minutes before treatment to maximize the response. Farber[22] uses quick stretch before resistance to increase the responsiveness of the muscle spindle. In addition, when a muscle contracts against resistance, it assumes a shortened length that causes the muscle spindles to contract so they readjust to the shorter length. This is called "biasing" the muscle spindle so it is more sensitive to stretch. Intermittent resistance graded to the desired motion is better than manual stretching for alleviating tight muscles.[51]

TAPPING. The tapping technique is done by tapping over the belly of a muscle with the fingertips. The therapist percusses 3 to 5 times over the muscle to be facilitated. This may be done before or during the time a patient is voluntarily contracting the muscle. This stimulus acts on the afferents of the muscle spindle and increases the tone of the underlying skeletal muscle.

VESTIBULAR STIMULATION. Vestibular stimulation is a powerful type of proprioceptive input.[18] The static labyrinthine system can be used to promote extensor patterns of the neck, trunk, and extremities.[62] The kinetic labyrinth can be used to elicit phasic subcortical responses, such as protective extension.[24] Jones and Watt[37] studied muscular responses to unexpected falls in human subjects. Their findings demonstrated that the vestibular system activates the antigravity muscles and their antagonist muscle before the stretch reflex of the muscle spindles.

The vestibular system is a divergent system that affects tone, balance, directionality, protective responses, cranial nerve function, bilateral integration, auditory-language development, and eye pursuits.[14,31,62] The vestibular system is stimulated during linear acceleration and deceleration in horizontal and vertical planes and angular acceleration and deceleration, such as spinning, rolling, or swinging. Vestibular stimulation can be either facilitory or inhibitory, depending on the rate of stimulation. Fast rocking tends to stimulate, whereas a slow rhythmical rocking tends to relax.[5]

INVERSION. Rood encouraged the use of the inverted position to alter muscle tone in selected muscles. In the inverted position the static vestibular system produces increased tonicity of the muscles of the neck, midline trunk extensors, and selected extensors in the limbs.[31] Tokizane[58] used human subjects to study the effects of head position on selected skeletal muscles. His findings indicated that extensor tone is maximized in certain muscles in the head-down position, whereas extensor tone is minimized in those muscles in the upright position. For best results, the head must be in normal alignment with the neck. If the neck is flexed or extended, the TNR will interfere with the response.[48]

Inversion should be used with extreme care for patients with cardiovascular diseases. As the head approaches a point below the level of the shoulders, baroreceptors in the carotid sinus are stimulated by blood pressure changes.[29] This produces a physiological response through the parasympathic nervous system and reduces blood pressure, decreases muscle tone, and promotes generalized relaxation. Inversion techniques can be combined with vibration or neck compression to change tone in selected muscles.[22]

THERAPEUTIC VIBRATION. Vibration may be defined as a series of rapid touch stimuli. Therapeutic vibration has been used for tactile stimulation, to desensitize hypersensitive skin, and to produce tonal changes in muscles.[22,31] Vibratory stimuli applied over a muscle belly activate the Ia afferent of muscle spindle, thereby causing contraction of that muscle, inhibition of its antagonist muscle, and supression of the stretch reflex (Fig. 14-11). This response is called the tonic vibration reflex and is best elicited with a high-frequency vibrator that delivers 100 to 300 cycles per second. A low-frequency vibrator that delivers 50 to 60 cycles per second can be used to fire subcutaneous encapsulated receptors called pacinian corpuscles.[61] These receptors send impulses along the dorsal columns to higher centers of the nervous system in which the vibratory sense is consciously perceived.[1] Pacinian corpuscles do not elicit the tonic vibration reflex but may play a role in the suppression of pain perception at the cutaneous level.[30,47]

Since vibration is a proprioceptive therapeutic modality, it has a short latency period and lasts as long as the stimulus is applied.[8-10] To elicit the tonic vibration reflex, the vibrator should be applied over the muscle belly, parallel to the muscle fibers. If the vibrator is placed over the tendon, it may conduct along the bone and stimulate adjoining muscles. The muscle should be on stretch or contracting[30] (Fig. 14-12). The vibrator should be applied with light pressure because

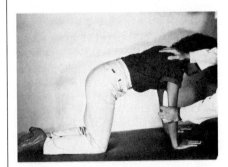

Fig. 14-11. Vibration combines with joint compression.

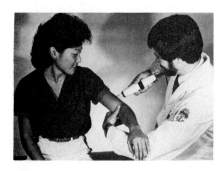

Fig. 14-12. Vibration with pressure to muscle insertion.

deep pressure is inhibitory and may interfere with the results. The duration of vibration should not exceed 1 to 2 minutes per application because heat and friction will result.[10] The position of the patient may also be a factor. The prone position may be best while vibrating flexor muscle groups, and the supine position may enhance extensor muscle groups.[8-10] Temperature may also be a factor when using vibration. For example, ice compresses applied to painful joints may slow nerve conduction and have a dampening effect on the tonic vibration reflex. However, if the patient is in a cool environment, it may increase the activity of the sympathetic nervous system, increase muscle tone, and maximize the tonic vibration reflex. When using vibration for cutaneous stimulation, it is best to have the patient in a warm environment because the skin receptors are at a lower threshold for firing.[22]

The results of vibration will also be influenced by the patient's response to the stimulus or his or her emotional state.[10] If the patient is depressed or angry, the tonic vibration reflex may be less effective than when the patient is calm. Certain medications such as muscle relaxants and barbiturates can block synaptic transmission at the myoneural junction or in the fusimotor system. These medications will also decrease the tonic vibration reflex.[8-10] Vibration should not be used with children less than 3 years of age. Vibration is a powerful stimulus and the CNS is not well myelinated in children.[63] In addition, vibration should not be applied near

joints in children, since it may interfere with bone cells in the growth (epiphyseal) plate.[30] In elderly individuals over 65 years of age, the skin is thinner and the blood vessels, bones, and organs are more susceptible to vibratory stimuli. With extrapyramidal or cerebellar lesions, vibration may increase tremors, promote irregular muscle tone, or impair the action of synergies.[8-10]

The electrical vibrator can be a useful tool when properly applied. More research needs to be done on vibration, and therapists should be properly trained before using vibration on patients with neurological dysfunction.

OSTEOPRESSURE. Pressure on bony prominences has been used with some success to facilitate or inhibit voluntary muscles.[51] It is not clear if the stimulus is affecting the nerve network in the periosteum of the bone or the subcutaneous pressure receptors (pacinian corpuscle) of the skin. According to Rood, osteopressure produces a slower reaction and needs to be preceded with a light moving touch stimulus. For example, if light moving touch is applied to dermatome C7 of the arm and pressure applied over the lateral epicondyle of the elbow, the arm will extend.[51] Pressure on the medial aspect of the calcaneous facilitates the lateral dorsiflexors, whereas pressure on the lateral calcaneous facilitates the medial dorsiflexors and inhibits the calf muscles.[52] The light moving touch is probably applied to dermatomes L3 and L4. This technique needs further research verification before it can be used as an effective treatment modality.

SPECIFIC INHIBITION TECHNIQUES USED IN TREATMENT
Neutral warmth

The neutral warmth technique most likely affects the temperature receptors of the hypothalamus and stimulates the parasympathetic nervous system.[53] Neutral warmth can be used for patients with hypertonia, particularly spasticity and rigidity. It may also be helpful for children who are hyperkinetic. The procedure has the patient assume a recumbent position while the entire body is wrapped in a cotton blanket or comforter for approximately 5 to 10 minutes. Neutral warmth pro-

vides a moderate amount of heat that is homeostatically compatible to the CNS. The patient usually feels relaxed and muscle tone is decreased.[21]

Gentle shaking or rocking

Gentle shaking or rocking is a generalized inhibitory technique that uses light compression of the cervical vertebrae and slow rhythmical circumduction of the head. The patient lies in the supine position and the therapist places the palm of the right hand under the occiput of the head. The left hand is positioned on top of the patient's head. The neck is held in slight flexion and head is slowly moved in a circumferential pattern (Fig. 14-13). As the head is moved slowly and rhythmically, light joint compression is applied down through the cervical vertebrae.[22] This motion may affect the proprioceptors of the neck and the vestibular apparatus. A similar technique can be applied to the shoulder and pelvic girdles to promote segmental relaxation of the upper and lower extremities. For the upper extremity the patient lies in a supine position, and the therapist places one hand under the scapula and the other hand on the anterior aspect of the shoulder. The scapula is slowly and rhythmically rotated. This works well for patients with a spastic scapula. It slowly relaxes and mobilizes the scapula so it can move along with the upper extremity.[22] To gently shake or rock the lower extremities, the patient assumes a prone position. The therapist places his or her hands on the pelvic crests and slowly rotates the pelvis from side to side. These procedures are continued until relaxation can be palpated in the upper or lower extremities.

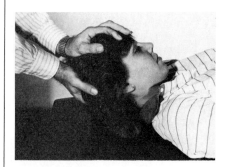

Fig. 14-13. Gentle shaking and rocking.

Slow stroking

Slow stroking has been described as an inhibitory technique. The client lies in the prone position while the therapist provides rhythmical, moving deep pressure over the dorsal distribution of the primary posterior rami of the spine. The therapist applies finger pressure on both sides of the spinous process to affect the nerve endings and sympathetic outflow of the autonomic nervous system. The stroking action is done slowly and continuously from the occiput to the coccyx. The hands are alternated so that as one hand reaches the bottom of the spine, the other is starting downward from the top. This procedure should not exceed 3 minutes, since it may cause a rebound phenomenon resulting in excitation of the sympathetic branch of the autonomic nervous system.

Slow rolling

The patient is placed in a sidelying position, however, the hemiplegic patient should first lie with the uninvolved side down. The therapist kneels behind the patient and places one hand on the rib cage and the other hand on the lateral aspect of the patient's pelvis (Fig. 14-14, *A*). The patient is rolled slowly from a sidelying position to a prone position and back again in a rhythmical fashion[21,22] (Fig. 14-14, *B*). In addition to rolling the entire body from lying on the side toward a prone position, the therapist can incorporate some slow rotational movements between the hip and the trunk. This technique should be done to both sides of the body. With some patients it is necessary to place a pillow between the knees or under the head to prevent friction and malalignment of the body.

Tendinous pressure

Manual pressure applied to the tendinous insertion of a muscle or across long tendons produces an inhibitory effect.[4,31] This technique has a dramatic effect on spastic or tight muscle groups in which the tendons are accessible to the forces of pressure. Pressure provided by hard surfaces are preferable to soft surfaces.[17] Therefore many therapists use a hard cone in the hand with the tapered end toward the thumb side to inhibit the flexors.[21] A hard surface over the anterior aspect of the forearm is inhibitory to the extrinsic flexors of the hand.[52] This principle has been used in a number of orthotic devices to manage muscle imbalance and contractures produced by spasticity. It is postulated that the pacinian corpuscle is responsible for the inhibition of the muscle.[59] The Golgi tendon organ, however, may also play a role in this response, because it is located in the musculotendinous insertions and monitors tendon tension.[43]

Light joint compression (approximation)

Joint compression of body weight or less can be used to inhibit spastic muscles around a joint.[52] This technique may be used with hemiplegic patients to alleviate pain and to temporarily offset the muscle imbalance around the shoulder joint.[22] The patient can be sitting or lying in the supine position. The therapist places one hand over the shoulder and the other hand under the patient's flexed elbow joint. The arm is abducted 35° to 45° and a compression force is applied through the longitudinal axis of the humerus.[4] This force should be the approximate body weight

or less. This procedure compresses both the glenohumeral joint and the articulation between the humerus and ulna. Moreover, if applied properly, this technique compresses two joints but has the most dramatic effect on the shoulder. Once the muscles begin to relax, the therapist can slowly and gently circumduct the humerus in small circles to reduce pain and stiffness in the shoulder joint.[22] Joint compression of the shoulder and elbow joints can also be achieved when the patient is in the on-elbows position.[57] Light joint compression is also beneficial when applied through the longitudinal axis of wrist and elbow joints.[22] The therapist places one hand behind the elbow and places the patient's forearm in midposition, the wrist joint is extended, and compression is applied through the heel of the patient's hand. Joint compression has its greatest effect during the time the stimulus is applied.[60]

Maintained stretch

Rood has recommended positioning hypertonic extremities in the elongated position for various periods to cause lengthening of the muscle spindles.[52] The rationale for this is to reset or "bias" the afferents of the muscle spindle to a longer position so they are less sensitive to stretching. Rood does not advocate the use of passive stretch for tight muscles. Instead, she recommends maintained stretch in the lengthened position for the stronger agonist muscle to increase the threshold of the muscle spindles. The antagonist muscle is then facilitated by cutaneous stimulation to offset the muscle imbalance.[51] Rood also used autogenic inhibition through the Golgi tendon organ to reciprocally facilitate the antagonist muscle.[49,52] However, new information indicates the secondary ending may also be causing this response. This is done by asking the patient to briefly contract a muscle before it is voluntarily moved to a lengthened position.

Rocking in developmental patterns

In keeping with the developmental sequence and the concept of mobility superimposed on stability, Rood encouraged movement as the patient gains

A   B

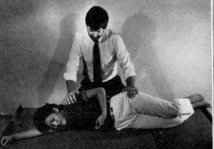 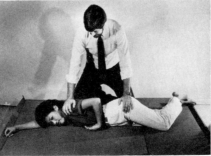

Fig. 14-14. A and B, Slow rolling.

mastery of the static position.[57] Developmentally, the patient must first assume and be able to achieve a static position and then integrate coordinated movements while holding that pattern. Rood refered to this as the development of "skill." For example, in the quadruped position, the patient shifts weight to a three-point stance so one hand is free to reach forward to grasp and explore. Movement may begin by shifting the weight forward and backward. The shifting may progress to side to side and diagonal patterns as the patient becomes comfortable with the rhythmical movements.[22] Hemiplegic patients are assisted in the quadruped position by achieving stability of the involved elbow (see Fig. 14-10) when the therapist applies pressure and stretch to the triceps brachii and anconeus. As the therapist applies compression that is greater than body weight to facilitate cocontraction, the pressure exerted on the extended wrist and heel of the hand inhibits the wrist flexors. Light moving touch over the dorsum of the hand is done to promote finger extension.[57] Rocking in the quadruped position should first be done with the neck in a straight normal relationship to the body so the proprioceptors of the neck do not influence the tonicity of the limbs.[32] As the patient moves in an anteroposterior plane, the shoulder and pelvic girdles are being mobilized. Later on in treatment the therapist may want to incorporate flexion, extension, and rotation of the neck as a reflex inhibiting measure.[45]

SPECIAL SENSES FOR FACILITATION OR INHIBITION

Rood has suggested the use of olfactory and gustatory stimuli to facilitate cranial nerves and to influence the autonomic nervous system.[52,57] In principle pleasant odors, such as vanilla and banana oil, may have a calming effect or evoke strong moods. Unpleasant odors, such as sulfur and fresh horseradish, can produce primitive protective responses, such as sneezing or choking.[22] Rood has used noxious substances, such as ammonia or vinegar, to affect the trigeminal nerve, which activates the muscles of mastication.[57]

Warm liquids may be calming to the oral musculature, whereas sweet foods or sour tastes can stimulate the salivary glands.[29] As with other stimuli the intensity of warm liquids and sweet and sour tastes can be gauged to facilitate or inhibit the CNS. Rood did not provide specific guidelines for the stimulation of special senses.[57]

The importance of using many sensory modalities in the rehabilitation of neurological dysfunction is emphasized by several therapists.[5,22,31] In theory, the CNS retains its capacity to produce adaptive changes to stimuli throughout life.[16,63] Bach-y-Rita[6] has suggested that a process called "sensory substitution" can compensate for the loss of a particular sensory modality. Sensory substitution is the process in which a blind individual uses the tactile sense instead of vision in reading braille. Another example is the stroke patient who sees four objects on a table and with the eyes closed can identify the objects correctly by using the sense of touch alone. Farber[22] refers to this phenomenon as "cross-modal" stimulation. Regardless of what it is called, the ability to learn and relearn depends on the integration of sensory input. Rood's basic hypothesis, that sensory stimulation can elicit specific motor responses, continues to gain credence in the realm of physical medicine and rehabilitation.

APPLICATION OF THE ROOD APPROACH IN OCCUPATIONAL THERAPY

The occupational therapist uses the techniques previously described primarily to prepare the patient for purposeful activities. Patients who have undergone severe neurological damage usually do not have voluntary control over their muscles. The motor responses exhibited by the patient may begin with primitive reflexive motions. Therefore the therapist may need to begin with the ontogenetic developmental patterns. During this phase of rehabilitation, the therapist must carefully select the pattern to be trained and control extraneous conditions. Next, the desired motor patterns should be done passively by the therapist and reinforced by sensory stimulation. The motor patterns should be repeated until the patient can actively perform the pattern in a slow, accurate manner. The speed of the movement should not be increased until

precision is accomplished. The therapist should avoid fatiguing the patient and should not allow incorrect patterns to develop. Thousands of correct repetitions may be necessary before the speed and force of contraction are increased.[38,39] As the patient gains mastery of a motor pattern, the therapist should introduce purposeful activities into the repertoire. Hence, as mentioned earlier, a basic tenet of the Rood approach is that activity should be purposeful. The introduction of purposeful activities adds meaning and relevance to the endeavor. Routine exercises and neurophysiological technique alone can become redundant and the patient may reach a plateau too early in the therapeutic progression.

Ontogenetic motor patterns with activities

SUPINE WITHDRAWAL. The therapist may use an activity that promotes elbow flexion or shoulder adduction. The patient may squeeze an accordion or a large balloon to add resistance and reinforce the pattern. An easel or macrame frame may be set up in such a way that the patient can lie supine, reach forward toward the midline, and paint an oil painting or tie cords for plant hangers. Certain leather-work projects or numerous minor crafts could be manipulated in this pattern. The incentive for the patient is an end product that can adorn his or her room or be given to a "significant other."

ROLL OVER. The roll-over pattern can be promoted by placing an object on either side of the patient so he or she has to visually fixate on the object and roll to reach for it. It is best to minimize extraneous demands and external stimuli in the room so the patient can concentrate on the task at hand. The therapist may begin the roll-over pattern by having the patient lie on an equilibrium board that can be slightly tilted to one side to remove some of the gravitational demands. Objects, such as cassette tape recorders or a remote control for a television or video game, can provide an incentive to roll, reach, and manipulate an object.

PIVOT PRONE. The pivot-prone position is a stability pattern that places demands on the proximal extensor muscles. Scooter board activities are ideal for this pattern because the patient must lift the extremities against gravity. The scooter board may be equipped with a rope and pulley system so the board can accelerate and decelerate forward and backward. This linear movement (forward and backward) stimulates the vestibular apparatus and enhances the tonicity of the extensor muscles. The prone-extension pattern (pivot prone) can also be reinforced with activities that provide light resistance. The patient can lie prone on a soft bolster (suspended or on a mat) and manipulate strings attached to bells or talking toys. The object of this activity is to entice the patient into looking up so his or her neck extends and the arms pull backward away from the midline axis.

NECK COCONTRACTION. Neck cocontraction can be reinforced by positioning the patient in the prone position on a firm surface, such as a table. The head and neck should extend off the end of the table so the weight is distributed on the patient's chest region. In this position the patient can suck through a straw to pick up objects and transfer them from one container to another. The object of the sucking action is to reinforce neck cocontraction. For an advanced activity, table tennis balls marked with numbers could be place in a pan of water. The object would be to pick up these balls by sucking through the straw. The score board can be positioned on the wall in front of the patient so he or she has to extend the neck and look up to see the score.

ON ELBOWS. A patient on his or her elbows is in a position that is conducive to many activities. The patient may be positioned on a mat in front of a video game monitor. The control handle is placed near the midline so the patient can use either hand to manipulate the controls. This activity provides concentration and fine eye-hand manipulation as the patient bears weight on the elbows. A number of minor crafts, games, and puzzles can be integrated into this pattern.

ALL FOURS (QUADRUPED). The quadruped position does not allow freedom of the hands for manipulation unless the patient can shift weight to a three-point stance. Thus if the patient can support his or her body weight on the knees and one hand, the patient can use one hand to draw or manipulate objects. In an effort to produce mobility in the quadruped position, the patient can support half of his or her body weight on a scooter board. For example, the hands and anterior part of the body can rest on the scooter board while the lower extremities provide forward propulsion. This activity does not provide coordination and reciprocal movements between the upper and lower extremities but does afford mobility and exploration of the environment. In addition, when the knees are resting on the scooter board and the upper limbs are used for propulsion, the patient is receiving some of the benefits of inversion.

STATIC STANDING. Standing provides the best position for activities of daily living (ADL) and purposeful activities. In this position, the arms are free to explore and manipulate while the task of weight bearing is placed on the legs. The patient can begin with light resistive activities on a high bench and proceed to resistive crafts, such as woodworking, leather crafts, or ceramics. As the patient develops stability in standing and in activities that require weight shift and equilibrium, the responses can be integrated into the repertory of motor skills.

WALKING. Walking is the skilled level of mobility. The upright bipedal position requires an integration of many components of the CNS. The physical therapist will usually undertake the responsibility of gait training, whereas the occupational therapist provides purposeful activities to encourage walking for ADL, such as grocery shopping, visiting neighbors, or facilitating the cardiovascular system. The occupational and physical therapists should work closely together on walking skills so the patient can receive a well-coordinated treatment plan.

REVIEW QUESTIONS

1. List the four goals of the Rood approach.
2. Differentiate between the motor responses elicited by the TNR and TLR.
3. What are the three major reactions produced by sensory stimulation?
4. Describe the four rules for sensory stimulation.
5. List the four sequences of motor development.
6. Describe the eight ontogenetic motor patterns.
7. Differentiate between exteroceptive and proprioceptive stimulation.
8. Which size nerve fibers carry pain, temperature, and light touch?
9. Which nerve fibers carry conscious and subconscious proprioceptive messages?
10. Contrast the functions of the stabilizer and mobilizer muscles.
11. How often is the light touch stimulus applied and what happens if it is applied too often?
12. How long should fast brushing be applied to the skin?
13. Why should fast brushing be applied according to dermatomal segments?
14. List the skin areas where fast brushing is contraindicated.
15. Describe the uses of C icing, A icing, and autonomic icing and the principle motor responses elicited by each.
16. Discuss the advantages of proprioceptive stimulation over cutaneous stimulation.
17. How is heavy joint compression differentiated from light joint compression?
18. Describe how inversion is used as a therapeutic modality.
19. Explain how therapeutic vibration can be used to activate muscles and cutaneous receptors.
20. Discuss three methods of reducing muscle tone.

REFERENCES

1. Abbruzzese, G., et al: Excitation from skin receptors contributing to the tonic vibration reflex in man, Brain Res. **150**:194, 1978.
2. Afifi, A., and Bergman, R.: Basic neuroscience, Munich, 1980, Verlag Urban und Schwarzenberg.
3. Alpern, M., Lawrence, N., and Wolsk, D.: Sensory processes, Belmont, Calif., 1976, Brooks/Cole Publishing Co.

4. Ayres, J.: The development of sensory integrative theory and practice, Dubuque, Iowa, 1974, Kendall/Hunt Publishing Co.

5. Ayres, J.: Sensory integration and learning disorders, Los Angeles, 1972, Western Psychological Services.

6. Bach-y-Rita, P.: Sensory substitution in rehabilitation of the neurological patient, Oxford, England, 1983, Basil Blackwell Publisher, Ltd.

7. Barr, M.L.: The human nervous system, ed. 2, New York, 1974, Harper & Row, Publishers, Inc.

8. Bishop, B.: Vibratory stimulation. I. Phys. Ther. 54:1273, 1974.

9. Bishop, B.: Vibratory stimulation. II. Phys. Ther. 55:29, 1975.

10. Bishop, B.: Vibratory stimulation. III. Phys. Ther. 55:139, 1975.

11. Bishop, B.: Spasticity: it's physiology and management, Parts I, II, and III, Phys. Ther. 57:4, 1977.

12. Buchwald, J.: Exteroceptive reflexes and movement, Am. J. Phys. Med. 46:121, 1967.

13. Clark, B.: The vestibular system. In Mussen, P.H., and Rosenzweig, M.R., editors: Annual review of psychology, New York, 1970, Harper & Row, Publishers, Inc.

14. Clark, R.: Clinical neuroanatomy and neurophysiology, ed. 5, Philadelphia, 1975, F.A. Davis Co.

15. Chusid, J.G.: Correlative neuroanatomy and functional neurology, ed. 18, Los Altos, Calif., 1982, Lange Medical Publications.

16. Colavila, F.: Sensory changes in the elderly, Springfield, Ill., 1978, Charles C Thomas, Publisher.

17. Dayhoff, N.: Re-thinking stroke: soft or hard devices to position hands? Am. J. Nurs. 7:1142, 1975.

18. DeQuiros, J.B.: Diagnosis of vestibular disorders in the learning disabled, J. Learning Disabilities 9:50, 1974.

19. Eldred, E.: The dual sensory role of muscle spindles, Phys. Ther. 45:290, 1965.

20. Eldred, E.: Peripheral receptors: their excitation and relation to reflex patterns, Am. J. Phys. Med. 46:69, 1967.

21. Farber, S.: Sensorimotor evaluation and treatment procedures for allied health personnel, Indianapolis, 1974, Indiana University and Purdue University Medical Center.

22. Farber, S.: Neurorehabilitation: a multisensory approach, Philadelphia, 1982, W.B. Saunders Co.

23. Fox, J.U.D.: Cutaneous stimulation effects on selected tests of perception, Am. J. Occup. Ther. 18:53, 1964.

24. Fukuda, T.: Studies on human dynamic postures from the viewpoint of postural reflexes, Acta Otolaryngol. 161(suppl.):8, 1961.

25. Fulton, J.F.: Physiology of the nervous system, vol. 179, ed. 3, New York, 1949, Oxford University Press, Inc.

26. Gardner, E.: Fundamentals of neurology, ed. 6, Philadelphia, 1975, W.B. Saunders Co.

27. Gilman, S., and Winans, S.: Essentials of clinical neuroanatomy and neurophysiology, ed. 6, Philadelphia, 1982, F.A. Davis Co.

28. Goldberg, S.: Clinical neuroanatomy made ridiculously simple, Miami, 1979, Medical Master, Inc.

29. Guyton, A.: Structure and function of the nervous system, Philadelphia, 1972, W.B. Saunders Co.

30. Hagbarth, K.E., and Edlund, G.: The muscle vibrator: a useful tool in neurological therapeutic work, Scand. J. Rehabil. Med. 1:26, 1969.

31. Heininger, M., and Randolph, S.: Neurophysiological concepts in human behavior, St. Louis, 1981, The C.V. Mosby Co.

32. Hellebrandt, F., Schade, M., and Carns, M.: Methods of evoking the tonic neck reflexes in normal human subjects, Am. J. Phys. Med. 41:89, 1962.

33. Hellebrandt, F., et al.: Tonic neck reflexes in exercises of stress in man, Am. J. Phys. Med. 35:144, 1956.

34. Henderson, A., and Coryell, J.: The body senses and perceptual deficit. Proceedings of the occupational therapy symposium, Boston, 1973.

35. Hirt, S.: The tonic neck reflex mechanism in the normal human adult, Am. J. Phys. Med. 46:362, 1967.

36. Huss, A.J.: Sensorimotor approaches. In Hopkins, H., and Smith, H., editors: Willard and Spackman's occupational therapy, Philadelphia, 1978, J.B. Lippincott Co.

37. Jones, G.M., and Watt, D.: Muscular control of landing from unexpected falls in man, J. Physiol. (Lond.) 219:729, 1971.

38. Kottke, F.: From reflex to skill: the training of coordination, Arch. Phys. Med. Rehabil. 61:551, 1980.

39. Kottke, F., Stillwell, K., and Lehmann, J.: Krusen's handbook of physical medicine and rehabilitation, ed. 3, Philadelphia, 1982, W.B. Saunders Co.

40. Matthews, P.B.C.: Muscle spindles and their motor control, Physiol. Rev. 44:219, 1964.

41. McCloskey, D.I.: Kinesthetic sensibility, Physiol. Rev. 58:763, 1978.

42. Montague, A.: Touching: the significance of the skin, ed. 2, San Francisco, 1978, Harper and Row, Publishers, Inc.

43. Moore, J.: The Golgi tendon organ and the muscle spindle, Am. J. Occup. Ther. 28:415, 1974.

44. Murray, M.P.: Gait as a total pattern of movement, Am. J. Phys. Med. 46:290, 1967.

45. Payton, R., Hirt, E., and Newtown, G., editors: Scientific basis for neurophysiologic approaches to therapeutic exercise: an anthology, ed. 2, Philadelphia, 1978, F.A. Davis Co.

46. Pedretti, L.W.: Occupational therapy: practice skills for dysfunction, St. Louis, 1981, The C.V. Mosby Co.

47. Pertovaara, A.: Modification of human pain threshold by specific tactile receptors, Acta Physiol. Scand. 107:339, 1979.

48. Roberts, T.: Neurophysiology of postural mechanisms, New York, 1967, Plenum Publishing Co.

49. Rood, M.: Occupational therapy in the treatment of the cerebral palsied, Phys. Ther. Rev. 32:220, 1952.

50. Rood, M.: Neurophysiological reactions as a basis for physical therapy, Phys. Ther. Rev. 34:444, 1954.

51. Rood, M.: Neurophysiological mechanisms utilized in the treatment of neuromuscular dysfunction, Am. J. Occup. Ther. 10:4, 1956.

52. Rood, M.: The use of sensory receptors to activate, facilitate and inhibit motor response, automatic and somatic, in developmental sequence. In Sattely, C., editor: Approaches to the treatment of patients with neuromuscular dysfunction, Dubuque, Iowa, 1962, Wm. C. Brown Book Co., Publishers.

53. Schmidt, R.: Fundamentals of sensory physiology, New York, 1978, Springer-Verlag, Inc.
54. Smythies, J.R.: Brain mechanisms and behavior, ed. 2, New York, 1970, Academic Press, Inc.
55. Spicer, S.D., and Matyas, T.A.: Facilitation of the tonic vibration reflex (TVR) by cutaneous stimulation, Am. J. Phys. Med. **59:**223, 1980.
56. Stejskal, L.: Postural reflexes in man, Am. J. Phys. Med. **58:**1, 1979.
57. Stockmeyer, S.: An interpretation of the approach of Rood to the treatment of neuromuscular dysfunction, NUSTEP proceedings, Am. J. Phys. Med. **46:**900, 1967.
58. Tokizane, T., et al.: Electromyographic studies on tonic neck, lumbar and labyrinthine reflexes in normal persons, Jpn. J. Physiol. **2:**30, 1951.
59. Trombly, C.A., and Scott, A.D.: Occupational therapy for physical dysfunction, Baltimore, 1977, Williams & Wilkins.
60. Vallbo, A., et al.; Somatosensory proprioceptive and sympathetic activity in human peripheral nerves, Physiol. Rev. **4:**59, 1979.
61. Werner, J.: Neuroscience: a clinical perspective, Philadelphia, 1980, W.B. Saunders Co.
62. Wilson, V.J., and Paterson, B.W.: The role of the vestibular system in posture and movement, In Mountcastle, V. editor: Medical physiology, ed. 14, St. Louis, 1979, The C.V. Mosby Co.
63. Yakovlev, P., and Lecours, A.: Regional development of the brain in early life, vol. 3, Oxford, 1967, Minkowski Blackwell Scientific Publication.

CHAPTER 15

Movement therapy

THE BRUNNSTROM APPROACH TO THE TREATMENT OF HEMIPLEGIA

LORRAINE WILLIAMS PEDRETTI

The material presented in this chapter is summarized primarily from *Movement Therapy in Hemiplegia*[3] by Signe Brunnstrom, a physical therapist who developed this treatment approach from her research and extensive work with hemiplegic patients.

The theoretical foundations, treatment goals, and methods are intended as an overview and introduction to some of the procedures that the new practitioner may find helpful. To learn the details of the treatment approach and additional procedures the reader is referred to the original source for further study.

THEORETICAL FOUNDATIONS

Following cerebrovascular accident (CVA) resulting in hemiplegia, the patient progresses through a series of recovery steps or stages in fairly stereotyped fashion (Table 15-1). The progress through these stages may be rapid or slow, and recovery may be arrested at any stage.

In effect, an "evolution in reverse"[3,5] occurs after neurological disease. Afferent-efferent mechanisms developed in early phylogenesis are retained in man but are inhibited in the developmental process. The basic limb synergies seen in hemiplegic patients are primitive spinal cord patterns[2] of flexion and extension, reminiscent of amphibian patterns of movement, which have been retained through the evolutionary process.[3]

The flexor synergy of the upper limb consists of scapular adduction and elevation, shoulder abduction and external rotation, elbow flexion, forearm supination, wrist flexion, and finger flexion. Elbow flexion is the strongest component, and shoulder abduction and external rotation are the weakest (Fig. 15-1). The extensor synergy consists of scapula abduction and depression, shoulder adduction and internal rotation, elbow extension, forearm pronation, and wrist and finger flexion or extension. Shoulder adduction and internal rotation are the strongest components of the extensor synergy, and elbow extension is the weakest component (Fig. 15-2).

In the lower limb the flexor synergy consists of hip flexion and abduction and external rotation, knee flexion, ankle dorsiflexion and inversion, and toe extension. Hip flexion is the strongest component, and hip abduction and external rotation are the weakest components. The extensor synergy is composed of hip adduction, extension, and internal rotation; knee extension; ankle plantar flexion and inversion; and toe flexion. Hip adduction, knee extension, and ankle plantar flexion are the strong components, whereas hip extension and internal rotation are weaker. These patterns are modified in man through the

Table 15-1
Motor recovery following cerebrovascular accident[3]

Stage	Characteristics		
	Leg	Arm	Hand*
1	Flaccidity	Flaccidity; inability to perform any movements	No hand function
2	Spasticity develops; minimal voluntary movements	Beginning development of spasticity; limb synergies or some of their components begin to appear as associated reactions	Gross grasp beginning; minimal finger flexion possible
3	Spasticity peaks; flexion and extension synergy present; hip knee-ankle flexion in sitting and standing	Spasticity increasing; synergy patterns or some of their components can be performed voluntarily	Gross grasp, hook grasp possible; no release
4	Knee flexion past 90° in sitting, with foot sliding backward on floor; dorsiflexion with heel on floor and knee flexed to 90°	Spasticity declining; movement combinations deviating from synergies are now possible	Gross gasp present; lateral prehension developing; small amount of finger extension and some thumb movement possible
5	Knee flexion with hip extended in standing; ankle dorsiflexion with hip and knee extended	Synergies no longer dominant; more movement combinations deviating from synergies performed with greater ease	Palmar prehension, spherical and cylindrical grasp, and release possible
6	Hip abduction in sitting or standing; reciprocal internal and external rotation of hip combined with inversion and eversion of ankle in sitting	Spasticity absent except when performing rapid movements; isolated joint movements performed with ease	All types of prehension, individual finger motion, and full range of voluntary extension possible

*NOTE: Recovery of hand function is variable and may not parallel the six recovery stages of the arm.

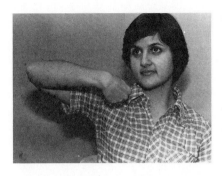

Fig. 15-1. Flexor synergy of upper limb in hemiplegia.

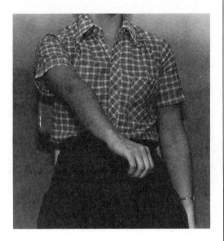

Fig. 15-2. Extensor synergy of upper limb in hemiplegia.

influence of higher centers of nervous system control during development. After CVA, they return to their primitive, stereotyped character. When the influence of higher centers is disturbed or destroyed, primitive and pathological reflexes, such as the tonic neck reflex (TNR), tonic lumbar reflex, and tonic labyrinthine reflex (TLR), reappear, and normal reflexes, such as the deep tendon reflexes (DTR), become exaggerated. These reflexes were present at an earlier phylogenetic period and therefore may be considered "normal" when, as in hemiplegia, the central nervous system (CNS) has regressed to an earlier developmental stage.[3]

The Brunnstrom approach to the treatment of hemiplegia is based on the use of motor patterns available to the patient at any point in the recovery process. It enhances progress through the stages of recovery toward more normal and complex movement patterns.

Brunnstrom sees synergies, reflexes, and other "abnormal" movement patterns as a "normal" part of the process the patient must go through before normal voluntary movement can occur. Synergistic movements are used by normal persons all of the time, but they are controlled, occur in a wide variety of patterns, and can be modified or stopped at will. Brunnstrom maintains that the synergies appear to constitute a necessary intermediate stage for further recovery. Gross movement synergies of flexion and extension always precede the restoration of advanced motor functioning following hemiplegia.[3] Therefore during the early stages of recovery (stages 1 to 3) Brunnstrom maintains that the patient should be aided to gain control of the limb synergies and that selected afferent stimuli (TNR, TLR, cutaneous and stretch stimuli, and positioning and associated reactions) can be advantageous in helping the patient to initiate and gain control of movement. Once the synergies can be performed voluntarily with some ease, they are modified, and simple to complex movement combinations can be performed (stages 4 and 5) that deviate from the stereotyped synergy patterns of flexion and extension.[3]

The advisability of using pathological and primitive reflexes and movement patterns to effect motion is challenged by some experts.[1] It is argued that no pathological responses should be used in training for fear that by repeated use the efferent pathways will become too readily available for use at the expense of normal pathways.[2,3]

DEFINITIONS OF TERMS

Some definitions of terms are necessary to comprehend the discussion of treatment principles that follows.

A *limb synergy* of flexion or extension, seen in hemiplegia, is a group of muscles acting as a bound unit in a primitive and stereotyped manner.[3,6] The muscles are neurophysiologically linked and cannot act alone or perform all of their functions. If one muscle in the synergy is activated, each muscle in the synergy responds partially or completely. The patient then cannot perform isolated movements when bound by these synergies.

Associated reactions are movements seen on the affected side in response to voluntary forceful movements in other parts of the body.[3] Resistance to flexion movements of the normal upper extremity usually evokes a flexion synergy or some of its components in the affected upper extremity. By the same token resistance to extension on the sound side evokes extension on the affected side. In the lower extremities the responses are reversed. Resisted flexion of the normal limb evokes extension of the affected limb and vice versa.[6]

Homolateral limb synkinesis appears to be a mutual dependency between the synergies of the affected upper and lower limbs. The same or similar motion occurs in the limb on the same side of the body. For example, efforts at flexion of the affected upper extremity evoke flexion of the lower extremity.[3,6]

The mirroring of movements attempted or performed on the affected side by the unaffected side, perhaps in an effort to facilitate the movement, is called *imitation synkinesis.*[3]

Several specialized reactions can be noted in the hemiplegic hand. These are the proximal traction response, grasp reflex, instinctive grasp reaction, instinctive avoiding reaction, and Souques' finger phenomenon. The *proximal traction response* is elicited by a stretch to the flexor muscles of one joint of the upper limb, which evokes contraction of all flexors of that limb, including the fingers. It may therefore be used to elicit the flexion synergy. To elicit the *grasp reflex* deep pressure is applied to the palm and moved distally over the hand and fingers, mostly on the radial side. The responses are complex but in general there is adduction and flexion of the digits. The *instinctive grasp reaction* is differentiated by Brunnstrom from the grasp reflex. It is a closure of the hand in response to contact of a stationary object with the palm of the hand. The person is unable to release the object-stimulus once the fist has been closed.

A hyperextension reaction of the fingers and thumb in response to forward-upward elevation of the arm is the *instictive avoiding reaction.* Brunnstrom reported that, with the arm in this position, stroking distally over the palm and attempting to reach out and grasp an object resulted in an exaggeration of the reaction. The automatic extension of the fingers when the shoulder is flexed is known as *Souques' finger phenomenon* and can be observed in some but not all hemiplegic patients. Brunnstrom found that although this phenomenon may not be exhibited, the elevated position of the affected arm is a favorable one for the facilitation of finger extension.[3]

MOTOR EVALUATION OF HEMIPLEGIC PATIENT

Brunnstrom[3] in *Movement Therapy in Hemiplegia* described an evaluation procedure that assesses muscle tone, stage of recovery, movement patterns, motor speed, and prehension patterns of the upper extremity.

The evaluation is based on the recovery stages after the onset of hemiplegia. The test requires the client to perform motor acts that are graduated in complexity and require increasingly finer neuromuscular control. Thus the degree of recovery of the CNS can be evaluated.

Progress through the recovery stages is gradual, and signs of two stages may be apparent at any given time in the client's recovery. Since it is not possible to establish an absolute demarcation between one recovery stage and the next, the client may be classified as stages 2 and 3 or 3 and 4, for example. This indicates that the client is progressing from one stage to the next. The upper extremity evaluation portion of the Hemiplegia Classification and Progress Record is presented in Fig. 15-3. The reader should refer to this while reading the directions for test administration, which have been summarized from *Movement Therapy in Hemiplegia*.

Gross sensory testing

The sensory evaluation precedes the motor evaluation and includes assessment of passive motion sense and touch localization in the hand. Tests of passive motion sense of the shoulder, elbow, forearm, wrist, and fingers are carried out by procedures similar to those described in Chapter 9. Results are recorded on the first and second pages of the form (shown in Fig. 15-3, *A* and *B*).

Fingertip recognition is evaluated by asking the subject to localize touch stimuli to specific fingers. The subject is seated with forearms pronated and resting on a pillow in the lap. The test is given with the vision occluded after a rehearsal in full view. The palmar surface of the fingertips is lightly touched with a pencil eraser in a random sequence. The subject must indicate which finger is being touched. Results are recorded on the second page of the form (in Fig. 15-3, *B*).

Motor tests, upper extremity[3]

The subject is classified in stage 1 when no voluntary movement of the affected arm can be initiated. The examiner should move the limb passively through the synergy patterns and assess the degree of resistance to passive movement. The subject should be asked to attempt movement during these maneuvers. During recovery stage 1 the limb will be predominantly flaccid and will feel heavy, there will be little or no resistance to passive movement, and the subject will be unable to initiate or effect any movement voluntarily. At this time the subject is likely to be confined to bed and be too weak for extensive evaluation.

During recovery stage 2 spasticity begins to increase, and the limb synergies or some of their components may be evoked on voluntary effort or as associated reactions. The flexor synergy usually appears first.[3] The examiner may again move the limb passively, alternating between flexor and extensor synergy patterns. The examiner should ask the subject to "help" in the movements. Thus it is possible to assess the degree of spasticity and whether the subject's voluntary efforts are evoking any movement responses.

During recovery stage 3 spasticity is increased and may be marked. The limb synergies or some of their components are performed voluntarily. The subject may remain at this stage for a long period of time. Severely involved hemiplegics may never progress beyond it. The pectoralis major, pronators, and wrist and finger flexors may be very spastic, causing limited performance of their antagonists.

The subject is seated, and the complete flexor synergy is demonstrated by

the examiner. The subject is asked to perform the movement pattern with the unaffected side to ascertain that the directions were understood. The subject is then asked to perform the movement pattern with the affected side after a command, such as "Touch your ear" or "Touch your mouth," which gives purpose and direction to the effort.

A similar procedure is used to evaluate performance of the extensor synergy. The subject is asked to reach forward and downward to touch the examiner's hand, which is held between the subject's knees.

The responses may be influenced by the predominant spasticity seen in components of each of the synergies. For instance, the very spastic pectoralis major and elbow flexors may predominate during the subject's efforts and result in the subject reaching across the thorax to touch the opposite shoulder.

The status of the synergies is recorded on the evaluation form in terms of the active joint range achieved for each motion in the pattern. The joint ranges are estimated and recorded as 0, ¼, ½, ¾, or full range.

When the subject has reached recovery stage 4, there is a decrease in spasticity, and the subject is capable of performing gross movement combinations that deviate from the limb synergies. Brunnstrom chose three movements to represent stage 4. These are (1) placing the hand behind the body to touch the sacral region, (2) raising the arm forward to 90° of shoulder flexion with elbow extended, and (3) pronating and supinating the forearm with the elbow flexed to 90° and stabilized close to the side of the body. The subject performs all of the movements while seated, and as in all test items, no facilitation is allowed. During the test for pronation-supination, bilateral performance is allowed so that the examiner can make a comparison of the two sides.

Further decrease of spasticity and ability to perform more complex combinations of movement characterize recovery stage 5. The subject is relatively free of the influence of the limb synergies and performs the stage 4 movements with greater ease. Three movements chosen to represent stage 5 are (1) raising the arm to 90° of shoulder abduction with the elbow extended and

HEMIPLEGIA CLASSIFICATION AND PROGRESS RECORD

Upper limb-test sitting

Name _____ Age _____ Date of onset _____ Side affected _____

Date _____

____ Passive motion sense: Shoulder _____ Elbow _____

____ Pronation-supination _____ Wrist flexion-extension _____

____ 1. NO MOVEMENT INITIATED OR ELICITED _____

____ 2. SYNERGIES OR COMPONENTS FIRST APPEARING. Spasticity developing _____
____   Flexor synergy_____
____   Extensor synergy_____

____ 3. SYNERGIES OR COMPONENTS INITIATED VOLUNTARILY. Spasticity marked _____

A

FLEXOR SYNERGY		ACTIVE JOINT RANGE		REMARKS
Shoulder girdle	Elevation			
	Retraction			
Shoulder joint	Hyperextension			
	Abduction			
	Extension rotation			
Elbow	Flexion			
Forearm	Pronation			
EXTENSOR SYNERGY				
Shoulder	Pectoralis major			
Elbow	Extension			
Forearm	Pronation			
4. MOVEMENTS DEVIATING FROM BASIC SYNERGIES. Spasticity decreasing	Hand to sacral region			
	Raise arm forward-horizontally			
	Pronate-supinate elbow at 90 degrees			
5. RELATIVE IN-DEPENDENCE OF BASIC SYNERGIES. Spasticity waning	Raise arm sideways -horizontally			
	Raise arm over head			
	Pronate-supinate elbow extended			
6. MOVEMENT COORDINATION NEAR NORMAL. Spasticity minimal				

Continued.

Fig. 15-3. Hemiplegia classification and progress record. (From Brunnstrom, S.: Movement therapy in hemiplegia, New York, 1970, Harper & Row, Publishers, Inc.)

B

HEMIPLEGIA CLASSIFICATION AND PROGRESS RECORD

Upper limb-test sitting cont'd

Name _____

Date _____

SPEED TESTS FOR Classes 4, 5, 6   Strokes per 5 second

Hand from	Normal		
lap to chin	Affected		
Hand from lap	Normal		
to opposite knee	Affected		

___ Passive motion sense, digits _____

___ Fingertip recognition _____

___ Wrist stabilization   1. Elbow extended _____
for grasp
                           2. Elbow flexed _____

___ Wrist flexion   1. Elbow extended _____
and extension
___ Fist closed   2. Elbow flexed _____
___ Wrist circumduction _____

DIGITS

___ Mass grasp _____ Dynamometer test Normal _____ lb.
                                                     Affected _____ lb.

___ Mass extension _____

___ Hook grasp (handbag, 2 lb.) _____

___ Lateral prehension (card) _____

___ Palmar prehension (pencil) _____

___ Cylindrical grasp (small jar) _____

___ Spherical grasp (ball) _____ Catch _____ Throw _____

___ Indiv. thumb movements
hands in lap   1. Vertical movements _____
Ulnar side down   2. Horizontal movements _____

___ Individual finger movements _____

___ Button and unbutton shirt   Using both hands _____
___   Using affected hand only _____

___ Other skilled activities _____

Fig. 15-3, cont'd. Hemiplegia classification and progress record.

HEMIPLEGIA CLASSIFICATION AND PROGRESS RECORD

Trunk and lower limb

Name _____ Evaluation date _____

SUPINE

Passive   Hip_____ Knee_____
motion
sense   Ankle_____ Big toe_____

Flexor synergy_____

Extensor synergy_____

Hip: Abduction_____ Adduction_____

SITTING ON CHAIR	STANDING
Trunk balance (no back support)	With _____ Without _____ support Balance, normal limb sec.
Sole sensation Correct (no. of answers) Incorrect	Double scale (a) _____ (b)_____ reading†
Hip-knee-ankle flexion	Hip-knee-ankle flexion
Knee flexion-extension small range	Knee flexion-extension small range
Knee flexion beyond 90 degrees	Knee flexion hip extended
Ankle, isolated dorsiflexion	Ankle, isolated dorsiflexion
Reciprocal hamstring action*	Hip abduction knee extended

C

AMBULATION   Evaluation date _____

Brace?_____ Cane? _____ In parallel bars_____

Supported_____ Escorted_____ Alone_____

Arm in sling _____ Arm swings loosely_____ Elbow held flexed_____

Arm swings near normal _____

GAIT ANALYSIS   Evaluation date_____

STANCE PHASE	SWING PHASE
Ankle_____	_____
Knee_____	_____
Hip_____	_____

Walking cadence: Steps per min.   Speed: Feet per min.

*Inward and outward rotation at knee with inversion-eversion at ankle.
†Recorded as normal/affected; (a) preferred stance, (b) weight shift on affected limb.

Fig. 15-3, cont'd. Hemiplegia classification and progress record.

forearm pronated, (2) raising the arm forward, as in stage 4, but above 90° of shoulder flexion, and (3) pronating and supinating the forearm with the elbow extended. The third movement is performed with the arm in the forward or side horizontal position and is not isolated from shoulder internal and external rotation.

Individuals who progress to recovery stage 6 will be able to perform isolated joint motions and demonstrate coordination that is comparable or nearly comparable to that of the unaffected side. On close observation the trained observer may detect some awkwardness of movement, and there may be some incoordination when rapid movement is attempted. The subject may be evaluated while performing a variety of daily living tasks, provided that recovery of hand function has kept pace with recovery of arm function.

The tests of motor speed on the second page of the evaluation form (Fig. 15-3, *B*) may be used to assess spasticity during any recovery stage, provided the subject has enough range of active motion to perform the necessary movement. The tests are especially useful in stages 4, 5, and 6. The normal side is tested first for comparison, then, the affected side is tested. The two movements that are tested are (1) hand to chin and (2) hand to opposite knee. The subject is seated in a sturdy chair without armrests. The trunk should be stabilized against the back of the chair, and the head should be erect. The hand is closed, but not tightly, and rests in the lap. For the hand-to-chin test the forearm is at 0° neutral between pronation and supination. The examiner asks the client to bring the hand from lap to chin as rapidly as possible, first with the unaffected side and then with the affected side, and records the number of full back-and-forth movements accomplished in 5 seconds. If speed is slow because of marked spasticity, half movements may be counted. The same procedure is followed for the hand-to-opposite knee test, except that the forearm is positioned in full pronation on the lap. The hand is moved from the lap to the opposite knee, using full range of elbow extension. These two tests measure the spasticity of elbow flexors and extensors.

Wrist stabilization, which is automatic during normal grasp, is often lacking after a stroke. Therefore it is important to evaluate wrist stabilization during fist closure. This is done with the elbow both flexed and extended. During the recovery stages when the synergies are dominant, the wrist will tend to flex when the elbow flexes. The subject is asked to make a fist while the elbow is extended across the front of the body. The subject is then asked to make a fist while the elbow is flexed at the side of the body. Whether the wrist remains stabilized in the neutral position or extends slightly is observed. This test is followed by a request for wrist flexion and extension with the fist closed. The subject holds an object such as a wide (1¾ inches or 4.5 cm) dowel, in the hand and extends and flexes the wrist. This is done in the elbow-extended and elbow-flexed positions as on the previous test.

Circumduction of the wrist indicates significant recovery to the advanced stages. When evaluating the ability to perform this movement, the examiner should stabilize the forearm in pronation. The upper arm should be stabilized against the trunk.

Mass grasp is tested with a dynamometer, which measures pounds of pressure of grasp strength. The normal side is tested first, then the affected side is tested, and the results are recorded for comparison. Mass extension is evaluated by asking the subject to release and actively extend the fingers to the degree possible. Whether active extension was accomplished and the approximate amount of range achieved should be noted on the form. Active release to full range of extension is very difficult for many persons with CVA.

All types of prehension are evaluated in order of their difficulty. Everyday tasks that require the particular prehension pattern should be used. Hook grasp may be assessed by asking the subject to hold a handbag. Holding a card demands lateral prehension. Palmar prehension is required for grasping a pencil. Cylindrical grasp may be assessed by asking the subject to hold a small, narrow jar. Grasping a ball requires spherical grasp. The subject's

ability to catch and throw the ball may be observed. These are difficult activities for hemiplegics, since they require rapid grasp and release, coordination of the entire limb, and time-space judgment. In all the prehension tests the normal side should be observed first for purposes of comparison.

Individual thumb movements are evaluated with the subject's hand resting in the lap, ulnar side down. The normal side is observed first, then the affected side is observed. The subject is asked to move the thumb up and down (flexion-extension) and side to side (adduction-abduction).

Individual finger movements are evaluated by asking the subject to tap the index and middle fingers on the tabletop or on a pillow held in the lap. Isolated control of metacarpophalangeal (MP) flexion and extension and noted on the evaluation form.

Fine, coordinated use of the affected hand/arm and of both hands together usually is indicative of advanced recovery. Subjects who have succeeded well at the prehension tests may be asked to button and unbutton a shirt, first using both hands, then using the affected hand only. Other skilled activities, such as writing, threading a needle, removing a small bottle cap, and picking up and placing ¼-inch (0.6 cm) mosaic tiles, may be used to further test skilled hand use.

Motor tests, trunk and lower extremity

The portion of the evaluation form that outlines the trunk and lower extremity motor tests is shown in Fig. 15-3, *C*. To evaluate trunk and lower extremity function the patient is tested first in the supine position, then in the sitting position, and then in the standing position. If the patient is ambulatory, a gait analysis is made. Tests in the supine position include tests of passive motion sense, flexor and extensor synergies, and hip abduction and adduction. In the sitting position trunk balance, sole sensation, and specific movements of the lower limb are tested. These include hip-knee-ankle flexion, knee flexion and extension in small range, knee flexion beyond 90°, isolated ankle dorsiflexion, and reciprocal hamstring action (which is inward and outward rotation at the knee with inversion-eversion at the ankle). In the standing position balance and selected movements are evaluated. These are hip-knee-ankle flexion, knee flexion-extension in small range, knee flexion with the hip extended, isolated ankle dorsiflexion, and hip abduction with the knee extended. The lower extremity evaluation concludes with a gait analysis, including timed walking cadence.[3]

Testing the trunk and upper and lower limbs may be carried out by the physical therapist. In facilities where evaluation is coordinated between physical therapy and occupational therapy the physical therapist is primarily responsible for the trunk and lower limb testing, and the occupational therapist may test for upper extremity function. However, each therapist working with the patient must be aware of the test results and use an integrated approach in treatment. An integrated approach incorporates upper limb, trunk, and lower limb function, according to prescribed goals in exercises and activities.

GENERAL PRINCIPLES OF FACILITATING MOTOR FUNCTION

The goal of Brunnstrom's movement therapy is to facilitate the patient's progress through the recovery stages that occur after onset of hemiplegia (see Table 15-1). The use of the available afferent-efferent mechanisms of control is the means for attainment of this goal. Some of these mechanisms are summarized here.

Postural and attitudinal reflexes are used as means to increase or decrease tone in specific muscles.[6] For instance, changes in head and body position can influence muscle tone by evoking the tonic reflexes, such as the TNR, tonic lumbar reflex, TLR, and equilibrium and protective reactions. Associated reactions may be used to initiate or elicit synergies in the early stages of recovery by giving resistance to the contralateral muscle group on the normal side. Efforts at flexion synergy of the affected leg may be used to elicit a flexion synergy of the arm through homolateral limb synkinesis.

Stimulation of the skin over a muscle by rubbing with the fingertips produces contraction of that muscle and facilitation of the synergy to which the muscle belongs. An example is briskly stimulating the triceps muscle during other efforts at performance of the extension synergy, which enhances elbow extension and amplifies the synergy pattern. Muscle contraction is facilitated when muscles are placed in their lengthened position, and the quick stretch of a muscle facilitates its contraction and inhibits its antagonist. Resistance facilitates the contraction of muscles resisted. Synergistic movement may be augmented by the voluntary effort of the patient. Visual stimulation through the use of mirrors, videotape of self, and movement of parts can facilitate motion in some patients as can auditory stimuli in the forms of loud and repetitive commands to perform the desired movement.

The strongest component of one synergy will inhibit its antagonist through reciprocal innervation. It follows that if relaxation of the stronger or spastic muscle can be effected, it may be possible to evoke some activity in the weaker antagonist, which may appear to be functionless because of its inability to overcome the very spastic agonist.[2,6]

GENERAL TREATMENT GOALS AND METHODS

Before the initiation of any intervention strategies the occupational and physical therapists must make a thorough evaluation of the motor, sensory, perceptual, and cognitive functions of the adult hemiplegic. The motor evaluation yields information about stage of recovery, muscle tone, passive motion sense, hand function, sitting and standing balance, leg function, and ambulation. The treatment goals and methods summarized are directed primarily to the rehabilitation of the hemiplegic upper extremity. The point at which the therapist initiates treatment depends on the stage of recovery and muscle tone of the individual client.

Bed positioning[3]

Proper bed positioning begins immediately after the onset of the stroke when the patient is in the flaccid stage. During this period the limbs can be placed in the most favorable positions without interference from spastic muscles. Correct bed positioning is often the responsibility of the nurse; therefore it is essential that the physical therapist or occupational therapist provide information about the influence of the limb synergies on bed postures.

If left unsupervised, the lower limb tends to assume a position of hip external rotation and abduction and knee flexion. This posture is partly a result of mechanical influences on the flaccid limb, that is, the weight of the part tends to pull the hip into external rotation. On a neurological basis this position mimics the flexor synergy of the lower extremity. The advent of muscular tension in the flexor and abductor muscle groups of the hip and the flexor group of the knee contributes to the posture of the lower extremity as described above.

If the extensor synergy is developed in the lower extremity, a different position may be present. Spasticity of the extensor muscles usually exceeds that of the flexor muscles in the lower limb. In this case the posture of the lower extremity is characterized by extension and adduction at the hip, knee extension, and ankle plantar flexion. If adductor spasticity is severe, the patient may habitually place the unaffected leg under the affected leg, which allows the affected limb to adduct even more and results in a crossed-limb posture.

If the extensor synergy dominates in the lower limb, the recommended bed position in the supine position is slight flexion of the hip and knee maintained by a small pillow under the knee. Lateral support of the leg at the knee with pillows or a rolled blanket or bolster should be provided to prevent abduction and external rotation. The bed clothes should be supported to prevent them from resting on the foot. This will help prevent excessive ankle plantar flexion. The position of slight flexion at the hip and knee is beneficial because it has an inhibitory effect on the extensor muscles of the knee and ankle, counteracting the development of severe spasticity in these muscles, which hinders ambulation.

If the flexor synergy dominates in the lower limb, the knee must be maintained in extension. Hip external rotation can be prevented with supports as described above. The choice of bed position is determined on an individual basis. The position selected should be opposite the pattern of the greatest amount of muscle tone to effect the inhibition of excessive spasticity.

The affected upper extremity is supported on a pillow in a position comfortable for the patient. Abduction of the humerus in relation to the scapula should be avoided, since in this position the stabilizing action of the lower portion of the glenoid fossa on the humeral head is reduced and the superior portion of the joint capsule is slackened. This position can predispose the humeral head to downward subluxation. In handling the patient, traction on the affected upper extremity is to be avoided. The patient is instructed to use the unaffected hand to support the affected arm when moving about in bed.

Bed mobility[3]

Turning toward the affected side is easier for patients, since it requires little activity of the affected limb(s). The affected arm is placed close to the body and the patient rolls over the affected arm when turning. Turning toward the unaffected side requires muscular effort of the affected limbs. The unaffected arm can be used to elevate the affected arm to a vertical position over the face with the shoulder in 80° or 90° of flexion and the elbow fully extended. The affected lower extremity is positioned in partial flexion at the knee and hip and can be stabilized in this position momentarily by the therapist. The patient turns by swinging the arms and the affected knee across the body toward the unaffected side. The movements of the limbs assist in the turn of the upper body and pelvis. When control improves, the patient can carry out the maneuver independently in one smooth, continuous movement to turn from the supine position to the side lying position on the unaffected side.

Trunk movement and balance

One of the early goals in treatment is for the client to achieve good trunk or sitting balance. Most hemiplegic persons demonstrate "listing" to the affected side, which may result in a fall if the appropriate equilibrium responses do not occur. To evoke balance responses the therapist deliberately disturbs the client's erect sitting posture in forward-backward and side-to-side direction. This may be done while the client sits on a chair, edge of a bed, or mat table. The client is prepared for the procedure with an explanation and is pushed, at first, gently, then more vigorously. The client may support the affected arm by cradling it to protect the shoulder. This prevents the client from grasping the supporting surface during the procedure. Later the therapist initiates and assists the client with bending the trunk directly forward and obliquely forward. The client sits and supports the affected arm as previously described. The therapist's hands are held under the client's elbows. The therapist may use the knees to stabilize the client's knees if balance is poor. In this position the therapist guides the client while inclining the trunk forward and obliquely and attains some passive glenohumeral and scapular motion at the same time.

Trunk rotation is encouraged in a similar manner, with the therapist sitting in front of the client or standing behind and supporting the client's arms as before. Trunk rotation is first performed through a limited range and is gently guided by the therapist. The range is gradually increased. Some neck mobilization may be attained almost automatically during these maneuvers. As the trunk rotates, the client cradles the affected arm and swings the arms rhythmically from side to side to achieve shoulder abduction and adduction alternately as the trunk rotates. The shoulder components of the flexor and extensor synergies might be evoked during these procedures through the TNR and tonic lumbar reflexes.[3]

Shoulder range of motion

A second important early goal in treatment is to maintain or achieve pain-free range of motion (ROM) at the glenohumeral joint. There appears to be a relationship between the shoulder pain, so common in adult hemiplegics, and the stretching of spastic muscles around the shoulder joint. Traditional forced passive exercise procedures may actually produce this stretching and contribute to the development of pain. Such exercise is harmful and contraindicated. Once the client has experienced the pain, the anticipation of it increases the muscular tension that in turn decreases the joint mobility and increases the pain experienced on passive motion. Therefore the shoulder joint should be mobilized without forceful stretching of hypertonic musculature about the shoulder and shoulder girdle.

This is accomplished through guided trunk motion. The client sits erect, cradling the affected arm. The therapist supports the arms under the elbows while the client leans forward. The more the client leans the greater range of shoulder flexion can be obtained. The therapist guides the arms gently and passively into shoulder flexion while the client's attention is focused on the trunk motion. In a similar fashion the therapist can guide the arms into abduction and adduction while the client rotates the trunk from side to side. The TNR and tonic lumbar reflex facilitate relaxation of muscles during this maneuver. When the client is confident that the shoulder can be moved painlessly, active-assisted movements of the arm in relation to the trunk can begin.

First, the client moves both shoulders into elevation and depression and scapula adduction and abduction. These are then combined with glenohumeral movements. The arm is supported by the therapist from behind, with the shoulder between forward flexion and abduction, the elbow flexed less than 90°, and the wrist supported in slight extension. The therapist may ask the client to elevate the shoulders while tapping the upper trapezius with the fingertips. At the same time the therapist is assisting the client to elevate the arm as well. Active shoulder elevation will tend to elicit other components of the flexor synergy that in turn will tend to inhibit the strong adduction component of the extensor synergy (pectoralis major), allowing the therapist to elevate the arm into abduction by small degrees each time the client repeats the active shoulder girdle elevation. The procedure is repeated, and the therapist gives the appropriate verbal commands "pull up, let go." The abduction movement is at an oblique angle between forward flexion and full abduction. Sideward abduction with the arm in the same plane as the trunk is likely to be painful and should be avoided. Alternate pronation and supination of the forearm by the therapist should accompany the elevation and lowering of the arm throughout the procedure. The forearm should be supinated when the shoulder is elevated and pronated when the arm is lowered. Head rotation to the normal side inhibits activity in the pectoralis major muscle through the TNR. When abduction movement above the horizontal has been accomplished without pain, the client can be directed to reach overhead and straighten out the elbow if there has been sufficient recovery to do so. The client is directed to rotate the head to the affected side to facilitate the elbow extension while observing the movement of the arm.

These techniques result in increased ROM at the shoulder and also help the development of the flexor synergy. A small ROM in the path of the extensor synergy should be performed between the patient's efforts at flexion so that both synergies are developed. As training progresses, greater emphasis is placed on the development of the extensor synergy.

Shoulder subluxation

Glenohumeral subluxation appears to be a result of dysfunction of the rotator cuff muscles: supraspinatus, infraspinatus, teres minor, and subscapularis. Activation of these muscles in treatment is necessary if subluxation is to be minimized or prevented. Function of the supraspinatus muscle is particularly important for the prevention of subluxation. Slings have been used in an effort to hold the humeral head in the glenoid fossa, but they do not in any way activate the muscles needed to protect the integrity of the shoulder joint.[3] Recently, the use of slings has been found to be of little value, and slings may actually be harmful.[4] A more complete discussion of shoulder problems and slings appears in Chapter 16.

Upper limb training

The training procedures for improving arm function are geared to the client's recovery stage. During stages 1 and 2 when the arm is essentially flaccid or some components of the synergy patterns are beginning to appear, the aim is to elicit muscle tone and the synergy patterns on a reflex basis. This is accomplished through a variety of facilitation procedures. Associated reactions and tonic reflexes may be employed to influence tone and evoke reflexive movement. The proximal traction response may be used to activate the flexor synergy. Tapping over the upper and middle trapezius, rhomboids, and biceps may elicit components of the flexor synergy. Tapping over the triceps and stretching of the serratus anterior may activate components of the extensor synergy. Passive movement alternately through each of the synergy patterns is not only an excellent means for maintaining ROM of several joints but provides the client with proprioceptive and visual feedback for the desired patterns of early movement. Quick stretch to muscles and surface stroking of the skin over them are also used to activate muscles. These methods are not employed in any set order or routine but are selected to suit the particular responses of each individual client. Since the flexor synergy usually appears first, it may be useful to begin trying to elicit the flexor patterns. This should be followed immediately with facilitation of the extensor synergy components, since these tend to be weaker and more difficult to perform in later stages of recovery.[3,5]

When the client has recovered to stages 2 and 3, the synergies or their components are present and may be performed voluntarily. Spasticity is developing and reaches its peak in stage 3. During this period the aim is for the client to achieve voluntary control of the synergy patterns. This is accomplished by repetitious alternating performance of the synergy patterns, first with the assistance and facilitation of the therapist. Facilitation is provided through resistance to voluntary motion, verbal commands, tapping, and cutaneous stimulation. This is followed by voluntary repetition of the synergy patterns without the facilitation and,

finally, concentration on the components of the synergies from proximal to distal with, then without, facilitation. Bilateral rowing movements with the therapist holding the client's hands are a useful activity for reciprocal motion of the synergies that should be started during this time.[3,5]

The treatment aim during stages 4 and 5 is to break away from the synergies by mixing components from antagonistic synergies to perform new and increasingly complex patterns of movement. One means for accomplishing this goal is using skateboard or powder board exercises in arcs of movement to get elbow flexion, combined with shoulder horizontal adduction and forearm pronation, and alternating with shoulder horizontal abduction and elbow extension with forearm supination (Fig. 15-4). These same movement patterns may be used to perform the therapeutic activities just mentioned. Later the client may be able to perform the more complex figure eight pattern on the skateboard or powder board.

In the final recovery stages 5 and 6 increasingly complex movement combinations and isolated motions are possible. The aims in treatment are to achieve ease in performance of movement combinations and isolated motion and to increase speed of movement.

It should be noted that the hemiplegic upper extremity seldom makes a full recovery. If voluntary and spontaneous movement is possible, the client should be trained to use the limb as an assist to the sound arm to the extent possible in bilateral activities.

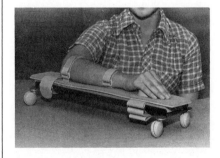

Fig. 15-4. Skateboard exercises for synergy or combined movement patterns in gravity-eliminated plane.

Hand training

Methods for retraining hand function are treated separately, since recovery of hand function does not always coincide with arm recovery. Hand retraining commensurate with the recovery status of the client should be carried out continuously through the treatment program.

The first goal of hand retraining is to achieve mass grasp. The proximal traction response and grasp reflex may be used to elicit early grasp movement on a reflex level. During the proximal traction response maneuver the therapist should maintain the client's wrist in extension and give the command "squeeze."

Because the normal association between wrist extension and grasp is disturbed, another important aim is to achieve wrist fixation for grasp. Wrist extension often accompanies the extensor synergy. Wrist extension can be evoked if the therapist applies resistance to the proximal palm or fist while supporting the arm in the position described earlier for elevation of the arm into abduction. Percussion of the wrist extensors with the elbow in extension and arm elevated and supported by the therapist can activate wrist extension. The proximal portion of the extensors are tapped, and the therapist directs the client to "squeeze" simultaneously. The commands to "squeeze" and "stop squeezing" are given at appropriate points in the facilitation procedures. During the wrist extension and fist closure the therapist carries the elbow forward into extension. During the wrist and finger relaxation the therapist carries the elbow back into flexion. While the client is maintaining fist closure, the therapist may withdraw the wrist support and give the command "hold." The therapist may continue tapping the wrist extensors while the client attempts to hold the posture. The goal is to synchronize the muscles for fist closure with wrist extension.

This procedure should be alternated with a command to "stop squeezing" and the wrist should be allowed to drop and fingers open while the elbow is moved into flexion. These steps are alternated and the wrist extension-fist closure is gradually performed with increasing amounts of elbow flexion so that the client can learn to grasp with wrist stabilization when the arm is in a variety of positions.

A third objective in hand retraining is to achieve active release of grasp. This is difficult, since there is usually a considerable degree of spasticity in the flexor muscles of the hand. A release of tension in the finger flexors, then, is primary to the achievement of any active finger extension. Active grasp should be alternated with manipulations to release tension in the flexors. The therapist sits facing the client and pulls the thumb out of the palm by gripping the thenar eminence. The forearm is supinated. The wrist is allowed to remain in slight flexion. The therapist maintains the grasp around the thumb and alternately pronates and supinates the forearm with emphasis on supination. Pressure on the thumb is decreased during pronation and increased during supination. Cutaneous stimulation is given to the dorsum of the hand and wrist when the forearm is supinated. This manipulation is likely to develop some tension in the finger extensors, and the fingers extend. The client may actually participate in opening the hand when the forearm is supinated. However, strong efforts on the part of the client may evoke flexion instead and should be avoided.

If this manipulation is inadequate, stretch of the finger extensors may be used. With the therapist and client positioned and the hand manipulated as just described, the therapist uses the free hand for distally directed, rapid stroking movements over the proximal phalanges of the affected hand. This causes momentary flexion of the MP joints, which then bounce back into partial extension. The stroking movement is performed so that the proximal, then distal interphalangeal (IP) joints are included. The movement is performed rapidly and continuously, causing rapid flexion and then bounce back of MP and IP joints. The fingers become extended, and the finger flexors are relaxed because they are reciprocally inhibited by the stretch reflex response in the extensors. If the flexors are stretched or stroking is performed over the palmar surface of the fingers, the spasticity will return to the finger flexors, and they will act to close the hand.[3] For this reason the fingers should not be pulled into extension.

Active finger extension may be further facilitated by the use of a finger extension exercise glove with rubber bands, which the client uses while the hand is manipulated into supination with the thumb pulled out of the palm as described earlier (Fig. 15-5).

Elevation above the horizontal position evokes the extensor reflexes of the fingers. After flexor spasticity has been decreased by the maneuvers just described, the therapist stands on the affected side and maintains the thumb in abduction and extension and the forearm in pronation. The fingers are kept in extension by pressure over the IP joints and stabilization of the fingertips. The grip on the thumb is released, and the arm is raised above the horizontal position. The therapist strokes distally over the IP joints with the heel of her hand. The fingers will extend or hyperextend, and the therapist gradually discontinues contact with the client's hand. If the client is ready, slight voluntary mental effort can be superimposed on the reflex extension which may bring about additional extension of the fingers.

If the forearm is supinated while the arm is elevated, thumb extension will be enhanced. The hand should be positioned overhead for this maneuver. To facilitate extension of the fourth and fifth fingers the forearm should be pronated as the arm is elevated and friction should be applied over the ulnar side of the dorsum of the forearm.

When reflex extension of the fingers is well-established, alternate fist opening and closing can begin. The arm is

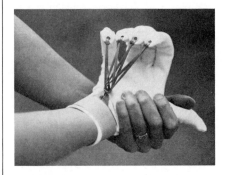

Fig. 15-5. Finger extension exercise glove.

lowered passively, and the elbow is flexed. The forearm and wrist are supported, and the client is asked to "squeeze" then "stop squeezing." As soon as the fingers relax, the manipulations to facilitate finger extension are carried out. These two steps are alternated, and the client's voluntary efforts are superimposed on the reflex activity so that the movements begin to assume a semivoluntary character. Semivoluntary finger extension is influenced by the position of the limb and appears to be linked to gross movements other than the synergy patterns.

Voluntary movements of the thumb appear when semivoluntary mass extension becomes possible. Once the flexor muscles have been relaxed, the hand can be placed in the client's lap, ulnar side down, and the client can attempt to move the thumb away from the first finger, a preliminary for lateral prehension. The therapist may stimulate the tendons of the abductor pollicis and the extensor pollicis brevis by tapping or friction at the point where they pass over the wrist to enhance the client's effort. The client can learn to "twiddle" the thumbs to attain further control of thumb motion. The client folds hands, wrists slightly flexed, and moves the thumbs around each other. Initially the normal thumb may push the other around, but the involved thumb may begin to participate actively. The willed effort, visual input, and sensory feedback from affected and unaffected sides contribute to the development of this movement. During the treatment sessions the client must be comfortable and relaxed. The client's willed efforts must be slight lest too much effort evoke a flexor rather than the extensor response that is desired. Excessive muscle tension in the limb and entire body must be avoided or finger extension will not occur.

Many adult hemiplegics never achieve good voluntary extension or coordinated fine hand motions. However, if semivoluntary extension can be well-established, voluntary extension usually follows, so that the client can open the hand in all positions.[3]

The accomplishment of palmar prehension and fine hand movements requires the achievement of voluntary opening of the hand, opposition of the thumb to the fingers, and ability to release objects in contact with the palm of the hand.

Lower limb training

Training procedures for the lower extremity are primarily the domain of the physical therapist. However, when training the patient in functional activities, the occupational therapist can use procedures that are in concert with the work of the physical therapist. To name a few examples, transfer training, dressing, toileting, and ambulating about in the occupational therapy clinic will involve motor activity of the lower limb. Therefore it is important for the occupational therapist to know which training procedures are in progress, which movement patterns are to be encouraged or inhibited, and which methods facilitate the desired gait pattern when assisting or accompanying the patient during functional tasks.

Lower limb training is directed toward restoring safe standing and the development of a gait pattern that is as nearly normal as possible. The goal is to modify the gross movement synergies and facilitate movement combinations that are more nearly like those used during normal ambulation. Lower limb training includes trunk balance and activation of specific muscle groups followed by gait training. The reader is referred to the original source for a detailed description of these training procedures.[3]

OCCUPATIONAL THERAPY APPLICATIONS

Controlled movements achieved in upper limb training will have more significance if the patient can use them for functional activities. Even with limited control the affected limb can be used in many ways to assist with function. Encouraging the use of the affected arm in everyday activities decreases the possibility of the patient functioning strictly as a one-handed individual.

During stages 3 and 4 when the client has voluntary control of the synergies and may begin to be able to use movement combinations that deviate from the synergies, the occupational therapist should help the client to use the newly learned movement for functional and purposeful activities. Some

of the activities that can be adapted to use the synergy patterns or gross combined movement patterns are skateboard or powder board exercises (Fig. 15-4), sanding, leather lacing, braid weaving, finger painting, sponging off tabletops, and using a push broom or carpet sweeper. Activities that demand too much cortical control and conscious effort on the part of the client will tend to increase fatigue and muscle tension and should be avoided.

Brunnstrom[3] described several possible uses for the flexor and extensor synergies in stage 3. The extensor synergy may be used to stabilize an object on a table while the unaffected arm is performing a task. Examples are stabilizing stationery while writing letters or stabilizing fabric for sewing. The extensor synergy may also be used to stabilize a jar against the body while unscrewing the lid or to hold a handbag or newspaper under the arm. When pushing the affected arm through the sleeve of a garment, the garment can be positioned so that the arm follows the path of the extensor synergy. (This requires that the forearm be pronated first, however, to facilitate elbow extension.) The flexor synergy or its components may be used to carry a coat or handbag over the forearm and to hold a toothbrush while the unaffected hand squeezes the toothpaste, for example. Bilateral pushing and pulling activities that alternate the paths of both synergies may be helpful for some patients. Examples of these are sweeping, vacuuming, and dusting. Such activities may be performed with the unaffected hand stabilizing the affected one. The affected hand may be more a hindrance than a help until greater control is gained. Strongly motivated patients will try to use available movements under the guidance and encouragement of the occupational therapist.

To promote transition from stage 3 to stage 4 movement combinations are facilitated and practiced in upper limb training. These movements are hand to chin, hand to ear on the same side and opposite side, hand to opposite elbow, hand to opposite shoulder, hand to forehead, hand to top of head, hand to back of head, and stroking movements from top to back of head and from dorsum of the forearm to the shoulder and toward the neck on the normal side. As soon as possible, these movement patterns should be translated to functional activities. Success at functional tasks increases motivation and establishes a purpose for the training. Also contact with body parts where sensation is intact is instrumental in guiding the hand to its goal. Examples of application of these movements to function are hand-to-mouth motions used in eating finger foods, combing hair, washing the face, washing the unaffected arm, and reaching the opposite axilla for washing or application of deodorant.[3] The therapist's role is to analyze activities for movement patterns that are possible for the patient to perform, and to select activities with the patient that have meaning and are interesting.

At this time the occupational therapist should stress the use of any voluntary movement of the affected limb in performance of activities of daily living. Using the arm for dressing and hygiene skills translates the movements to purposeful use. It should be borne in mind that the degree to which purposeful, spontaneous use of the arm is possible depends on the sensory status of the limb and not only on the motor recovery achieved.

If the patient surpasses stage 4, the number of activities that can be performed will increase, and more movement combinations will be possible. The involvement of the affected limbs in activities of daily living should be encouraged. The activities mentioned earlier can be performed now in their usual manner and can be graded to demand finer and more complex movement patterns. Loom weaving, block printing, gardening, furniture refinishing, leather tooling, rolling out dough, sweeping, dusting, and washing dishes are a few of the activities that may enlist the use of the affected arm purposefully if hand recovery is adequate.

REVIEW QUESTIONS

1. List the stages of recovery of arm function after CVA, as described by Brunnstrom.
2. List the motions in the flexor and extensor synergies of the arm, and draw stick figures to illustrate the positions.
3. What is the strongest component of the flexor synergy of the arm?
4. What is the weakest component of the extensor synergy of the arm?
5. What is the basis of the Brunnstrom approach to the treatment of hemiplegia?
6. For what purposes does Brunnstrom recommend the use of primitive reflexes and associated reactions in the early recovery stages after onset of hemiplegia?
7. Define or describe the following terms: limb synergy, associated reactions, imitation synkinesis, proximal traction response, grasp reflex, and Souque's finger phenomenon.
8. Describe or demonstrate the procedure that Brunnstrom recommended to maintain or achieve pain-free ROM at the glenohumeral joint.
9. What is the aim of treatment for functional recovery of the arm during stages 1 and 2? Stages 2 and 3? Stages 3 and 4?
10. List two treatment methods that could be used to achieve each of these aims.
11. Describe three activities other than those listed in the text that may be used in occupational therapy to enhance voluntary control of the flexor and extensor synergies.
12. What is the effect of the proximal traction response on muscle function?
13. Describe or demonstrate the procedure that Brunnstrom recommends to establish wrist fixation in association with grasp.
14. Describe the procedure that may be used to relax spastic finger flexion and facilitate finger extension.
15. Which muscle group is thought to play a significant role in maintaining glenohumeral joint stability?
16. Describe proper bed positioning for the patient with a dominant extensor synergy of the leg. What is the rationale for this position?

REFERENCES

1. Bobath, B.: Adult hemiplegia: evaluation and treatment, London, 1978, Heinemann, Ltd.
2. Brunnstrom, S.: Motor behavior in adult hemiplegic patients, Am. J. Occup. Ther. **15**:6, 1961.
3. Brunnstrom, S.: Movement therapy in hemiplegia, New York, 1970, Harper & Row, Publishers, Inc.
4. Cailliet, R.: The shoulder in hemiplegia, Philadelphia, 1980, F.A. Davis Co.
5. Perry, C.: Principles and techniques of the Brunnstrom approach to the treatment of hemiplegia, Am. J. Phys. Med. **46:**789, 1967.
6. Sawner, K.: Brunnstrom approach to treatment of adult patients with hemiplegia: rationale for facilitation procedures, Buffalo, 1969, State University of New York. Mimeographed.

CHAPTER 16

Neurodevelopmental treatment

THE BOBATH APPROACH TO THE TREATMENT OF ADULT HEMIPLEGIA

JAN ZARET DAVIS

This chapter introduces and orients the reader to the Bobath approach in the treatment of adult hemiplegia: neurodevelopmental treatment (NDT). It is designed to provide a basic foundation in the principles of treatment, describe treatment techniques, identify problems with the hemiplegic shoulder, and provide specific management of the painful shoulder. Those interested in expanding their knowledge in this area are directed to readings from the references, particularly *Adult Hemiplegia: Evaluation and Treatment* by Berta Bobath.[2]

Berta Bobath, a physical therapist, and her husband, Dr. Karel Bobath, have been developing special treatment techniques in London since World War II. This technique, often called NDT, is commonly used in the treatment of cerebral palsy and acquired adult hemiplegia. It is most effective when used in the 24-hour per day care of the patient. The principles of treatment can be followed by all those concerned with the patient's care. These include the nursing staff, occupational therapists, physical therapists, speech therapists, and family. It is ideal to begin treatment immediately during the acute stages of illness but treatment can be started and be effective at any time. The information and techniques described in this chapter are meant to be used specifically in the treatment of adult hemiplegia.

Rationale for use of neurodevelopmental treatment techniques with adult hemiplegics

The primary goal of NDT is to relearn normal movements. The techniques used are intended for more than just the movements of an arm or leg; they treat the person as a whole, encouraging the use of both sides. The client uses less adaptive equipment (for example, slings, braces, and canes) and is more able to move about freely with

normal muscle tone.[2] This creates a better atmosphere for the psychosocial adjustment to family and everyday living. The more normal a person appears to others, with less deformity from spasticity, the better he or she is accepted.

The Bobaths use specific techniques to decrease spasticity and inhibit abnormal patterns of movement. This suppression or inhibition of abnormal patterns (synergies) must be accomplished before normal, selective isolated movement can take place. It is impossible to superimpose normal movement on a person still being influenced by spasticity.[2]

The following are terms often used in describing the NDT techniques of Bobath. These are defined as they are used throughout this chapter.

Positioning
Rotation of trunk
"Placing"
Spasticity
Inhibition
Weight bearing
Scapular mobility
Normalization of tone
Postural reactions
    Righting reactions
    Equilibrium reactions
Protective extension

Some additional terms associated with this approach and their definitions are:

ASSOCIATED MOVEMENTS. Extraneous movements, which occur normally and are well coordinated, are seen in children and adults when new and difficult tasks are learned. The movements are the same types of movements of both limbs, and the activity of the limb not involved in the motor task reinforces that of the limb on the opposite side of the body involved in the motor task.[2]

ASSOCIATED REACTIONS. In the hemiplegic patient, forceful voluntary activity of the unaffected limbs can result in an apparent limb movement, a palpable increase in tone, and a wide-

spread increase in spasticity on the hemiplegic side. Associated reactions are abnormal and occur as a result of tonic reflexes or released postural reactions in muscles deprived of voluntary control. These reactions must be prevented in treatment, and therefore the patient should not use any part of his or her body with excessive effort.[2]

KEY POINTS OF CONTROL. Points on the body, usually proximal (for example, shoulder and pelvic girdles), which when handled by the therapist in a specific manner can be used to change part of an abnormal pattern to reduce spasticity throughout the body and to guide the patient's active movements. Spasticity of the limbs can be influenced and reduced from these key points of control.[2]

POSTURAL TONE. Postural tone is normal central nervous system (CNS) activation of large groups of muscles in patterns for the maintenance of posture. Normal postural tone is high enough to resist gravity and low enough to give way to movement.[2]

REFLEX INHIBITING PATTERNS. Patterns of movement, which are opposite to spastic patterns and guided by the therapist from key points of control, are used to inhibit abnormal motor activity and facilitate more normal motor activity.[2]

For more complete definitions and discussion the reader is advised to consult the original source.[2]

EVALUATION

The initial phase in treatment is the evaluation. To do an accurate evaluation the therapist should have a good understanding of normal development. "Normal postural reflex activity forms the necessary background for normal movements and functional skills. The *normal postural reflex mechanism* consists of a great number and variety of automatic movements which gradually develop along with the maturation of the infantile brain. For the purpose of assessment and treatment, three large groups of automatic reactions can be differentiated as follows:"[2]

1. Righting reactions: "The righting reactions are automatic reactions which serve to maintain and restore the normal position of the head in space and its normal relationsip with the trunk, together with the normal alignment of trunk and limbs."[2]

2. Equilibrium reactions: "Equilibrium reactions are automatic reactions which serve to maintain and restore balance during all our activities, especially when we are in danger of falling. Another important automatic reaction which is closely associated with the development of equilibrium reactions is the protective extension of the arms."[2]

3. Automatic adaptation of muscles to changes of posture: "In a normal person, the postural reflex mechanism controls the weight of a limb during movements both into and against gravity." It allows for smooth and well-controlled mobility against the forces of gravity. "The normal person does not relax when being moved—relaxation, unless fully supported, being a voluntary learnt ability. The limb can be 'placed.' It feels light to the examiner, follows the movement actively and is controlled throughout its whole range by adequate contraction of the antigravity muscles."[2]

An NDT evaluation includes the assessment of the previously mentioned reactions as well as sensation, motor pattern, and postural tone. The reader is referred to the original source[2] for a more complete discussion of the evaluation. The occupational therapist must also include an activities of daily living (ADL) and a perceptual evaluation in the assessment. The patient is evaluated by the therapist to see just what he or she can or cannot do. In evaluation emphasis is placed on the *quality of movement,* that is, the ways in which the patient moves, his or her coordination, movement patterns, tonus changes, and postural reactions rather than on muscles and joints.[2] It is important to understand what is "normal" and "abnormal" in the posture and movement of the body. Most patients will display at least one abnormal reaction following a cerebrovascular accident (CVA). Normal and abnormal movements are listed here for comparison.

Normal	Abnormal
Muscle tone at rest	Flaccidity, spasticity
Voluntary selective movement	Abnormal postural tone
Isolated control	Synergistic movement
Associated movements	Associated reactions
Postural reactions	Lack of or reduced equilibrium reactions

CHARACTERISTIC PROBLEMS OF ADULT HEMIPLEGIA

There are many components of normal movement. The adult hemiplegic patient often has many problems that either singularly or in combination can be debilitating. The following are some of the most common problems seen in adult hemiplegia:

1. Asymmetry. Asymmetry is the most common problem seen in hemiplegia. It may be caused by the imbalance of tone and reciprocal interaction of muscle groups. This is seen in the trunk, extremities and in the face. Asymmetry may also be influenced by any of the following listed problems.

2. Nonweightbearing. Most patients are afraid to bear weight on the affected side of their body. Instead of the weight being evenly distributed over both lower extremities, the weight is usually shifted to the nonhemiplegic side. In rare instances the patient may bear weight entirely on the hemiplegic side, finding it difficult to shift weight evenly over both lower extremities.

3. Fear. Fear may be the most debilitating factor of all for many patients. Fear magnifies other problems that cause the patient to be dependent rather than independent. Fear can be caused by loss of sensation, poor balance reactions, lack of protective extension (fear of falling), or perceptual or cognitive problems. Any change in the normal daily schedule can produce fear. Fear is also a major factor influencing spasticity.[5]

4. Sensory loss. Sensory loss may include loss of stereognosis, position sense, light, touch, and pressure. The functional potential of an extremity can be dependent on the sensation. Often one will see a patient whose extremity remains useless because of sensory loss even though he or she has good motor control.[2,5]

5. Neglect. Unilateral neglect can be quite complicated. It is often a combination of one or more of the following: sensory, perceptual, cognitive, or visual field cut (homonymous hemianopsia). Again the patient may have good motor recovery but not be able to use it functionally because of the neglect.[5]

There are a number of other problems related to CVA, such as aphasia, apraxia, and a variety of perceptual motor problems. These are discussed in Chapter 30.

MOTOR PROBLEMS

The two major motor problems in hemiplegia are flaccidity and spasticity. Flaccidity or hypotonus is most common at the onset of a CVA. During this time the patient is often passive, displaying low endurance and low tolerance to activity. This may last a few days or as long as several months. Even though the patient displays no movement in the affected extremities at this time, a proper treatment program can have a strong impact on the entire rehabilitation program.[2]

Spasticity or hypertonus is the motor problem most common and most difficult to treat following a CVA. If not treated correctly, spasticity can progress to the point where it makes independent living nearly impossible. Spasticity interferes with the patient's ability to move by interfering with selective motor function. It produces abnormal sensory feedback and contributes to weakness of the antagonist muscles. It can cause contractures, pain, and an all-consuming fear in many patients. Fear, pain, and spasticity are often so intertwined that a vicious cycle appears. The spasticity can cause an increase in pain, which can cause an increase in fear, which in turn increases the amount of spasticity.[5]

If preventive measures are taken to reduce pain and fear, the therapist has a
much better chance with the techniques
used to reduce spasticity. Other factors
that can influence the amount of spasticity are stress (either emotional or
physical), temperature, effort, and the
rate at which an activity is done.

The typical posture of the adult
hemiplegic patient (Fig. 16-1) is described as follows:

• Head. Lateral flexion toward the involved side with rotation away from
  the involved side.
• Upper extremity.
  1. Scapula—depression, retraction
  2. Shoulder—adduction, internal ro-
     tation
  3. Elbow—flexion
  4. Forearm—pronation
  5. Wrist—flexion, ulnar deviation
  6. Finger—flexion
• Trunk. Lateral flexion toward the involved side (trunk shortening).
• Lower extremity.
  1. Pelvis—posterior elevation, retrac-
     tion
  2. Hip—internal rotation, adduction,
     extension
  3. Knee—extension
  4. Ankle—plantar flexion, supina-
     tion, inversion
  5. Toes—flexion

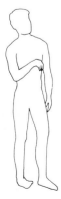

Fig. 16-1. Typical posture of hemiplegic adult in standing position. (Courtesy of Graphic Arts Department, Harmarville Rehabilitation Center,
Pittsburgh.)

The one fortunate characteristic
about spasticity is the fact that *it can be
influenced,* which means that therapists
can reduce or inhibit spasticity to some
degree. Normalization of muscle tone
(the inhibition of spasticity of the facilitation of flaccidity) may be accomplished by using one or more of the following techniques:[2,5,6]

1. Proper positioning
2. Weightbearing over the affected side
3. Trunk rotation
4. Elongation of the affected side
5. Shoulder protraction
6. Careful gradation of stimulation

These six points provide the foundation for treatment of the adult hemiplegic using the Bobath approach. As
previously stated, the techniques are
most effective and provide the best potential in rehabilitation when they are
started in the acute phase at the time of
admittance to the hospital. These techniques, however, can be used in any
phase throughout the treatment program.

TREATMENT

In each medical setting the roles of
occupational therapy and physical therapy may differ slightly. Yet the techniques described are imperative for
proper patient treatment, and all
professional services should be aware of
them and be able to apply them appropriately. The Bobaths strongly emphasize that the upper and lower extremities must not be separated.[2] The
occupational therapist must be constantly aware of the tonus, motor patterns, positions, and reflex mechanisms
of both the upper and lower extremities.

Tips for nursing, family, and staff

The following tips help the patient to
become more aware of the hemiplegic
side, to better integrate both sides of
the body, and to increase sensory stimulation to the hemiplegic side. By following these tips, some problems that
are characteristic of hemiplegia can be
prevented or minimized.

1. Room position.[4] The hemiplegic
   side of the patient should face the source
   of stimulation. The patient's hemiplegic side should face the door and
   be positioned so that the telephone,

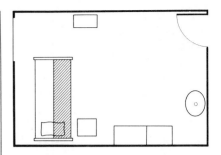

Fig. 16-2. Room arranged so that client
must turn to affected side. Shaded area
represents affected side of body.

the nightstand, the television, and
other stimulation encourages the patient to turn toward that side, thus
increasing integration of both sides
of the body (Fig. 16-2).
2. Always approach the patient from
   the hemiplegic side. The purpose of
   approaching the patient from the
   hemiplegic side is to encourage eye
   contact. Sometimes the patient has
   difficulty in turning the head and
   may need assistance in doing so.
   The therapist should simply assist
   the patient by firmly turning the
   head until he or she is able to establish eye contact. Family members
   can be encouraged to give tactile input to the patient by holding his or
   her hand or stroking his or her arm.
3. Naming. During nursing tasks, such
   as washing, each body part is named
   to increase its awareness.
4. Encourage independence. The patient should begin to assist in simple
   ADL. If the patient is unable to
   complete a task independently, the
   therapist can guide his or her hands.
   This will encourage the patient to
   learn to carry out the task sooner.[1]
5. Positioning. The patient should be
   properly positioned in bed or when
   sitting (see Figs. 16-3 to 16-6). The
   reasons that patients should be positioned in this manner are (1) weight-
   bearing inhibits spasticity, (2)
   weightbearing increases awareness of
   the hemiplegic side, and (3) lengthening of the hemiplegic side inhibits
   spasticity. There are three basic positions: lying on the affected side,
   lying supine, and lying on the unaffected side. Patients should be repositioned as often as nursing procedures require for the prevention of
   decubiti.

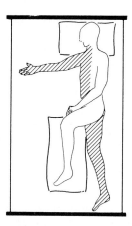

Fig. 16-3. Bed position when lying on affected side.

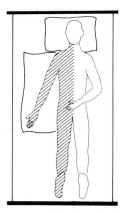

Fig. 16-4. Bed position when lying supine.

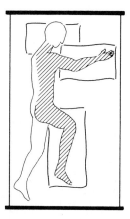

Fig. 16-5. Bed position when lying on unaffected side.

To position the patient on the hemiplegic side (Fig. 16-3),[2,5] the back of the patient should be parallel with the edge of the bed. The head is placed on the pillow symmetrically but not in extreme flexion. The shoulder is fully protracted with at least 90° of shoulder flexion (less than 90° encourages a flexion synergy). The forearm is supinated and the wrist is supported on the bed or can be slightly off the bed, which encourages wrist extension. The nonaffected leg is placed on a pillow. The affected leg is slightly flexed at the knee. A pillow can be placed behind the patient to keep him or her from rolling onto the back.

To position the patient in a supine position (Fig. 16-4),[2,5] the head is symmetrical on the pillow. The body and trunk are also symmetrical (to prevent the shortening of the hemiplegic side of the trunk). A pillow is placed under the affected shoulder, supporting the shoulder so it is at least level with the non-hemiplegic shoulder (it is common for the affected shoulder to be pulled back into retraction). The affected arm is fully supported with the elbow extended and the forearm in supination and entirely supported on a pillow in elevation. A small pillow can be placed under the hip to reduce retraction of the pelvis. *Do not place a pillow under the knees or a foot board at the end of the bed* (because this encourages knee flexion contractures and extension synergy of the lower extremity).

To position the patient on the non-hemiplegic side (Fig. 16-5),[2,5] the back should be parallel with the edge of the bed. The head is placed symmetrically on the pillow. The shoulder is in full protraction with the shoulder in at least 90° of flexion. The arm and hand are fully supported on a pillow. The wrist should not be allowed to drop off the pillow into flexion. The affected lower extremity is in hip flexion, knee flexion, and fully supported on a pillow. The foot and ankle must be supported to keep the foot from inverting.

To position the patient in a sitting position (Fig. 16-6), the trunk should be supported symmetrically in extension. The hips are flexed and knees extended. The arms are forward with the scapulae in protraction. The hands are clasped together with the hemiplegic

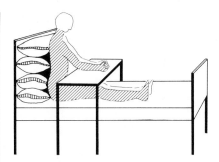

Fig. 16-6. Bed position when sitting upright.

thumb on top (see Fig. 16-18) and the entire forearm is supported on a bed table. This position of the arms will inhibit the flexion synergy.

THE OCCUPATIONAL THERAPY PROGRAM
Application of Bobath principles

The basic principles of the Bobath approach in the treatment of adult hemiplegia can be applied in all areas of the occupational therapy program. These include ADL, therapeutic activities, and home exercise programs. Following the initial evaluation of the patient, the therapist begins to formulate the treatment program. It is important that meaningful activities are selected that best meet the patient's needs and goals as well as therapeutic goals. Throughout the treatment session, the therapist must continually observe not only what the patient is doing, but also *how* he or she is doing it. The therapist is constantly aware of the position of the patient's upper and lower extremities. For example, if the therapist is working on reducing the tone in the upper extremity and the patient's lower extremity goes into an extension synergy, the lower extremity must be corrected before full inhibition of the upper extremity is obtained.

As stated previously, there are some specific techniques used to prevent spasticity from the beginning or reducing it once it is there. These are:

1. Proper positioning. In lying (see Figs. 16-3 to 16-5), the proper position has already been discussed. In

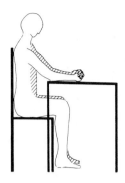

Fig. 16-7. Position when sitting in chair at table. Hands clasped in front, elbows extended, and entire forearm supported.

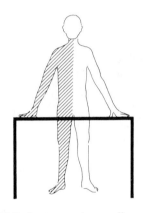

Fig. 16-8. Symmetry in standing with weight bearing on upper limbs.

sitting (Figs. 16-6 to 16-7), the patient should have the feet flat on the floor, ankles, knees, and hips in 90° of flexion, and trunk extended (no thoracic flexion). The head should be in midline and the arm fully supported when working at the table. In standing (Fig. 16-8) the head should be in midline, trunk symmetrical, and weight should be equally distributed on both lower extremities.

2. Weight bearing. Whether in lying (see Fig. 16-3), sitting (Fig. 16-9), or standing (see Fig. 16-8), the most effective method of normalizing tone is through weight bearing over the hemiplegic side. The effects are quite amazing. Patients typically

bear weight only on the nonhemiplegic side, encouraging abnormal postural tone. In all activities the therapist must constantly check to see whether or not the patient has weight over the affected side.

3. Trunk rotation (Fig. 16-10). Several things occur as a patient rotates the trunk. Rotation encourages weight bearing, elongation of the hemiplegic side, and provides vestibular input. Through trunk rotation, the patient not only helps to normalize tone but also learns to better integrate both sides of the body.

4. Elongation of the trunk on the affected side. Since it is typical for a hemiplegic patient to exhibit shortening (lateral flexion) on the affected side of the trunk, and this shortening (which is caused by hypertonicity) can affect the tone at the pelvis and shoulder girdle, it is important that the therapist reduce this tone. This can be accomplished in lying, sitting, or standing positions through proper positioning and the use of reflex inhibiting patterns as explained by Bobath.[2] A prolonged stretch will not only reduce tone in the proximal regions but will have an effect distally as well.

5. Shoulder protraction (Fig. 16-11). When working on the upper extremity, shoulder protraction will accomplish two goals. First, it helps to normalize tone, and second, it helps to maintain scapular mobility. When the patient pulls back into scapular retraction, an increase in tone in the flexor pattern can be detected throughout the extremity. Shoulder protraction is an effective method that is easily incorporated into the occupational therapy program.

6. Careful gradation of stimulation. Stimulation can refer to a number of things. Auditory stimulation will affect muscle tone. The therapist's voice, background noise, or any loud noise can produce an increase in muscle tone.[1] Tactile stimulation (including vibration and temperature) can also increase or decrease muscle tone depending on how it is applied and length of time. Stimulation can also be the rate (how fast) an activity or facilitation technique is performed.

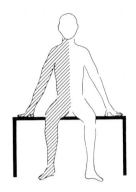

Fig. 16-9. Weight-bearing position of upper limbs in sitting position.

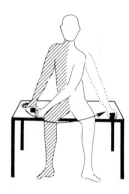

Fig. 16-10. Trunk rotation is practiced while patient bears weight on affected arm and transfers objects from one side of bench to other.

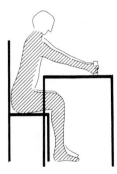

Fig. 16-11. Shoulder protraction demonstrated during bilateral activity of upper limbs.

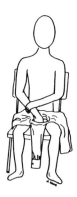

Fig. 16-12. Dressing training. Shirt positioned across patient's knees, arm hole visible, and sleeve dropped between knees.

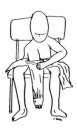

Fig. 16-13. Patient bends forward at hips (inhibiting extension synergy of lower extremity) and places affected hand into sleeve.

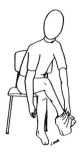

Fig. 16-14. Proper position while putting on pants and underclothes.

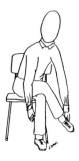

Fig. 16-15. Proper position while putting on shoes and socks.

Practical application in occupational therapy activities

DRESSING ACTIVITIES

Purpose. The patient learns to inhibit his or her own spasticity. The procedure breaks up typical hemiplegic patterns of lower extremity extension synergy and upper extremity flexion synergy. Using the NDT approach, dressing is learned faster than traditional, one-handed methods, especially for patients with perceptual problems. The patient learns to carry over techniques of inhibition into daily living skills.

Tips. The patient should not attempt to get dressed in bed. Instead, the patient should be seated on a (preferably normal) chair next to the bed. The therapist should *always* assist from the affected side. Always begin dressing with the hemiplegic side. The same sequence in dressing is maintained to increase learning.

PROCEDURE

Donning shirt (Figs. 16-12 and 16-13)

1. Position shirt across patient's knees with arm hole visible and sleeve between knees.
2. Bend forward at hips (inhibiting extension synergy of the lower extremity), placing affected hand in sleeve.
3. Arm drops into sleeve; shoulder protraction and gravity inhibit upper extremity flexion synergy.
4. Bring collar to neck.
5. Sit upright, dress nonhemiplegic side.
6. Button shirt from bottom to top.

Donning underclothes and pants (Fig. 16-14)

1. Clasp hands and cross affected leg over nonhemiplegic leg. (Therapist helps when needed.)
2. Release hands. Hemiplegic arm can "dangle" but should not be trapped in lap.
3. Pull pant leg over hemiplegic foot.
4. Clasp hands to uncross leg.
5. Place nonhemiplegic foot in pant leg (no need to cross legs). This is difficult, since the patient must bear weight on hemiplegic side.
6. Pull pants to knees.
7. While holding onto waistband, patient stands with therapist's facilitation.
8. Zip and snap pants.
9. Therapist facilitates patient returning to sitting position.

Donning shoes and socks (Fig. 16-15)

1. Clasp hands and cross legs (as before).
2. Put sock and shoe on hemiplegic foot.
3. Cross nonhemiplegic leg, put on sock and shoe.

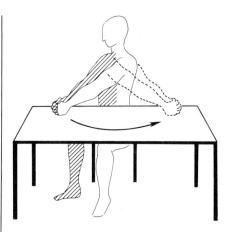

Fig. 16-16. Bilateral activity incorporating trunk rotation.

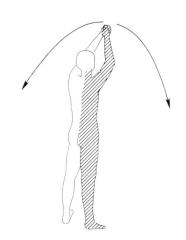

Fig. 16-17. Proper position in standing for activities incorporating bilateral use of upper extremities.

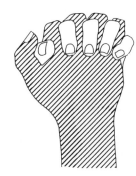

Fig. 16-18. During bilateral activity and when in sitting position, hands are clasped as shown. Shaded hand is affected one. NOTE: hemiplegic thumb is always on top.

THERAPEUTIC ACTIVITIES. Therapeutic activities that encourage weight bearing on the hemiplegic side (see Figs. 16-8 and 16-9) in sitting and standing positions must be included in the treatment program. The purposes of weight bearing are to provide proprioceptive input to the hemiplegic side, encourage more normal postural tone and balance reactions, decrease fear, reduce spasticity, and prevent contractures of the wrist and fingers.

Bilateral activities (Figs. 16-16 and 16-17) with hands clasped together (Fig. 16-18) are used to increase awareness of the hemiplegic side, increase sensory input to the hemiplegic side, bring the affected arm into the visual field, begin "purposeful" movement of the hemiplegic arm, discourage flexion synergy by protraction of the scapula and extension of the elbow and wrist, develop abduction of fingers and thumb that discourages spasticity of the hand, and teach the patient reflex inhibiting patterns that he or she can perform without any help.

The positions just described should be incorporated into all activities in occupational therapy. Each therapeutic activity can be done sitting or standing, depending on the level of the patient's progress. At every possible opportunity the patient should be treated in a normal chair (or standing) instead of the wheelchair to obtain maximal benefit.

The following two activity plans demonstrate how the Bobath principles can be applied to activities. Positioning of the patient, goals, therapist facilitation, common errors, correction, and variations are included. This format can be used to design many other activities.

THE SHOULDER IN HEMIPLEGIA

The variety of problems relating to the hemiplegic shoulder are often frustrating and confusing to the occupational therapist. Spasticity and pain can hinder the entire rehabilitation program. It is the responsibility of therapists to learn how to evaluate these problems and prepare a treatment program that is effective in dealing with them. It is important to understand the basic anatomy and functional mechanism of the shoulder girdle. Those interested in expanding their knowledge in this area are directed to readings

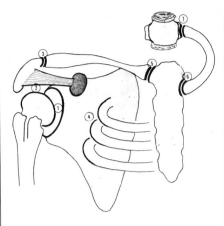

Fig. 16-19. Composite drawing of shoulder girdle. (Reproduced with permission from Cailliet, R.: The shoulder in hemiplegia, Philadelphia, 1980, F.A. Davis Co.)

from the references, particularly *The Shoulder in Hemiplegia* by Rene Cailliet.[3]

The shoulder girdle is made up of seven joints (Fig. 16-19): (1) glenohumeral, (2) suprahumeral, (3) acromioclavicular, (4) scapulocostal, (5) sternoclavicular, (6) costosternal, and (7) costovertebral.

To have full pain-free range of motion (ROM), all seven joints need to be working synchronously. The glenohumeral joint allows for considerable mobility but is unfortunately an unstable joint. It is dependent on the proper alignment of the scapula and humerus (for mechanical support) as well as the supraspinatus.

It is important to understand the relationship of the scapula to the humerus and its significance in pain-free shoulder flexion and abduction. When the arm is raised in forward flexion or abduction, the scapula must glide and rotate upward. The humerus and the scapula work in unison; more specifically, they work in a 2:1 ratio pattern. In other words, if the shoulder moves 90° of abduction, the humerus will move 60° while the scapula moves 30°. Another example might be 180° of shoulder flexion in which the humerus would move 120° and the scapula 60° (again, a 2:1 ratio).[3]

If for any reason the arm is raised in shoulder flexion or abduction without the scapula gliding along, joint trauma and pain can occur. It is imperative that the therapist is aware of this and should be taken into consideration dur-

ing ROM, ADL, transfers, and all other activities.

In the hemiplegic shoulder the muscles that move the scapula in downward rotation (rhomboids, latissimus dorsi, and levator scapulae) are often spastic. This makes it difficult for the scapula to glide upward, which is necessary for pain-free movement. The scapula must first be mobilized and the spasticity reduced to regain the ROM and allow for selective movement. The arm must never be fully raised before the scapula has been mobilized and the therapist can feel its gliding movements. Even in a flaccid arm the scapula can be influenced by spasticity of the rhomboids, trapezius, and latissimus dorsi. The techniques previously described will assist the therapist.

Because the hemiplegic shoulder is often pulled back into retraction, the emphasis of treatment is placed on protraction of the scapula. By protracting the scapula, the patient is able to reduce the hypertonicity of the upper extremity, allowing for more isolated movement and selective control. When the spasticity is too strong for the patient to obtain protraction of the shoulder, the therapist must assist. The therapist should use reflex inhibiting patterns to control and reduce spasticity. As Bobath stated, "The main reflex inhibiting pattern counteracting spasticity in the trunk and arm is the extension of neck and spine and external rotation of the arm at the shoulder with elbow extended. Further reduction of flexor spasticity can be obtained by adding extension of the wrist with supination and abduction of the thumb"[2] (Fig. 16-20).

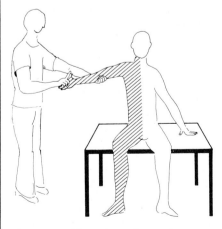

Fig. 16-20. Therapist assists patient to obtain reflex-inhibiting pattern for arm.

Occupational therapy application: activities

"BOWLING" WITH LIGHTWEIGHT BALL	LINOLEUM BLOCK PRINTING

"BOWLING" WITH LIGHTWEIGHT BALL

Positioning of patient
Sitting on chair or bench
Trunk and hips forward
Shoulders forward
Arm hanging down
Knees 90°

Common errors	Correction
Patient "braces" with unaffected arm, causing associated reactions.	Bring both arms forward.
Patient tries to swing arm too hard, increasing flexor spasticity.	Encourage light movements.
Patient uses back by sitting up rather than arm.	Keep patient forward.
Patient slides hemiplegic foot under instead of flat on floor.	Bring weight over hemiplegic side.

  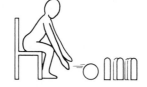

Goals
Symmetry of body
Bringing weight forward
Isolated control of shoulder flexion and wrist extension
Facilitation of finger extension
Shoulder protraction

What therapist does
Stands on hemiplegic side (one hand on hemiplegic shoulder, especially for patients with poor balance)
Guides patient through movement until moving independently
Stops patient if spasticity increases, repositions
Checks position throughout activity

Variations
Pins placed to left or right; encourages head rotation and compensation for neglect
Both hands clasped together to bowl
Size of ball
Box or crate as goal instead of pins
Number or color pins; makes game more challenging

LINOLEUM BLOCK PRINTING

Positioning of patient
Standing with table directly in front
Weight evenly distributed on both feet
Feet comfortably apart
Hands clasped around grip
Ink or paint on hemiplegic side

Common errors	Correction
Patient puts weight only on unaffected leg.	Stand closer to patient; use firmer contact.
Patient leans against table too much.	Help patient to find balance point.
Patient buckles knee.	Position therapist's leg to control patient's leg.
Patient presses unevenly or printing block pulls back.	Keep shoulder forward, support under elbow.

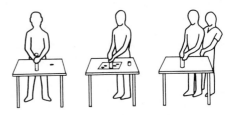

Goals
Trunk rotation
Increased standing (or sitting) tolerance
Increased awareness of hemiplegic side (good compensation training for hemianopsia)
Bilateral use of upper extremities
Increased shoulder protraction, elbow extension

What therapist does
Stands on patient's hemiplegic side
Places hands on patient's hips to facilitate weight bearing onto hemiplegic leg
Checks hands
Checks elbows for good extension

Variations
Shape and size of grip
Sitting instead of standing
Size of paper
Complexity of design
Placement of paint to increase trunk rotation
Stencil used to reduce complexity

Subluxation

Many professionals are particularly afraid of the subluxed shoulder. Numerous efforts are made to protect it and "prevent" it. Subluxation cannot be "prevented." If the muscles around the shoulder girdle, which are attached to the humerus, are weak enough, the shoulder will be subluxed. Slings do not help subluxation. They only keep the arm in a poor position and may contribute to pain and swelling. Subluxation itself does not cause pain. The pain is caused by the improper *handling* of a subluxed arm. Forcing the head of the humerus back into place can cause trauma and pain. Doing standard ROM procedures on an arm without a gliding scapula can also cause pain. Treatment of the subluxed arm should include proper sitting (see Figs. 16-6 and 16-7), weight bearing (see Figs. 16-8 and 16-9), and mobilization of the scapula and proper positioning in bed (see Figs. 16-3 to 16-6).

Slings

The application of a sling to the hemiplegic arm is a source of considerable controversy. However, it has been demonstrated over the past several years that "the commonly used hemiplegic sling has no appreciable effect on ultimate ROM, subluxation, pain, or peripheral nerve traction injury."[8] It has also been stated that "there is no need to support a pain free shoulder in order to prevent or correct subluxation since the sling does not prevent, improve, cure or reduce such a deformity."[7] The use of a sling on the hemiplegic arm can actually contribute to subluxation and lead to a painful, disabling condition called the shoulder-hand syndrome. It is important to realize that when a patient wears a sling, the arm is supported in a position that is typical of the typical hemiplegic posture and discourages the patient from using the arm either bilaterally or unilaterally. Even the sling previously described by the Bobaths[2] is *no longer being used*. It was found that this sling hindered the circulation of the arm and pushed the head of the humerus into lateral subluxation as well. There is no need to apply a sling to the hemiplegic arm.

The nonfunctional arm

Even if the upper extremity has no potential for functional use, the trunk and arm must be retrained for bilateral activity. At all times the arm should be in front of the body where it can be seen and not hanging down to the side. If emphasis is placed only on the unaffected arm, the client will lose potential for sensory and motor recovery of the affected arm.[2]

PREPARING THE PATIENT FOR HOME

The benefits of the treatment program will be lost if the client is not adequately prepared for returning home. This preparation should include prescribing a home exercise program, family education, and communication with the follow-up therapist if necessary. The hospital or clinic is a very secure setting, and it is very important that both the client and family feel comfortable and confident on their return home. The home exercise program is important to maintain mobilization and movement. The therapist should select exercises that can be done easily and correctly without assistance. If stress is used to complete the exercises, it is likely that the client will form "bad habits" and spasticity will increase.

After the selection of exercises the therapist must train the client in each of them. To encourage consistency the client should follow the same sequence of exercises each day. This should begin long before discharge from occupational therapy so that it is a well-established part of the daily routine.

Each exercise should be written down in the proper sequence. This should include how often they should be done, for example, twice a day; number of repetitions, for example, 10 times each; and diagrams if necessary.

Next the family should be trained so they are also well-acquainted with each exercise. Thus they can guide the home program properly. For best results in family teaching the occupational therapist should demonstrate tasks, explaining the importance; emphasize each major point, for example, position of arm and placement of hands; have the family work with the client under the therapist's guidance; and repeat instructions as often as needed until the family

and client are confident enough to do the exercises at home alone. Family education should include a home exercise program and ADL training in areas of dressing, eating, grooming, hygiene, bathing, transfers, and cooking. This program should also include instruction in proper positioning (lying, sitting, and standing) and proper use of equipment. Before discharge from the treatment center the therapist should give the family his or her name and work telephone number, set up a date for a reevaluation if necessary, and contact the therapist treating the client following discharge from the treatment facility to ensure proper carry over.

General treatment principles[5]

1. Never exercise—*retrain!* The brain knows patterns and movements, not muscles and bones.
2. Start and finish a treatment session with something positive, something the patient can do well.
3. Use slow, controlled movements—fast movements can increase spasticity.
4. The patient must find the treatment useful, purposeful, and meaningful.
5. Do not magnify pain by dwelling on it.
6. If the patient thinks there has been no progress, it may be caused by memory loss.
7. Proper sequence of activities leads to success.
8. After spasticity is inhibited, follow with a purposeful movement—put it to use! Do not inhibit spasticity unless you plan to use the limb.
9. Do not ask a patient who is influenced by spasticity to relax—he or she cannot.
10. Encourage the patient to look at his or her arm.
11. Tell the patient when he or she has done a movement correctly so the client can *feel* it.
12. It is of great importance to train proprioceptive, tactile, and spatial sensation.
13. Discourage stressful or excessive efforts of the sound arm, which increase associated reactions of the affected arm.
14. Ask for "automatic movements" to reduce stress. The patient then will think about the activity rather than the arm.
15. If spasticity starts, *stop!*
16. The patient often has to relearn movements, even on his "good" side.

Popular misconceptions about adult hemiplegia[5]

1. Shoulder subluxation causes pain.
2. A person with hemiplegia has a normal side.
3. Slings prevent shoulder subluxation.
4. The harder the client tries, the better the client will get.
5. Strength is more important than control.
6. Hemianopsia is the primary reason for neglect of the hemiplegic side.
7. Hemiplegia of long standing cannot be changed.
8. Return of sensation is totally dependent on the lesion.
9. Walking is enough of a rehabilitation goal.
10. If the affected arm has no functional use, forget it.
11. An arm with an intravenous drain in place is an immobilized arm.

SUMMARY

The NDT approach was developed by Karel and Berta Bobath. It may be effectively used with a wide variety of CNS dysfunctions but is most widely known for its application in treatment of cerebral palsy and adult hemiplegia.

The NDT approach is based on normal neuromotor development and function. Its primary goal is to enhance the relearning of normal movement patterns. Special techniques of positioning and motion are used to inhibit spasticity, abnormal patterns of movement, and abnormal reflex activity.

Emphasis is on treating the client as a whole rather than using an isolated approach to treatment of the arm, leg, or trunk. Quality of movement, control, and coordination are developed through the treatment techniques rather than muscle strength and joint motion per se.

Sensory reeducation and involvement of the family in the rehabilitation program are important elements in this approach to treatment.

REVIEW QUESTIONS

1. What is the fundamental or primary goal of the NDT approach?
2. List three advantages of this approach stated in the text.
3. What are the elements of an NDT evaluation?
4. List four factors that can cause or increase spasticity.
5. Describe the vicious cycle that may occur that contributes to the maintenance of spasticity.
6. What are some of the factors that contribute to the neglect of the hemiplegic side?
7. Describe the positions that Bobath recommends to reduce this neglect in sitting and standing.
8. What are the purposes of trunk rotation? Bilateral activities?
9. Describe recommended positioning and mobilization procedures used to prevent shoulder pain and severe spasticity around the shoulder and shoulder girdle.
10. How is subluxation treated in the NDT approach?
11. What is the role of the occupational therapist in preparing the patient to go home?
12. Why does Bobath stress scapula protraction in positioning and movement of the hemiplegic arm?
13. According to the NDT approach how should the hemiplegic arm be positioned when the client is seated? What is the rationale for this position?
14. Describe and assume the typical posture of the adult hemiplegic.
15. What is meant by "trunk shortening?" What is its cause?
16. Why is the common hemiplegic sling contraindicated?

REFERENCES

1. Affolter, F.: Perceptual processes as prerequisites for complex human behavior, Bern, Switzerland, 1980, Hans Huber A.G.
2. Bobath, B.: Adult hemiplegia: evaluation and treatment, London, 1978, William, Heinemann, Ltd.
3. Cailliet, R.: The shoulder in hemiplegia, Philadelphia, 1980, F.A. Davis Co.
4. Cash, J.: Neurology for physiotherapists, London, 1977, Faber & Faber, Ltd.
5. Davies, P.: Treatment techniques for adult hemiplegia, study course, Bäderklinik, Valens, Switzerland, 1979.
6. Eggers, O.: Occupational therapy in the treatment of adult hemiplegia, London, 1982, William Heinemann Medical Books, Ltd.
7. Friedland, F.: Physical therapy. In Licht, S., editor: Stroke and its rehabilitation, Baltimore, 1975, Williams & Wilkins.
8. Hurd, M.M., Farrell, K.H., and Waylonis, F.W.: Shoulder sling for hemiplegia: friend or foe? Arch. Phys. Med. Rehabil. 55:519, 1974.

CHAPTER 17

The proprioceptive neuromuscular facilitation approach

NANCY D. THOMPSON

This chapter presents an overview of proprioceptive neuromuscular facilitation (PNF), which is a system of therapeutic exercise based on normal motor behavior. It includes methods for facilitating motor learning that are useful to all persons.[25]

The purpose of this chapter is to outline and present the principles and representative procedures of PNF and to convey to students of physical dysfunction a significant philosophy. PNF stimulates more than muscle control. It involves the therapist and another human being with the ideas of potential, cooperation, challenge, coordination, and function.

To understand PNF knowledge of anatomy, kinesiology, neurophysiology, normal development, motor behavior, and motor learning is essential. Many of the principles and procedures of PNF are applicable to functional activities that are in the domain of occupational therapy. In order for occupational therapists to apply PNF supervised classroom practice and clinical training by a qualified instructor are necessary. Individual study and PNF courses should include methods that integrate the head, trunk, and all extremities.[24]

If occupational therapists are to apply the principles and methods of PNF or any of the sensorimotor approaches to activities, it is necessary for them to understand the approaches and each approach's principles, rationale, and methods.[18]

There is a great need for activity analysis within the frame of reference of sensorimotor approaches in occupational therapy. Occupational therapists who apply these approaches can effectively participate in the continuum of treatment from facilitation-inhibition techniques and preparatory exercise to purposeful activity.[18]

HISTORY

Kabat,[25] neurophysiologist and physician, conceived of PNF as a treatment for paralysis. He worked on its development from 1946 to 1951 at what is now the Kaiser Foundation Rehabilitation Center in Vallejo, California.[15]

Knott and Voss,[25] physical therapists, expanded Kabat's ideas to an approach to therapeutic exercise.[25] They applied its principles and procedures to the evaluation and treatment of patients with neurological and orthopedic conditions.[21] By refining applications of PNF to mat, gait, and self-care activities they provided a means for occupational and physical therapists to design individual treatment plans based on normal human motion and development. Although no specific procedures have been developed since 1951,[15] a wide variety of applications have progressed to meet the needs of selected patients.*

THEORETICAL FOUNDATION

"In developing the techniques of the method, Kabat relied upon his knowledge of the physiology of Sherrington."[25] In addition, the work of Gellhorn, Coghill, McGraw, Gesell, and Pavlov among others was used as supportive evidence for the approach.[4,25]

A unique feature of the PNF approach is the use of specific spiral and diagonal patterns of movement that are based on normal developmental motor patterns and occur in normal motor performance.[26] "From extensive observation, it is apparent that the fundamental mass movement patterns are all diagonal movements rather than straight movements."[8] Diagonal patterns were first observed in normal individuals. They were modified by trial and error for use in treatment. Patterns were used because they facilitate the patient's ability for movement and for stabilization and therefore for function.

---

*References 3, 5, 9-15, 20-28.

Thus Kabat considered neurophysiology, motor behavior, mass movement patterns, and motor learning as fundamental to PNF.

In 1954 Ayres, an occupational therapist, summarized her analysis of PNF with the following statement:

It seems that the fundamental organization of the neuromuscular system is based on function. When something disturbs that fundamental organization, it is reasonable to presume that treatment might well be based on function—on activities simulating simple, normal, life-like processes utilizing neurophysiological mechanisms recognized for the integrative role they play. This approach is found inherently in the techniques of occupational therapy. However, even though this sounds very logical, it has not been found to be entirely practical.[1]

There is little doubt that the neurophysiological rationale exists for much of PNF as it is currently applied.[4,6,7,15,21] However, the current body of knowledge is incomplete, and the "success" of some techniques is difficult to explain.

PRINCIPLES OF TREATMENT

The principles of treatment are based on normal growth and development. The more the therapist understands about normal development, the more insight the therapist brings to patient treatment.

It is essential that the student of PNF understand and continue to review the principles of PNF. Voss presented the following principles during the Northwestern University Special Therapeutic Exercise Project (NUSTEP) in 1966.[25]

First principle

The first principle is also the philosophy of the PNF approach. It states that "all human beings have potentials that have not been fully developed."[25] This concept underlies the treatment of the patient. PNF emphasizes ability rather than disability and taps the abilities and potentials of the patient in such a way as to reduce dysfunction.[25]

Second principle

"Normal motor development proceeds in a cervicocaudal and proximodistal direction." This principle is fundamental in treatment.[25]

Third principle

"Early motor behavior is dominated by reflex activity. Mature motor behavior is reinforced or supported by postural reflexes."[25] Because development proceeds from reflex activity toward selective motor control, reflex mechanisms are used to reinforce the voluntary efforts of the patient.[25]

Fourth principle

"Early motor behavior is characterized by spontaneous movement."[25] An infant's movements fluctuate between flexion and extension. This rhythmic and reversing character of movement remains throughout life. Spontaneous movement in early development proceeds toward the development of the ability to perform deliberate, goal-directed activity. Performance of functional tasks relies on the ability to reverse the direction of movement.[25]

Fifth principle

"Developing motor behavior is expressed in an orderly sequence of total patterns of movement and posture."[25] These patterns require an orderly sequence of interaction between movements of the head, neck, trunk, and extremities.[25]

Sixth principle

"The growth of motor behavior has cyclic trends, as evidenced by shifts between flexor dominance and extensor dominance."[25] The reciprocal relationship between flexion and extension is established by shifts between a dominance of one or the other until motor control develops.[25] In treatment flexor or extensor dominance can be facilitated until the patient attains a functional balance between flexion and extension.

Seventh principle

"Normal motor development has an orderly sequence, but lacks step by step quality."[25] In the treatment of the patient the next phase may begin before the previous one is complete. The patient will benefit from an approach that overlaps the performance of total patterns.

Eighth principle

"Normal movement and posture are dependent upon 'synergism' and a balanced interaction of antagonists."[25] In treatment prevention and correction of imbalances between antagonistic pairs of movements, reflexes, muscles, and components of joint motions are objectives.

Ninth principle

"Improvement of motor ability is dependent upon motor learning."[25] Motor learning ranges from the conditioning of responses to the mastery of complex voluntary motor acts. In treatment patients are challenged according to their abilities and needs. The therapist selects appropriate sensory cues and uses techniques of facilitation to place demands for appropriate motor activity. Procedures may be used singly or in combination.[25]

Tenth principle

"Frequency of stimulation and repetitive activity are used to promote and for retention of motor learning, and for the development of strength and endurance."[25] Such activity might include structured self-exercise programs, use of weights and pulleys, or resisted functional activities. Occupational therapy can be the logical source for the quality of functional activities needed to enhance the goals just mentioned.

Eleventh principle

"Goal-directed activities coupled with techniques of facilitation are used to hasten learning of total patterns of walking, ascending and descending stairs, and of self-care activities."[25] When facilitation procedures and goal-directed activities are combined, they hasten learning of total patterns and skilled activities. To meet patient needs PNF procedures are superimposed on

functional tasks. For example, a progression from assisted to resisted diagonal 1 flexion, lower extremity pattern on a hemiplegic patient may be used while teaching the patient how to lift the wheelchair footrest in preparation for transfer; also a rhythmic stabilization of the lower trunk while the patient comes to a standing position may enhance all transfers.

PHILOSOPHY OF TREATMENT

In their textbook on PNF Knott and Voss[15] stated that the philosophy of treatment using techniques of PNF is based on the ideas that all human beings respond in accordance with demand; that existing potentials may be developed more fully; that movements must be specific and directed toward a goal; that activity is necessary for the best development of coordination, strength, and endurance; and that the stronger body parts' strengthening of weaker parts through cooperation leads toward a goal of optimal function.

Kabat stated that, after sufficient recovery of function from facilitation, emphasis must be placed on training of habit patterns of motor activity that incorporate the newly recovered voluntary movements into routine activities and essential skills. He further stated that, when the restored motions are used routinely in proper habit patterns of gait, posture, self-care, and hand skills, recovery of function may be expected to be permanent without further facilitation, because the habitual routine motor activities are themselves therapeutic for the involved muscle groups.[7]

A recent development in therapeutic exercise appears to be an effort to integrate PNF with other well-known systems. Sullivan, Markos, and Minor.[21] authors of *An Integrated Approach to Therapeutic Exercise*, stated that their method does not constitute a new approach. Rather, it provides students and clinicians with the common terminology required "to recognize and evaluate the component parts of a therapeutic exercise procedure."[21] These components are procedure, activity, technique, and elements; they are defined in the following sections. Using an integrated approach the practitioner is free to think generically about cause and effect. Therapists may become conceptually fluent in therapeutic exercise as a whole instead of being encumbered during one treatment session with translations of the approaches of Brunnstrom, Bobath, Rood, and PNF. Although beyond the scope of this text, the reader is alerted to this promising approach in the hope that therapists' understanding and application of treatment might be more objective, efficient, comprehensive, and easily shared through practice, documentation, and research.

TREATMENT PLANNING

Treatment planning is a process that includes evaluation, analysis of data, development of a treatment plan, patient treatment, and patient reevaluation.[21] The result is a treatment plan designed for the individual patient. The key to effective treatment planning is the quality of communication the therapist has with others about the treatment procedures, rationale, and outcomes. The documentation of treatment may be recorded in patient charts, on forms, or in problem-oriented progress notes.

The general sequence of evaluation in the PNF approach is from proximal to distal. It includes *proximal functions* related to breathing; oral functions; facial motions; and movement responses to visual, auditory, and tactile stimuli. *Head and neck patterns* are followed by evaluation of upper trunk, upper extremities (proximal, intermediate, and distal movements), lower trunk, and lower extremities (proximal, intermediate, and distal movements). *Combined patterns* reveal the level of coordination between the extremities and the trunk. The *developmental activities* are based on the postures and movements of the developmental sequence. Often they are a major factor in determining where treatment should begin. They may be combined with the stages of motor control to enhance functional goals, and performance can be recorded on a chart like the one shown in Fig. 17-1. Finally, *self-care activities* including transfers and activities of daily living (ADL) are observed. If the patient is challenged by a realistic environment, the therapist can contrast the ability to perform patterned movement with the ability to complete a functional task. For example, while at the rehabilitation center, a woman with a neurological condition is able to perfom upper trunk patterns and has been trained in bathroom ADL. When she goes home, an inconsistency in performance becomes apparent. The patient is still able to perform trunk patterns, but her endurance, balance, and self-care skills prove inadequate when confronted with the increased challenge of wheelchair mobility on carpeted floors and poor bathroom access. The therapist must reevaluate the patient's performance in the living environment and adjust the treatment plan. If the inconsistency persists, further evaluation of cognitive functions, sensory deficits, endurance, balance, coordination, and motivation is indicated.

TREATMENT PROCEDURES

This section presents a description of some PNF treatment procedures. A full discussion of each is beyond the scope of this chapter. PNF procedures are fully discussed and clearly illustrated in *An Integrated Approach to Therapeutic Exercise*,[21] and the second edition of *Proprioceptive Neuromuscular Facilitation*.[15] Sullivan, Markos, and Minor[21] described the procedures in three units: activities, techniques, and elements.

N = Level of control normal

P = Level of control present but quality is poor

O = Level of control absent

Activities	Stages of motor control				
	Mobility	Stability	Controlled mobility	Static dynamic	Skill
Rolling	N	N	N	N	P
Sitting	N	N	P	P	O
Prone on elbows	N	N	N	P	O
Quadruped	N	N	P	P	O
Modified plantigrade	N	N	P	O	O
Standing	N	P	P	O	O

Evaluation of a patient with variations in motor ability

Fig. 17-1. Chart for recording level of motor control. (From Patricia Sullivan, Prudence Markos, Mary Alice Minor: An integrated approach to therapeutic exercise-theory and clinical application, p. 190, Reprinted with permission of Reston Publishing Company, Inc., A Prentice-Hall Company, 11480 Sunset Hills Road, Reston VA 22090.)

A

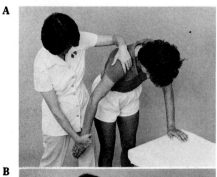

B

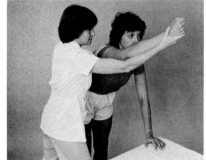

Fig. 17-2. A, Starting position for
D_1UE extension going to flexion. **B,**
Starting position for D_1UE flexion
going to extension.

Activities

Activities of a procedure refer to the
postures of the developmental sequence
and the movements that occur within
those postures. Activities also include
trunk patterns and bilateral and unilateral extremity patterns.[21] Unless otherwise specified, the term *trunk pattern* is
used to include head and neck patterns.

DEVELOPMENTAL SEQUENCE.
Combinations of trunk and extremity
patterns can facilitate the mobility, stability, controlled mobility, and skill involved in each stage of the developmental sequence. The sequence of
developmental movements and postures
includes side lying and rolling, sitting,
pivot prone, prone on elbows, quadruped, bridging, kneeling, half kneeling, modified plantigrade (Fig. 17-2),
standing, and walking.[21] PNF patterns,
techniques, and elements (sensory cues)
are applied in each sequence to improve
muscle control for progress to the next
sequence. They promote the overlapping quality of normal development.

**UNILATERAL EXTREMITY PAT-
TERNS.** Extremity patterns are labeled
as diagonal 1 or diagonal 2, by flexor or

extensor direction as determined by the
movement of the shoulder or hip, and
by the direct involvement of the upper
or lower extremity. Patterns are usually
learned in the following order: unilateral, bilateral, and trunk patterns. The
therapist who understands unilateral
patterns will recognize more clearly
how they combine during bilateral and
trunk patterns. Once learned, the patterns are often applied in the reverse

order to gradually increase the challenge to the patient. Unilateral patterns
represent the most intense muscle activity.[21] Therapists need to know which
muscle groups are activated in each pattern. Although the same muscle groups
may function in several patterns, there
is an optimal pattern of facilitation of
individual muscles.[15,21]

Examples of functional activities follow each unilateral extremity pattern to

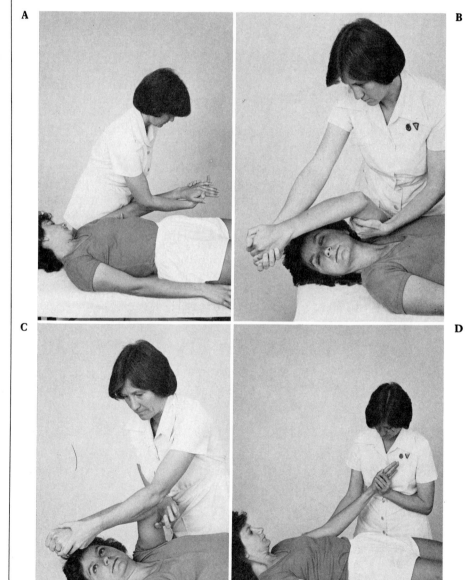

Fig. 17-3. D_1UE, supine. **A,** D_1UE extension going to flexion. **B,** D_1UE
flexion. **C,** D_1UE flexion going to extension. **D,** D_1UE extension.

help the reader visualize the components. The therapist needs to be able to identify patterns in normal activities and patient-care activities. Functional activities use partial diagonals; this further challenges the therapist's ability to identify and understand patterned movement. Unilateral extremity patterns include the following diagonals.

Diagonal 1 upper extremity.[15,21] As the arm moves up and across the chest into flexion, the fingers and wrist flex and radially deviate; the thumb adducts; the elbow flexes or remains extended throughout the movement pattern; the shoulder flexes, adducts, and externally rotates; the scapula elevates, abducts, and upwardly rotates (Fig. 17-3, *A* and *B*). This portion of diagonal 1 upper extremity (D_1UE) is used when putting on a right earring with the left hand, screwing in a light bulb above and in front of self, or reaching up and across the chest to adjust a pillow.

To complete the D_1UE pattern the arm moves down and away from the chest into extension. The fingers and wrist extend and deviate to the ulnar side. The thumb abducts, and the elbow extends or remains extended throughout the movement pattern. The shoulder extends, abducts, and internally rotates, and the scapula moves into depression, adduction, and downward rotation (Fig. 17-3, *C* and *D*).

The extension components of D_1UE occur during activities, such as reaching down to pick up a briefcase on the same side, reaching toward the wheelchair brake on the same side, or reaching down to adjust a car radio on the same side.

Diagonal 2 upper extremity.[15,21] As the arm moves up and away from the chest into flexion, the fingers and wrist extend and radially deviate; the thumb extends; the elbow extends or remains extended throughout the movement; the shoulder flexes, abducts, and externally rotates; and the scapula elevates, adducts, and upwardly rotates (Fig. 17-4, *A* and *B*).

The sequence of the diagonal 2 upper extremity D_2UE can be observed as a person reaches to a higher level while rope climbing, as children enthusiastically raise their hands at school, or as a hitchhiker signals for a ride.

To complete the D_2UE pattern the arm moves down and across the chest into extension. The fingers and wrist flex and deviate to the ulnar side. The thumb opposes the fingers. The elbow flexes or remains extended throughout the movement pattern. The shoulder extends, adducts, and internally rotates, and the scapula moves into depression, abduction, and downward rotation (Fig. 17-4, *C* and *D*). The extension components of D_2UE are seen as a baseball pitcher throws a ball or as a tennis player makes a serve.

Upper extremity patterns can be performed in many postures, including supine, prone, sitting, quadruped, and modified plantigrade. The techniques and elements outlined in the following discussion can be superimposed on these patterns according to the desired goals.

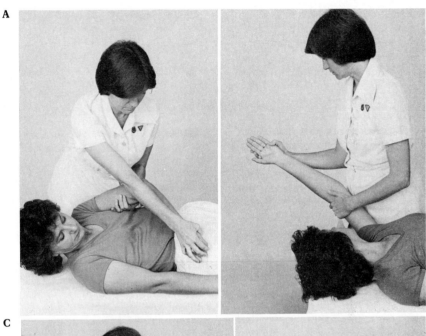

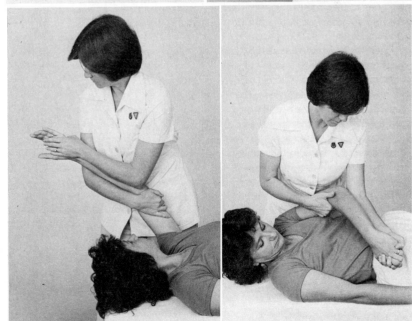

Fig. 17-4. D_2UE, supine. **A,** D_2UE extension going to flexion. **B,** D_2UE flexion. **C,** D_2UE flexion going to extension. **D,** D_2UE extension.

Diagonal 1 lower extremity.[15,21] The diagonal 1 lower extremity (D_1LE) patterns are the same proximally as the upper extremity patterns. As the leg moves forward and across the midline into flexion, the ankle and toes dorsiflex and invert; the knee may extend or may remain extended throughout the movement pattern; the hip flexes, adducts, and externally rotates; and the pelvis protracts. This portion of the D_1LE pattern is seen when a football player kicks a field goal.

To complete the D_1LE pattern the leg moves behind and away from the midline into extension. The ankle and toes evert and plantar flex. The knee flexes or remains extended throughout the movement pattern. The hip extends, abducts, and internally rotates. The pelvis retracts. This sequence is used in preparation for stepping backward up to a curb or in preparation for kicking a ball.

Diagonal 2 lower extremity.[15,21] The D_2LE patterns combine different rotational components. As the leg moves forward and away from the midline into flexion, the ankle and toes dorsiflex and evert; the knee extends or remains extended throughout the movement pattern; the hip flexes, abducts, and internally rotates; and the pelvis elevates. This portion of the D_2LE pattern is seen as the track athlete brings one leg forward and over the top of a hurdle.

To complete the D_2LE pattern the leg moves behind and toward the midline into extension. The ankle and toes plantar flex and invert. The knee flexes or remains extended throughout the movement pattern. The hip extends, adducts, and externally rotates. The pelvis moves into depression. This sequence is used when a soldier moves one foot behind the other in preparation for an "about face" maneuver.

BILATERAL EXTREMITY PATTERNS. Bilateral patterns combine both of the upper or lower extremities in simultaneous exercise. The following

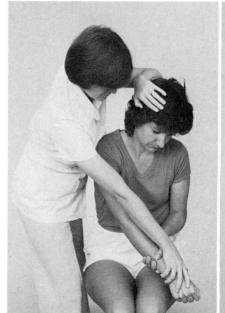 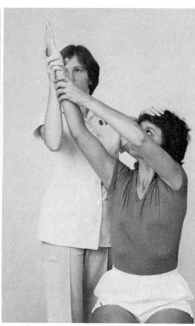

Fig. 17-5. Lifting, seated with manual contacts on head and wrist (manual contacts may vary). **A,** Starting position of lift to the right. **B,** The arms move bilaterally and asymmetrically (leading arm in D_2 and assisting arm in D_1) into flexion; the head, neck, and upper trunk extend with rotation to the right.

descriptions of PNF activities (in reduced type) are excerpts from *An Integrated Approach to Therapeutic Exercise.**

Bilateral symmetrical patterns (BS)
The bilateral performance of one diagonal pattern (D_1 or D_2) by either both upper or both lower extremities. Movement of both extremities occurs simultaneously in the same direction—that is, both limbs flex or extend together.

Reciprocal symmetrical patterns or bilateral reciprocal (BR)
The reciprocal performance of one diagonal pattern (D_1 or D_2) by either both upper or both lower extremities. Movement of both extremities occurs in different directions—that is, one limb flexes while the other extends in the same diagonal pattern.

Bilateral asymmetrical patterns (BA)
The bilateral performance of the two diagonals (D_1 and D_2) by either both upper or both lower extremities. Movement of both extremities occurs simultaneously in the same direction—that is, both limbs flex or extend together.

*From Patricia Sullivan, Prudence Markos, Mary Alice Minor: An integrated approach to therapeutic exercise-theory and clinical application, pp. 13-14, Reprinted with permission of Reston Publishing Company, Inc., A Prentice-Hall Company, 11480 Sunset Hills Road, Reston, VA 22090.

Reciprocal asymmetrical or crossed diagonal patterns (RA, CD)
The reciprocal performance of the two diagonal patterns (D_1 and D_2) by either both upper or both lower extremities. Movement of both extremities occurs simultaneously in different directions—that is, one limb flexes in D_1 while the other extends in D_2.

TRUNK PATTERNS. Upper trunk patterns are made up of asymmetrical upper extremity patterns combined with head, neck, and upper trunk movement. They include the chop and the lift. Lower trunk patterns are usually performed in the supine or sitting positions but are also applicable during activities of the developmental sequence. Like upper trunk patterns, these patterns also combine asymmetrical extremity patterns.

Upper trunk
CHOP:
An upper trunk flexion pattern that combines bilateral asymmetrical extensor patterns of the upper extremities—for example, chopping to the right combines D_1 extension of the right upper extremity and D_2 extension of the left upper extremity. Chopping may be easier for the patient to perform than bilateral asymmetrical patterns because the body-on-body contact results in a closed kinematic chain.

LIFT:

An upper trunk extension pattern that combines bilateral asymmetrical flexor patterns of the upper extremities—for example, lifting to the right combines D_2 flexion of the right upper extremity and D_1 flexion of the left upper extremity. Lifting may be easier for a patient to perform than bilateral asymmetrical patterns because the body-on-body contact results in a closed kinematic chain (Fig. 17-5).

Lower trunk

LOWER TRUNK FLEXION (LTF):

A lower trunk flexor pattern combines bilateral asymmetrical flexor patterns of the lower extremities . . . (Fig. 17-6).

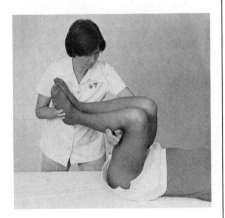

Fig. 17-6. Lower trunk flexion with rotation to left.

LOWER TRUNK EXTENSION (LTE):

A lower trunk extensor pattern that combines bilateral asymmetrical extensor patterns of the lower extremities. . . . As with the upper trunk patterns, there is a closed kinematic chain in both lower trunk patterns resulting from the body-on-body contact of the two legs in approximation with each other (Fig. 17-7).

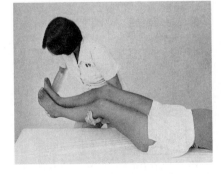

Fig. 17-7. Lower trunk extension with rotation to right.

Techniques

PNF techniques are superimposed on the patterns and the developmental sequence to promote desired types of muscular contractions for the achievement of functional goals. They may also be used with traditional exercise, to increase range of motion, strengthen muscles, and minimize pain. Techniques are used in conjunction with the four stages of motor control: mobility, stability, controlled mobility, and skill.[21] The techniques that are most useful in the training of functional tasks are outlined in this discussion.

RHYTHMIC INITIATION. Rhythmic initiation is used to promote mobility in patients with hypertonicity or with motor planning dysfunction. Movement of the body part progresses from assistive to active-assistive to active-resistive.[21] For instance, a patient with Parkinson's disease holds a comb and is asked to relax and let the therapist move it. The therapist repeats the movement slowly and rhythmically and says to the patient in a soothing voice, "Now you do it with me." When some active control becomes evident, mild resistance is applied to facilitate increased mobility. Then the therapist can say, "Now you take it up there all by yourself."

AGONISTIC REVERSAL. Agonistic reversal promotes mobility, controlled mobility, and skill by facilitating reversal of movement.[21] Agonistic reversal is used to help a person learn to slowly lower the arm after bringing a spoon to the mouth. This technique is effective when applied through increments of range in the spastic extremity while attempting to remove a wheelchair armrest, for example.

REPEATED CONTRACTION. Repeated contraction emphasizes movement on one side of the joint to promote strengthening of specific muscles.[21] The quadriplegic patient with poor triceps works on reaching the wheelchair lock as the therapist applies repeated contractions. Use of quick stretch delays fatigue and assists the muscle contraction.

HOLD-RELAX. When there is muscle tightness on one side of the joint, hold-relax promotes relaxation and mobility. It is particularly useful when the

immobility is a result of pain.[21] Hold-relax could be applied in preparation for dressing activities in the patient with a burn and an axillary release.

CONTRACT-RELAX. When there is limitation of motion on one side of the joint, contract-relax promotes relaxation and mobility. It is contraindicated in the presence of pain because of the type of movements used.[21] Contract-relax would be useful as a relaxation technique for the patient with a hemiplegic lower extremity before putting on pants.

RHYTHMIC STABILIZATION. Rhythmic stabilization uses resisted isometric contractions to promote stability (cocontraction) and stabilized motion (controlled mobility).[21] Rhythmic stabilization is applied at different points in the D_1UE pattern to help the patient who has difficulty stabilizing the fork-to-mouth sequence.

Elements

Elements are superimposed on activities and techniques to provide sensory input for facilitation or inhibition of a response. These sensory cues result from proprioceptive stimulation via muscle spindles, Golgi tendon organs, and joint receptors; exteroceptive stimulation via touch and pressure; and auditory and visual stimulation.

Precautions and contraindications are carefully considered and the patient must be monitored for undesirable effects.[21] Application of these elements is quite specific in PNF and is fully described in the references listed at the end of this chapter. Skilled application of these elements within the approach requires study and supervised practice. PNF elements include quick stretch, resistance, manual contacts, visual input, and verbal commands.

APPLICATIONS OF PNF IN OCCUPATIONAL THERAPY

The principles of PNF and the goals of occupational therapy are complementary. The complementary factors include the focus on the ability to perform rather than to compensate with assistive devices, the use of the developmental sequence, the use of the principles of motor learning, and the use of normal patterns of movement. Diagonal patterns can be applied to activities, since they are normal functional patterns of motion.[17]

There is no specific approach for the direct clinical application of PNF to occupational therapy modalities. The occupational therapist must work with the physical therapist, understand the principles and methods of PNF, and apply these within the performance of activity after careful activity analysis.

PNF may be an appropriate choice of treatment in many instances. Suggested applications in occupational therapy are listed under each of the five features identified as unique to PNF by Voss.[26] The five features are human motion, training of coordination, use of maximal resistance, battery of techniques, and tone of voice.

Human motion

"Human motion occurs in mass movement patterns which are spiral and diagonal in nature."[26] These patterns are specific movements in which each joint of a body segment contributes three components of motion. These are flexion and extension combined with abduction or adduction and external or internal rotation. These patterns allow easy elicitation of stretch reflexes. When positioned in the lengthened range of an agonistic or desired pattern, maximal muscle tension in the segment is achieved.[26]

Many everyday activities require diagonal patterns that can be used to enhance motor learning and to reinforce facilitated patterns. When performing a functional task, the pattern often becomes modified. Some examples of diagonals that occur in activities outlined by Myers[17] are listed in the following discussion.

D_1UE can be seen in the everyday activities of combing or brushing hair (opposite side), washing face, brushing teeth, eating, reaching down and pulling up pants, reaching for wallet, balancing, picking things up from floor, and pushing up to stand.

D_2UE is demonstrated when reaching up for objects, holding an umbrella, brushing or combing hair (same side), pulling a light cord, reaching to pull up pants or zipper (opposite side), and ironing.

Bilateral asymmetrical patterns are used in dressing, washing face (one hand assisting the other), sweeping, making a bed, golfing, and ironing.

Bilateral symmetrical patterns are used while lifting a box and placing it, lifting a cake into the oven, and washing the face (using both hands).

The integration of bilateral patterns with appropriate trunk movement can be facilitated in bed activities, wheelchair activities, and dressing.

Patterns performed in the supine, sitting, modified plantigrade, or standing positions prepare the proximal segment for fine hand activities, since multiple muscles are involved in the positioning or movement of even one finger. Facilitation of the entire segment is considered, since the challenge of hand control often exceeds the patient's capacity to supervise using totally voluntary observation and regulation.[16] Mat work using combined patterns may help prepare the proximal segment for performance of skilled life tasks.

Proper use of patterns can enhance patient transfers and self-care. Physical therapy and occupational therapy might overlap in teaching ADL before, during, and after therapeutic pool class.

Woodworking including sawing, planing, filing, sanding, or driving nails may be adapted to achieve facilitation through mass patterns. Weaving, using a punching bag, and wedging clay across the body are other possibilities for mass diagonal patterns.[1]

Toys and games can be excellent for offering the kind of feedback and repetition necessary for rapid motor learning. Those that encourage diagonal movements include shuffleboard, darts, hammering games, push toys, and throwing toys.[1]

Tasks placed diagonally in relation to the patient promote the performance of diagonal patterns.[17] "Functional patterns and patterns of facilitation may differ."[24] When isolated facilitation is the goal, activities requiring grasp and grasp-release must correspond to the appropriate pattern.[24]

Training of coordination

"Training of coordination within patterns of a segment and between segments."[26] Patterns are combined in appropriate ways and at the appropriate time. They are selected when the therapist analyzes motor performance and plans the treatment program accordingly.

Treatment often should begin with trunk patterns or bilateral motion because it is developmentally lower and influences the head, neck, and trunk to help movement of the extremities.[17] The therapist may accomplish this by first superimposing functional tasks on the total pattern of movement and posture (the developmental sequence). Then the therapist increases the patient's challenge by progressing treatment to use combinations that are more difficult, such as trunk or bilateral patterns and finally unilateral patterns. For example, chopping and lifting are performed by the hemiplegic patient to promote trunk balance in preparation for learning to apply a wheelchair brake. PNF overlaps with other sensorimotor approaches in using the stages of motor control and the developmental sequence. Mobility and stability must be integrated before the patient becomes functional in a sequence. Any PNF procedure may be superimposed on these overlapping areas. Occupational therapy applications are limited only by the imagination and skill of the therapist, bearing in mind that there may be times when PNF is not practical.

Occupational therapy departments should be equipped with low mat tables and wall pulleys. The increasing incidence of combined physical therapy and occupational therapy departments solves this problem in some instances.[19] For those patients who can perform a diagonal with normal distal to proximal timing, self-exercise involving preparatory trunk and bilateral upper extremity patterns may precede and facilitate a unilateral self-care activity. An example of such a sequence might proceed as follows: A patient who has had a stroke sits in a wheelchair with side at arm's length from the wall pulleys and pulls with both hands in an unresisted lifting pattern. The patient progresses to a bilateral symmetrical pattern with two pounds resistance. After a rest the patient attempts toothbrushing using a toothbrush with a built-up handle.

Training coordination by combining patterns often proceeds using an indirect approach followed by a direct approach. For example, a patient with a healing thenar skin graft is allowed to perform only active thumb motions. The treatment goal is the achievement of functional opposition, and a prefunctional activity is underway. The short-term goal of active thumb abduction might be indirectly achieved with a resisted upper trunk pattern progressing to a resisted unilateral pattern, such as chopping and D_1UE with the forearm as the distal manual contact. Progress to a direct approach might include repeated contractions followed by a functional pinching activity.

Patients with perceptual deficits and unilateral denial problems benefit from activities that cross the midline and increase body awareness. Combined patterns place gradually increasing perceptual demands on patients. Occupational therapy activities provide a source of the repetition necessary to duplicate normal development.

Use of maximal resistance

"The use of maximal resistance or adjusted resistance (promotes) irradiation of impulses within a pattern, from head and neck and trunk to extremities, or in a reverse sequence."[26] Manual resistance may be employed during various phases of dressing or other self-care tasks. For example, the therapist resists the head and to a lesser degree the forearm of a patient who is pulling up a sock, thus resisting the flexion pattern. The opposite movement (extension) may also be resisted in preparation for pulling up the sock (see contract-relax).

Assessment of the patient's functional strength and normal timing (distal to proximal for free-moving segments and proximal to distal for fixed segments) is possible using graded maximal resistance in a pattern. This is an efficient method for reevaluating short-term goals. Documentation of the quality of the movement sequence is important.

Ideally, the treatment program includes activities that superimpose recuperation and skill on preceding activities that facilitate or relax. Once a patient can perform a pattern with normal timing, irradiation (spread of muscle activity within a pattern) and reinforcement (irradiation between body segments)[15] are accomplished by resisting functional tasks using mat activities, wall pulleys, dental dam, or suspension sling. This equipment might also be used to resist selected patterns in preparation for unresisted functional activities.

Some patients are not candidates for supervised exercise. PNF principles may then be applied by resisting various phases of self-rewarding occupational tasks to increase repetition of desired movements and to maintain patient interest, motivation, and cooperation.

As a final suggestion, resisted patterns may produce the overflow needed to stimulate vital and related functions.

Battery of techniques

"Battery of techniques or procedures which are superimposed upon movement or posture (enhance) performance and (promote) motor learning."[26] These include certain elements, such as manual contacts. The range of techniques and elements varies according to the voluntary effort the therapist is able to elicit from the patient.[26]

Contact stimulation and stretch are useful when stimulating vital functions and related functions. Manual contacts might be applied generally to facilitate voluntary movement by exerting pressure over the appropriate muscle belly. Direct manual contacts are used to facilitate scapular mobility or stability when the therapist's hands are placed on the scapula being exercised. Indirect manual contacts are used to segmentally facilitate mobility when the therapist touches the leg behind the knee and requests the patient to use the same foot to lift the wheelchair footrest.

Manual contacts must be learned in conjunction with each pattern. They may interfere with occupational therapy activities and require modification.[17]

Contact stimulation is usually manual but may be obtained from adaptations, such as built-up handles, weighted bags, cuff weights, or artificial grasping devices.[1]

Tone of voice

"Use of tone of voice (increases) or (decreases) stress."[26] There seems to be a direct relationship between verbal command volume and magnitude of muscle contraction.[6] Voss[26] stated that loud tones of voice are used to promote movement and softer tones are used to encourage stability. Verbal commands may be used during performance of preparatory patterns and during performance of activities, and the tone may be selected to enhance the desired effect. Preparatory and action commands are learned in conjunction with each PNF procedure. They vary according to the patient's age and ability to cooperate, are used during the learning phase, and may be repeated to stimulate maximal effort.[15]

PNF is consistent with criteria for therapeutic application of activity; it is goal directed, has significance at some level to the patient, requires patient involvement, is geared to the improvement of function, is adaptable and gradable, and is selected as a result of the therapist's professional judgment based on proper knowledge and training.[2] The potential to apply PNF to a wider range of activities than is currently being carried out in practice is great.[18]

PNF provides a way to analyze activities in terms of diagonal patterns.[17] The organization of occupational therapy procedures that could link PNF to self-rewarding activities is the challenge to occupational therapists. Self-rewarding activities promote the feedback and repetition that are the keynotes of motor learning. Developing clinical applications for PNF is one way that occupational therapy can enhance motor learning and help the patient close the gap between neuromuscular and functional reeducation.

SUMMARY

This chapter introduces the occupational therapy student to PNF as an approach to treatment. A review of this information should prepare students for further study by outlining PNF procedures and suggesting occupational therapy applications. The understanding and use of PNF procedures during functional activities seem a "natural and logical extension of their use in neuromuscular re-education."[3] Despite the lack of formal research in this area, applying PNF to occupational therapy appears to be gathering momentum.

REVIEW QUESTIONS

1. List the movements that take place during D_2UE (elbow extended).
2. Which unilateral pattern would be selected to facilitate thumb opposition?
3. Discuss five principles of PNF.
4. Why are spiral or diagonal movements used to promote functional reeducation?
5. How does the developmental sequence relate to PNF?
6. How do the stages of motor control relate to PNF and the evaluation of the patient?
7. Name some equipment that might be used to resist patterns once the patient demonstrates normal timing.
8. How can PNF help the occupational therapist in activity analysis?
9. Name two self-care activities that use D_1UE.
10. Discuss the proprioceptive elements as they are applied in PNF.
11. Describe rhythmic stabilization and how it promotes cocontraction.
12. Which PNF technique is useful when range of motion is limited because of muscle tightness on one side of a joint?
13. Name three types of adaptations that might provide contact stimulation.
14. List seven postures and movements of the developmental sequence on which PNF procedures are superimposed.
15. List five elements or sensory cues and techniques of facilitation that are used to facilitate motor learning.

REFERENCES

1. Ayres, A.J.: Proprioceptive facilitation elicited through the upper extremities. III. Specific application to occupational therapy, Am. J. Occup. Ther. **9**:121, 1955.
2. Hopkins, H.L., Smith, H.D., and Tiffany, E.G.: Therapeutic application of activity. In Hopkins, H.L., and Smith, H.D., editors: Willard and Spackman's occupational therapy, ed. 6, Philadelphia, 1983, J.B. Lippincott Co.
3. Humphrey, T.L., and Huddleston, O.L.: Applying facilitation technics to self-care training, Phys. Ther. Rev. **38**:605, 1958.
4. Huss, A.J.: Overview of sensorimotor approaches. In Hopkins, H.S., and Smith, H.D., editors: Willard and Spackman's occupational therapy, ed. 6, Philadelphia, 1983, J.B. Lippincott Co.
5. Ionta, M.K.: Facilitation technics in the treatment of early rheumatoid arthritis, Phys. Ther. Rev. **40**:119, 1960.
6. Johansson, C.A., Kent, B.E., and Shepard, K.F.: Relationship between verbal command volume and magnitude of muscle contraction, Phys. Ther. **63**:1260, 1983.
7. Kabat, H.: Proprioceptive facilitation in therapeutic exercise. In Licht, S., editor: Therapeutic exercise, ed. 2, Baltimore, 1961, Williams & Wilkins.
8. Kabat, H.: Studies on neuromuscular dysfunction. In Payton, O.D., Hirt, S., and Newton, R.A., editors: Neurophysiologic approaches to therapeutic exercise, Philadelphia, 1977, F.A. Davis Co.
9. Knott, M.: Report of a case of Parkinsonism treated with proprioceptive facilitation technics, Phys. Ther. Rev. **37**:229, 1957.
10. Knott, M.: Avulsion of a finger with protracted disability, Phys. Ther. Rev. **38**:52, 1958.
11. Knott, M.: Bulbar involvement with good recovery, J. Am. Phys. Ther. Assoc. **42**:38, 1962.
12. Knott, M.: Neuromuscular facilitation in the treatment of rheumatoid arthritis, Phys. Ther. **44**:737, 1964.
13. Knott, M., and Barufaldi, D.: Treatment of whiplash injuries, Phys. Ther. Rev. **41**:573, 1961.
14. Knott, M., and Mead, S.: Facilitation technics in lower extremity amputations, Phys. Ther. Rev. **40**:587, 1960.
15. Knott, M., and Voss, D.E.: Proprioceptive neuromuscular facilitation, ed. 2, New York, 1968, Harper & Row, Publishers, Inc.
16. Kottke, F.J.: Therapeutic exercise to develop neuromuscular coordination. In Kottke, F.J., Stillwell, G.K., and Lehmann, J.F., editors: Krusen's handbook of physical medicine and rehabilitation, ed. 3, Philadelphia, 1982, W.B. Saunders Co.
17. Myers, B.: Proprioceptive neuromuscular facilitation: treatment of the hemiplegic patient, Workshop, Mills Hospital, San Mateo, Calif., Sept. 24, 1983.
18. Pedretti, L.W.: Proprioceptive neuromuscular facilitation, Lectures, delivered at San Jose State University, San Jose, Calif., 1982-1983.
19. Rud, A.M.: Combining physical therapy and occupational therapy departments: a survey—clinical management in physical therapy, Am. Phys. Ther. Assoc. **3**:1, 1983.
20. Smith, W.D.: Combining wall pulleys and mat activities to total pattern movements, Phys. Ther. **54**:746, 1974.
21. Sullivan, P.E., Markos, P.D., and Minor, M.A.D.: An integrated approach to therapeutic exercise: theory and clinical application, Reston, Va., 1982, Reston Publishing Co., Inc.
22. Torp, M.J.: Adaptations of neuromuscular facilitation technics, Phys. Ther. Rev. **36**:577, 1956.
23. Torp, M.J.: An exercise program for the brain injured, Phys. Ther. Rev. **36**:644, 1956.
24. Voss, D.E.: Proprioceptive neuromuscular facilitation: application of patterns and techniques in occupational therapy, Am. J. Occup. Ther. **13**:191, 1959.
25. Voss, D.E.: Proprioceptive neuromuscular facilitation. In Bouman, H.D., editor: An exploratory and analytical survey of therapeutic exercise: Northwestern University special therapeutic exercise project (NUSTEP), Baltimore, 1967, Williams & Wilkins.
26. Voss, D.E.: Proprioceptive neuromuscular facilitation: the PNF method. In Pearson, P.H., and Williams, C.E., editors: Physical therapy services in the developmental disabilities, Springfield, Ill., 1972, Charles C Thomas, Publisher.
27. Voss, D.E., Knott, M., and Kabat, H.: The application of neuromuscular facilitation in the treatment of shoulder disabilities, Phys. Ther. Rev. **33**:536, 1953.
28. Whitaker, E.W.: A suggested treatment in occupational therapy for patients with multiple sclerosis, Am. J. Occup. Ther. **6**:247, 1950.

CHAPTER 18

Wheelchairs and wheelchair transfers

LORRAINE WILLIAMS PEDRETTI
GREGORY STONE

WHEELCHAIRS

The wheelchair (Fig. 18-1) provides a comfortable and efficient mode of ambulation for those persons whose physical dysfunction makes walking impossible or impracticable. Others who ordinarily walk with supportive devices such as canes or crutches may find a wheelchair helpful when daily activities require speed or physical endurance that would be overtaxing. A wheelchair, for such persons, can enrich life experiences by making activities, such as trips to shopping centers, theaters, amusement parks, and sight-seeing vacations, possible.

In a sense the wheelchair becomes an extension of the self or the body.[5] The user must learn to manage the wheelchair skillfully, safely, and efficiently; learn to measure space and judge speed and distance with the wheelchair; adapt to viewing the world from a different eye level; and cope with the symbolic meaning of the device to the individual and the society.

The collapsible wheelchair enables the attainment of a normal life pattern.[11] Wheelchair accessibility in the community and in public buildings has improved significantly in recent years. Curbs, building entrances, restrooms, buses, airports, airplanes, restaurants, and concert halls have been adapted to accommodate the wheelchair user. Consequently, there are many more wheelchair users about in the community and their presence is no longer rare or unusual.[11]

The wheelchair is an aid to recreation and socialization. Those who are skillful wheelchair users participate in sports, dance, and dramatic productions.[11]

Occupational and physical therapists are usually responsible for measuring the client for a wheelchair, recommending the wheelchair style and accessories that are most appropriate for the client's life-style, and for teaching wheelchair safety and mobility. An individualized wheelchair prescribed for the unique needs of the client is essential to promoting maximal physical independence.

Wheelchair size

Wheelchairs are available in three major sizes: (1) standard or adult size, (2) intermediate or junior size, and (3) children's size. The standard adult size is suitable for most adults. It can be obtained with a wider (20 inches or 50.8 cm) or narrower (16 inches or 40.6 cm) than standard seat width 18 inches or 45.7 cm) to accommodate wide and narrow adults. The intermediate or ju-nior size is suitable for small adults and older children. The children's size is suitable for children less than age 6.[2]

The unprescribed wheelchair is potentially hazardous. Yet "it has been estimated that 80-95 percent of the wheelchairs sold are obtained without professional guidance or prescription." The hazards of the unprescribed wheelchair include undue fatigue, potential trauma, secondary deformity, and failure to achieve optimal function.[11] To effect the best comfort and use efficiency the wheelchair should fit the person who will use it. Therefore the occupational or physical therapist should measure the client, as a preparatory step to completing a wheelchair prescription. Fig. 18-2 illustrates the wheelchair selection chart section of the Everest and Jennings, Inc. wheelchair prescription form. The complete prescription comprises a section for recording the client's measurements and for indicating the selection of wheelchair modifications and accessories.[3]

WHEELCHAIR MEASUREMENT. When properly fitted the wheelchair should conform to the following specifications[5]:

1. The seat width should be 2 inches (5 cm) wider than the widest point across the client's hips or thighs. This is to prevent pressure of the body against the sides of the chair. If braces are worn, the measurement across the hips should include the braces.

2. The seat depth should be 2 or 3 inches (5 to 7 cm) less than the distance from the rear of the buttocks to the inside of the bent knee. The purposes are to distribute weight evenly along the thighs, thus relieving pressure on the buttocks, and to prevent pressure in the popliteal area.

3. To obtain the correct footrest and seat height adjustment, these must be evaluated together. Leg length measurement is taken from the heel

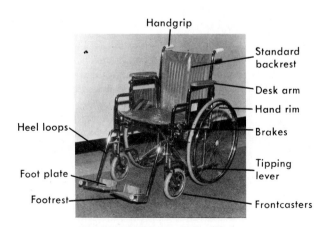

Fig. 18-1. Standard adult wheelchair with detachable desk arms and detachable swing-away footrests.

WHEELCHAIR SELECTION CHART

Wheelchair Specialists:

(1) Using either the "Premier," "Universal" or "Traveler" column, review all major component areas of the wheelchair.
(2) After selecting the correct feature variations, place an "X" in the space provided.
(3) When all selections have been made, transfer the CODE designator to the chart at the bottom of the page.
(4) When the chart has been filled in, it will automatically display the correct sequence of alpha-numeric designators used in the Everest & Jennings Wheelchair model numbers. Refer to Price List for Basic Wheelchair Prices.

	Premier Code	Universal Code	Traveler Code
BASIC WHEELCHAIR TYPE			
"PREMIER" model	P ☐		
"UNIVERSAL" model		U ☐	
"TRAVELER" model			T ☐
CASTER SIZE			
5" diameter (12.5 cm) TT, PST, PSP only	5 ☐	5 ☐	5 ☐
8" diameter (20.3 cm)	8 ☐	8 ☐	8 ☐
CHAIR SIZE (Basic) Seat Width x Depth			
Inches Centimeters			
Adult 18" x 16" 45.72 x 40.64	A ☐	A ☐	A ☐
Narrow Adult 16" x 16" 40.64 x 40.64	N ☐	N ☐	N ☐
Slim Adult 14" x 16" 35.56 x 40.64		S ☐	
Junior 16 16" x 16" 40.64 x 40.64	J ☐		
Junior 13 16" x 13" 40.64 x 33.02	K ☐		
Growing Chair 14" x 11½" 35.56 x 29.21	G ☐		
Childs Chair 14" x 11½" 35.56 x 29.21		C ☐	
Tiny Tot 12" x 11½" 30.48 x 29.21	T ☐	T ☐	T ☐
Pre-School Tot 12" x 10" 30.48 x 25.40		PST ☐	
Pre-School Pediatric 10" x 8" 25.40 x 20.32		PSP ☐	
FRAME STYLE			
Amputee	A ☐		
Outdoor	U ☐		
Indoor	T ☐		
SPECIAL CONSTRUCTION			
Active Duty Lightweight	LD ☐		
Active Duty Lightweight (Tall)	LT ☐		
Lightweight (Standard)	LW ☐		LW ☐
Low Seat (17½" high)(44.45 cm)	SL ☐	HE ☐	
Low Seat Lightweight (17½" high)(44.45 cm)	LL ☐	HL ☐	
Tiny Tot-Hi seat (20" high)(50.80 cm)	SH ☐		
Tiny Tot-Lo seat (17" high)(43.18 cm)	SL ☐		
SPORTSMAN	SM ☐		
PATHFINDER, Lightweight		LD ☐	
COMPANION		LC ☐	
WIDE SEAT (20" wide)(50.80 cm)		WS ☐	
ARM STYLE			
Non-Detachable			
Standard	200 ☐	200 ☐	200 ☐
No arm, no socket	210 ☐		
Offset, full length	230 ☐		
Offset, desk length	240 ☐		
Detachable			
Regular, full length	250 ☐	250 ☐	250 ☐
Regular, desk length	260 ☐	260 ☐	260 ☐
Adj-height, full length	25A ☐	25A ☐	25A ☐
Adj-height, desk length	26A ☐	26A ☐	26A ☐
Wrap-Around, full length	25W ☐		
Wrap-Around, desk length	26W ☐		
Adj-height, Wrap-Around, full length	25C ☐		
Adj-height, Wrap-Around, desk length	26C ☐		
Sportsman, full length	25S ☐		
Sportsman, desk length	26S ☐		
Sportsman, sloped	27S ☐		

	Premier Code	Universal Code	Traveler Code
DRIVE (OTHER THAN STANDARD)			
One-Arm Drive, Right arm	31R ☐		
One-Arm Drive, Left arm	31L ☐		
Power Drive, 12 volt, Micro-Switch			
Right hand control	34R ☐		
Left hand control	34L ☐		
Chin control (See Accessories)			
Power Drive, 24 volt, Proportional Indoor			
Right hand control	3NR ☐		
Left hand control	3NL ☐		
Power Drive, 24 volt, Proportional			
Right hand control	3PR ☐		
Left hand control	3PL ☐		
Chin control (See Accessories)			
BACK (OTHER THAN STANDARD)			
Sectional-Detachable	44 ☐		
Specify height above seat:			
12½" (31.75 cm) _____			
14½" (36.83 cm) _____			
16½" (41.91 cm) _____			
18½" (46.99 cm) _____			
20½" (52.07 cm) _____			
Semi-Reclining (30 degree recline)	41 ☐	41 ☐	41 ☐
Full Reclining (90 degree recline)	47 ☐	47 ☐	47 ☐
Hinged Back	46 ☐		
HEAVY DUTY CONSTRUCTION			
14" wide seat (35.56 cm)	614 ☐		
16" wide seat (40.64 cm)	616 ☐		
18" wide seat (45.72 cm)	618 ☐		
(The following require Offset or Detachable Arms)			
19" wide seat (48.26 cm)	619 ☐		
20" wide seat (50.80 cm)	620 ☐		
21" wide seat (53.34 cm)	621 ☐		
22" wide seat (55.88 cm)	622 ☐		
23" wide seat (58.42 cm) [Price on]	623 ☐		
24" wide seat (60.96 cm) [request]	624 ☐		
FRONT RIGGING			
No Front Rigging — No brackets	7XX ☐		
Tiny Tot (1 piece footrest)	7TT ☐	7TT ☐	
Indoor Chair (vertical hanger)	72T ☐		
Footrest with permanent hanger	720 ☐		
Footrest, Swinging-Detachable (Pin)		760 ☐	760 ☐
Footrest, Swinging-Detachable (Cam)	770 ☐		
Legrest (Elev), Swinging-Det. (Pin)		764 ☐	764 ☐
Legrest (Elev), Swinging-Det. (Cam)	774 ☐		
Legrest (Elev), Low Pivot			

CUSTOM MODIFICATIONS — "PREMIER" ONLY

Seat Width _____   Arm _____   Back _____
Seat Depth _____   Height _____   Height _____
Seat Height _____   Front Rigging _____ Min. _____ Max. _____

Model Code	Caster Size	Chair Size	Frame Style	Special Const.	Arm Style	Drive Method	Back Style	Heavy Duty	Front Rigging	Basic Wheelchair Price
P										
U										
T										

PAGE THREE

Fig. 18-2. Wheelchair selection chart from Everest and Jennings, Inc. Wheelchair prescription form. (Reproduced with permission, Everest and Jennings, Inc., Camarillo, Calif.)

of the shoe or the heel of the foot if shoes are not to be worn to under the thigh, just behind the bent knee. Seat height is determined by adding 2 inches (5 cm) to this measurement.[5] The correct adjustments will result in a clearance of 1 inch (2.5 cm) of height and 1½ inches (3.8 cm) of depth under the thighs, while the step plates clear the floor by at least 2 inches (5 cm) for safety. If a wheelchair cushion is to be used, this must be considered when measuring for seat height and footrest adjustments. Special seat heights are available for unusually tall persons.

4. The wheelchair armrest helps in maintenance of posture and balance and provides a comfortable support for the arms. The armrest height should be approximately 1 inch (2.5 cm) more than the distance from the seat level to the bottom of the elbow when flexed to 90°. When the armrest is properly fitted, the client's shoulders should not be elevated nor should the client lean to meet the armrests. If a cushion is to be used, this must be considered when measuring for arm height. Adjustable height arms are available and could be more economical than ordering special custom arms, in some cases.[5]

5. The current trend is for back rest height to be as low as possible. The backrest height required will depend on the extent of the disabiity and the amount of back support required. It should provide support that is adequate for physical needs and activity requirements.[5] The height of the standard seat back is 4 inches (10 cm) less than the distance from the seat level to the posterior aspect of the axilla when the shoulder is flexed to 90°. The seat back should provide support to the client's back, help to maintain posture, and permit free arm movement without irritation. If full trunk support is required, semi-reclining or reclining seat backs or a headrest extension is available.

It is possible to fit most wheelchair users with one of the manufacturers' standard sizes. However, custom modifications are possible at some additional expense to accommodate individual needs.[5]

Wheelchair selection

A wide variety of combinations of wheelchair features are available. Therefore it is essential to select a chair that will best meet the client's needs, having only those features that are necessary for optimal function.[2]

Besides proper fit of the wheelchair several other factors should be considered before the wheelchair prescription is completed and the wheelchair is ordered. The diagnosis, prognosis, age, size, weight, safety factors, method of transfer, mode of propulsion, expense, life-style of the client, and environments in which the wheelchair is to be used are also important considerations.[2] These factors influence selection of the type of frame, wheels, and special accessories.

The outdoor (universal) frame with the large wheels in the rear and 8-inch front casters is the most frequently recommended frame for the majority of wheelchair users. It is designed for indoor and outdoor use and is easily modified.[6]

The client with a bilateral lower extremity amputation may benefit from the amputee frame. On this type the large wheels are set further back than on the outdoor frame to improve balance. Since the client's weight is centered more to the rear of the chair, this frame type prevents tipping over backward.[6]

The indoor (traveler) frame has the large wheel in front and the casters in the rear. It is primarily for indoor use and has many disadvantages in maneuverability, as compared to the outdoor frame. It may be more useful for individuals with limited range of motion (ROM), however.[4,6]

Wheelchair construction is designed in standard, heavy-duty, or lightweight models, depending on weight, endurance, strength, and activities of the wheelchair user.

Propelling a wheelchair may be accomplished in a variety of ways, depending on the physical capacities of the user. The standard drive (see Fig. 18-1) has the hand rims attached directly to the large wheels. These are operated by pushing-pulling motions of the arms and by grasp. This is the most common type of propulsion and assumes sufficient grasp, arm strength,

and physical endurance to propel the chair and body weight for daily living.[6]

When grasp strength is inadequate but there is sufficient arm strength and motion, a hand rim with projections may be ordered (Fig. 18-3). The chair is operated by pushing the heel of the hand against the hand rim projections to push the large wheels. This type of operation is often used by quadriplegics with good arm function but inadequate grasp strength.

The one-arm drive has both hand rims on the same side of the chair (Fig. 18-4). The outer rim, which is slightly smaller than the inner one, operates the opposite wheel. The inner one is attached directly to the wheel on the same side.[6] This propulsion system is

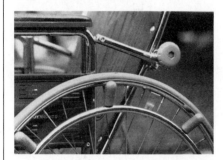

Fig. 18-3. Hand rim projections on wheelchair hand rim.

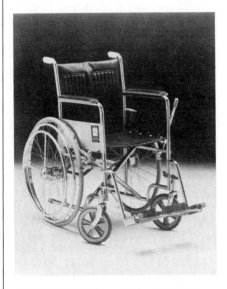

Fig. 18-4. One-arm drive wheelchair. (Reproduced with permission, Everest and Jennings, Inc., Camarillo, Calif.)

used by individuals with only one functional upper extremity and lower extremity involvement such as in triplegia. It may be used by individuals with hemiplegia in some instances. However, they can benefit from a hand and foot method of wheelchair propulsion, using a standard wheelchair (Fig. 18-5).

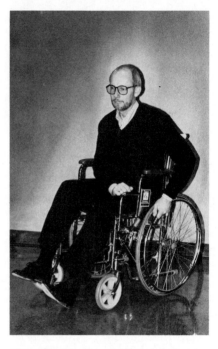

Fig. 18-5. Persons with hemiplegia can propel standard wheelchair by using unaffected arm and leg.

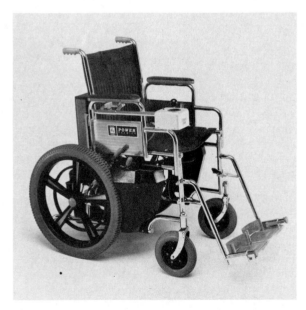

Fig. 18-6. Electric or power-driven wheelchair. (Reproduced with permission, Everest and Jennings, Inc., Camarillo, Calif.)

For those with severe disability and minimal use of the arms the power drive or electric wheelchair is the choice if some independence is to be achieved (Fig. 18-6). The usual system has a control box that can be located near either hand, with a single stick lever projecting from it. The wheelchair is operated by pushing the lever in different directions to effect the desired movement. If upper extremity function is insufficient for this control system, the controls can be adapted for operation by head, chin, mouth, elbow, foot, or toe.[6]

There are many wheelchair accessories available. Some of the major accessories and their benefits are discussed here.

Armrests come in fixed, fixed offset, desk, and detachable styles. The fixed armrest is a continuous part of the frame and is not detachable. It limits proximity to table, counter, and desk surfaces and prohibits side transfers. Fixed offset armrests give extra width for those wearing casts or braces without increasing the overall width of the chair. Desk armrests have a "step" in the front to permit fitting under desk or table surfaces. Detachable armrests permit side transfers.[6]

Footrests may be standard, swinging detachable, or swinging detachable and elevating. The standard footrests are fixed to the wheelchair frame and do not move. They prohibit getting close to counters and may make some types of transfers more difficult. The swinging detachable footrests can be moved to the side of the chair or removed entirely from the chair. They allow a closer approach to bed, bathtub, or counters, and when removed, reduce the overall wheelchair length and weight for easy loading into a car. They lock into place when on the chair with a lever-type locking device. They are recommended for most wheelchair users. The footrest step plates may have heel loops, heel loops with ankle straps, or toe loops. The heel loops prevent the foot from slipping backward off the step plate. The toe loops or ankle straps help to control involuntary motion and maintain the position of the foot on the step plate.[6]

Elevating footrests are recommended to aid circulation or when disability necessitates periodic rest. They might be appropriate when knee flexion is limited or lower extremity edema is a problem.[2] They are usually used when the wheelchair has a reclining backrest.[6]

Backrests are standard or reclining. These may be fully reclining or semireclining. A headrest extension can be added to any backrest to give greater trunk support. The backrest may be obtained in detachable or zip-open styles that allow for a rear transfer.

A reclining or semireclining backrest might be a feature selected for patients who have postural hypotension, as in a spinal cord injury.[2]

Wheelchair tires are usually solid. Pneumatic tires are available as well, primarily for rough and uneven surfaces.[6] They are more difficult to use indoors than the solid tires. Some wheelchair users who are active in the outdoors choose to have two wheelchairs to meet their needs.

Some type of cushion is usually used on the wheelchair seat. Sensory loss necessitates the use of a cushion 4 inches (10 cm) thick to aid in the prevention of pressure sores.[2] These cushions come in a variety of styles and may be made of foam rubber or filled with water, gel, or air.[2,11] Seat boards under the cushions can improve lower extremity posture. A horseshoe-shaped cushion with the opening positioned at the back of the wheelchair seat can provide an area of noncontact between the cushion and the sacral-coccygeal area, which is so vulnerable to pressure sores.[2]

Before the wheelchair is selected, the therapist(s) should make a home evaluation to ascertain wheelchair accessibility and maneuverability. Deep pile carpets, doorsills, stairs, arrangement of furniture and appliances, floor plan, and entrance can influence wheelchair use in the living place. Modifications to the home, as well as to the wheelchair, may need to be considered. In some instances a change of living place is necessary to accommodate the wheelchair.

If a ramp needs to be installed to allow the wheelchair user to enter and exit, it should be 1 foot of length for every inch of stair height of the home entrance. At this incline the wheelchair user can usually manage the ramp safely and independently.

The life-style of the wheelchair candidate should also be considered. Is the user going to be active in sports and outdoor activities? If so heavy-duty construction and pneumatic tires should be considered. Is the patient going to be involved primarily in indoor work and leisure? If so the universal construction should be adequate. Does the patient have limited arm strength or endurance? Then the lightweight construction may be the best choice.

These are some of the important considerations before wheelchair prescription and selection.

When the type, size, and features of the wheelchair have been selected, it is most desirable for the client to try a wheelchair of similar size and features before his or her own chair is ordered. Many rehabilitaion facilities have a sample group of wheelchairs available for trial use. These should include chairs of various sizes with special features, such as detachable armrests and footrests, reclining backrests, desk arms, and swing-away legrests. If the client is allowed to use a wheelchair most similar to the one prescribed, the staff can best evaluate the selection and make any necessary adjustments in the prescription before the actual purchase. If sample chairs are not available, it may be possible to rent a wheelchair from a local rehabilitation equipment

company for a trial period.[2] The process of wheelchair selection and prescription should be carefully guided by the professionals working with the client and the family to obtain a wheelchair that fits properly, provides comfort and increases mobility, and is adequate for the client's life-style.

Psychology of the wheelchair

The wheelchair evokes feelings and attitudes in its user and observers. It has a functional and symbolical meaning to the user and symbolical meaning to the observer.[11] These feelings, attitudes, and meanings may be negative (evoke fear, threat, and concepts of total disablement) or positive (evoke feelings of special status and greater mobility and environment control). The therapist who is responsible for wheelchair training will need to understand the meaning of the wheelchair to the client and may have to facilitate a change of attitude from negative to positive in some clients and those closest to them. The understanding therapist can facilitate the client's physical and psychological adjustment to life in a wheelchair.

Some clients readily accept and tolerate the wheelchair. They see it as a necessity that meets specific physical and functional needs and that improves their functioning. Others become attached to the wheelchair because it is easier and less taxing than ambulation and may cling to the use of the wheelchair even when it is no longer necessary or desirable. Still others regard the wheelchair as a "punishment," following the disability, which is the primary "punishment."[11]

It is difficult for some clients to accept the wheelchair as a necessary part of their rehabilitation. They may regard it as a sign of complete disability and total surrender. This attitude can be related to the symbolical meaning of the wheelchair to the client, to nonacceptance of the disability, or to an unrealistic assessment of physical capacities. Such clients require support and encouragement and can benefit from extended trials with the wheelchair to learn the benefits of decreased fatigue, increased safety, mobility, and function and should have realistic confrontations with the reactions of family, friends, and the public.

Often clients consider the wheelchair as a status symbol and may value it as much as a car is valued. The possibility of shiny chrome, special upholstery colors, and extra gadgets makes a given wheelchair special and affords its user status in some social groups.[11]

Wheelchair safety

Elements of safety for the wheelchair user and an assistant are as follows:

1. Brakes should be locked during all transfers.
2. Step plates should never be stood on and should be up during transfers.
3. In most transfers it is an advantage to have footrests swung away if possible.
4. If an assistant is pushing the chair, he or she should be sure that the client's elbows are not protruding from the armrests and hands are *not* on the hand rims. If approaching from behind to assist in moving the wheelchair, the assistant should inform the client of this intent and check the position of the feet and arms before proceeding.
5. If the assistant wishes to push the client up a ramp, he or she should move in a normal, forward direction. If the ramp is negotiated independently, the client should lean slightly forward while propelling the wheelchair up the incline.[7]
6. If the assistant wishes to push the client down a ramp, he or she should tilt the wheelchair backward by pushing the foot down on the tipping levers to its balance position, which is a tilt of approximately 30°. Then the assistant should ease the wheelchair down the ramp in a forward direction, while maintaining the chair in its balance position. The assistant should keep his or her knees slightly bent and the back straight.[7] The assistant may also move down the ramp backwards while the client maintains some control of the large wheels to prevent rapid backward motion. This approach is useful if the grade is relatively steep. Ramps with only a slight grade can also be managed in a forward direction if the assistant

maintains grasp and pull on the hand grips, and the client again maintains some control of the big wheels to prevent rapid forward motion. If the ramp is negotiated independently, the client should move down the ramp facing forward while leaning backward slightly and maintaining control of speed by grasping the hand rims. Gloves are recommended to reduce the effect of friction.[7]

7. An assistant can manage ascending curbs by approaching them forward, tipping the wheelchair back, and pushing the foot down on the tipping levers, thus lifting the front casters onto the curb and pushing forward. The large wheels then are in contact with the curb and will roll on with ease as the chair is lifted slightly onto the curb.

8. To descend the curb using a forward approach the wheelchair is tilted backward, and the large wheels are rolled off the curb in a controlled manner, while the front casters are tilted up. When the large wheels are off the curb, the assistant can slowly reduce the tilt of the wheelchair until the casters are once again on the street surface. The curb may be descended using a backward approach. The assistant can move him or herself and the chair around as the curb is approached and pull the wheelchair to the edge of the curb. Standing below the curb, the assistant can guide the large wheels off the curb by slowly pulling the wheelchair backward until it begins to descend. After the large wheels are safely on the street surface, the assistant can tilt the chair back to clear the casters, move backward, lower the casters to the street surface, and then turn around.

With good strength and coordination, many clients can be trained to manage curbs independently. To mount and descend a curb, the client must have a normal grip, good arm strength, and good balance. Quadriplegic patients with lesions at T1 and below may achieve this skill. To mount the curb, the client tilts the chair onto the rear wheels and pushes forward until the front wheels hang over the curb, then

lowers them gently. The client then leans forward and forcefully pushes forward on the hand rims to bring the rear wheels up on the pavement. To descend a curb, the client should lean forward and push slowly backward until the rear and then the front wheels roll down the curb.[1]

The ability to lift the front casters off the ground and balance on the rear wheels is a useful skill and will expand the client's independence in the community for curb management and in rural settings for movement over grassy, sandy, or rough terrain. Clients who have good grip, arm strength, and balance can usually master this skill and perform safely. The technique involves being able to tilt the chair on the rear wheels, balance the chair on the rear wheels, and move and turn the chair on the rear wheels. The client should not attempt to perform these maneuvers without instruction and training in the proper techniques, which are beyond the scope of this chapter. The reader is referred to the references for specific instructions on teaching these skills.[1]

TRANSFER TECHNIQUES

The major and most obvious purpose of transfers is to move a client from one surface to another. Transfer techniques for moving the client specifically from wheelchair to bed, chair, toilet, or bathtub are included in this section. Assuming that a client has some physical incapacity, it will be necessary for the therapist to assist in or supervise a transfer. Many therapists question which transfer to employ or feel perplexed when a particular one does not succeed with the client. It is important to remember that each client, therapist, and situation is different. The techniques outlined here are not all-inclusive but are basic ones. Each must be adapted for the particular client and his or her needs.

Preliminary concepts

It is important for the therapist to be aware of the following concepts when selecting and carrying out transfer techniques:

1. The therapist should be aware of the client's assets and deficits, especially his or her physical and cognitive abilities.

2. The therapist should know his or her own assets and limitations and whether he or she can communicate clear, sequential instructions to the client.

3. The therapist should be aware of and employ correct moving and lifting techniques.[12] The following are adapted from the guidelines of the Sister Kenny Institute*:
   a. Maintain broad base of support by standing with feet apart (shoulder's width), knees flexed, and one foot slightly forward. Head and trunk should remain upright.
   b. Maintain center of gravity by carrying, supporting, or lifting others as close to the body as possible.
   c. Lift with the legs, not the back.
   d. Avoid spine rotation; move the feet to turn.
   e. Know personal limitations: do *not* lift alone if in doubt.

4. The therapist should be acutely aware of the safety aspects of transfers.
   a. Maintain all equipment in proper order and state of repair.
   b. Stabilize or lock all surfaces, including wheelchairs, beds, or chairs.
   c. Employ a transfer belt securely fastened around the client's waist.
   d. Clear the work area by removing wheelchair footrests and legrests when possible and armrests when appropriate.

5. The therapist should employ the following basic principles applicable to most transfers:
   a. Stabilize surfaces (for *safety*).
   b. Equalize heights of surfaces as much as possible.
   c. Unless otherwise necessary position wheelchair to bed, chair, or toilet at optimal angle of approximately 60°.
   d. Support the client using a transfer belt. If necessary to hold onto the client, support the client around his or her back with an open hand.

---

*Yates, J., and Lundberg, A.: Moving and lifting patients: principles and techniques, Minneapolis, 1970, Sister Kenny Institute.

e. Avoid grasping the client's arm, as, in general, this offers poor support.

f. Always explain the transfer procedure to the client so that both client and therapist are working toward the same goal.

It is important for the therapist to be familiar with as many types of transfers as possible so that he or she can resolve each situation as it arises. Some excellent resources regarding transfers, which go beyond the scope of this text, are included in the references.[1,8-10,12]

Directions for some transfer techniques that are most commonly employed in practice are outlined later. The standing-pivot transfers and the seated-sliding transfers to bed, chair, toilet, and bathtub are included. Many classifications of transfers exist, based on the amount of therapist participation. Classifications can range from dependent, where the client is unable to participate and the therapist moves the client, to independent, where the client moves himself or herself while the therapist merely supervises or observes. In general, progression of therapist participation should begin with active assistance, then gradually the assistance is

withdrawn if and when the client's abilities and performance improve.

Standing-pivot transfers

The standing-pivot transfer requires that the client is able to come to standing and pivot on one or both feet. It is most commonly used with those clients who have hemiplegia, hemiparesis, or general loss of strength or balance.

WHEELCHAIR-TO-BED ASSISTED TRANSFER (Fig. 18-7). The procedure for accomplishing the wheelchair-to-bed assisted transfer with client and therapist is as follows:

1. The therapist positions the wheelchair at an approximately 60° angle next to the bed, which should be on the client's stronger side.
2. The therapist sets the brakes and removes the footrests.
3. The therapist positions the client's feet (with shoes on) securely on the floor 6 to 10 inches (15.2 to 25.4 cm) apart, directly below and slightly behind knees.
4. The therapist applies the transfer belt.
5. The therapist should be sure the client knows the transfer procedure.

6. The therapist positions him or herself in front of the client on the affected side, stabilizing the client's foot and knee with his or her own.
7. The therapist asks the client to lean forward so that the shoulders are above the knees.
8. The therapist grasps the transfer belt at the client's back and lifts by extending his or her knees and hips, *not* the back!
9. At the same time the client pushes on the armrest(s) and straightens the lower extremity or extremities.
10. The client comes to a complete standing position.
11. The client pivots on the unaffected foot, as the therapist pivots and repositions his or her rear foot.
12. The client reaches for the bed and sits as the therapist flexes his or her knees and hips to lower the client, avoiding the use of his or her back for this maneuver.
13. The therapist then ensures that the client is firmly and safely seated on the bed and assists the client to recline.
14. The therapist removes the transfer belt.

A   **B**   **C**

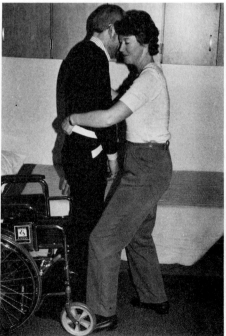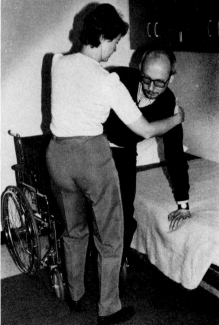

Fig. 18-7. A, Wheelchair and client are prepared for transfer, and therapist is positioned to assist client to stand. **B,** Client is standing, and therapist assists client to pivot to prepare to sit down on bed. **C,** Client pivots, reaches for bed, and sits as therapist assists.

A

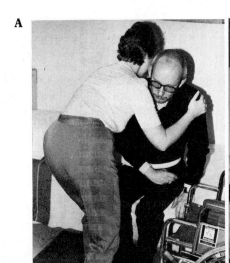

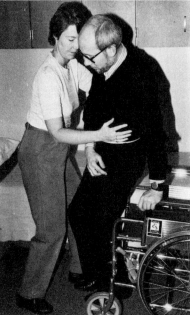

B

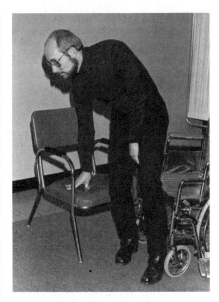

Fig. 18-8. A, Client is seated on bed ready to move toward wheelchair. Therapist is positioned to assist. **B,** Client has stood and pivoted, reaches for wheelchair armrest, and lowers body into wheelchair.

Fig. 18-9. Client, in midtransfer, reaches for seat of chair, pivots, and lowers body to sitting.

BED-TO-WHEELCHAIR TRANSFER

(Fig. 18-8). The bed-to-wheelchair transfer procedure is essentially the same as the wheelchair-to-bed assisted transfer, except for the following points:

1. The client is positioned on the edge of the bed, sitting with feet securely on the floor. The therapist should be aware of the bed's instability and the possibility of the client slipping from its edge.
2. It is more difficult for the client to come to a standing position, since there is no armrest, and it is difficult to push off from the soft bed.
3. After coming to a standing position and pivoting, the client reaches for the armrest to assist in sitting.
4. After the client is sitting, the therapist removes the transfer belt, fastens the seat belt (if used), and repositions the footrests.

WHEELCHAIR-TO-CHAIR AND RE-TURN TRANSFER

(Fig. 18-9). The wheelchair-to-chair and return transfer is similar to the transfer to bed, as described earlier, except for the following differences:

1. The therapist and the client should be aware that the chair may be light and less stable than a bed.

2. When lowering to the chair, the client reaches for the *seat* of the chair. The client avoids reaching for the armrest or back of the chair, since this may cause the chair to tip over.
3. When moving from the chair to the wheelchair, the client pushes with arm(s) from the seat of the chair as he or she comes to standing.
4. Standing from a chair is often more difficult if the chair is low or seat cushions are soft. It is wise to select a chair that is as near as possible to the height of the wheelchair. Secure and firm cushions may be added to chairs that are lower.

WHEELCHAIR-TO-TOILET AND RETURN TRANSFER

(Fig. 18-10). In general, the wheelchair-to-toilet and return transfer is a very difficult transfer for both the therapist and the client because of the confined space of most bathrooms, compounded by the client's usual and justified fear of transferring to the slick and small surface area of a toilet seat. Problems that may arise include the following:

1. It may be necessary to position the wheelchair at a greater angle than 60°, often even facing the toilet, requiring up to a 180° pivot.

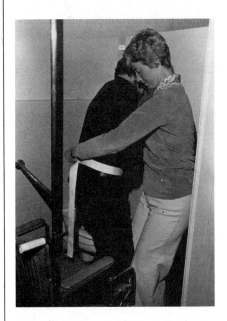

Fig. 18-10. Standing pivot transfer to toilet.

2. It may not be possible to position the wheelchair so that a hemiplegic client moves *toward* the strong side.
3. The confined quarters may force both the therapist and the client to assume foot positions of less than optimal stability.
4. The client may have to reach for and sit on the toilet seat, but therapist and client should be aware of the instability of the hinged seat.

A   B   C

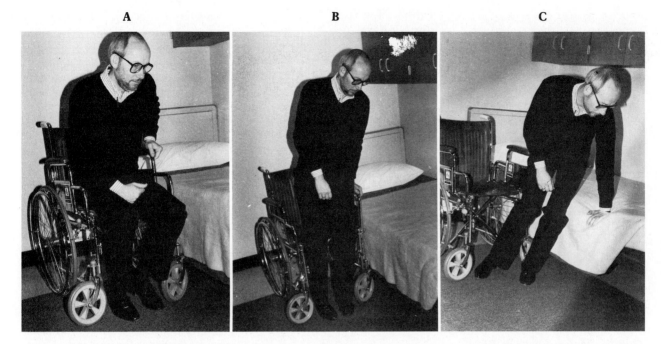

Fig. 18-11. A, Client is properly positioned and leaning on armrest, ready to stand. **B,** Client comes to standing position and begins to pivot. **C,** Client reaches for bed and lowers body to sitting position.

Some comments should be made concerning removal of lower clothing for toilet use. There are advantages and disadvantages of removing clothing before the transfer or after being seated on the toilet. *Before* the transfer waist closures may be loosened so that trousers and underwear can be lowered when coming to standing. Skirts or dresses may be rolled up and tucked into the belt. This can present problems, since it is often difficult to lower clothing when standing or clothing dropped to knees-ankles may encumber the pivot. *After* the transfer, clothes may be removed when seated on the toilet. This, however, requires leaning and hip-hiking (often difficult for the client), and the clothes may get wet in the bowl. No simple solutions are available, except for therapist and client to discover the best and safest method for them.

INDEPENDENT PIVOT TRANSFER (Fig. 18-11). All of the transfers just discussed may be accomplished by the client independently; the obvious difference here is that the client does *all* of the tasks. An independent transfer from one surface to another requires the client to perform the following steps:

1. Position wheelchair and set brakes.

2. Flip up or remove footrests.
3. Scoot forward in chair.
4. Position feet directly below and slightly behind knees at 6 to 10 inches (15.2 to 25.4 cm) apart.
5. Lean forward so that shoulders are over the knees, and look up.
6. Push down with the arm(s) on the armrest(s) while extending the knees and hips.
7. Come to a complete standing position and pivot.
8. Reach for the stable area of a bed, chair, or toilet, and sit.
9. Unlock the wheelchair and reposition (if necessary) to be ready for the return transfer.

Seated-sliding transfers

Seated-sliding transfers are best suited for those individuals who cannot bear weight on the lower extremities or who are too unstable to accomplish a standing transfer. The transfers require the ability to use the upper extremities and are most often employed with persons who have lower extremity amputations or paraplegia or those who have quadriplegia with adequate upper extremity function.

In the previous section on standing-pivot transfers each was first discussed

as a therapist assisted the transfer. Subsequently the independent transfer was outlined. In this section the techniques will be discussed from the point of view of the therapist *supervising* the transfer. Active assistance will be assumed to be minimal. Initial assistance might include helping the client to move his or her body by lifting on the transfer belt or ensuring that the client does not fall or injure him or herself.

It is assumed that all proper lifting, moving, and *safety* techniques are employed. In general, use of additional equipment is discouraged so that the client may learn to perform as independently as possible. With these transfers, however, instruction often begins with the use of a sliding board that is eventually eliminated if and when the client has become stronger and more stable and confident in his or her transfer abilities. NOTE: The client may initially manifest poor balance and decreased strength, which will require more assistance from the therapist. In general, the therapist should position him or herself in front of the client to offer both physical and psychological support by holding on to the client's transfer belt (Fig. 18-12).

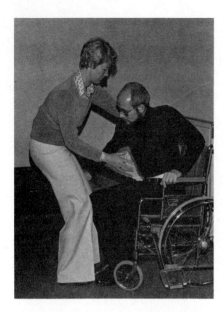

Fig. 18-12. Client and wheelchair are positioned and transfer board has been placed under buttocks and on edge of bed.

WHEELCHAIR-TO-BED AND RE-TURN TRANSFER WITH SLIDING BOARD (Fig. 18-13). The wheelchair-to-bed transfer with a sliding board can be accomplished by using the following procedure:

1. The client positions the locked wheelchair next to the bed at a 60° to 90° angle.
2. The client removes the armrest of the wheelchair that is nearest the bed.
3. The client slips the transfer board under buttocks, as shown, and bridges the board securely across to the bed.
4. The client then lifts his or her body by pushing down with one hand on the sliding board and the other hand on the seat or arm of the wheelchair.
5. Then by lifting the buttocks from the surface the client moves on the board toward the bed in a series of small shoves or moves.
6. When secure on the bed surface, the client removes the sliding board and lifts his or her legs onto the bed.

To return the following procedure is used:

1. The client sits on the edge of the bed with the feet on the floor for stability (if the bed is low enough).
2. The sliding board is positioned under the buttocks and bridged to the wheelchair.
3. Again, in a series of small moves, the client lifts his or her body weight and edges to the wheelchair seat.

NOTE: In moving from the wheelchair to the bed or return there is a tendency for the weaker, less stable client to pitch forward or backward. Also, this transfer is made more difficult if surfaces are of unequal heights.

WHEELCHAIR-TO-BED AND RE-TURN TRANSFER WITHOUT SLIDING BOARD (Fig. 18-14). There are two recommended techniques if the client is stronger and more stable and does not require the use of a sliding board.

The first technique, similar to the transfer just discussed, is as follows:

1. The client positions the locked wheelchair at a 60° to 90° angle next to the bed with the armrest nearest the bed removed.

A   B   C

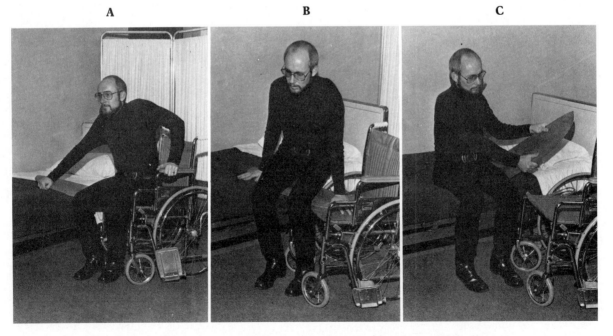

Fig. 18-13. A, Client moves across board toward bed. **B,** Client is on middle of transfer board, lifting weight from surface. **C,** Client reaches bed and removes transfer board.

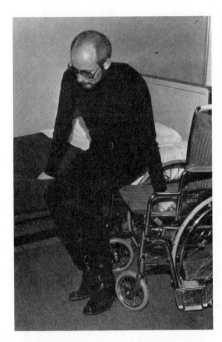

Fig. 18-14. Client has pushed up and is shifting from wheelchair to bed without transfer board.

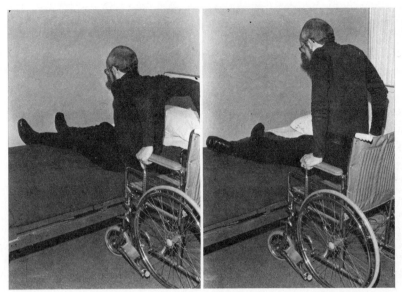

Fig. 18-15. A, Client is positioned and ready to move backward into wheelchair. **B,** Client pushes up and pulls body back into wheelchair.

2. The client positions him or herself in the wheelchair as close to the bed as possible.
3. The client places one hand on the seat or armrest of the chair (seat preferred for stability) and the other hand approximately 12 to 18 inches (30.5 to 45.7 cm) onto the bed surface.
4. The client pushes his or her body weight up from the seat and swings the buttocks onto the bed.
5. The process is reversed to return.

The second technique is a forward-backward approach, whereby the locked wheelchair is positioned directly facing and touching the edge of the bed. This technique, more easily used to move from the bed to the wheelchair, is as follows (Fig. 18-15):

1. The client sits on the bed with the back toward the wheelchair.
2. The client places a hand on each armrest.
3. The client pushes his or her body up and over into the seat of the wheelchair.

WHEELCHAIR-TO-CHAIR AND RE-TURN TRANSFER. The wheelchair-to-chair and return process is very similar to the wheelchair-to-bed transfer. In general, it is best accomplished when the client can transfer without using a sliding board, since a chair allows less room for maneuverability. This transfer is also further complicated because a chair is less stable or secure than a bed. The steps are as in the first seated-sliding transfer described earlier. This transfer is easier than a bed transfer if the chair used is hard, straight back type and is of equal height to the wheelchair.

WHEELCHAIR-TO-TOILET TRANS-FER (Fig. 18-16). The wheelchair-to-toilet transfer is also like the first wheelchair-to-bed transfer described earlier if the wheelchair can be positioned next to or at an acute angle to the toilet. In some instances a second method is employed, whereby the wheelchair is positioned facing the toilet as closely as possible. Then by performing a forward-backward transfer the client slides directly on and off the toilet, facing the rear or tank end of the bowl.

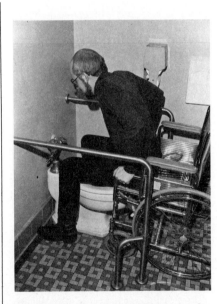

Fig. 18-16. Forward-backward transfer to toilet.

Wheelchair-to-bathtub, standing or seated, transfers (Fig. 18-17)

The bathtub transfer is more dangerous than others because the bathtub is considered one of the most hazardous areas of the home. It is *not* recommended that a client transfer directly from the wheelchair to the floor of the bathtub but rather from the wheelchair

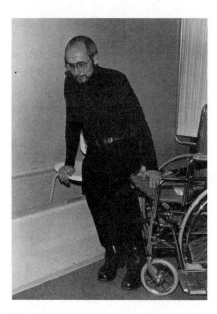

Fig. 18-17. Seated transfer from wheelchair to bathtub chair. Legs are lifted into bathtub following transfer.

to either a commercially produced bathtub chair or a well-secured straight back chair placed in the bathtub. Therefore whether a standing or sliding transfer is employed, the technique is basically similar to a wheelchair-to-chair transfer. However, the transfer is further complicated by the confined space, the slick bathtub surfaces, and the bathtub wall between the wheelchair and the bathtub seat.

If a standing pivot transfer is employed, it is recommended that the locked wheelchair be placed at a 60° angle to the bathtub if possible. The client should stand, pivot, sit on the bathtub chair, and *then* place the lower extremities into the bathtub.

If a seated transfer is used, the wheelchair is placed next to the bathtub with the armrest removed. The client should then slide to the bathtub chair (with or without a sliding board). In some instances more capable clients may transfer to the edge of the bathtub and then to the bathtub chair or even the bathtub floor. This obviously requires greater strength and balance and good judgment on the part of the client.

In general, the client may exit by first placing his or her feet securely outside the bathtub on a nonskid floor surface *and then* performing a standing or seated transfer back to the wheelchair.

Dependent standing transfer (Fig. 18-18)

The dependent standing transfer is more specifically designed for use with the individual who has virtually no functional ability. Its purpose is to move the client from surface to surface. The transfer is used with the highly involved quadriplegic client. The requirements are that the client be cooperative and willing to follow the instructions. The therapist should be keenly aware of correct leverage and lifting techniques, as well as his or her own physical abilities and limitations.

If performed incorrectly, this is a potentially dangerous transfer for both the therapist and the client. Therefore this should be first practiced with able individuals and *initially* employed with the client only if standby assistants are available. The procedure is as follows:

1. The therapist positions the locked wheelchair at a 60° angle to the bed.
2. The therapist positions the client's feet together directly under the knees.
3. The therapist then stabilizes the client's feet by placing his or her feet laterally to each of the client's feet.

A   B   C

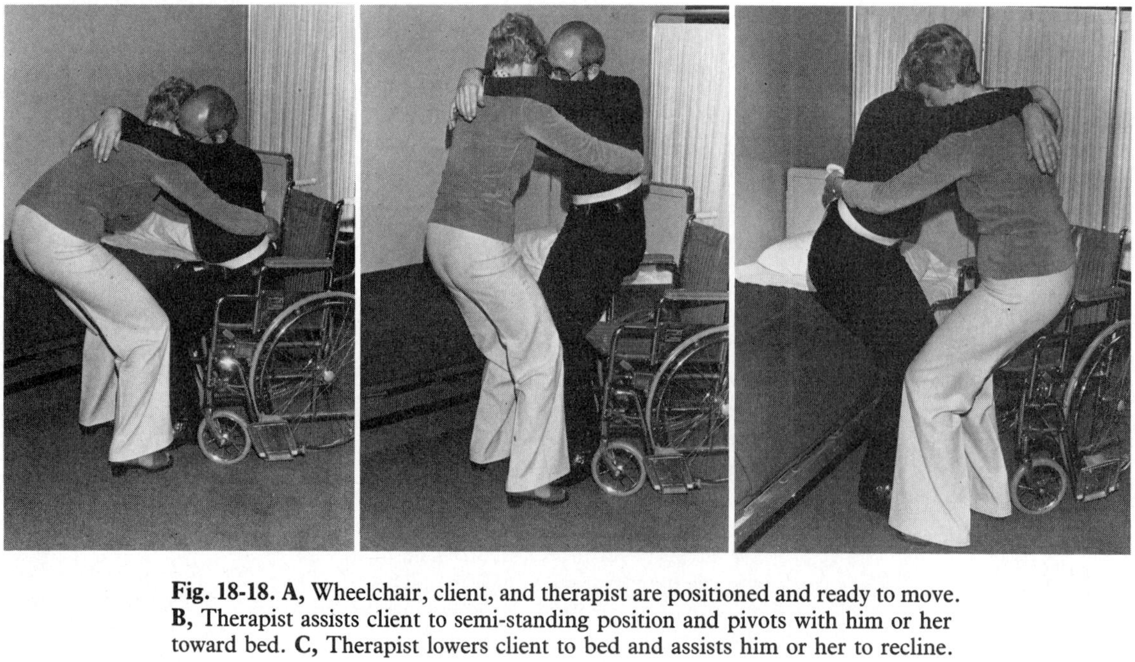

Fig. 18-18. A, Wheelchair, client, and therapist are positioned and ready to move.
B, Therapist assists client to semi-standing position and pivots with him or her toward bed. **C,** Therapist lowers client to bed and assists him or her to recline.

4. The therapist then stabilizes the client's knees by placing his or her knees toward the anterolateral aspect of the client's knees.
5. The therapist assists the client to lean forward over the knees with the arms draped securely over the therapist's shoulders.
6. The therapist grasps the transfer belt with both hands toward the midline of the back, positioning him or herself and the client as close together as possible.
7. The therapist then rocks gently forward and backward with the client to gain momentum.
8. On the count of three, as the client rocks forward, the therapist extends his or her knees and hips while lifting the belt to bring the client up from the seat, taking care *not* to lift with the back. The therapist stabilizes the client's feet and knees with his or her feet and knees.
9. At this point one of two actions take place. Either the therapist comes to a standing position with the client, pivots in place, and flexes the knees and hips to lower the client to the bed or, without coming to a full stand but using the previously gained momentum, the therapist pivots the client from the wheelchair to the bed in a semi-seated position.
10. The therapist secures the client on the bed, assists him or her to recline, and lifts his or her feet onto the bed.

This transfer can be adapted to move a client from one surface to another. It is recommended that transfers to other surfaces be attempted only when the therapist and the client feel secure with this first procedure.

SUMMARY

A wheelchair that fits well and can be managed safely and easily by its user and an attendant is the most significant factor in the client's ability to perform activities of daily living with maximal independence.[5] Each wheelchair user must learn the capabilities and limitations of the wheelchair and safe methods of performing ADL. If there is an assistant, he or she needs to be thoroughly familiar with safe and correct techniques of handling the wheelchair and the client.

Transfer skills are among the most important activities that must be mastered by the physically disabled person. The ability to transfer increases the possibility of mobility and travel. Yet transfers can be hazardous. Safe methods must be learned and followed.[7] Several basic transfer techniques are outlined in this chapter. There are additional methods and more detailed training and instructions available, as cited previously.

It should be recognized that many wheelchair users with exceptional abilities have developed unique methods of wheelchair management. Although such innovative approaches may work well for the individual who has devised and mastered them, they cannot be considered basic procedures that can be learned by everyone.[7]

REVIEW QUESTIONS

1. If the wheelchair is properly fitted, what is the correct seat width?
2. What is the danger of having a wheelchair seat that is too deep?
3. What is the mimimal distance for safety from the floor to the bottom of the wheelchair step plate?
4. List three types of wheelchair frames and the general uses of each.
5. Describe three types of wheelchair propulsion systems and when each would be used.
6. What are the advantages of detachable desk arms and swing-away footrests?
7. Discuss the factors for consideration before wheelchair selection.
8. Name and discuss the rationale for at least three general wheelchair safety principles.
9. Describe or demonstrate how to descend a curb in a wheelchair with the help of an assistant.
10. Describe or demonstrate how to descend a ramp in a wheelchair with the help of an assistant.
11. List four safety principles for correct moving and lifting technique during wheelchair transfers.
12. Describe or demonstrate the basic standing-pivot transfer from wheelchair to bed and wheelchair to toilet.
13. Describe or demonstrate the wheelchair-to-bed transfer, using a sliding board.
14. What is meant by the "balance position" of the wheelchair?
15. List and discuss three possible attitudes of client's toward their wheelchairs as outlined in this chapter.

REFERENCES

1. Bromley, I.: Tetraplegia and paraplegia: a guide for physiotherapists, ed. 2, London, 1981, Churchill Livingstone.
2. Ellwood, P., Jr.: Prescription of wheelchairs, In Kottke, F.J., Stillwell, G.K., and Lehmann, J.F.: Krusen's handbook of physical medicine and rehabilitation, ed. 3, Philadelphia, 1982, W.B. Saunders, Co.
3. Everest and Jennings, Inc.: Wheelchair prescription (form), Camarillo, Calif., 1978, Everest and Jennings, Inc.
4. Everest and Jennings, Inc.: Modification and accessory analysis (form), Camarillo, Calif., 1979, Everest and Jennings, Inc.
5. Everest and Jennings, Inc.: Wheelchair prescriptions: measuring the patient (Booklet no 1), Camarillo, Calif., 1979, Everest and Jennings, Inc.
6. Everest and Jennings, Inc.: Wheelchair prescriptions: wheelchair selection, (Booklet no 2), Camarillo, Calif., 1979, Everest and Jennings, Inc.
7. Everest and Jennings, Inc.: Wheelchair prescriptions: safety and handling (Booklet no 3), Camarillo, Calif, 1983, Everest and Jennings, Inc.
8. Ford, J.R., and Duckworth, B.: Physical management for the quadriplegic patient, Philadelphia, 1974, F.A. Davis Co.
9. Hale, G., editor: The source book for the disabled, London, 1979, Paddington Press, Ltd.
10. Kamenetz, H.L.: The wheelchair book, Springfield, Ill., 1969, Charles C Thomas, Publisher.
11. Pezenik, D., Itoh, M., and Lee, M.: Wheelchair prescription. In Ruskin, A.: Current therapy in physiatry, Philadelphia, 1984, W.B. Saunders Co.
12. Yates, J., and Lundberg, A.: Moving and lifting patients: principles and techniques, Minneapolis, 1970, Sister Kenny Institute.

CHAPTER 19

Mobile arm support and suspension slings

LORRAINE WILLIAMS PEDRETTI

The mobile arm support and the suspension sling are both devices that support the upper extremity in a plane parallel to the floor and facilitate some useful arm motion in the presence of significant muscle weakness.

MOBILE ARM SUPPORTS

The mobile arm support (MAS) may also be called a balanced forearm orthosis or a ball bearing feeder.[6] It is usually mounted on the wheelchair, but it can be mounted on a table or working surface or more rarely on a belt at the level of the iliac crest. It consists of a forearm trough that supports the user's forearm and a pivot and linkage system under the trough. This system can be preset and adjusted so that the user can produce elbow and shoulder motion with slight motions of the trunk or shoulder girdle[1] (Fig. 19-1).

The MAS is adjusted so that gravity is used to assist weak muscles. Various adjustments are possible, and these are individualized to suit the needs of the particular client. The MAS provides assistance for shoulder and elbow movement by using gravity to aid lost muscle power. It provides a large, usable range of arm motion over the tabletop that would otherwise not be available to the client. It helps support, assist, and strengthen weakened musculature and enables clients to perform simple activities of daily living (ADL) and recreational and avocational activities that they could not perform without them.[7]

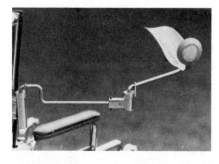

Fig. 19-1. Mobile arm support mounted on wheelchair.

Candidates for use of the MAS

Generally those clients with disabilities that result in muscle weakness but intact coordination, such as poliomyelitis, cervical spinal cord injuries, Guillain-Barré syndrome, muscular dystrophy, and amyotrophic lateral sclerosis are candidates for MAS. When there is moderate to severe muscle weakness in the upper extremities (muscle grades 0 to fair (F) at the elbow and grades 0 to F at the shoulder) and limited endurance for sustained movement, the MAS could increase function.[7]

The client must have a source of muscle power to initiate movement of the MAS. This may be at the neck, trunk, shoulder, or leg. There must be adequate, pain-free range of motion (ROM) as follows: (1) shoulder flexion to 90°, abduction to 90°, external rotation to 30°, and internal rotation to 80°; (2) elbow flexion from 0° to 140°; (3) full forearm pronation from midposition and supination to midposition; and (4) hip flexion from 0° to 95°.[7]

The client must have sufficient coordination to cope with and control movement of the freely swinging arms of the MAS. Involuntary movement precludes effective use.[7] There must be adequate trunk and neck stability provided by the client's own muscle power or by outside support. A consistently stable sitting posture and good body alignment are key factors in the successful use of the MAS. The MAS works best when the user is sitting in an upright position. Successful use decreases as the user reclines. A recline of 30° is about maximum for successful use, and in this position there are some limitations in use.[7] Sitting tolerance and balance and gadget tolerance[6] must be adequate to engage in the training program and, later, make use of the MAS worthwhile.[2]

There must be sufficient motivation to use the MAS and enough frustration tolerance to persevere at the training program until use is mastered.[2] It is important that the client know the pur-

pose in using the MAS. The client should be aware that the motion provided will strengthen muscles and that the device may not necessarily be for permanent use.[7] Motivation to take care of personal needs, eat independently, or enjoy avocational activities that would otherwise be impossible can be a determining factor in acceptance and mastery of the MAS. Successful experience with the MAS can be a motivating factor.[6,7]

Parts of the MAS and their functions[6,7]

The parts of a standard MAS are shown in Fig. 19-2. There are several types of MAS. Additional attachments and assisting devices are available to suit individual needs.[6,7] The semireclining, adjustable *bracket assembly* holds the MAS to the wheelchair. It supports the proximal arm and controls the height of the MAS. It can be adjusted to assist horizontal movement at the shoulder and elbow. It may be adapted for use in the reclining position, but the upright position is most desirable.[2,7] The standard *proximal swivel arm* permits horizontal abduction and horizontal adduction at the shoulder and contains the distal ball bearings. Both the bracket assembly and the proximal ball

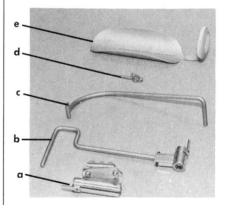

Fig. 19-2. Parts of MAS. *a,* Bracket assembly with stop. *b,* Proximal swivel arm and proximal ball bearing housing with stop. *c,* Distal swivel arm. *d,* Rocker arm assembly. *e,* Forearm trough.

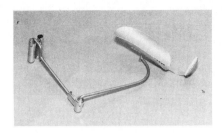

Fig. 19-3. Mobile arm support.

bearing housing have stops that can be set at any position on the circumference of the housing unit to limit horizontal motion. The proximal ball bearing housing on the proximal swivel arm can also be tilted so that gravity assists elbow flexion or extension.[7]

The *distal swivel arm* permits forearm motion in the horizontal plane. It supports the rocker arm assembly and forearm trough. Attached to the forearm trough is the *rocker arm assembly*. It is positioned in the distal swivel arm and permits vertical (hand-to-mouth) motions. It swivels to produce added horizontal motion. The *forearm trough* supports the forearm. It offers stable elbow support but may limit elbow extension. The elbow dial can be bent to produce adjustments for comfort and vertical motion.[7] Fig. 19-3 illustrates an assembled mobile arm support.

How the MAS works

The client must have adequate muscle power to activate the mobile arm support. Some source of power at the neck, trunk, shoulder girdle, shoulder, and elbow may serve alone or in combination to operate the mobile arm support. Some controlling muscle in both elbow and shoulder is necessary if the user is to have control of motions in the horizontal plane over the lapboard.[7]

The mobile arm support allows horizontal and vertical motions. The device assists horizontal motions across the tabletop. Vertical movement allows tabletop-to-face activity. To assist horizontal motion the bracket assembly and the proximal ball bearing housing on the proximal swivel arm can be adjusted to produce an inclined plane in the direction of horizontal abduction or horizontal adduction, as the need may be. Gravity then assists motion to the low

point in the plane, and muscular effort must be exerted to return the arm to the high point of the plane.[7]

Adjustments for vertical motions are somewhat more complex. The rocker arm assembly is fastened to the underside of the forearm trough and acts as the fulcrum of this first class lever. There are several holes in the length of the forearm trough so that the fulcrum can be moved toward or away from the elbow (force end). Any force applied by the user proximal to the fulcrum lifts the weight of the hand and anything in the hand toward the face. Shoulder elevation and depression are used to effect the vertical motions of the forearm trough. The distance of the fulcrum from the elbow will determine whether the mechanical advantage is on the load side (hand) or force side (elbow) of the lever.[7]

Adjustment and checkout of the MAS[3,7]

To adjust the MAS the therapist must find the best position for the client in the wheelchair, choose the correct bracket assembly for the arm being fitted, since the right and left are not interchangeable, and set the height of the bracket to position the whole MAS at the proper height for the client. The forearm trough is then fitted to the client. It is balanced for maximal range and force in vertical motion. The bracket is adjusted for maximal range and force in horizontal motion at the glenohumeral joint. The therapist must then tilt the distal bearing, if necessary, to produce the maximal range and force in horizontal motion at the elbow joint. The therapist should then reevaluate range and force of combined horizontal motions of the glenohumeral and elbow joints and reevaluate the vertical motion of the trough. Some clients may require special attachments, such as straps, to stabilize the forearm in the trough.[7]

The following questions can serve as a guide for the therapist to determine the correctness of fit and adjustments of the MAS.[3]

1. Are the client's hips set back in the chair?
2. Is the spine in good vertical alignment?
3. Does the client have lateral trunk stability?

4. Is the chair seat adequate for comfort and stability?
5. Is the client able to sit upright?
6. If the client wears hand splints, does the client have them on?
7. Does the client meet requirements for passive ROM?
8. Are all the screws tight?
9. Is the bracket tight on the wheelchair?
10. Are all arms and joints freely movable?
11. Is the proximal arm all the way down in the bracket?
12. Is the bracket at the proper height so that the shoulders are not forced into elevation?
13. Does the elbow dial clear the lapboard when the trough is in the "up" position?
14. When the trough is in the "up" position, is the client's hand as close to the mouth as possible?
15. Can the client obtain maximal active reach?
16. Is the trough short enough to allow wrist flexion?
17. Are the trough edges rolled so that they do not contact the forearm?
18. Is the elbow secure and comfortable in the elbow support?
19. Is the trough balanced correctly?
20. In vertical motion is the dial free of the distal arm?
21. Can the client control motion of the proximal arm from either extreme?
22. Can the client control motion of the distal arm from either extreme?
23. Can the client control vertical motion of the trough from either extreme?
24. Have stops been applied to limit range, if necessary?
25. What is the client's maximal reach in front of the body (measured from the bracket)?
26. What is the distance between the two extremes of the horizontal arc?
27. What is the client's vertical range (in degrees)?
28. What is the maximal weight the client can lift from the lapboard to the face?
29. What is the distance from the hand to the mouth when the trough is in the "up" position?

Training in use of the MAS

The therapist should be sure that supports are fitting well and adjusted correctly before attempting to instruct the client in their use. If two MASs are used, the client should practice with one at a time until each is mastered. Bilateral use of MASs requires considerable practice. Early use includes training in vertical motions (external and internal rotation of the shoulder). External rotation is accomplished by depressing the shoulder to elevate the hand, shifting the body weight to the side of the MAS, rolling the shoulder back, tilting or turning the head toward the side of the device, or leaning backward. Internal rotation is accomplished by gravity, elevating the shoulder on the same side as the mobile arm support, shifting the body weight to the opposite side from the device, rolling the shoulder forward, tilting and turning the head to the opposite side from the MAS, or leaning forward. Work is started on horizontal adduction and abduction with the trough balanced at midposition. Then the client can proceed to practice these motions with the trough at various heights between wheelchair tray and head. Practice progresses to include elbow flexion and extension with the trough at various heights. Activities that are designed to offer practice in the use of MASs are typing on an electric typewriter, turning book pages, dialing the phone, playing the chord organ, and playing games, such as checkers, chess, cards, and puzzles.

The MAS offers the client with significant upper extremity weakness the necessary assistance to make maximal use of minimal muscle power. Once assembled, fitted, and adjusted it enables the client to perform a variety of self-care and avocational activities that promote self-esteem, a sense of independence, and pleasure in doing. The reader is referred to the references for more comprehensive discussion of MASs and their use.[2,6,7]

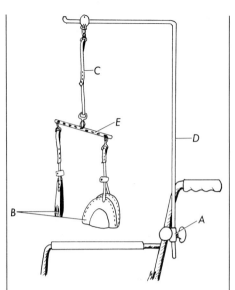

Fig. 19-4. Suspension sling. *a*, Bracket. *b*, Arm cuff. *c*, Suspension strap. *d*, Suspension rod. *e*, Horizontal supporting device for cuffs. (Reproduced after modification with permission from Occupational Therapy Department, Rancho Los Amigos Hospital, Downey, CA.)

SUSPENSION SLINGS

The suspension sling supports the upper extremity in a plane parallel to the floor. The suspension sling is used to facilitate horizontal movement during activity or exercise in which the force of gravity on the movement of the upper extremity needs to be minimized[4] (Fig. 19-4).

Parts of the suspension sling

A bracket holds the suspension rod to the back of the wheelchair. The bracket is constructed so that it can be adjusted to keep the top of the suspension rod parallel to the floor. It also allows for adjustments in height. The suspension sling is hung from the suspension rod with a spring or a strap. The length of the suspension device determines the height of the sling in relation to the user's body. The suspension device also swivels to eliminate friction or twisting and to allow maximal mobility. If a spring suspension is used, it adds to the amount of motion that the user can produce in the sling but may decrease coordination.

The cuffs of the suspension sling are fastened to a horizontal metal device that has holes along its entire length.

These allow the cuffs of the sling to be placed for optimal balance to assist vertical or horizontal motions of the arm. A forearm trough, as used on the mobile arm support, is sometimes substituted for the arm cuffs shown in the illustration, and the assembly is referred to as a suspension feeder.[4]

Use of the suspension sling

In many instances the suspension sling can be used with clients who have the same diagnoses as just cited, although somewhat greater muscle power is required for effective use. In addition, it is often used in stroke rehabilitation to reinforce specific movement patterns and to facilitate functional use of the affected arm.[5] Use of the suspension sling may be initiated with enabling exercise to establish patterns of horizontal abduction and adduction, hand-to-body movements, and hand-to-face movements. Use may then progress to activities, such as eating, face care, braid weaving, finger painting, mosaic tile work, writing, typing, leather lacing, and some types of needlework.

REVIEW QUESTIONS

1. What kinds of clients are good candidates for use of the MAS (in terms of disability or muscle grades)?
2. What kinds of clients are poor candidates for use of the MAS? Why?
3. List the five criteria a client must meet to use the MAS successfully.
4. Describe how the MAS works (refer to parts and their functions, how the device is activated, and how it is adjusted so that gravity assists movement).
5. What kinds of activities can be performed with the MAS that could not be performed without it?
6. List the three major steps in training the client to use MAS.
7. List two ways external rotation motion can be accomplished.
8. List two ways internal rotation motion can be accomplished.
9. What are some activities that are good for practicing use of the MAS?
10. What is the primary purpose of the suspension sling?

11. List three purposeful activities that may be performed by clients with significant upper extremity dysfunction while using a suspension sling. Can you think of some that were not listed in the text?

REFERENCES

1. Bender, L.F.: Upper extremity orthotics. In Kottke, F.J., Stillwell, G.K., and Lehmann, J.F.: Krusen's handbook of physical medicine and rehabilitation, ed.3, Philadelphia, 1982, W.B. Saunders Co.
2. Dicus, R.G.: Mobile arm supports, part 1, film, Downey, Calif., 1970, Rancho Los Amigos Hospital, S.R.S. Service Dept. (Available at the Instructional Resources Center, San Jose State University.)
3. Rancho Los Amigos Hospital: Check-out sheet for feeders. In Marshall, E.: Occupational therapy management of physical dysfunction, Loma Linda, Calif., 1976, Department of Occupational Therapy, School of Allied Health Professions, Loma Linda University. (Distributed by Fred Sammons, Inc., Box 32, Brookfield, Ill., 60513.)
4. Rancho Los Amigos Hospital: Suspension feeders and slings: parts and their functions. In Marshall, E.: Occupational therapy management of physical dysfunction, Loma Linda, Calif., 1976, Department of Occupational Therapy, School of Allied Health Professions, Loma Linda University. (Distributed by Fred Sammons, Inc., Box 32, Brookfield Ill., 60513.)
5. Ruskin, A.: Understanding stroke and its treatment. In Ruskin, A., editor: Current therapy in physiatry, Philadelphia, 1984, W.B. Saunders Co.
6. Thenn, J.E.: Mobile arm support: installation and use, San Jose, Calif. 1975, Self-published. (Distributed by Fred Sammons Inc., Box 32, Brookfield, Ill., 60513.)
7. Wilson, D.J., McKenzie, M.W., and Barber, L.M.: Spinal cord injury: a treatment guide for occupational therapists, Thorofare, N.J., 1974, Charles B. Slack, Inc.

CHAPTER 20

Hand splinting

LORRAINE WILLIAMS PEDRETTI

The purposes of this chapter are to introduce the reader to the basic principles of hand splinting and to enable him or her to construct and evaluate two hand splints through the use of a self-instruction program.

It is important for the occupational therapist to understand the principles of hand splinting and to be able to construct some types of hand splints. The occupational therapist is usually the professional who works most closely with hand rehabilitation. Therefore the therapist is depended on to analyze hand dysfunction, make suggestions for splinting needs, evaluate splint performance, and train the client in the use of the splint.[4,7] The occupational therapist may determine when the goals of splinting have been achieved, recommend changes in the splint, or see that its use is discontinued.[4]

Temporary splints made of high- and low-temperature thermoplastic materials are often made by the occupational therapist. These splints are usually used in treating temporary conditions of muscle weakness and joint limitation. They may be used to prevent or correct deformity, substitute for lost muscle power, and assist weak muscles in normal patterns of motion.

Splints required for long-term use to treat permanent conditions are often made of metal and should be referred to a certified orthotist for design and construction.[1,8]

NORMAL HAND FUNCTION

The occupational therapist must understand normal hand function and hand-to-upper extremity relationships to perform splint design and construction accurately and effectively.

The normal hand has many assets, several of which cannot be replaced or helped with splints. The normal hand is capable of mobility and stability at all joints. Splinting can provide one or the other but usually not both.[3,7] The normal hand has strength and skill in a wide variety of grasp and prehension patterns.[3,7] Splinting may assist in only one or two patterns, such as palmar prehension or grasp.[3] The normal hand has considerable dexterity and can move in a quick, accurate manner. The use of a splint may aid in the ultimate recovery of dexterity, but while the splint is being worn, dexterity is hindered or limited. Sensation is a major asset of the normal hand. The normal hand has the ability to sense pain and temperature and interpret qualities of objects, such as size, weight, and texture. Splinting can do nothing to aid sensation and actually limits sensation during wear.[2,7]

The normal hand has unique padding on the palm and fingertips that contributes to the effectiveness of grasp and pinch. Splinting may limit or hinder the function of this unique padding. The hand is supplied with complex blood-vascular and lymphatic systems. Effective splinting and splint use can aid good circulation, whereas poor splinting can limit circulation. Finally the hand has cosmetic significance in that, after the face, it is a primary organ of expression. After splinting a more cosmetically acceptable hand may be achieved, but during splinting the hand is less cosmetically appealing.[7]

The joints of the upper extremity must have adequate range of motion (ROM) to ensure normal hand function. This will allow the hand to reach the object or perform the activity. Joints of the hand and arm must have stability and the ability to be fixed or to cocontract at any point in their ROM. The hand and arm must have enough muscle power for the reaching, placing, performing, or holding that is required by the task to be done.[4]

Wide ranges of shoulder motions are critical to placing the hand at some distance from the body, such as extending over the head and reaching behind and out to the side of the body. A lesser degree of shoulder motion is essential for hand-to-mouth and hand-to-body activities such as toileting and combing hair.[4]

To perform hand-to-face activities the elbow must have full range of flexion. Full extension is required if activities at some distance from the body are to be accomplished such as putting on socks or reaching to high shelves. Pronation and supination are essential for placing the hand at the correct angle for holding or activity performance.

Lesser ROM at the wrist is required for basic hand function. More important is the wrist's stability. For the hand to function maximally it should be possible to stabilize the wrist at any point in its ROM and make fine adjustments in the degree of wrist motion. This ability to stabilize and make fine adjustments in the wrist contributes to the fine coordination possible in the hand. Wrist extension is most important, since finger flexion and grasp are best performed with the wrist in extension. If the wrist is flexed, grasp will be limited and the arches of the hand will tend to flatten.

Prehension and grasp are the primary functions of the hand. Hand movements are complex and occur in smooth sequence and combinations. However, it is possible to reduce these movements to several basic types of prehension and grasp.[4]

Types of prehension and grasp[3,4,7] (Fig. 20-1)

FINGERTIP PREHENSION (Fig. 20-1, *A*) Finger tip prehension, contact of the thumb pad with that of the index or middle fingers, is used to pick up small objects, such as pins, nails, and buttons, and to fasten buttons and snaps and hold a needle for sewing. It requires very fine coordination.

PALMAR PREHENSION (Fig. 20-1, *B*). Palmar prehension, also called "three-jaw chuck grip" or "palmar tripod pinch,"[4] is the contact of the thumb pad with the middle and index fingers. It is the most common type of prehension and requires a high level of coordination. It is used to pick up and hold small square, cylindrical, or spherical objects, such as a marble, pen, or small cube, and is the prehension pattern used for holding a pen or eating utensil.

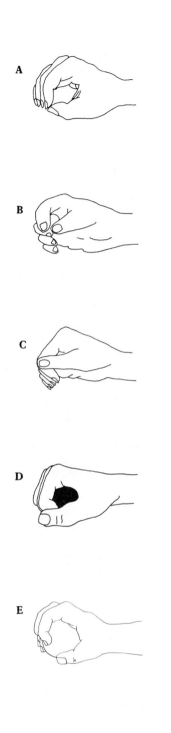

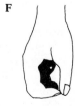

Fig. 20-1. Basic types of prehension and grasp. **A,** Fingertip prehension. **B,** Palmar prehension. **C,** Lateral prehension. **D,** Cylindrical grasp. **E,** Spherical grasp. **F,** Hook grasp.

LATERAL PREHENSION (Fig. 20-1, *C*). During lateral prehension the thumb pad is in contact with the lateral surface of the index finger at the middle or distal phalanx. For this to be a functional prehension pattern the thumb and index finger must have good stability, and the first dorsal interosseous muscle must have good to normal strength. The fourth and fifth fingers must act as a support to the index and middle fingers. Lateral prehension is used for turning a key or thumbscrew, carrying a plate or teacup, and winding a watch. It is a stronger type of prehension than fingertip or palmar prehension and requires less coordination to perform.

CYLINDRICAL GRASP (Fig. 20-1, *D*). The cylindrical grasp is the position the normal hand assumes when holding objects, such as a tumbler, rail, hammer, or pot handle. The object is stabilized against the palm by the fingers, which close or flex around it. Intrinsic and thenar muscle strength are essential to the power of this grasp. It is one of the earliest grasp patterns, occurring reflexly in infants and developing later into voluntary gross grasp.[4]

SPHERICAL GRASP (Fig. 20-1, *E*). The spherical grasp, also called "ball grasp," is the position the normal hand assumes when grasping a small rubber ball, such as a tennis ball. The five fingers are flexed around the object and hold it against the palm, which is in an arched position. It is used to hold balls, apples, oranges, and round doorknobs. Its power depends on the stability of the wrist and finger joints and the strength of the intrinsic and extrinsic muscles of the hand.

HOOK GRASP (Fig. 20-1, *F*). The hook grasp is the position the normal hand assumes when carrying a briefcase or similar bag handle. The grip can be accomplished entirely by the fingers. The thumb remains outside the fingers and is relatively passive. It acts simply to close the hook, but its presence and power are not essential to hook function. The hook grasp requires strength and stability of the interphalangeal (IP) joints, primarily. The metacarpophalangeal (MP) joints and the wrist remain in the neutral position and need not be completely stabilized. This type of grasp is used to carry heavy objects,

such as pails, suitcases, and shopping bags, and may also be used to pull open drawers and cabinets with hardware that require four fingers to hook to pull them.

Arches of the hand[3,4] (Fig. 20-2)

There are three arches of the hand that must be considered when making splints. There are the metacarpal and carpal transverse arches and the longitudinal arch.

METACARPAL TRANSVERSE ARCH. The metacarpal transverse arch lies across the distal metacarpal heads at a slightly oblique angle. The second and third metacarpal bones are relatively stable elements in the arch, whereas the fourth and fifth metacarpal bones are the more mobile elements. The normal arch increases as the hand is used functionally. The dexterity and function of the fingers are dependent on the mobility and flexibility of this arch. Grasp function will be impaired if the mobility of the metacarpal bones is limited and if the transverse arch is flattened or prevented from increasing during functional use. These conditions can be caused by poor positioning of the hand in the splint, poorly constructed or ill-fitting splints, intrinsic paralysis, edema, and scarring and contracture of the dorsal skin of the hand.[4]

The metacarpal transverse arch should be considered in splinting, since

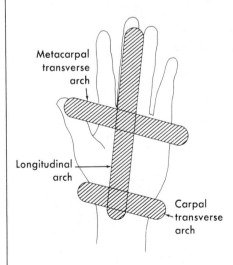

Fig. 20-2. Arches of hand.

the splint should be designed to maintain the normal arch of the hand and allow the arch to increase during hand use. If the metacarpal transverse arch is flattened, the thumb will be unable to oppose the fingers and thus hand function will be considerably impaired.

CARPAL TRANSVERSE ARCH. The carpal transverse arch is located at the wrist. It is troughlike and is formed by the annular ligaments and carpal bones. It provides the mechanical advantage to the finger flexor tendons by acting as the fulcrum.

LONGITUDINAL ARCH. The longitudinal arch follows the long lines of the carpal and metacarpal bones at a slightly oblique angle and primarily involves the third finger. The carpal and metacarpal bones are the fixed units, and the fingers through their flexion and extension abilities are the mobile units. This flexibility allows for a wide range of prehension patterns. The function of the longitudinal arch can be disturbed by intrinsic paralysis, poor hand positioning, edema, scarring of the dorsal skin, and adhesions of extensor tendons or bony obstructions.[4]

Creases of the hand (Fig. 20-3)

The palmar skin is tough and not very pliable or mobile. These qualities allow for stability and fixation of the palmar skin during motion and grasp. The palm has several skin creases that can act as guides in individual design and fitting of splints.

Splints should not obstruct the distal palmar crease if full MP flexion is to be allowed. The thenar crease must not be obstructed if opposition is to occur or if the hand is to be in the position of function. The wrist creases are good points for locating the wrist strap if the splint is to remain in a good position and not slide forward.[4]

Dual obliquity of the hand[3]

Because of the arches of the hand and the successive decrease in length of the metacarpals from the radial to the ulnar side of the hand, objects grasped in the hand are held at two oblique angles. The first is an oblique angle formed by the decreasing length of the metacarpals. An object held using cylindrical grasp with the hand in full pronation will be parallel to the metacarpal heads and *not* parallel to the axis of the wrist joint (Fig. 20-4, *A*). The second oblique angle is formed by the

transverse metacarpal arch and the mobility of the fourth and fifth metacarpals when the hand is used. Because of the arch and the metacarpal mobility, an object grasped with a cylindrical grasp will be higher on the radial side than on the ulnar side of the hand and thus *not* parallel to the floor when the hand is in full pronation[3] (Fig. 20-4, *B*).

When making hand splints, these two oblique angles must be considered. The radial side of the splint must be longer or more distal than the ulnar side, and the splint must be higher on the radial side than on the ulnar side[3] (Fig. 20-5)

Position of function (Fig. 20-6)

The functional position of the hand is a position similar to that which the hand assumes when grasping a ball. The wrist is in 20° to 30° of extension. The transverse metacarpal arch is

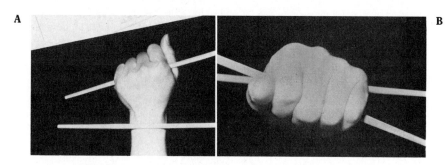

Fig. 20-4. Dual obliquity of the hand. **A,** Oblique angle of metacarpal heads in relation to axis of wrist joint. **B,** Oblique angle of metacarpal heads from radial to ulnar side of hand. (Reproduced with permission, George Wu, M.D., San Francisco.)

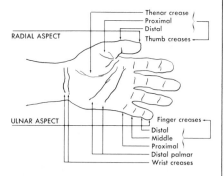

Fig. 20-3. Palmar creases of hand. (Reproduced with author's permission from Malick, M.H.: Manual on static hand splinting, Pittsburgh, Harmarville Rehabilitation Center.)

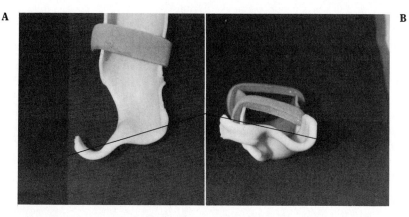

Fig. 20-5. A, and **B,** Distal end of cock-up splint demonstrates dual obliquity.

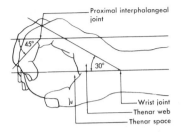

Fig. 20-6. Position of function, lateral view, right hand. (Reproduced with author's permission from Malick, M.H.: Manual on static hand splinting, Pittsburgh, Harmarville Rehabilitation Center.)

rounded. The thumb is in abduction and is in opposition to the pads of the four fingers. The metacarpal joints are flexed to about 30° and the proximal interphalangeal (PIP) joints are flexed to about 45°.[4,6]

The functional position of the hand may be described as the midposition of the ROM of every joint. In this position there is equal tension of all musculature, and the muscles are in the best mechanical position for efficient function.

The functional position is an important concept, since it is usually desirable to splint the hand in a position as near the functional position as possible.[3,7] Placing the hand in the functional position alone will improve its performance and decrease the possibility of developing deformity in many instances.

Position of rest (Fig. 20-7)

The position of rest is slightly more relaxed than the position of function. It is similar to the position the normal

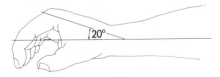

Fig. 20-7. Position of rest. (Reproduced with author's permission from Malick, M.H.: Manual on static hand splinting, Pittsburgh, Harmarville Rehabilitation Center.)

hand assumes when resting passively on a tabletop. The wrist is in 10° to 20° of extension. All finger joints are slightly flexed. The thumb is in partial opposition and abduction, and the thumb pad faces the pad of the index finger. The metacarpal, carpal, and longitudinal arches are maintained when the hand is in the position of rest.[4] The hand is often splinted in this position in a static resting splint if joint rest or prevention of deformity is desirable in conditions such as peripheral nerve injuries and rheumatoid arthritis.

PRINCIPLES OF HAND SPLINTING
Types of splints

There are two types of hand splints—static and dynamic. *Static splints* have no moving parts. It is usually desirable to hold the involved part in a functional position or as close to a functional position as is physically possible. The antideformity splint for the burned hand (see Fig. 22-5) and the postoperative flexor tendon splint (see Fig. 24-10) are two examples of exceptions to this rule. To the extent possible, the client should be able to perform daily living tasks while wearing the splint. This of course depends on the type of splint and its purpose. Some splints necessarily eliminate most or all functioning. The use of the functional position in splinting will help to ensure the ability to perform activities of daily living (ADL) when the splint is removed even if function is not possible when the splint is being worn. However, the physician's requirements regarding the position of the hand for splinting may vary with the diagnosis and purposes of the splint. These requirements must be considered when designing splints, and the therapist with the physician must plan for facilitating the regaining of maximal function following the splinting period.[3]

All splints should be designed to meet the client's physiological and functional needs. The splint must achieve the desired purposes while not creating dysfunction. All static splints must be removed periodically for exercise of the affected part, and the client should be encouraged to use the part as frequently as possible while wearing the splint.[4]

Static splints may be used for three major purposes. The first purpose is for protection of weak muscles. A static splint can protect weak muscles from overstretching and therefore prevent their antagonists from contracture. Prevention of overstretching muscles weak because of temporary paralysis is important to ensure good function when nerve and muscle recovery occurs.

The second major purpose of static splints is for support. A joint may be supported or immobilized for resting purposes, as in rheumatoid arthritis, or for healing purposes, as in tendon lacerations and skin grafting. The function of the hand can often be improved if the wrist is supported in extension. Therefore a simple static wrist cock-up splint can improve finger function for grasp and prehension.

The third major purpose of static splinting is for prevention or correction of deformity. The splint may be designed to force the involved joint into correct or near correct alignment, such as the protective ulnar drift splint used in rheumatoid arthritis.[6]

The *dynamic hand splint* has a static base and one or more moving parts. Thus the same splint may incorporate both static and dynamic elements. Some parts may be supported in their best anatomical position for function, whereas other parts are assisted in movement by the dynamic features of the splint. The splint is designed to apply a relatively constant force on a part as it moves. It provides mobility to the joints with control on the direction and degree of motion. This splint is designed to assist weak muscles or substitute for lost muscle power.[5]

Movement in dynamic splints may be effected by another part of the body or available muscle group, as in the wrist-driven flexor hinge splint, also called the wrist-hand orthosis (Fig. 20-8), or by springs, pulleys, and rubber bands, as in the long opponens splint with MP stop and extensor assist (Fig. 20-9), or by an external power source, such as an electronic or pneumatic unit.[2,3,5,9]

A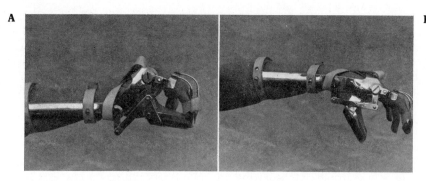

Fig. 20-8. Wrist-hand orthosis. **A,** Prehension effected by wrist extension. **B,** Release of prehension effected by relaxation of wrist extension.

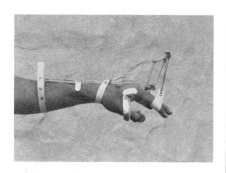

Fig. 20-9. Long opponens splint with MP stop and extensor assist.

General guidelines for splint design and fitting

The wrist is the key joint of the upper extremity in relation to hand function. Wrist stability is essential to optimal function of hand muscles, and wrist extension is critical to forceful grasp and prehension patterns. When the wrist is flexed because of pain, paralysis, or deformity, the long extensor tendons stretch, the metacarpal transverse arch flattens, and the thumb drifts into the plane of the palm of the hand. To prevent this nonfunctional position and potential deformity from developing, the wrist should be splinted in slight extension. There are exceptions, of course, depending on the particular dysfunction, limitations already present at the wrist, degree of paralysis, and goals of hand splinting. Individual variations in wrist positioning will depend on these factors and should be determined by the therapist in concert with the supervising physician.

The MP joints are the key joints of the fingers. Their ability to flex and be stabilized at any point in their range of flexion is critical to grasp and prehension. When the MP joints are hyperextended, the IP joints flex as a result of the stretch placed on the long flexor tendons of the fingers in this position. If the MP joints are allowed to remain in hyperextension for a prolonged period, clawhand deformity may ultimately develop. In the extended or hyperextended position the MP joints will become limited in their ROM or immobilized because of shortening and thickening of the collateral ligaments. These ligaments are at their shortened length when the MP joints are extended.[7] If the collateral ligaments develop contractures caused by poor positioning, MP flexion may be difficult or impossible even if recovery of muscle function occurs. If splinted, the MP joints should be positioned between 30° and 80° of flexion depending on the particular dysfunction and the goals of splinting.

The thumb is the most valuable element of the hand. One or two other fingers and the thumb will make a more functional hand than four fingers and no thumb. Thumb opposition is critical to all of the prehension patterns. It acts as a flexible force in strong grasp patterns. It must be possible for the thumb to rotate at the carpometacarpal (CMC) joint if true opposition of thumb pad to finger pads is to take place. Hand splints are often used to stabilize and position the thumb properly for some grasp and prehension patterns.[7] In some instances splints may be used to assist thumb extension, abduction, or opposition.[5]

The normal hand can perform a wide variety of prehension and grasp patterns, which have already been reviewed. The finer prehension patterns require minimal strength and flexibility in the hand, whereas grasp patterns require more strength and flexibility in the hand. The grasp and prehension patterns that may be provided by hand splinting are determined by the muscles that are functioning, potential and present deformities, and how the hand is to be used.[7]

Pronation and supination are valuable in positioning the hand at the desired angle for function. Full pronation is required if the hand is to perform adequately. Supination to midposition is sufficient for adequate function.

The carpal and metacarpal transverse arches are critical to hand function. Motion and opposition of the thumb and little finger, ability to grasp round or large objects, convergence of the fingers during flexion, and strength or pressing with the palm are dependent on these arches.[7] The arches must be maintained if the hand is splinted. Flattening of the MP transverse arch will place the hand in a nonfunctional position and will severely limit the types of grasp and prehension possible.

Purposes of splints[7]

A hand splint may be prescribed and fitted for more than one purpose. If there is limited joint motion, the splint may be a positioning or corrective device, and more function may not be achieved until the ROM is improved. In such instances performance of hand skills may be greater without the splint, although not necessarily in the most desirable patterns of motion. A splint may be a positioning device to enhance function during the day and a corrective device at night.

The ultimate and idealistic goal of hand splinting is to assist in the development of as near a normal hand as possible. The following are some specific goals of hand splinting:

1. Prevent deformity caused by joint tightness or muscle contracture. Contracture of muscles whose antagonists are weak or paralyzed can

be prevented by placing the muscle at its resting length in the functional position and facilitating motion through the splint or passively.

2. Protect weak muscles from overstretching so that maximal efficiency will be obtained when the muscle regains its function. This goal is related to number 1.

3. Prevent increased muscle imbalance by providing assistance to the weaker muscle group, for example, using rubber bands, to pull the part through the full ROM. This will enable weak muscles to work and allows active ROM.

4. Strengthen weak muscles by providing assistive motion first. Assistance is gradually decreased as muscle function improves. The goal is related to number 3. The MP extensor assist or opponens assist are examples of splints with these purposes.

5. Correct or prevent deformity by maintaining the ROM gained in forced stretching exercise or maintaining corrected alignment of joints.

6. Provide temporary support for a painful part while permitting motion of uninvolved segments. An example is the wrist cock-up splint to support an arthritic wrist while allowing some hand function.

7. Prepare the hand for future surgery to approximate the position or motions to be gained by surgery and provide the needed ROM and strength, if possible.

8. Place the hand in the correct or appropriate position after burn, surgery, trauma, or skin grafting.

9. Aid in the development of a useful tenodesis tightness in the long finger flexors for the wrist-driven flexor hinge splint.

10. Transfer power from one joint to another for increased function. An example is the wrist-driven flexor hinge splint, where wrist extension effects palmar prehension and wrist flexion effects release through the splint. Later with the controlled development of some finger flexor tightness many clients can discard this splint and use the tenodesis action of the hand for some prehensile function.

11. Substitute for permanently paralyzed muscles through the use of external power such as electricity or the carbon dioxide muscle. An example of this type of splint is the battery-driven flexor hinge splint and the Rancho electric arm.[9]

12. Encourage use of normal movement patterns, prevent substitutions, and facilitate muscle reeducation. These purposes may be achieved by placing the part in a functional position and providing as near a normal range as possible. Return of function will be facilitated by use of the hand in coordinated movement patterns. Proper position and motion will aid returning muscles to work to their maximal potential but will have no effect on reinnervation of the muscle itself.[7]

Limitations of hand splints

Motion and sensation are intimately related in hand and upper extremity function. Sensory information and feedback from the parts are essential to normal motion. A person with severely limited sensation will have limited motor function even if muscles are normal or near normal. Splinting cannot aid in the restoration of sensation. Splints reduce the amount of sensory information being received from the part. The possibility of the development of pressure points and the resultant skin breakdown from splints is greater in the person with sensory deficits. Such clients must be taught how to compensate for and guard the affected part through the use of vision. The therapist and the client must be responsible for vigilant precautions against the adverse effects of splinting.

A splint cannot provide both mobility and stability of a joint, as in the normal hand, at the same time. Therefore a choice for one or the other must be made in relation to the dysfunction, purposes of splinting, potential deformities, and use of the hand.

The cosmetic appearance of the hand can be improved by splinting. However, during splint wear or use the hand may be less cosmetically appealing. This may influence the client's acceptance and use of the device.[7]

Precautions of splinting

Of greatest importance is the prevention of the adverse effects of immobilization. Prolonged immobility from splinting or positioning can produce limitations in joint ROM and ultimately joint stiffness and immobility. All static splints must be removed about every 2 hours, and active or passive exercise must be performed at splinted joints unless contraindicated by surgery, infection, or trauma.

Joints that do not require splinting should not be limited or immobilized by the splint. All joints proximal and distal to the splinted joint(s) should be used actively or exercised passively if active motion is not possible.

To ensure that proper fit and comfort have been achieved, the splint should be removed after short periods of wear (½ to 1 hour), and the part should be checked for indentations of the skin, redness, edema, pain, and changes in the degree of joint mobility.

The splint should be evaluated periodically for fit and function. The frequency of evaluation will depend on the disability and the purposes of the splint. For example, a splint for the burned hand should be evaluated at least daily, whereas one that is used during regeneration of a radial nerve could be evaluated weekly or at each patient visit. The therapist must determine if the splint is achieving the desired goals, making no difference, or possibly increasing dysfunction or deformity.[4,7]

Criteria for assessing splints

Certain general criteria can be outlined to estimate the practicality of splint construction by the occupational therapist. Static splints should be fitted soon after injury, surgery, or disease. They should be simple in design, easily adjustable, lightweight, cosmetically pleasing, and comfortable and should offer adequate support to achieve the objectives of the splint. It should be possible to fabricate the splint in a reasonable period. The splint should be inexpensive when materials and the therapist's time for construction are considered.[4] The splint should be neat, durable, and easy to clean.

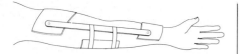

Fig. 20-10. Three-point elbow extension splint illustrates points of pressure proximal and distal to elbow joint and over it to increase or maintain extension.

For function the splint should follow the natural contours of the hand and arm as closely as possible without causing pressure areas. If the splint is to be lined or padded, this must be allowed for when first molding the splint by padding the client's arm.

The arches of the hand must be maintained, and the normal padding of the fingers and the hypothenar and thenar eminences must not be flattened. Joints should be positioned in correct anatomical alignment, and the hand should be positioned in or as nearly as possible to the position of function unless contraindicated.[7,9] In dynamic splints the joints of the splint should be lined up with the normal axes of anatomical joints. The therapist should be aware of and check the splints for shifts in position, which therefore change their function and support of the part.

If the splint is used for progressive increase of joint motion, three points of pressure should be used (Fig. 20-10).[7,11]

INDEPENDENT SPLINT CONSTRUCTION: A SELF-INSTRUCTION PROGRAM

This self-instruction program was designed to enable the reader to construct two simple static splints frequently fabricated by occupational therapists. These are the volar wrist cock-up splint and the resting splint. The wrist cock-up splint may be used to immobilize the wrist in a functional position while allowing finger function. It is used for rheumatoid arthritis, if rest or stabilization of the wrist is desirable, and also to protect the wrist and finger extensors from overstretching when there is muscle weakness producing the wrist-drop position.

The resting splint is worn for similar purposes but immobilizes the thumb and fingers as well as the wrist in the position of rest or function. It may be modified to the antideformity position required for splinting the hand with dorsal burns. In this position the wrist is at neutral, the MP joints are flexed to approximately 80°, and the IP joints are in full extension. The thumb is midway between radial and palmar abduction to maintain full stretch on the thumb web space.

The resting splint is sometimes used to prevent contractures of the hand with flexor spasticity. When the client wears the splint, no hand function is possible. Therefore it is often worn when the client is at rest or asleep or is worn on one side at a time if bilateral splinting is required.

Steps in making a hand splint independently

Study the preceding sections of this chapter and review the illustrations of grasp, prehension, hand creases, position of function, and position of rest. Then begin construction of the splint using the following steps:

1. Decide which type of splint is to be constructed.
2. Make a pattern for the splint according to the directions.
3. Follow the directions for splint construction.

SUPPLIES NEEDED. For making the splint pattern the following supplies will be needed:

1. Strip of paper towel 18 to 20 inches (45.7 to 50.8 cm) long
2. Twelve-inch flexible ruler
3. Soft pencil or felt tip pen
4. Scissors

For molding the splint the items listed here will be required:

1. Piece of low-temperature thermoplastic material, such as Orthoplast or Kay-Splint, 8 × 12 inches* (20.3 × 30.5 cm)
2. Marking crayon on stylus
3. Large scissors*
4. Heat gun*
5. Shallow pan filled with water ¾-inch (1.9 cm) deep, candy thermometer, and range or hot plate as heat source or thermostatically controlled rectangular, electric frying pan*

6. Tongs*
7. Pot holder or oven mitts*
8. Two Ace bandages or stockinette tubing*
9. Edger for smoothing splint edges*

For applying straps two or three prefabricated, self-adhesive Velcro straps with D rings* and a pair of scissors are needed.

MAKING A PATTERN FOR A SPLINT. The following are instructions for making a pattern for two basic types of hand splints. The reader is directed to choose *one* and construct a splint, making the pattern for the splint selected and constructing the splint on another person.

GENERAL INSTRUCTIONS FOR ALL TYPES OF PATTERNS[8]

1. Position the affected hand and forearm palm down on a long piece of paper towel. The fingers should be adducted and the wrist should be in a neutral position with the thumb against the index metacarpal and finger.
2. Draw a line around the hand, forearm, and thumb, keeping the pencil perpendicular to paper at all times.
3. With the hand still in place mark the wrist joint and the MP joints of the fingers on the radial and ulnar sides of the hand. Mark the MP joint of the thumb. Mark the ulna styloid and the olecranon of the elbow (Fig. 20-11).
4. Measure on the volar surface of the forearm from the distal wrist crease to the elbow crease and mark this distance on the tracing of the forearm, using the marks for the wrist joint as the point of reference.[3] Later when you are ready draw the splint pattern around this hand tracing.

---

*These items are available from Fred Sammons, Inc., Box 32, Brookfield, Ill., 60513.

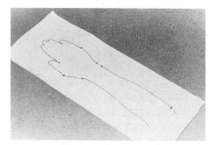

Fig. 20-11. Tracing of subject's arm marked to indicate location of joints.

Resting splint pattern[8] (Fig. 20-12)

1. On the tracing of the hand, beginning at the MP joint of the index finger, draw a line ½ inch (1.3 cm) around hand tracing, ending at the wrist on the ulnar side (line a). Extend the line on the radial side straight down to the CMC joint of the thumb and extend it another ½ inch (1.3 cm) (line b).
2. Measure the width of the thumb and add ¼ inch (0.6 cm) to this measurement. Mark this distance inward from line b at MP joint of index finger. Draw a line from this mark toward the wrist (line c). This line should be parallel to line b and equal in length to the length of the thumb from the tip of the MP joint plus ½ inch (1.3 cm). Taper this line inward slightly at the top and round the bottom.
3. From the elbow crease measure to the distal wrist crease and calculate two thirds of this distance.[3] Draw a line across the forearm at this point, indicating the length of the splint trough (line d). Extend this line on either side of the forearm tracing, to a distance equal to one half of the depth of the forearm at this level.
4. Beginning at a distance equal to one half the depth of the forearm on the ulnar side and on the radial side of the wrist, draw two lines extending to meet line d on each side of the forearm (line e). Taper these lines outward to accommodate for the increasing depth of the forearm as it moves proximally.
5. Cut pattern out and fit to hand, adding or trimming as necessary for proper fit. Cut along line c for the thumb support. Round out all sharp edges.

Proper fit

1. Hand section should not extend more than ½ (1.3 cm) around hand or thumb.
2. Narrowest point at wrist should be about the width of the wrist.
3. Sides of trough should extend halfway up the sides of the forearm at all points.

Wrist cock-up splint pattern[8] (Fig. 20-13)

1. Draw a line connecting the MP joint marks across the palm of the drawing. Extend this line 1 inch (2.5 cm) lateral to radial side and extend ¾ inch (1.9 cm) beyond ulnar side of the hand (line a).
2. Draw a line ¾ inch (1.9 cm) down from the radial side of line a (line 1) and another line on the ulnar side of line a, extending past the ulna styloid and parallel to the ulnar side of the arm (line 2).
3. To mark the thenar eminence measure the thumb from the tip to the MP joint and subtract ½ inch (1.3 cm). Using this measurement making an X in toward the palm from the MP joint of the thumb (3).
4. Draw a curved line (line b) from line 1, arching through the X (3), and end at the wrist.
5. Repeat steps 3, 4, and 5 of the resting splint pattern.
6. Ulna styloid should not be under the splint trough. Cut a notch in the splint to accommodate the ulna styloid if it is a potential pressure point (c).

Proper fit

1. Ulnar side of the splint at hand should extend halfway up the side of the hand.
2. Top of the splint should not prevent full flexion of MP joints (splint should fall just below distal palmar crease).

3. Radial side of top of splint should curve around the hand ½ to ¾ inch (1.3 to 1.9 cm) on the radial side.
4. Opposition and abduction of the thumb should have full ROM (move thumb into this position and check pattern).
5. Narrowest point at wrist should be slightly wider than the width of the wrist.
6. Sides of trough should extend halfway up the sides of the forearm at all points except at the wrist, where they should be slightly beneath the halfway line.

DIRECTIONS FOR USING LOW-TEMPERATURE THERMOPLASTICS IN THE CONSTRUCTION OF HAND SPLINTS[3,10]

1. Low-temperature thermoplastic materials soften when exposed to heat. Sources of heat used to soften them are hot water, ovens, or heat guns. Use hot water in a shallow flat pan or the heat gun as sources of heat. These materials soften at 130° to 160° F (54.4° to 71.1° C). If heated too hot or reheated more than two times, they may tend to shrink, stretch, or change their molding characteristics. Read directions for material in use carefully before proceeding.
2. Trace the pattern on the thermoplastic before it is heated, using the marking crayon or stylus (Fig. 20-14).
3. Place the thermoplastic, with the tracing on it, in a shallow pan of water or in the electric frying pan that has been heated to the temperature recommended by the manufacturer. Be sure the water is not boiling! Use a candy thermometer to monitor water temperature.
4. Within 1 or 2 minutes the material will have softened and can be removed from the hot water with tongs for cutting.

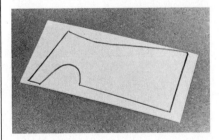

Fig. 20-14. Splint pattern traced on thermoplastic.

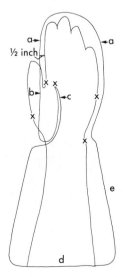

Fig. 20-12. Resting splint pattern.

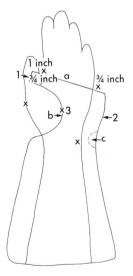

Fig. 20-13. Cock-up splint pattern.

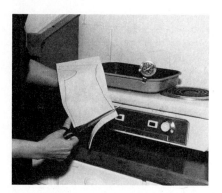

Fig. 20-15. Cutting splint out of thermoplastic.

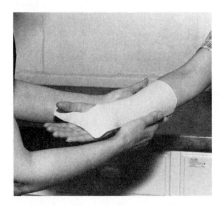

Fig. 20-16. Molding thermoplastic on forearm.

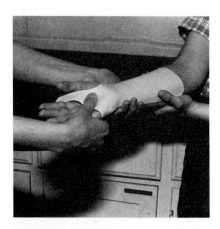

Fig. 20-17. Thumb pressed into concavity of palm to attain metacarpal palmar arch.

5. Low-temperature thermoplastics do not retain the heat and usually can be handled easily while cutting. With ordinary household shears cut the pattern out of the material, rounding all sharp corners. Since the material sets in 5 to 10 minutes after is has been removed from the heat, it may be necessary to place it back in the hot water very briefly before molding (Fig. 20-15).

6. It is usually possible to mold the material directly over the skin without harm. However, to prevent risk of burn or for hypersensitivity to heat the part may be wrapped with one layer of Ace bandage or a piece of stockinette tubing may be applied to the arm where the splint will be molded.

7. Place the softened material over the arm. Support the arm in the desired position. Mold the thermoplastic around the forearm (Fig. 20-16).

8. If it is not possible to hold the thermoplastic in position on the forearm while molding the hand section (and later when the splint sets), wrap an Ace bandage *loosely* on the subject's arm to mold the material in place. Be careful *not* to wrap too tightly or twist the splint on the forearm while wrapping.

9. While holding the forearm section in place (the subject may help do this), press a thumb into the concavity of the palm to be sure to get the contour of the arch of the hand into the splint. Be sure the subject's wrist is extended between 10° and 30° when this is done (Fig. 20-17).

10. Have the subject abduct and oppose the thumb to the little finger to get a fold in the thermoplastic that will mark the medial border of the thenar eminence (Fig. 20-18).

11. Then with the thumb moved out of the way roll this edge over. Mold the radial extension through the thumb web space and flat against the dorsum of the hand (Fig. 20-19).

12. Also have the subject flex the MP joints and roll over the distal end of the splint. These rolls give the splint strength, provide a smooth edge against the skin, and should be formed to allow for full flexion of MP joints and full opposition of the thumb (Fig. 20-20).

13. If necessary, resoften the proximal end of the splint and roll over this end ⅛ to ¼ inch (0.3 to 0.6 cm) as well.

NOTE: If the thermoplastic sets before the desired contours are formed, it is possible to reheat all or part of the splint and remold as desired. If reheating is necessary after the basic contours of the splint are formed, remove the splint, which is set, from the subject's arm and spot heat at the desired area

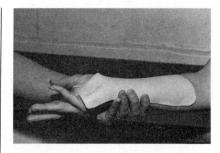

Fig. 20-18. Subject opposing thumb to little finger to attain medial fold on thenar eminence.

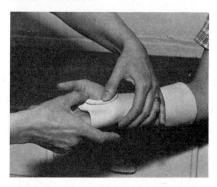

Fig. 20-19. Therapist rolls over thenar edge of splint.

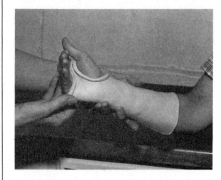

Fig. 20-20. Subject flexes MP joints, and therapist rolls over distal edge of splint.

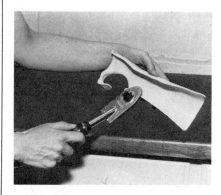

Fig. 20-21. Edger is used to smooth edges of splint.

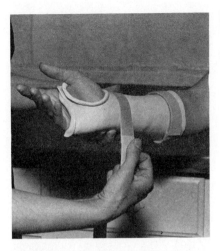

Fig. 20-22. Self-adhesive Velcro straps are applied to splint.

only by dipping the small area in the hot water; using the spot heater tip on the heat gun; or pouring small amounts of very hot tap water over the desired area with a cup, repeatedly, until the area is softened. When the desired pliability is reobtained, replace the splint on the subject's arm and remold. This same procedure can be followed if it is necessary to trim some material from the splint.

14. After the splint has been molded to the exact form desired, smooth any rough edges of the splint with the edger. Heat the edger to "medium" and touch it lightly to the splint, using gently strokes (Fig. 20-21).

NOTE: Too much heat or pressure will cause the thermoplastic to melt along the edges, and its appearance gets worse instead of improving.

Attaching straps to the splints

1. Using two Velcro self-adhesive straps place one strap on the splint at the proximal end and the other strap over the wrist, but not on top of the ulna styloid, which is a potential pressure point.
2. A third strap may be placed on the splint around the hand just proximal to the MP joints (Fig. 20-22).

EVALUATION OF SPLINT CONSTRUCTION. Finished splints may be evaluated for molding technique, function, fit, and appearance. Both the wrist cock-up and the resting splints should be evaluated for molding technique and fit by the following criteria:

1. Is the splint smoothly molded?
2. Is the trough twisted, or is it well-aligned to the forearm?
3. Are all of the corners rounded?
4. Are the straps correctly placed to afford stability and avoid pressure points?
5. Do the sides of the trough extend about halfway around the forearm at all points?
6. Does the splint fit loosely enough to prevent pressure areas along edges and over bony prominences?
7. Is there evidence of pressure (redness, soreness, or edema) after ¼ to ½ hour of wear?

Appearance of both the wrist cock-up and the resting splints may be evaluated according to the following criteria:

1. Is the thermoplastic material clean and free of bumps, dents, cuts, and ridges?
2. Are the straps clean and attached straight?
3. Does the splint have a neat appearance that would be acceptable for wear?

For function the resting splint may be evaluated by the following criteria:

1. Are the arches of the hand maintained?
2. Is the hand splinted in a resting position, that is, with the wrist in 10° to 30° extension, MP joints in 20° to 30° flexion, IP joints in 10° to 15° flexion, and thumb in palmar abduction and opposition, aligned with index finger?

The cock-up splint may be evaluated for function by the following criteria:
1. Are the arches of the hand maintained?
2. Does the splint allow full ROM at the MP joints?
3. Does the splint allow full, normal opposition to the little finger?
4. Is the wrist positioned in 10° to 30° of extension?
5. Can the subject use the hand for grasp and release while wrist stability is maintained?

SUMMARY

This chapter presents an overview of normal hand function and basic principles of hand splinting. Instructions for the construction of two hand splints are outlined. This information is intended as an introduction to splinting for the novice, and the reader is referred to the references[2-5] for further study of the subject.

REVIEW QUESTIONS
1. What is the role of the occupational therapist in hand splinting?
2. List five assets of the normal hand.
3. Describe the relationship of shoulder, elbow, and wrist function to hand use.
4. Which type of prehension is used to pick up a straight pin?
5. Which type of prehension is used to turn a key in a lock?
6. Which type of grasp is used to hold a tumbler?
7. What is the role and importance of the metacarpal transverse arch in hand function?
8. What happens to hand function if this arch is flattened?
9. In which position are the muscles of the hand at the best mechanical advantage to function efficiently?
10. Describe and demonstrate the dual obliquity of the hand. Why is it an important consideration in hand splinting?
11. Name two major classifications of splints. Give one example of each.
12. How are the adverse effects of immobilization by splinting best prevented?
13. What is the optimal position for splinting the wrist?
14. What effect does wrist flexion have on hand function?
15. Why is it important to splint the MP joints in some flexion if these joints are to be splinted?
16. What is the optimal position for splinting the thumb?
17. Describe six purposes of splinting.
18. List and describe three limitations of splints.
19. What are the factors that influence the practicability of splint construction by the occupational therapist?
20. List six general rules for achieving optimal fit and function of the splint.
21. Describe the purposes of the resting and wrist cock-up splints.

REFERENCES

1. Bender, L.F.: Upper extremity orthotics, In Kottke, F.J., Stillwell, G.K., and Lehmann, J.F.: Krusen's handbook of physical medicine and rehabilitation, ed. 3, Philadelphia, 1982, W.B. Saunders Co.
2. Fess, E.E., Gettle, K.S., and Strickland, J.W.: Hand splinting: principles and methods, St. Louis, 1980, The C.V. Mosby Co.
3. Kiel, J.H.: Basic hand splinting: a pattern designing approach, Boston, 1983, Little, Brown & Co.
4. Malick, M.: Manual on static hand splinting, vol. 1, rev. ed., Pittsburgh, 1972, The Harmarville Rehabilitation Center.
5. Malick, M.: Manual on dynamic hand splinting with thermoplastic materials, Pittsburgh, 1974, The Harmarville Rehabilitation Center.
6. Melvin, J.L.: Rheumatic disease: occupational therapy and rehabilitation, Philadelphia, 1977, F.A. Davis Co.
7. Principles of hand splinting, Downey, Calif. 1962, Occupational Therapy Department, Rancho Los Amigos Hospital. Mimeographed, unpublished.
8. Splinting manual, Jamaica Plain, Mass., 1972, Occupational Therapy Department, Lemuel Shattuck Hospital. Mimeographed, unpublished.
9. Trombly, C.A., and Scott, A.D.: Occupational therapy for physical dysfunction, Baltimore, 1977, Williams & Wilkins.
10. Von Prince, K.: Orthoplast splint construction, San Jose, Calif., 1971, special study, Department of Occupational Therapy, San Jose State College. Mimeographed, unpublished.
11. Willis, B.: The use of orthoplast isoprene splints in the treatment of the acutely burned child: preliminary report, Am. J. Occup. Ther. **23**:57, 1969.

PART 4

TREATMENT APPLICATIONS

CHAPTER 21

Amputations and prosthetics

LORRAINE WILLIAMS PEDRETTI

Limb loss can result from disease, injury, or congenital causes. Congenital amputees or those whose amputations occurred very early in life grow and develop sensorimotor skills and self-images without the amputated part. The individual who incurs amputation of a part in adolescence or adulthood is confronted with the task of adjusting to the loss of a part that was well-integrated into the body scheme and self-image.

These two types of amputees present somewhat different problems for the rehabilitation worker.[4] This chapter will be limited to discussion of the adult with acquired above-elbow (AE), below-elbow (BE), or lower extremity (LE) amputations.

Physical therapy is usually responsible for the preprosthetic preparation and prosthetic training of the LE amputee. Occupational therapy may be useful to the LE amputee for functional use training, standing and walking tolerance, and prevocational explorations. The preprosthetic and prosthetic training of the upper extremity (UE) amputee, on the other hand, is usually the primary responsibility of the occupational therapist. Psychosocial adjustment, controls and use training, wearing tolerance, and prevocational

assessment are important aspects of the occupational therapy program.[4]

ETIOLOGY

Amputations may result from trauma, peripheral vascular disease, thrombosis, embolism, and cancer.[2,4] The most common reason for UE amputations in adults is trauma, and LE amputations are most frequently the result of peripheral vascular disease.[2]

SURGICAL MANAGEMENT

The surgeon attempts to preserve as much tissue as possible during the amputation procedure. During and after surgery it is a primary goal to form the stump in a way to maintain maximal function of the remaining tissue and obtain a result that will allow maximal use of the prosthesis. Blood vessels and nerves are cut and allowed to retract so that they do not cause pain in the stump when the prosthesis is used. In any amputation the muscles involved in the function of the amputated part are affected by the loss.

A closed or open surgical procedure may be performed. The open method allows drainage and minimizes the possibility of infection. The closed method reduces the period of hospitalization but also reduces free drainage and increases the risk of infection. In either

case the stump that results must be strong and resilient. It must be possible to fit the prosthesis socket to the stump snugly and comfortably, since the amputee will be exerting much pressure on the stump when using the prosthesis.[4]

SPECIAL CONSIDERATIONS AND PROBLEMS

There are several factors and potential problems that can affect the outcome of the amputee's rehabilitation. Stump length, skin coverage, stump edema, hypersensitivity, rate of healing, infections, and allergic reactions to the prosthesis are some of the physical problems that can affect the fitting and use of the prosthesis.

The loss of feedback sensation from the amputated part is one of the major problems that confronts the amputee. The amputee must rely on visual and proprioceptive sensory feedback to control the use and function of the prosthesis. Sensation in the stump is functionally lost when the prosthesis is applied. An ill-fitting socket or a stump that is not well formed at the distal end can cause pain and discomfort when the prosthesis is worn. Besides the loss of normal sensation the amputee must become accustomed to new sensations as well. The pressure of the stump inside the socket and the feeling of the harnessing system must be accommodated.[4] Neuromas and phantom sensation or pain are two problems that may interfere with use of the prosthesis. The neuroma is nerve tissue growing into scar tissue that causes pain in the area when it is pressed or moved. It is treated by surgical excision or ultrasound therapy. The stump socket may be fabricated to accommodate the neuroma.[7]

Phantom sensation is a common experience among amputees. It is the sensation of the presence of the amputated part or a distal portion of it. The phantom sensation may be present for life or may eventually disappear. Phantom sensation does not usually interfere with good prosthetic usage. A much less common phenomenon that can prohibit good use of the prosthesis is phantom pain. In this condition the amputated limb is not only perceived as present but is painful as well.[7]

Surgical revision of the stump is sometimes necessary to alleviate the discomfort. Phantom sensations occur most frequently in crush injuries and are usually felt as distal parts, that is, a hand or foot, rather than the entire extremity. Supportive counseling and early use of the stump with a temporary or permanent prosthesis are effective measures for dealing with phantom sensations.[4] The therapist can allay the client's fears about these phenomena by offering information, support, and reassurance, unless the therapist considers these fears an indication of some mental imbalance. It is best not to dwell on discussion of phantom sensation but rather to focus on prosthetic training and the advantages of using a prosthesis. The appearance of phantom pain or overconcern with phantom sensation may require the intervention of a psychiatric specialist who may work with the client or provide advice to the occupational therapist.[7]

PSYCHOLOGICAL ADJUSTMENT

Amputation is likely to be accompanied by a profound psychological shock. Reactions are less severe in clients who have been well prepared for amputation surgery and more severe in persons who have experienced sudden traumatic injury that causes or necessitates amputation. The amputee may manifest depression, hostility, denial, or feelings of futility. Older persons may demonstrate postoperative confusion whereas younger persons may have a sense of mutilation or emasculation. The amputee will need a lot of reassurance during the preoperative, postoperative, and rehabilitative phases of care.[2]

Loss of a body part necessitates a revision of the body image. The amputee must accept the new body image. Such adjustment will have a beneficial effect on prosthetic training, since the amputee must integrate the prosthesis into the body scheme. The prosthesis must become part of the self before it can be used most effectively. Difficulties with acceptance of body scheme change may cause difficulties in prosthetic training.[4]

LEVELS OF AMPUTATION AND FUNCTIONAL LOSSES IN THE UPPER EXTREMITY (Fig. 21-1)

The higher the level of amputation the greater the functional loss of the part, and the more the amputee must depend on the prosthesis for function and cosmesis. The higher level amputations require more complex and extensive prostheses and prosthetic training. The more complex prostheses can be more difficult to operate and use effectively.[4]

The shoulder forequarter and shoulder disarticulation (SD) amputations will result in the loss of all arm and hand functions. The short AE amputation will result in the loss of all hand, wrist, and elbow functions and rotation of the shoulder. The long AE and elbow disarticulation amputations will result in loss of hand, wrist, and elbow functions, but good shoulder function will remain. The short BE amputation will result in loss of hand and wrist function, forearm pronation and supination, and reduction in the force of elbow flexion. Shoulder function will be intact and good. The long BE amputation will result in loss of hand and wrist function and most of the forearm pronation and supination. Elbow function and force of elbow flexion will be good. The wrist disarticulation will result in complete loss of hand and wrist function and about 50% loss of pronation

and supination. Amputations below the wrist across the metacarpal bones are called transmetacarpal or partial hand amputations. Functions of all the joints of the arm are intact, and there may be some hand function available, depending on whether the thumb was amputated or left intact.

Many types of prostheses are available for each level of amputation. Each prosthesis is individually prescribed according to the client's needs and lifestyle and is individually fitted and custom-made.[4]

Myoelectrical control of prostheses is a recent development and has been steadily gaining in clinical use over the past several years. Such a prosthesis uses signals from muscle contraction within the stump to activate a battery-driven motor that operates specific component functions of the prosthesis. It is possible to operate the cosmetic hand, wrist rotation, and elbow flexion and extension with myoelectrical controls. Both conventional and myoelectrical controls may be used within the same prosthesis in some instances.[5]

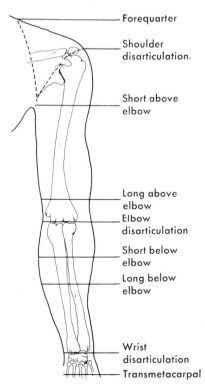

Fig. 21-1. Levels of UE amputation.

Candidates for myoelectrical prostheses are selected for potential success in mastering control and use of the device. Extrinsic factors essential to success with the myoelectrical prosthesis are the proximity of prosthetist, adequate funding sources, available prosthetic training, and appropriateness of the device to the amputee's vocation. Before the prosthesis is prescribed, the level of amputation, limb condition, amount of muscle power, and control of the remaining limb and body are evaluated to determine the appropriateness of the candidate.[5]

ACCESSORIES AND COMPONENT PARTS OF THE UE PROSTHESIS (Fig. 21-2)
Terminal device

Two types of terminal devices (TDs) that are available are the hook and the cosmetic hand. These may be either voluntary-opening or voluntary-closing in design.

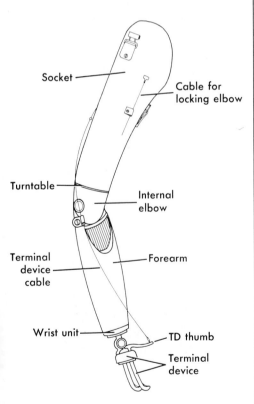

Fig. 21-2. Component parts of standard AE prosthesis. (Adapted from Santschi, W., editor: Manual for upper extremity prosthetics, ed. 2, Los Angeles, 1958, University of California Press.)

The voluntary-opening TD opens when the amputee exerts tension on the control cable, which connects to the "thumb" of the TD. When tension is released, rubber bands, springs, or coils close the fingers of the TD. The voluntary-opening type is the most frequently prescribed.[7]

The voluntary-closing TD is also activated when tension is applied to the control cable. The tension effects locking and maintaining the grasp force on the object in the desired position.

The hook TD may be made of aluminum or steel. It may have canted or lyre-shaped fingers and usually has a neoprene lining for the protection of the objects grasped and for the prevention of slippage. It is the most functional and most frequently prescribed and used TD. Several types of hooks are available to meet the individual needs of the amputee. The farmer's and carpenter's hooks allow for ease in handling tools, and narrow-opening hooks may be used for handling fine objects (Fig. 21-3). On the hook TD, the number of rubber bands controls the amount of grasp pressure. Training usually begins with one rubber band, and the number increases to three to four rubber bands as training progresses.

The cosmetic TD, designed to duplicate the amputee's hand as nearly as possible, is available in addition to the hook. One type of cosmetic hand that is used primarily for its appearance is the flesh-colored glove, which covers a par-

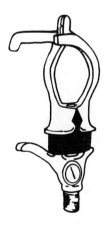

Fig. 21-3. "Farmer's hook," Dorrance model 7, heavy-duty stainless steel.

tial hand. It may be used to hold light objects or position objects by pushing or pulling. Another type of cosmetic hand is the functional hand, which may be attached to the wrist unit and activated by the same control cable that operates the hook. It comes in voluntary-opening and voluntary-closing types. The thumb of the functional hand is prepositioned manually in either of two positions to accommodate small or large objects. The fingers are controlled at the metacarpophalangeal (MP) joints by the prosthesis control cable, and palmar prehension between the thumb and these two fingers is possible through the control system. A natural-looking plastic glove fits over the mechanical hand.[4]

Wrist unit

The wrist unit joins the TD to the forearm socket. There are three basic types of wrist units. These are the friction, locking, and oval types. The wrist unit allows prepositioning of the TD to accommodate the task to be performed. It serves as a disconnecting unit so that TDs may be interchanged. The locking unit allows wrist flexion by manual operation or with the aid of another object, such as the edge of a table. It is usually used by the bilateral amputee for facilitating activities close to the body. The friction unit requires prepositioning of the TD manually or with the aid of another object. There is a rubber washer in the unit that creates the friction sufficient to hold the TD, as it was prepositioned, against moderate loads.[4,7,8]

The oval unit is used with the wrist disarticulation prosthesis. It minimizes the length of the components so that the prosthesis will match the length of the sound arm more closely.

The wrist unit is usually selected for its ability to meet the use needs of the amputee in daily living and vocational activities.[4]

Elbow unit

The elbow unit on the AE prosthesis allows the maximal range of motion (ROM) possible, locking of the elbow in various degrees of motion, and prepositioning of the prosthesis for arm rotation by a manual control friction turntable unit.

A spring-loading device is available for the elbow unit. This device allows the amputee to preset the spring by winding the device so that the amount of effort needed to flex the elbow is reduced by the assistance of the spring mechanism. The spring tension can be set to different levels by the degree to which the device is wound. The tension is reduced by releasing a small pin. The spring-loading device is helpful for lifting heavy loads and for accommodating a short AE stump.[8]

The BE prosthesis has flexible metal or leather hinges that allow amputees with longer stumps to use the available normal pronation and supination.

A rigid metal hinge with a step-up mechanism is available for the short BE stump. It allows the amputee to achieve a range of elbow flexion that would otherwise not be possible. The forearm socket and TD flex 2° for every 1° of flexion of the stump through this mechanism.

The forearm socket on the AE prosthesis provides the connection between the wrist and elbow units. It contains the wrist unit and TD and is fabricated to fit the arm length requirements of the individual amputee. The forearm lift loop, which allows the amputee to flex the prosthesis forearm, is fastened to this forearm socket.[7]

Upper-arm cuff

The upper-arm cuff is used on the BE prosthesis to increase stability and control of the prosthesis and provide an anchor point through which the cable passes to the TD. It prevents the control cable from floating freely and incorporates the elbow hinges to hold the forearm socket to the harness.

Socket

The forearm socket for the BE amputee is made of plastic resins and may have a single or double wall. The socket must be anchored stably on the stump to allow the wearer full power and control of the prosthesis. The BE stump socket may be constructed to allow any remaining pronation and supination to be used. The single wall socket is used when the outside diameter of the distal end of the stump is sufficient to permit tapering to the wrist

unit. The double wall socket is used when the stump is too short or slender to achieve the desired contour or tapering. The inner wall conforms to the stump and the outer wall gives the required length and contour for the forearm replacement. A rotation unit that fastens to the inner socket and rotates inside the outer shell may be used to increase the remaining pronation and supination. This unit is driven by the forearm stump and has a step-up ratio of $2:1$.[4,7]

The AE stump socket is a double wall unit. There is a locking elbow unit laminated onto the socket. The elbow unit provides elbow flexion, extension, and locking at various points in the ROM by the control cable system. The socket must fit snugly and firmly but allow full ROM at the shoulder.[4,7]

Cable and components

The cable is made of stainless steel and is contained in a flexible stainless steel housing. It is fastened to the prosthesis by a retainer unit made of a base plate and a retainer butterfly or a housing crossbar and a leather loop. A ball or ball swivel fitting at one end of the cable attaches it to the TD while a T bar or hanger fittings at the other end attach it to the harness.[3,7]

Harness

The purposes of the harness are to suspend the prosthesis and to provide the anchor point for the control cables. The figure eight Dacron harness is a commonly used design, although others are available. Extra straps may be

added to the figure eight as needed.[3,4,7] The higher the level of amputation the more complex the harnessing system. The amount of muscle power and ROM loss may necessitate variations in the harness design. Fig. 21-4 illustrates the lateral and medial aspect of an AE prosthesis.

Stump sock

A stump sock of knit wool, cotton, or Orlon-Lycra is usually worn by the amputee. It absorbs perspiration and protects from potential discomfort or irritation that could result from direct contact of the skin with the socket of the prosthesis. It accommodates volume change in the stump and aids with fit and comfort of the stump in the socket.[4,8]

THE UE PROSTHETIC TRAINING PROGRAM
Preprosthetic training

During the period between the amputation and the fitting of the prosthesis the amputee is engaged in a training program designed to promote stump shrinkage, desensitize the stump, maintain ROM of proximal joints, and increase the strength of the stump and proximal muscles. In addition, aiding in adjustment to the loss and achieving independence in self-care are important aspects of the training program.[6]

During the preprosthetic period the amputee should be encouraged to use the sound arm to perform activities for daily living (ADL). If the dominant arm was amputated, special training may be required for the nondominant

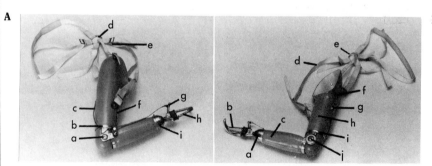

Fig. 21-4. **A,** Lateral side of AE prosthesis. *a,* Elbow unit. *b,* Turntable. *c,* Control cable. *d,* Harness ring. *e,* Figure 8 harness. *f,* Elbow lock cable. *g,* TD thumb. *h,* Hook TD. *i,* Wrist flexion unit. **B,** Medial side of AE prosthesis. *a,* Wrist unit. *b,* Hook TD. *c,* Forearm. *d,* Harness. *e,* Harness ring. *f,* Control cable. *g,* Baseplate and retainer. *h,* Socket. *i,* Turntable. *j,* Spring-load device.

limb to assume the dominant role. Practice in writing and activities requiring dexterity and coordination may be helpful in the retraining process.[4,7] Most amputees change dominance to the sound extremity automatically.

During the preprosthetic period the client may be counseled about the acceptance of the amputation and about the prosthesis and its benefits. It is important for the therapist to be aware of what the amputation and the prosthesis may mean to the client. It is also important to consider whether the client's primary need is function or cosmesis in selecting the prosthesis and presenting it to the amputee.

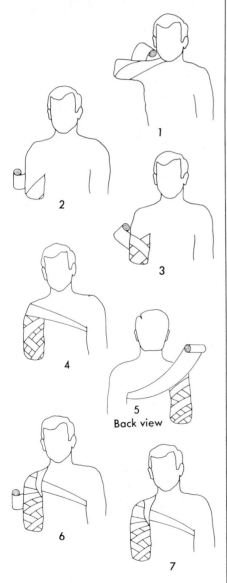

Fig. 21-5. Steps in stump bandaging for AE amputee.

With medical approval stump exercises may be commenced. These are designed to encourage use of the stump, maintain ROM of joints proximal to the amputation site, and strengthen muscles of the arm and shoulder. Many of these muscles will ultimately be used to operate the prosthesis, so strength and endurance are the desired results of training.

The loss of weight of the amputated part will cause a shift in the body's center of gravity. Early exercise programs geared toward correcting faulty body mechanics can help to prevent muscular atrophy, scoliosis, and compensatory curves, which can result from this shift in the center of gravity.

The client is encouraged to move and use the stump as much as possible during the healing period. After complete healing the stump is massaged. This increases circulation, aids with desensitization, reduces swelling, and discourages adhesions from scar tissue. It helps the patient overcome fear of handling the stump.

Stump shrinkage and shaping are effected with Ace bandaging of the stump several times a day. The bandage is applied from the distal to the proximal end of the stump. The bandage must be applied smoothly, evenly, and not too tightly[4,7] (Fig. 21-5).

Small utensils may be strapped to the stump to encourage its functional use. A temporary prosthesis fashioned of plaster or leather may be applied to the stump. This enhances early use of the stump for function and helps to accustom the amputee to prosthesis wear and use. Bilateral activities should be encouraged during the preprosthetic period. The early use of a temporary prosthesis may aid in psychological adjustment and increase the possibility of the acceptance and use of the prosthesis by the amputee.

Checkout of the prosthesis

When the prosthesis is received, it is checked by the members of the rehabilitation team to ensure that it is functioning efficiently, is mechanically sound, and meets prescription requirements. The prosthesis is checked for fit and function against specific mechanical

standards that were developed from actual tests on prostheses worn by amputees. Ranges of motion with the prosthesis on and off are compared. Control system function and efficiency, TD opening in various positions, degree of slippage of the socket on the stump under various degrees of load or tension, compression fit and comfort, and force required to flex the forearm are several of the factors that are measured against prescribed standards during the initial checkout.[7] The following methods and standards for the prosthesis checkout were adapted primarily from Wellerson.[7]

To perform a prosthetic checkout the therapist needs a spring scale (50 pound, 23 kg); ruler; goniometer; tape measure; masking tape; small woodblock (½ inch by ¾ inch by ½ inch or 1.3 cm by 1.9 cm by 3.8 cm); and three special, short adaptor cables to connect the scale to the hook or hand TD and harnessing system; a pencil; and a looped, leather strap.

Checkout of BE prosthesis

ROM. The therapist checks for range of elbow flexion with the prosthesis off and then with the prosthesis on. The ROM of elbow flexion should be the same in each case or lacking no less than 10° except if there are joint or muscle limitations.

Pronation and supination of the BE stump are measured by positioning the stump in neutral rotation and marking a vertical line on the end with the skin pencil. The line is used as a point of reference for goniometer placement and reading of ROM. The measurement is repeated with the prosthesis on. The TD is positioned in neutral rotation, and the TD thumb can be used as a point of reference for goniometer placement. Forearm rotation with the prosthesis on should be no less than 50% of the rotation possible without the prosthesis. This is true for long BE and wrist disarticulation amputations. Very short BE stumps will have little usable forearm rotation.

CONTROL SYSTEM EFFICIENCY. The amputee is positioned with the arm at the side and the elbow flexed to 90°. The TD should be in neutral rotation, and the small woodblock is placed between its fingers. The TD should have no less than 3 pounds (1.4 kg) of pressure (three rubber bands on the voluntary-opening type). The cable is then disconnected from the TD, and the spring scale is attached to the terminal device with a special adapter cable. The therapist stands behind the amputee and applies force to the scale in the same direction as force is applied by the regular control cable. The force on the scale is read at the moment that the finger of the TD begins to move away from the woodblock. Three readings are taken, and the cable of the prosthesis is then reconnected to the TD. This cable is then disconnected from the harness at the back, and the spring scale is connected to the proximal end of the control cable, using a special adapter cable. Once again force is applied to the control cable in its direction of pull, and three readings are taken. If the procedure was done correctly and the mechanism is not faulty, the readings should not deviate from one another by more than a half pound (0.2 kg). One reading is selected. The control system efficiency is calculated by dividing the force at the cable into the force at the TD. The efficiency should be 70% or better.

$$E = \frac{\text{Force at TD}}{\text{Force at control cable}}$$

TD OPENING AT 90° ELBOW FLEXION. With elbow flexed to 90° the amputee is asked to open the TD fully. The opening is measured with the ruler. The TD should have full opening in this position.

TD OPENING AT MOUTH AND FLY. The TD opening is measured as just described with the TD near the mouth (elbow fully flexed) and again near the fly of the trousers (elbow extended). The amputee should be able to achieve 70% to 100% of TD opening in these two positions.

TENSION STABILITY. The prosthesis is straightened to the side of the body. The scale is hooked over the TD, or the scale is hooked to the leather strap used around the wrist of the cosmetic hand. The stump or stump sock is marked with the skin pencil at the level of the upper rim of the socket.

Force is then applied straight down on the scale until it reads 50 pounds (23 kg). The top of the socket pulls away from the pencil mark, and the distance from the pencil mark to the top of the socket is measured. A 50-pound (23-kg) force should not displace the socket more than 1 inch nor should it cause failure of any part of the prosthesis or harness. An alternative method is to measure the distance from the medial or lateral epicondyle to a specific point at the top edge of the socket before and during the application of the force.

COMPRESSION FIT AND COMFORT. The amputee flexes the elbow to 90° and places the back of the elbow against a firm support, such as a wall. The therapist holds the TD, pushes the prosthesis toward the wall, and also pushes down on the TD. These forces should cause no discomfort or pain to the amputee. When the prosthesis is removed, there should be no irritation, blisters, abrasions, or signs of pressure.

Checkout of AE prosthesis

STUMP ROM WITH PROSTHESIS. With the prosthesis on and the elbow locked the amputee is instructed to move the stump (humerus) into shoulder flexion, extension, abduction, and internal and external rotation. The ROM of each of these is measured with a goniometer. Minimal standards for shoulder ROM with the prosthesis on are: flexion, 90°; extension, 30°; abduction, 90°; and rotations, 45°.

FLEXION OF MECHANICAL ELBOW. While the amputee is not wearing the prosthesis, the therapist flexes the mechanical elbow and measures the ROM with the goniometer. The ROM should be at least 135°. The forearm should not be flexed more than 10° when the mechanical elbow is resting in extension.

The amputee is then instructed to put the prosthesis on and actively flex the mechanical elbow. The range of active flexion is measured with the goniometer and should not be less than 135°.

SHOULDER FLEXION REQUIRED TO FLEX THE MECHANICAL ELBOW. While wearing the prosthesis, the amputee is instructed to slowly flex the shoulder, flexing the mechanical elbow.

With the goniometer the therapist measures the amount of shoulder flexion that is required to fully flex the mechanical elbow. This measurement should not exceed 45°.

FORCE REQUIRED TO FLEX THE ELBOW. While the amputee wears the prosthesis, the therapist tapes the TD closed and makes sure the elbow is unlocked. The therapist then attaches the special cable adapter and the spring scale to the control cable at the point where it attaches to the harness. The therapist supports the forearm in 90° flexion, and the upper arm is stabilized in adduction. The therapist then pulls the scale along the normal line of the cable, slowly releasing the forearm so that it remains at 90°. The therapist continues pulling the spring scale until some further elbow flexion is apparent. The force at the moment of this additional flexion should be noted. The force required to flex the mechanical elbow should not be more than 10 pounds (4.5 kg).

LIVE LIFT. The therapist tapes the TD closed, and the amputee flexes the forearm to 90° without locking the elbow. The scale is hooked over the prosthesis a distance of 12 inches (30.5 cm) from the axis of the elbow joint. It may be necessary to use the leather loop strap over the prosthesis at the correct distance. The therapist pulls straight down on the scale while the amputee resists the pull. The scale is read when the forearm slips below 90° flexion. It should be possible for the amputee to resist a force of at least 3 pounds (1.4 kg) at 12 inches (30.5 cm) from the elbow axis.

CONTROL SYSTEM EFFICIENCY. The prosthetic elbow is locked, and the control cable should be disconnected from the TD. The spring scale is attached to the hook thumb or the cosmetic hand by the adapter cable. The small woodblock is placed between the fingers of the TD. The therapist stands behind the amputee and pulls on the scale in the same direction as the pull normally exerted by the control cable. The force required to just move the TD away from the woodblock is recorded after three trials. If the procedure was done correctly and the mechanics of the prosthesis are not faulty, the readings on the three trials should not deviate more than one-half pound from one another. The cable is then reconnected to the TD.

With the elbow flexed to 90° and locked the control cable is disconnected from the harness at the back. The small woodblock is placed between the fingers of the TD as before. The scale is attached to the T bar of the control cable by use of a special adapter cable. The humerus is stabilized in adduction at the side of the trunk. The therapist exerts force on the spring scale, pulling in the same direction as the regular control cable. There should be three trials and three readings taken. One reading is selected to designate the force required to open the TD. The control system efficiency should be greater than 50%. This is calculated by dividing the force measured at the cable into the force measured at the TD.

$$E = \frac{\text{Force at TD}}{\text{Force at control cable}}$$

TD OPERATION AT 90° ELBOW FLEXION. The amputee flexes the TD to 90°, locks the elbow, and then actively operates the TD. The therapist measures TD opening with the ruler. The amputee should obtain full TD opening in this position.

TD OPERATION AT MOUTH AND FLY. The same procedure just described for elbow flexion at 90° is used, except the measurements are taken in full elbow flexion with elbow locked (TD at mouth) and an elbow extension with elbow locked (TD at fly of trousers). The TD opening is measured in both positions, and at least 50% of full opening should be obtained.

INVOLUNTARY ELBOW LOCKING. With the elbow unlocked the amputee is asked to walk a short distance, swinging the prosthesis as in normal arm swing during gait. The therapist faces the amputee and asks the client to abduct the prosthesis to 60°. There should be normal arm swing during ambulation without elbow locking, and with the arm abducted to 60° the elbow should not lock involuntarily.

MOVEMENT OF THE TD DURING ELBOW LOCKING. The therapist stands directly in front of the amputee and holds the end of a ruler at the lateral aspect of the waist and horizontal to the floor. The amputee is asked to flex the elbow to 90° without locking it and is instructed to hold the TD on top of the ruler, touching the therapist's waist and then actively locking the elbow. The TD should not move more then 6 inches (15.2 cm) from the original position. An alternative method would be to measure with a goniometer the amount of shoulder extension required to lock the TD.

TENSION STABILITY. With the prosthesis extended at the side of the body the elbow is locked. The scale is hooked over the TD, or the leather loop strap may be used around the wrist of the cosmetic hand with the scale hooked to the strap. The stump or stump sock is marked with the skin pencil at the level of the top edge of the socket. The therapist pulls straight down on the scale until it reads 50 pounds (23 kg). The socket should not pull more than 1 inch (2.5 cm) away from the pencil mark, and there should be no failure of any part of the prosthesis or harness. An alternative method is to measure the distance from the acromion to a specific point on the top edge of the socket before and during the application of the force.

FIT AND COMFORT. The amputee flexes the elbow to 90° and locks the elbow. The client is instructed to abduct the stump to 60° and then rotate the humerus. The amputee should be able to control the prosthesis during this motion. The socket should not slip around the stump.

With the forearm flexed to 90° and the elbow locked the scale is hooked over the prosthesis at a distance of 12 inches (30.5 cm) from the axis of the elbow joint. The amputee is instructed to resist the pull of the scale as force is applied from the lateral direction. The procedure is then repeated with the scale positioned on the medial side of the TD and the force applied from a medial direction. It should be possible for the amputee to withstand 2 pounds (0.9 kg) of pull at 12 inches (30.5 cm) in both medial and lateral positions. If the prosthesis has a turntable, it should be adjusted to withstand at least 2 pounds (0.9 kg) of pull.

With elbow flexed to 90° and locked the amputee rests the forearm on a table. The client is then instructed to force the stump down into the socket.

The elbow is then moved off the table, and the therapist pushes down on the TD and instructs the amputee to resist the push. There should be no pain or discomfort during these maneuvers. When the prosthesis is removed, the stump should not appear discolored or irritated.

The prosthesis checkout also includes a technical inspection of the prosthesis to determine correct length, fit, and mechanical function of all of its parts. Various forms have been devised to record all of the information for the complete checkout of the prosthesis. The initial checkout is done before prosthetic training is started, and the final checkout is done following all revisions and adjustments of the prosthesis and during or following prosthetic training.

Common considerations in training

The amputee should be instructed in stump hygiene and care of the stump sock in the early phase of the prosthetic training program. The stump and armpits should be washed daily and blotted dry. Underarm deodorant or deodorant powder should be applied every day. At least six stump socks of cotton, wool, or Orlon-Lycra should be obtained. A clean stump sock should be worn every day. The socks should be washed daily and squeezed out, not wrung, gently. The sock is placed on a flat surface to dry and spread out gently to its original dimension and contours. A T shirt for men and an underblouse for women are recommended for wear under the harness. These will absorb perspiration and protect the skin from irritation in the axillae and across the back. Stump socks and undergarments may need to be changed twice a day in very warm weather.[7,8]

The amputee should learn the names and functions of the parts of the prosthesis. This is important so that the amputee can communicate with the therapist, physician, or prosthetist, using terminology understood by all. It is especially important if the amputee is having difficulties with the prosthesis or if it is in need of repairs. The amputee then is trained in donning and removing the prosthesis with ease.[7,8]

Training the unilateral BE amputee

DONNING AND REMOVING THE PROSTHESIS. The amputee dons the stump sock with the sound arm. To apply the prosthesis the amputee places it on a table or bed and pushes the stump between the control cable and Y strap from the medial side into the socket. The harness is placed across the shoulder on the amputated side, and the opposite axilla loop is allowed to dangle down the back. The sound hand reaches around the back and slips into the axilla loop. The amputee then slips into the harness as if putting on a coat. The shoulders are shrugged to shift the harness forward and into the correct position.

To remove the prosthesis the amputee slips the axilla shoulder strap off on the sound side with the TD and then slips the shoulder strap off on the amputated side. The harness is then slipped off like a coat.[6]

TD CONTROL. Scapula abduction and glenohumeral flexion on the amputated side are the motions necessary to operate the TD. The therapist takes the movable finger on the TD and opens it, holding it to show the amputee that the control cable in back is slack. The therapist then pulls the prosthesis forward, so that the amputee's shoulder is in a flexed position and releases the TD, asking the amputee to maintain the tension on the control cable (Fig. 21-6). This will hold the TD open. The amputee is then asked to gradually move the shoulder back into extension, releasing the tension on the control cable and allowing the TD to close. The therapist will then hold one hand at the back of the amputee's stump and passively move the humerus into flexion (Fig. 21-7).[8] The therapist returns the stump to the neutral position at the amputee's side. During this procedure the amputee watches the TD operate and gains a sense of the tension on the prosthesis control cable. The amputee then repeats the motions without the therapist's assistance and verbalizes the actions that occurred during operation.

This same procedure is repeated, except that scapula abduction is used as the control motion. The therapist stands in front of the amputee and passively draws the shoulders together,

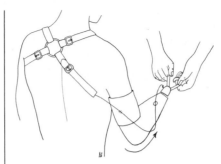

Fig. 21-6. Therapist pulls prosthesis forward, which opens TD, asks amputee to maintain tension on control cable, and then releases hands.

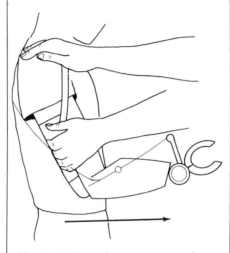

Fig. 21-7. Therapist moves stump forward to attain cable tension and TD opening.

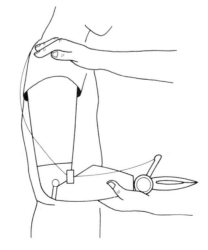

Fig. 21-8. Therapist passively flexes elbow to cause slackening of control cable.

rounding the back. The amputee feels and observes the effect of the motion on the TD and repeats the motion actively. This procedure is again repeated, using scapula depression as the control motion. The therapist instructs the amputee to hold the humerus at the side with the elbow extended. The therapist places one hand directly under the TD and asks the amputee to push down and push the hand away. The amputee again feels and observes the effect on the TD and repeats the movements, verbalizing the actions that are occurring.

If the forearm stump is more than 50% of the normal forearm length, pronation and supination should be practiced. The therapist stands behind the amputee and asks the client to flex the elbow to 90°. The therapist holds the amputee's elbow adducted to the side of the body, and the amputee pronates and supinates the forearm stump, observing the effect on the TD. The amputee then repeats the motion without assistance. The therapist then instructs the amputee to repeat all of these motions in one continuous sequence in both sitting and standing positions until they are smooth and natural.[7]

The amputee will then be instructed to open and close the TD in a variety of ranges of elbow and shoulder motion. TD opening and closing should be accomplished easily with the elbow extended, and at 30°, 45°, 90°, and full elbow flexion, as well as with the arm overhead, down at the side, out to the side, and leaning over to the floor level.[8]

Training the unilateral AE amputee

ELBOW CONTROLS. After learning to don and remove the prosthesis as just described, the AE amputee is instructed in elbow controls. Learning to flex the mechanical elbow is the first step in the training process. The therapist places one hand on the amputee's shoulder and the other on the forearm. The therapist passively flexes the prosthesis into full elbow flexion for the amputee, noting that the control cable is slackened by this maneuver (Fig. 21-8). The therapist then flexes the amputee's shoulder forward and asks the amputee to hold this position while the

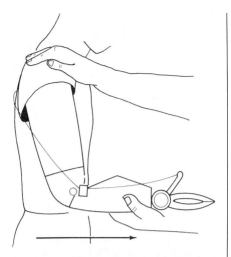

Fig. 21-9. Forearm is moved forward, which causes tension on control cable, to maintain elbow flexion.

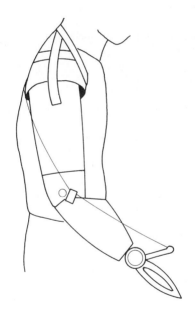

Fig. 21-10. Amputee relaxes stump to allow controlled extension of forearm.

therapist releases his or her hands (Fig. 21-9). The amputee gains a sense of the control cable tension across the scapula from this maneuver. The amputee is then asked to relax the stump to the side of the body once again, slowly allowing the forearm to extend (Fig. 21-10). This procedure is repeated by asking the amputee to flex the humerus and abduct the scapula to accomplish elbow flexion and relax the stump back slowly into shoulder extension to

achieve elbow extension. This is repeated until the amputee gains enough control of cable tension to accomplish elbow flexion and extension smoothly and with ease.[8] The therapist should be aware of the possible need for adjustment of the prosthesis and should consult with the prosthetist if this need becomes apparent.

The therapist then teaches elbow locking by placing one hand on the amputee's shoulder and the other hand on the TD. The therapist passively pushes the humerus into hyperextension with the elbow flexed thus locking the elbow (Fig. 21-11). The therapist brings the arm back to the neutral position and removes his or her hands from the prosthesis, demonstrating that the elbow mechanism is locked. The therapist repeats this maneuver, demonstrating that the elbow is now unlocked. The amputee is then asked to lock the elbow by moving the humerus into hyperextension and rolling the shoulder forward, using scapular depression and abduction at the same time to lock the elbow. This control motion may be difficult to master. It requires practice and the development of a "proprioceptive memory." The same motions are used to unlock the elbow mechanism. The amputee is then asked to practice locking and unlocking the elbow in various ranges of elbow flexion and extension until full flexion and extension are obtained[8] (Fig. 21-12).

TD CONTROL. Once elbow controls have been mastered, TD control training can begin. With the elbow locked the same motions of shoulder flexion and scapula abduction that were used to flex the forearm can now be used to control the TD. The amputee is instructed to lock the elbow, first at 90°, and perform the control motions to open the TD. The sequence of elbow flexion, elbow locking, TD operation, elbow unlocking, and elbow extension is repeated at various points in the range of elbow motion from full extension to full flexion.[6,8]

Once elbow controls are achieved, the therapist should show the amputee how to position the forearm in internal or external rotation. The elbow is flexed to 90°; then the amputee is instructed to rotate the forearm to the desired degree of internal or external rotation by

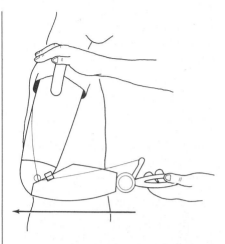

Fig. 21-11. Therapist pushes humerus into hyperextension to lock elbow.

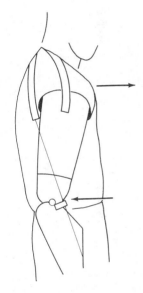

Fig. 21-12. Shoulder is rolled forward, scapula abducted, and humerus hyperextended to lock or unlock elbow at various points in ROM.

passively moving the forearm medially (toward the body) or laterally (away from the body).

Use training for AE and BE amputees

Once controls of the prosthesis are mastered, use training is commenced. The first stage in use training is prepositioning the TD. This involves rotating the TD to the best position to grasp an object or perform a given activity. The BE amputee is instructed to rotate the

Table 21-1
Use training suggestions for the unilateral UE amputees[3,4,7]

Activity	Suggestion	
	Sound arm	Prosthesis
Dressing		
Tie shoes	Use one-handed methods or elastic shoelaces	
	Tie double knot, complete bow	Hold one loop of bow
Tie necktie	Manipulate knot	Hold and stabilize short end of necktie
Don shirt, blouse	Insert in sleeve second, adjust shirt	Insert in sleeve first
Button and unbutton shirt or blouse	Manipulate buttons	Hold fabric taut
Button shirt cuff on sound arm	Hold cuff fabric taut	Button, using amputee buttonhook, if necessary
Don trousers	Tuck in shirt; fasten waist; zip zipper	Hold trousers up; hold bottom of zipper
Hang clothes on hanger	Place hanger in garment and hang in closet	Hold garment
Feeding		
Cut meat	Cut with knife (procedure may be reversed)	Hold fork with handle resting on TD thumb
Butter bread	Hold bread (procedure may be reversed)	Spread butter (TD at neutral, knife stabilized between TD fingers and over thumb)
Fill glass	Hold glass	Turn faucet handle
Open bottle	Open, remove, or unscrew cap	Stabilize carton or bottle
Carry tray	Hold one side of tray	Hold other side of tray, TD in neutral position
Sharpen pencil	Hold pencil	Operate crank
Read book	Turn pages	Hold book
Open envelope	Tear or cut open	Hold envelope
Home management		
Open jar	Unscrew lid	Hold jar
Wash dishes	Hold dish	Hold dish mop or sponge
Dry dishes	Hold dish	Hold towel
Iron	Maneuver iron	Stabilize and adjust garment
Use egg beater	Turn handle	Stabilize beater
Use mop or broom	Guide or push implement	Hold implement
Hammer nail	Use hammer	Hold nail
Hygiene and grooming		
Shave (safety razor)	Insert blade; shave	Hold razor
Apply toothpaste	Hold tube and turn (procedure may be reversed)	Hold cap
Communication and environmental hardware		
Use phone	Dial phone; write message	Hold receiver
Write	Hold pen (if dominant arm); hold paper (if nondominant arm)	Hold pen with TD in 90° pronation (if dominant arm); hold paper (if nondominant arm)
Type	Use one-handed method	Hold typing stick with TD in 90° pronation to operate keys, space bar, and shift key

TD into the desired degree of pronation or supination to accomplish the activity. For the AE amputee this involves flexing and locking the elbow and rotating the turntable to the desired degree of rotation before prepositioning the TD. The goal of prepositioning the TD should be to allow the amputee to approach the object or activity with as near normal a movement as one would with a normal hand and to avoid awkward body movements used to compensate for poor prepositioning.[6]

Along with prepositioning, prehension training should begin, first using large, hard objects, such as blocks, cans, and jars, and progressing to soft, then to crushable objects, such as rubber balls, sponges, paper boxes, cones, and paper cups. These objects should be placed at various heights and positions that demand prepositioning and opening and closing the TD, elbow flexion, and locking and unlocking, at various heights.[8]

A training board with common household hardware attached or actual hardware found in the training facility may be used as the next step in use training. Items, such as a pencil sharpener, door lock, padlock and key, jar and lid, and bottle opener, should be used to challenge the amputee. The amputee should be encouraged to use a problem-solving approach to these and other tasks to determine the best position for the TD and an appropriate use of the sound arm and the prosthesis in bilateral activities (Table 21-1). The prosthesis should be regarded as an assistive device and not as a primary member.

Use training should progress to performance of necessary ADL. The amputee is encouraged to analyze and perform the activities of personal hygiene and grooming, dressing, feeding, home management, communication and environmental hardware, avocation, and vocation as independently as possible. The therapist may help the amputee analyze and accomplish a task when needed or aid in task achievement through the use of a special method or gadget or repetitious practice to achieve the desired level of speed and skill.[7]

Prevocational evaluation may be included in the use training phase of the rehabilitation of the amputee. The therapist will need to assess the client's potential for returning to a former occupation or consider a change of occupation. Work tolerance may need to be improved through the use of increasingly long periods at job samples. Alternate but related occupations may be considered or training or education for new jobs may be necessary. Home management skills and child care should be included as part of the amputee's assessment when appropriate to life roles.[4]

Duration of training

The average adult unilateral BE amputee who is otherwise healthy and well-adjusted will require approximately 6 to 10 hours of training to master control and use of the prosthesis for daily living. The unilateral AE amputee, under the same conditions, will require approximately 15 to 25 hours of training.

The initial training session should be about 1 hour long, and subsequent sessions should steadily increase in time duration in accordance with the client's increasing tolerance for the prosthesis, capabilities in use of the prosthesis, and physical endurance for activity until a full day of wear can be tolerated.

When controls training and initial use training are mastered and wearing tolerance is 1 to 4 hours, the amputee is first allowed to take the prosthesis home for an overnight trial so that the therapist can check for problems and correct faulty use habits before they become well established. Use of the prosthesis over the weekend should follow before the amputee makes the prosthesis a part of his regular daily life.[7]

THE LE AMPUTEE

The preprosthetic exercise program, prosthetic fitting, and ambulation training for the LE amputee are usually carried out by the physical therapist. However, occupational therapy can play an important role in the amputee's rehabilitation.

Stump conditioning in the preprosthetic training period, through purposeful activity, can be carried out in occupational therapy if the amputee has a temporary prosthesis applied at the time of surgery or through the use of a temporary pylon or working prostheses described by Jones[1] in *An Approach to Occupational Therapy*. These devices, which can be constructed according to the specifications described by Jones, can be adapted for use on the floor loom, bicycle jigsaw, and treadle-operated machines. Use of the stump with the pylon or working prosthesis can promote circulation and healing, strengthen stump and proximal musculature, maintain joint ROM, and afford the amputee the senses of pressure, position, motion, and weight that may be similar to the actual prosthesis. In addition, the pylon or working prosthesis can be used to build standing tolerance when used with the stand-up table or can be worn while performing activities that require standing.

When the prosthesis is actually received and adequate ambulation skill has been achieved, the LE amputee can be engaged in ADL, such as dressing, hygiene and grooming, and home management tasks. Transfer and transportation skills may be an integral part of the occupational therapy program. Assessment of the client's vocational role and the need for change or modification should be part of the occupational therapy evaluation.

The temporary pylon or working prosthesis cannot be used until there is sound healing of the surgical site. Clients whose amputations resulted from circulatory disorders may need special adaptations, such as additional padding around the stump or the use of an above knee device on a below-knee amputee, to prevent undue pressure on vulnerable blood vessels and circulatory compromise. These devices should be used only when medical clearance is obtained. Their benefits and the effects of use should be evaluated after every treatment session. Signs of circulatory disturbance and spasms are contraindications for their use.[1]

Sample treatment plan

Case study

Mr. K. is 41 years old. He is a member of a minority group who has lived in poverty all of his life. He is intellectually limited, although some of this may be a result of a poor educational advantage. Mr. K. recently sustained a left AE amputation because of a traumatic injury. The stump is well healed, and there is good stump shrinkage. There are no medical complications.

Mr. K. is receiving state aid, and a prosthesis and vocational training have been authorized for him. He has done janitorial work and tobacco picking in the past. He reads the basic vocabulary necessary for everyday life at home and in the street (for example, signs and simple newspaper headlines). When employed Mr. K. is a steady and hard worker. He is married and has four children, all living at home. His interests are watching television, playing cards, and light gardening.

The client is accepting the prosthesis and is no longer depressed about the loss of his arm. Strength in the stump musculature is good to normal. He was referred to occupational therapy as an outpatient for prosthetic training and vocational evaluation. He will be scheduled for daily treatment sessions.

TREATMENT PLAN

A. **Statistical data.**
1. Name: Mr. K.
   Age: 41
   Diagnosis: Traumatic injury to left arm
   Disability: Left AE amputation
2. Treatment aims as stated in referral:
   Prosthetic training
   Vocational evaluation

B. **Other services**
Medical
Social service
Vocational counseling
Sheltered employment and community social groups (possibly)

C. **OT evaluation.**
Strength: Manual muscle test to muscles of stump
ROM: Left shoulder, test
Sensation (touch, pain, temperature) of end of stump: Test
Physical endurance: Observe
Manual dexterity, unilateral: Observe
Speed of movement and motor planning skill: Observe
Judgment: Observe
Problem-solving skills: Observe
Language skills: Observe
Potential work skills: Observe, test
Work habits and attitudes: Observe
Self-care independence: Test, observe
Independent travel: Observe or test

D. **Results of evaluation.**
1. Evaluation data.
   a. Physical resources.
      (1) Shoulder strength: G to N
          Rotators: G
          Flexors: N
          Extensors: N
          Adductors: G
          Abductors: N
      (2) ROM: All ranges normal
   b. Sensory-perceptual functions. Stump sensation (touch, pain, temperature): intact
   c. Cognitive functions. Limited reading skills prohibit following written directions. Client needs assistance with problem solving but succeeds with some verbal guidance.
   d. Psychosocial functions. Client tends to be quiet, cooperative, and compliant. He socializes when drawn into group interaction, but is somewhat hesitant and shy in interactions with therapist. He appears to be well motivated for prosthesis use and wear and return to employment.
   e. Prevocational potential. Client appears to have potential for unskilled work similar to that which was performed in the past. Janitorial tasks, assembly work, and simple use of tools will be part of the last phases of the prosthesis use training program.
   f. Functional skills. Mr. K. is performing most self-care activities independently, using the sound right arm, except for bilateral activities, such as cutting meat, buttoning shirt, applying deodorant, carrying large objects, and typing shoes. He needs some assistance in analyzing methods for one-handed performance.
2. Problem identification.
   a. Weakness in left shoulder rotators and adductors
   b. Limited problem-solving skills
   c. Partial self-care dependence
   d. Loss of vocational role, family provider
   e. Inability to use AE prosthesis

E Specific OT objectives	F Methods used to meet objectives	G Graduation of treatment
With daily exercise the strength of shoulder rotators and adductors will increase from good to normal	Progressive resistive exercise (PRE) to shoulder adductors, using wall pulleys; PRE to shoulder rotators, using weighted cuffs on stump; client holds stump in 90° shoulder flexion, then 90° shoulder abduction and rotates shoulder internally and externally	Increase resistance by adding weight; increase number of repetitions from 10 to 30 per day
The client will achieve proficiency in stump care within the first week of the treatment program, so that stump care is carried out independently on a daily basis at home	Washing and drying stump; application and removal of stump socks; washing out stump socks; daily change of stump socks	Decrease amount of direction and assistance as proficiency is achieved
The client will know the names and functions of all the parts of the prosthesis by the end of the first week of training	Teach names and functions of parts of prosthesis; review repetitively during remainder of first week of training	
The client will be able to put on and remove the prosthesis smoothly and efficiently within 5 minutes at the end of the first week of training	Repetitive application and removal of prosthesis for practice	Decrease amount of supervision and assistance
The client will achieve proficiency in controls of elbow flexion, elbow locking, and TD opening and closing, so that each control motion is performed when needed with little or no hesitation by the end of the second week of training	Practice in elbow flexion control, elbow locking, and TD opening and closing; practice in performing these tasks in sequence	From need for assistance and direction to *independent* functioning, increase time spent in training sessions and wearing prosthesis
The client will be able to preposition the TD when using practice objects, so that he can preposition the TD and pick up 75% of the objects with little or no hesitation by the end of the second week of training	Grasp and release of objects of various weights, textures, sizes, and shapes in a variety of positions, for example, cans, jars, wood cylinders, blocks, pencils, door knob, and cabinet handles	Grasp and release large, hard objects to soft, light objects; progress from table surface to grasp and release at side, overhead, and on floor
The client will achieve moderate skill in performance of bilateral ADL, so that he is performing 75% of these activities independently at home within the fourth week of training	Fasten trousers; handle wallet; tie shoes; clean fingernails; apply deodorant; tie necktie; button shirt; use phone; cut food	Increase number of simple to complex activities client is expected to perform; decrease amount of supervision and assistance
The client's potential for employment will be evaluated during the fifth and sixth weeks of the training program so that specific information about potential work skills, work habits and attitudes, and work tolerance can be conveyed to the vocational counselor	Janitorial work—floor cleaning, emptying trash Assembly jobs—electronic parts assembly Use of hand tools in light woodwork, such as sawing, hammering, drilling, using a screwdriver, planing, and sanding	Increase complexity and speed of work, time spent at work samples, and amount of manipulation required of prosthesis; decrease amount of instruction and supervision

H. Special equipment.
1. Ambulation aids.
   None required
2. Splints.
   None required
3. Assistive devices.
   Amputee buttonhook to button right shirt cuff

REVIEW QUESTIONS

1. What do the following abreviations mean?
   a. AE
   b. TD
   c. BE
2. Which arm function is lost and which functions are maintained in a long BE amputation?
3. Name two common problems of amputees that can interfere with prosthetic training. How is each solved?
4. What are the purposes of preprosthetic training?
5. Describe activities and exercises suitable for the preprosthetic period.
6. List the five major steps in prosthetic training.
7. What is the sequence of training in learning controls of the AE prosthesis?
8. What is the sequence of training in learning use of the prosthesis?
9. What motion of the arm accomplishes elbow locking on the AE prosthesis?
10. Before an AE amputee can operate the TD, what must be do?
11. What motions accomplish TD opening?
12. How is the TD prepositioned by the amputee?
13. Name two types of TDs. Which is more frequently prescribed and used?
14. How is use training graded?
15. When is the proper time for the amputee in a prosthetic training program to take his prosthesis home?
16. The best position for the TD when holding a coffee cup is at _____°
    _____.
17. When using an eggbeater, the _____ holds the top of the beater while the _____ cranks the handle.
18. Describe the role of occupational therapy in the rehabilitaion of LE amputees.

REFERENCES

1. Jones, M.S.: An approach to occupational therapy, ed. 2, London, 1964, Butterworth & Co. Ltd.
2. Larson, C.B., and Gould, M.: Orthopedic nursing, ed. 8, St. Louis, 1974, The C.V. Mosby Co.
3. Santschi, W.R., editor: Manual of upper extremity prosthetics, ed. 2, Los Angeles, 1958, University of California Press.
4. Spencer, E.A.: Amputations. In Hopkins, H.L., and Smith, H.D., editors: Willard and Spackman's occupational therapy, ed.5, New York, 1978, J.B. Lippincott Co.
5. Spencer, E.A.: Functional restoration:Amputations and prosthetic replacement. In Hopkins, H.L., and Smith, H.D., editors: Willard and Spackman's occupational therapy, ed. 6, Philadelphia, 1983, J.B. Lippincott Co.
6. Trombly, C.A., and Scott, A.D.: Occupational therapy for physical dysfunction, Baltimore, 1977, Williams & Wilkins.
7. Wellerson, T.L.: A manual for occupational therapists on the rehabilitation of upper extremity amputees, Dubuque, 1958, Wm. C. Brown Co., Publishers.
8. Wright, G.: Controls training for the upper extremity amputee, film, San Jose, Calif., Instructional Resource Center, San Jose State University.

CHAPTER 22

Burns

SHIRLEY W. CHAN
LORRAINE WILLIAMS PEDRETTI

The skin is the largest organ of the body and primarily functions as an environmental barrier. It prevents foreign organisms from invading the body, reduces loss of essential body fluids, assists in control of body temperature, regulates heat loss, and serves as a sensory organ. Anatomically the skin consists of two layers: the epidermis, a nonvascular layer made up of epidermal cells, and the dermis, a network of capillaries, sweat glands, sebaceous glands, nerve endings, and hair follicles.[2]

In a burn injury the skin and possibly the underlying structures are damaged, causing a destruction of the environmental barrier. It is one of the most severe forms of trauma to the body, and it can be a life-threatening injury in severe cases.

Burns are categorized as thermal, chemical, and electrical. Thermal injuries can be caused by flame, steam, hot liquid, and hot metals.[2] The extent and severity of the injury depend on the amount of skin surface area involved and the depth of the burn. Although burns are often accidental, it is known that children, the elderly, the physically handicapped, and the mentally unstable are high-risk groups.

Possible disabilities that can result from a burn injury include (1) loss of joint motion because of contractures of scar tissue;(2) loss of muscle strength caused by disuse or nerve involvement; (3) loss of sensation resulting from destruction of the sense receptors in the skin or concomitant nerve damage; (4) loss of body parts, especially common to fingers; (5) disfigurement; and (6) associated injuries, such as loss of vision, neurovascular damage, and fractures.

The injury can result in serious psychosocial problems that the rehabilitation team should be aware of and deal with in their treatment of the patient.

These include depression and withdrawal; adverse reactions to disfigurement; anxiety and uncertainty about the ability to resume work, family, community, and leisure roles; financial difficulties; and concern about being accepted by family and friends.

MEDICAL MANAGEMENT

Following the burn injury the extent and depth of the burn must be medically evaluated to determine its severity. The patient's age, general health, past medical history, part of the body involved, and other associated injuries are important factors in determining the severity of the burn injury.[6]

The percentage of the burn surface area is usually measured by the rule of nines in persons over 16 years of age. The measurements are modified for children to accommodate the difference in proportion of limbs to trunk to head. The rule of nines is used to estimate the total body surface area (TBSA) that has been injured. It divides the body surface into areas of 9% or multiples of 9%[6] (Fig. 22-1).

The depth of the burn is measured by degrees or thickness of the skin injured. This is determined primarily by

appearance of the wound and the presence of sensation, such as pain.[2] With a first-degree burn, such as a sunburn, only the epidermis in involved and damage is minimal. The wound is quite painful, characteristically erythematous and dry but without vesicles. It usually heals by itself in 1 week without scarring. Treatment usually consists of minor measures to relieve discomfort and prevent infection.[1]

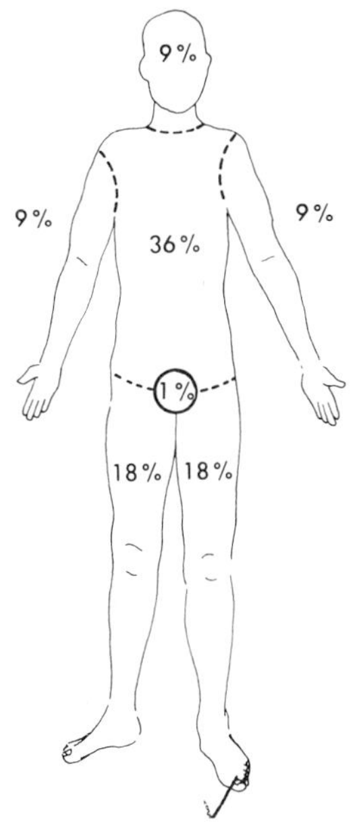

With a second-degree burn, also referred to as partial thickness burn,[1,6] the epidermis and some portion of the dermis is injured. These burns may be superficial or deep depending on the thickness of the dermis involved. The wound is painful, erythematous, possibly exudative with vesicles, and there is subcutaneous edema.[1,6] Healing occurs as a result of regeneration from epithelium-lined skin appendages, which are the hair follicles and sebaceous and sweat glands. A superficial second-degree wound will epithelialize in about 10 to 14 days without scarring. A deep second-degree wound requires 3 to 4 weeks to epithelialize and may require skin grafting. Scarring will occur, and if the burn is over a joint, contracture may also develop. Infection can convert the second-degree burn to a third-degree burn.[1]

The third-degree burn, or full thickness burn, destroys the entire epidermis and dermis down to the subcutaneous tissue.[1] There may be muscle, tendon, or bone damage as well,[6] which is sometimes referred to as a fourth-degree burn. The burn is not painful, since all nerve endings have been destroyed. The wound is leathery and can be pearly white or charred with considerable subcutaneous edema.[2] Spontaneous healing is not possible, and regeneration of the epidermis is only at the margins of the wound. Skin grafting is required to promote wound healing and minimize scarring and contracture.[1]

Fig. 22-1. Rules of nines.

Treatment procedures described in this chapter are modeled after those used at the Bothin Burn Center of Saint Francis Memorial Hospital, San Francisco.

COURSE OF RECOVERY

The course of recovery from a burn injury can be divided into three phases: (1) shock or emergent phase; (2) acute or infection phase; and (3) rehabilitation phase.[1,2]

Shock phase

The shock phase is the first 2 to 3 days immediately after the injury. During this period there is increased permeability of blood vessels, causing rapid leakage of protein-rich fluid to extravascular tissue thus resulting in intravascular hypovolemia.[1,6,7] The lymphatic system, which would normally carry away the excess fluid in the tissues, becomes overloaded,[6] causing subcutaneous edema. Fluid resuscitation, using intravenous fluid, such as Ringer's lactate solution, is extremely essential in this phase to replace venous fluid and electrolytes.[7]

The fluid volume required is determined by various formulas based on the extent of the burn and the weight of the patient.[1,6] The rate of fluid infusion is monitored by pulse rate, urinary output, central venous pressure, hematocrit, and state of consciousness.

In case of circumferential full thickness burns, the edema can produce a rise in interstitial pressure sufficient to impair capillary filling of the distal portion of the extremity, causing limb ischemia.[2] Escharotomy, or incision of the eschar (necrotic tissue), is performed to relieve such pressure and is usually painless because of the destroyed nerve endings. In deep wounds a fasciotomy or an incision down to the fascia is occasionally needed for adequate pressure relief.

Inhalation injury is a common secondary diagnosis with thermal injury, especially in facial burns, and is a major cause of mortality in burn patients. When there is objective evidence of inhalation injury, bronchoscopy, arterial blood gas, and chest x-ray examinations are used to confirm the diagnosis. Treatment usually includes giving the patient high flow oxygen and intravenous steroids. Nasotracheal intubation and ventilatory support may be required along with vigorous respiratory therapy and nasotracheal suctioning. A tracheostomy is generally not performed unless absolutely necessary.[16]

Daily hydrotherapy is carried out in the Hubbard tank or tub to allow thorough cleansing of the wound as well as the uninvolved areas and to allow a total assessment of the wound and enable exercising without restriction of dressings.[2] Debridement may be initiated to remove debris and loose epidermis. Topical and systemic antibiotic therapy may also be initiated.[1]

Acute phase

The acute phase follows immediately after the shock phase and continues until the burn wounds are nearly healed. During this period vulnerability to wound infection, sepsis, and septic shock is especially great, and treatment is focused on promoting healing and minimizing infection. Burn wound colonization begins at the moment of injury, and by the fourth day the normal bacterial flora can be replaced by gram-negative organisms, such as *Pseudomonus aeruginosa*, which lives on dead tissue.[1,15] Wound cultures and biopsies are performed routinely to monitor the severity of the infection, since it can convert into sepsis when there is systemic bacterial penetration.[7] Septic shock is a state of circulatory collapse, a cardiovascular response to bacteria and their by-products (endotoxins), and the result can be fatal. The syndrome is characterized by ischemia, diminished urine output, tachycardia, hypotension, tachypnea, hypothermia, disorientation, or coma.[1]

Infection is treated with topical and systemic antibiotics. Some of the commonly used topical antibiotics are silver sulfadiazine cream, nitrofurazone (Furacin), povidone-iodine, polymyxin B sulfate, Neosporin, and mafenide acetate (Sulfamylon cream).

Debridement is also carried out to remove eschar and can be done chemically using topical ointments, such as proteolytic enzymes (Travase and Collagenase), which act enzymatically to digest dead tissue, or mechanically with forceps and scissors, dressings, or surgically.

Eschar must be removed completely to allow healing and for skin grafting to be successful. There are three types of skin grafts: (1) xenograft, (2) homograft, and (3) autograft. A xenograft or heterograft is processed pigskin, and a homograft or allograft is processed human skin from another person. These are used as biological dressings to provide temporary wound coverage and pain relief. Autograft is a surgical procedure in which skin is harvested from an unburned area of the patient (donor site) and applied to the clean granulating tissues of the burn wound (graft site). With proper care, the donor site will reepithelialize by itself and the skin graft is permanent once it "takes."

Adequate nutrition is absolutely essential during this phase, since the metabolic rate of the burn patient is greatly increased and the protein, vitamin, mineral, and calorie needs are correspondingly increased. Protein is essential for wound healing and must be provided in substantial amounts. Nutritional requirements are calculated based on the TBSA and patient's admission weight. Calorie and protein counts and the patient's weight are monitored daily to ensure proper intake. If the patient is unable to meet individual requirements through diet, high protein and calorie supplements are given either orally or through a nasogastric tube. Intravenous hyperalimentation is occasionally necessary.

Since burn injuries and treatment procedures are often painful, narcotic analgesia is often used liberally.[7] Relaxation and imagery techniques are also employed to reduce stress and anxiety. The amount of narcotic analgesia given will be gradually decreased as the wound heals, and patients usually require minimal pain medications on discharge.

During the shock and acute phases positioning, splinting, and exercising are an integral part of the total treatment program and are carried out consistently to prevent contracture and deformity and to maintain range of motion (ROM).

Rehabilitation phase

The third phase of recovery is the rehabilitation phase. This is the postgrafting period when the patient is medically stable. The goals of treatment are maximal self-care independence, prevention of deformity, contracture, and hypertrophic scarring, recovery of strength and ROM, preparation for discharge from the hospital, vocational exploration, and psychosocial adjustment.

The rehabilitation team is composed of the physician, psychiatrist or psychologist, physical and occupational therapists, nurse, dietitian, social workers, art and play therapists, recreational therapist, vocational counselor, patient, and family. The team works closely together to help the patient achieve individual rehabilitation goals.

During this phase patient and family education is especially important so that the patient can be familiar with his or her care in preparation for discharge. Patient education is done by the entire team, and the family is asked to observe and practice assisting the patient with his or her care. Visiting nurses are particularly helpful in assisting the patient and the family through the initial period following discharge to readjust to the home environment. Reassessment on an outpatient basis is carried out routinely by the team to ensure progressive recovery. If reconstructive surgery is necessary to correct excessive scarring and joint contracture, the patient will need to return for a short hospital stay.

THE ROLE OF OCCUPATIONAL THERAPY
Pregrafting stage

During the initial stage following a burn injury medical management is of utmost importance for the survival of the patient, and the goal of occupational therapy is primarily prophylactic in nature, such as preventing contractures, deformities, and loss of ROM and strength. As the patient recovers and progresses toward the rehabilitation phase, he or she will require less medical intervention, and occupational and physical therapy become the main focus of the treatment program to assist the patient in returning to the previous level of function. Although the role delineation between occupational and physical therapy differs in each facility, it is essential that the two disciplines work closely together and communicate frequently in a team approach so that the patient benefits from the skills and viewpoints of both disciplines.

The occupational therapy evaluation should be completed soon after admission and a treatment program should be established early. This is so that a baseline of the patient's level of functioning can be obtained, rapport can be established, and the patient can get accustomed to the therapy procedures as part of the daily routine. Pertinent information, such as type, percentage, depth, and location of the thermal injury, other secondary diagnoses, past medical history, functional ability before the injury, and psychosocial status can be obtained from the medical history and through a patient interview. Active and passive ROM of affected and unaffected extremities should be measured or estimated without dressings if possible. Any preexisting contractures or deformities should be noted. Muscle strength can be estimated through observation of functional activities. Initially manual muscle testing is not indicated in the involved extremities, since it could cause excessive bleeding and increased pain.

In cooperation with the aims of the other members of the rehabilitation team, the treatment aims of occupational therapy are to prevent deformity and joint contractures, prevent loss of ROM and strength in affected and unaffected parts, achieve maximal self-care independence possible at this stage, and provide psychological support.

Treatment is conducted in a sterile environment, using aseptic techniques, so the therapist must be familiar with infection control procedures.

To prevent contractures and deformity, a splinting and positioning regimen is indicated when there is a burn over a joint, especially over a flexor surface.[11] This should be established soon after admission. The principle of positioning is to maintain the affected extremities in antideformity positions or keep them extended and abducted, since the position of comfort is the position of contracture. Elevating the extremities at the same time will also decrease dependent edema. Positioning techniques are listed in Table 22-1.

Some of the commonly used positioning devices are (1) foam head donut for patients with anterior neck burns to prevent excessive pressure on the occiput, since pillows are not allowed, (2)

foam ear protector to prevent pressure on a burned ear, (3) arm trough to keep shoulders abducted, (4) bed extension for prone positioning, and (5) foot board to keep ankles at a neutral position when supine. Pillows are often used to elevate the extremities.

Splinting plays an important role in maintaining antideformity positions. Splints should not be fabricated until approximately 12 hours after the injury to allow edema to occur, and they are made of low-temperature thermoplastics molded on the patient over the dressings. Splints should be thoroughly cleaned and dried before each application and their fit should be reevaluated at least daily. Revisions are made as often as needed.[6] The splint should be labeled with the patient's name and body part to ensure proper application and to prevent cross-contamination.

Depending on the area involved some splints that may be used to maintain antideformity positions are the neck conformer (Fig. 22-2), axillary or airplane splint (Fig. 22-3), elbow or knee conformer (Fig. 22-4), antideformity hand splint (Fig. 22-5), cock-up splint, three-point extension splint for the elbow or knee, and ankle or foot drop splint. All splints should be removed at least two to three times daily to allow wound cleansing, dressing changes, and exercising the involved joints.

In addition to splinting and positioning the occupational therapy program should include active ROM excerises. Exercising during dressing changes or hydrotherapy is also beneficial, since friction from dressings and bandages is eliminated, thus allowing more joint excursion.[6] Several short sessions of active or gentle passive ROM exercise with five to seven repetitions of each motion are often more effective than a single long session, especially for patients with major burns. Slow, complete motions are encouraged rather than short, jerky movements.

If there are deep second- or third-degree dorsal burns of the hands and fingers, fist making and passive proximal interphalangeal (PIP) flexion should not be performed to protect the extensor mechanism.[8] Progressive resistive exercises may be used for unaffected areas

Table 22-1
Antideformity positioning and splinting[6,15]

Body part and splint	Position		
	Supine	Prone	Side lying
Neck Neck conformer, soft cervical collar	Slight extension; no pillow, except small roll behind neck and/or foam head donut may be used	Extension; small role under forehead or head turned to side	Extension; pillows can be used to maintain position as needed
Shoulders Axillary or airplane splints	Abducted at least 90° with slight internal rotation	Same as for supine position	Position free shoulder at or near 90° flexion
Elbows Elbow conformer, three-point extension splint	Position in full extension and forearm in supination when anterior surface is involved	Alternate between 40° flexion and full extension	Extension; splints may be used to maintain extended position
Wrist and hand Antideformity splint	Splint to maintain antideformity position or maintain wrist extension by placing roll between thumb and fingers; elevate above heart level	Same as for supine position	Splint to maintain antideformity position
Hips No splints used	Extension with approximately 15° of abduction to separate thighs	Same as for supine position	Alternate extension of hips
Knees Three-point extension splint or knee conformer	Extension; splinting if knee, posterior thigh, or leg are burned	Extension; same as for supine position	Alternate extension of knees
Ankles and feet Footboard, foot drop splints	Ankles at neutral position with no pressure at heel and the plantar surface supported; foot drop splint to maintain position; elevate part	Hang feet over edge of mattress to maintain the position	Maintain neutral position; splint if necessary; keep pressure off malleoli

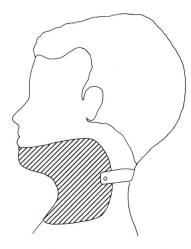

Fig. 22-2. Neck conformer splint to prevent flexion contracture of neck skin.

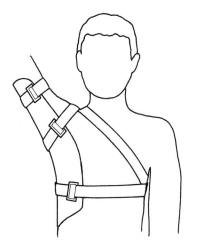

Fig. 22-3. Axillary or airplane splint to prevent adduction contracture of shoulder.

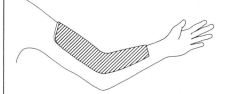

Fig. 22-4. Elbow conformer splint to prevent elbow flexion contracture.

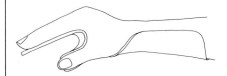

Fig. 22-5. Antideformity splint for dorsal burn of hand to prevent clawhand deformity.

to maintain strength and ROM but are generally avoided for burned areas until good skin coverage is evident. This is to prevent capillary trauma and bleeding during a crucial and tenuous period of healing.

Although physical therapists are generally responsible for gait training, it is important that occupational therapists be aware of the precautions for lower extremity burns as well. When there is lower extremity involvement, elastic bandage wraps must be applied before the patient is allowed to dangle the feet or to ambulate to support the capillary bed in the new granulating tissue and to prevent edema. Elastic bandage wraps should be applied from the metatarsal heads, including the heel, to the groin in figure eight or spiral patterns. Static standing or dangling the feet should be avoided, but if it is necessary, such as when shaving at the sink, the patient should be instructed to take steps in place to improve circulation. The lower extremities should be elevated as soon as the patient returns to bed or sits down. Should there be burns on the soles of the feet, weight bearing on the feet should be eliminated entirely, which includes bridging in bed, standing, and ambulating, until the soles of the feet are healed.

Simple craft activities and self-care activities that are within the patient's ability may be used to encourage purposeful use of affected parts, promote independence, enhance self-esteem, and divert attention from the dysfunction to functional capacities.[11] For patients with hand burns adaptive equipment, such as built-up utensils, may be necessary. Patients who are intubated will need an alphabet board, since they cannot communicate verbally.

The occupational therapist needs to offer the patient reassurance and psychological support. Physical proximity to other people and facilitation of the relationship between the patient and important others in his or her life can help to overcome feelings of revulsion and aversion to self.

Grafting stage

Since it is essential to immobilize and minimize pressure to the new graft after an autograft procedure, additional splints and positioning devices may be needed. It is important that the occupational therapist discuss postoperative positioning needs with the physician and nurses before surgery so that splints and positioning devices are readily available immediately after the surgical procedure. The joints proximal and distal to the graft site are generally immobilized for 5 to 7 days to allow the graft to "take."[5] Gentle active ROM exercise can then commence with the physician's consent and should be done without dressings to avoid shearing on the new graft. At 7 to 10 days, the patient is allowed to exercise with the dressings on, and active, assisted exercises can be started. As the graft heals, the treatment can progress to include resistive exercises and use of exercise equipment, such as reciprocal pulleys. Active exercise to donor sites is generally permitted after 2 to 3 days if there is no excessive bleeding. Lower extremity donor sites are treated similarly to lower extremity burns, and therefore elevation and wrapping with elastic bandage are used. In lower extremity autografts the patient is not allowed to ambulate for 10 days. With the physician's consent the patient is then encouraged and assisted to ambulate for short distances and thus slowly increase his or her endurance. Wrapping with an elastic bandage, elevation, and avoidance of static stance are particularly important to protect the graft.

Throughout the grafting stage, active and resistive exercise to the uninvolved extremities should be continued if possible to maintain ROM and strength. Environmental stimulation, self-care, and avocational activities should be continued and increased if possible, commensurately with the patient's physical abilities and tolerance level.

Depending on the parts involved, activities that can be used include leather lacing, ceramic tile work, peg games, and puzzles.[5] Activities that require irritating substances or potentially hazardous tools or equipment, such as clay modeling or woodworking should be avoided.[13]

Postgrafting stage

When the grafts heal and activity level increases, the patient is in the rehabilitation phase.

During this phase a more thorough occupational therapy evaluation can be carried out with greater emphasis on assessment of performance skills.

Active and passive ROM measurements should be taken. Muscle strength can be measured by the manual muscle test, although this should be done only if the graft has taken well and with extreme caution when applying resistance on skin surfaces. Endurance and performance of self-care and home management activities should be evaluated, including the need for assistive devices.[3]

Home visits may be needed, depending on the patient's independence, social situation, and home environment. Psychological adjustment should be assessed by observation, interview, and consultation with other members of the rehabilitation team, especially the psychologist or psychiatrist and the social worker. Some patients may require driving evaluation. Evaluation of vocational potential should be undertaken in the later stages of rehabilitation if residual dysfunction necessitates a change in former vocational role.[3]

During the rehabilitation phase the treatment aims are to (1) familiarize the patient with necessary care in preparation for discharge from the hospital, (2) increase ROM of affected joints, (3) improve strength and physical endurance for return to community and employment, (4) prevent hypertrophic scarring, (5) achieve independence in activities of daily living (ADL), (6) explore vocational potential, and (7) aid psychological adjustment, including the restoration of self-confidence, social adjustment, and community reentry.[3]

Because of the damaged or destroyed sebaceous glands, artificial lubrication to the healed area is necessary. A lubricant is applied at least twice daily while massaging the scars in a circular fashion. This will assist in softening the scars and is especially beneficial when done before exercising. It is also a form of desensitization. Sunlight exposure to the involved area should be avoided, since the new skin is more prone to sunburn and hyperpigmentation. The patient should be encouraged to use the involved extremities during functional activities. An active resistive exercise and therapeutic activity program should be established so that they can be carried out after discharge from the hospital.

Simulated work activities or work sample testing may be used to evaluate vocational potential. Training in self-care and home management activities and use of assistive devices as needed are carried out. Training in mobility, transfers, and ambulation is appropriate if wheelchair or other ambulation aids are required.

Hypersensitivity of burned areas may be decreased through the self-application of handling, touch, and pressure stimuli, and activities using tools and materials may be graded from soft to hard. This must be done with extreme caution to avoid blistering and breakdown of the newly healed skin.

Pressure splints, bandages, and pressure garments are used to prevent hypertrophic scarring.[3] The occupational therapist is often responsible for the measurement, ordering, and fitting of the pressure garments[5] and for patient instruction regarding their application and care. These are designed to conform to the burned part with the desired amount of pressure at different points in the garment.[13] They are used from approximately 2 weeks after grafting and have proved to be effective in reducing hypertrophic scars and contractures.

The occupational therapist should maintain a supportive and reassuring approach, yet not give excessive or false praise or demonstrate pity. Activities that require gradually increasing amounts of decision making, responsibility, and initiative can increase self-determination and self-confidence.

Splinting at this stage is used to correct deformities, increase ROM, and apply extra pressure to problem areas. Static and dynamic splints may be used, depending on the need. Night-time splinting allows functional use of the extremity during the day and prevents contractures at rest. Outpatient follow-up visits are important to assess the patient's progress and monitor for new problems that may arise. Reassessment of ROM, scars, effectiveness of the pressure garments, splints, home program, activity level, ADL independence, and psychosocial readjustment should be carried out every 6 to 8 weeks for 1 year or sometimes longer. Driving evaluation and prevocational assessment may also be needed. More frequent outpatient occupational therapy may be necessary to provide a more structured treatment program for complications and special needs. This decision is made by the physician and the occupational therapist on an individual basis.

COMPLICATIONS OF BURN INJURY
Heterotopic ossification

Heterotopic ossification is a calcium deposit in a joint, frequently at the elbow, that causes progressively limited joint excursion with a stiff endpoint and considerable joint pain. It occurs more commonly in circumferential burns of the extremities, and the therapist should be aware of its early signs. If they appear, the physician should be notified. It has been found that positioning the elbow in 5° to 10° of flexion instead of full extension can help decrease potential disability. Once it has developed, active ROM exercise to the joint should be carried out frequently but only within the pain-free range. Use of splints and passive stretching to the involved joint should be discontinued. The condition may resolve itself with time or surgical intervention may be required.

Peripheral nerve injury

Peripheral nerve injury can result from improper splinting, awkward positioning, and prolonged immobilization. Frequent reassessment of the patient's neurological status is advisable and notice should be taken of any signs, such as decreased muscle strength or sensation.

Decubitus ulcer

Decubitus ulcers are caused by excessive pressure, usually over a bony prominence, for a prolonged period of time. They can be prevented by proper positioning, frequent change of position, and devices, such as foam donuts and water bags, placed under areas where excessive pressure is anticipated.

Hypertrophic scarring, contracture formation, and pressure therapy

Most burn wounds have a satisfactory flat appearance on healing. However, it can worsen with time because the healed burn wound does not become elevated until 1 to 2 months after basic wound coverage. The process of healing of burn wounds is conducive to the formation of hypertrophic scars and concomitant contractures. The following are characteristics of a hypertrophic scar:

1. *Marked increase in vascularity.* A scar that remains hyperemic at the end of 2 months following healing and becomes progressively firmer will become hypertrophic.
2. *Marked increase in fibroblasts, myofibroblasts, collagen, and interstitial material.* The contractile properties of fibroblasts, myofibroblasts, collagen, and interstitial material may exert sufficient force to cause contractures, and the burn wound will shorten until it meets an opposing force.
3. *Voluntary muscle contraction.* Most patients prefer to assume a flexed, adducted position for comfort. This permits the new collagen fibers in the wound to fuse together. The collagen becomes compact and piled up in whorls and nodules, which results in scar contracture. New hypertrophic scar, which is made of collagen, is easily influenced by mechanical forces. Because collagen linkage is less stable in new scars, it will readily respond to pressure and splinting. Early and consistent intervention using pressure garments and splinting to prevent hypertrophic scarring and contracture formation is the treatment of choice.[9]

Pressure garments are indicated for all donor sites, graft sites, and burn wounds that need more than 2 to 3 weeks to heal spontaneously. Pressure can be applied when the open area is smaller than 1 inch (2.5 cm) in diameter. Pressure garments should provide approximately 35 mm Hg pressure to the involved area and must be worn continuously and consistently for 23 hours a day to be effective. They should be removed only for bathing and changing into a clean set. Both custom-made garments and ready-made garments are available commercially.* Ready-made garments are often used temporarily while waiting for custom-made garments to be fabricated. All custom-made garments need to be measured and ordered following the special instructions of each company. The companies will provide order forms and instructions on request. Elastic bandages are sometimes used as an alternative form of pressure.

Some of the most commonly used garments are the face mask, chin strap, vest, sleeve, glove, gauntlet, panty brief, waist height support, knee height support, and anklet (Fig. 22-6). Willis[17] described and illustrated a variety of Jobst garments. Generally two of each garment are ordered to allow for laundering. Because of the resilient construction of the fabric, it is essential that the garments are hand washed with pure soap and air dried in the shade. Use of washing machines, dryers, and direct heat should be avoided to prolong the life of the garments. If they are cared for properly, the garments will last approximately 3 months before a new set is needed. Children will need replacements more frequently resulting from their growth and active life-style.

Pressure should be applied to the burned area for approximately 6 to 12 months or until the scarring process is complete. Donor sites and sites of reconstructive surgery can also benefit from pressure therapy for 2 to 3 months. When the scar matures, there is resolution of the hyperemia, the area is flat and soft to the touch, and wrinkles appear when gently squeezed. When scar maturation occurs, the patient is instructed to remove the pressure garments or to reduce the time spent wearing them until they are no longer needed.

---

*Custom-made garments are available from the Jobst Institute, Inc. in Toledo, Ohio and Bio-Concepts, Inc. in Phoenix, Arizona. Ready-made garments are available from Genetic Laboratories, Inc. in St. Paul Minnesota and from Tubigrip, which is distributed by Mark One Health Care Products, Inc. in West Point, Pa.

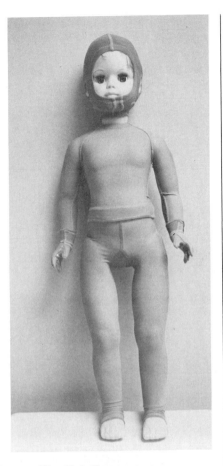

Fig. 22-6. Pressure garments.

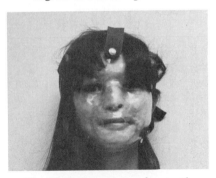

Fig. 22-7. Transparent face mask.

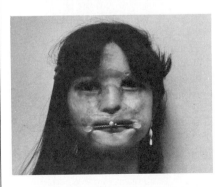

Fig. 22-8. Microstomia device.

For facial hypertrophic scars, the standard treatment used to be the elastic face mask. However, because of the multiple openings for the eyes, nose, and mouth and the contours of the face, it was found that the ordinary face mask does not provide adequate pressure in the central area of the face. In recent years the transparent face mask (Fig. 22-7) made with a high temperature material, Uvex, has been used. This provides more adequate pressure than the elastic face mask and is more cosmetically acceptable, since it is transparent and the patient's face and expression can be seen.[10] Transparent face masks are custom-made by therapists and orthotists at many burn centers throughout the country. Burns around the oral area can lead to microstomia, or "small mouth," caused by tight scars around the mouth. Mouth stretching exercises are essential and a microstomia device (Fig. 22-8) that acts as a mouth splint is commercially available.[4]*

THE BURNED HAND

A burn injury of the hand requires special consideration, since it is a common injury. It can result in serious dysfunction if not treated appropriately. These inujuries are primary concerns of the occupational therapist.[6]

Dorsal burns are more common than those on the palmar surface. A dorsal burn can result in a clawhand deformity. A contracture of the skin on the dorsal surface of the hand will tend to flatten the metacarpal transverse arch and pull the metacarpophalangeal (MP) joints into hyperextension with associated flexion of the interphalangeal (IP) joints, and the thumb will assume the adducted and extended position. The wrist may be pulled into flexion and radial deviation.[6] The extensor tendons, which lie superficially on the dorsum of the hand, are especially vulnerable to injury as they cross the proximal interphalangeal (PIP) joint. The central slip of the extensor tendon, inserting at the PIP joint, may rupture. If this occurs, a boutonnière deformity can result.[6,12]

---

*One type, the microstomia prevention appliance, can be obtained from the Microstomia Prevention Appliance, Inc., Iowa City, Iowa and is available in several sizes.

Serious palmar burns are uncommon because of the thickness of the palmar skin and because the hands are used instinctively to protect the face or body.[15] Palmar burns usually result from direct contact with a hot object, electricity, or chemical substance. The deformity that could result from the palmar burn is severe flexion and adduction contractures of the fingers and thumb.[15]

Treatment of the dorsal burn

The elements of treatment of a dorsal burn of the hand consist of active exercise, or active-assisted exercise if the patient is incapable of active motion, splinting, and elevation of the hand above heart level from the first day after the injury occurs. Elevation can be done by securing a tube stockinette over the arm to a position above the elbow and attaching the other end as high as possible to an intravenous stand. Another method, less effective when there is severe edema, is to rest the hand on pillows. When the dorsum of the fingers are burned, the hand is splinted in the antideformity position,[6] which is 0° to 30° of wrist extension, 45° to 70° of MP flexion, complete PIP and distal interphalangeal (DIP) extension, and extension and palmar abduction of the thumb.[12] This position prevents contracture of the collateral ligaments and intrinsic muscles, protects the central slip of the extensor tendon over the PIP joint from rupture, and maintains the dorsal skin and thumb web space fully stretched. The splint is applied over the dressing with a bias-cut stockinette or rolled gauze. The splint should be wrapped securely, particularly across the PIP joints, but not so tightly as to inhibit circulation. This will prevent the hand from slipping on the splint, which could cause the hand to assume a clawhand position.[6] Hand position should be checked at least daily and the splint should be remolded when necessary. If the fingers are spared, a cock-up splint with 0° to 30° of wrist extension is adequate.

In first-degree or superficial second-degree burns splinting may not be necessary unless there is edema and resulting tendency to revert to the claw position. Active exercise is initiated on the first day with no restrictions of motion. Fist making is allowed, and the patient is encouraged to use the hand functionally.

In moderate to deep second- to third-degree burns continuous splinting is necessary during the edema phase except during exercise periods and dressing changes. When edema has subsided, the splint is removed for periods of supervised functional activities and exercise during the day to encourage motion. To protect the extensor mechanism, passive PIP flexion and fist making are contraindicated, and the patient should be made aware of this. ROM exercise is modified so that active PIP and DIP flexion exercises are allowed if the MP joints are stabilized in extension, and MP flexion exercise is done with the IP joints extended. Full finger extension and abduction and wrist and thumb motions are allowed. The patient is encouraged to perform ADL, such as self-feeding, brushing teeth, and marking hospital menus. Adaptive equipment, such as built-up utensils and pen, is needed to avoid excessive stretching of the extensor tendons. Continuous splinting is maintained until full coverage of dry skin over the MP and PIP joints is visible. At this time, fist making is allowed and encouraged. Other hand activities, such as squeezing a foam ball, manipulating therapy putty, simple hand crafts, writing, dowel sanding, and muscle strengthening exercises are performed.[12] A pressure glove is necessary and should be ordered as soon as the hand has good dry skin coverage. A thorough hand evaluation should be administered to obtain baseline data. The hand evaluation should include passive and active ROM, strength, sensation, coordination, and functional testing.

Treatment of the palmar burn

The treatment of the full thickness palmar burn also involves splinting, positioning, and exercise. The antideformity position is 0° to 20° of wrist extension, full extension and abduction of the fingers, and extension and radial abduction of the thumb.[6,12] A volar or dorsal pancake splint can be used to maintain the hand in this position, and a bulky dressing is used to keep the fingers abducted. An alternative is the banjo splint applied to the dorsum of the hand. Dressmaker's hooks, glued to each fingernail with a polymer adhesive, allow the fingers to be held in gentle traction by fastening rubber bands from each of them to the distal end of the splint.[14] There is no contraindication to fist making or to ordinary ROM exercise. Functional use of the hand should be encouraged as tolerated. Guidelines for applying pressure garments are the same as for the dorsal burn of the hand.

When there is a circumferential burn of the hand, the dorsal and palmar antideformity splints can be used alternately.

Some of the common complications of hand burns are web space contracture, tendon adhesion, finger flexion contracture, and boutonnière deformity, which is sometimes accompanied by a sharp abduction and rotation contracture usually seen in the fifth digit. Splinting, exercise, and pressure devices are needed. Finger web spacers can be ordered from companies that make custom-made pressure garments* or can be inexpensively made by using foam inserts between fingers under the pressure glove to provide extra pressure to each web space involved. A dynamic finger extension splint with a lumbrical bar is often used to increase PIP and DIP extension while preventing hyperextension of the MP joint. A dynamic MP flexion splint, which is made by attaching rubber bands and finger cuffs at the volar surface of a cock-up splint, is also commonly used to increase ROM. Surgical intervention is often needed to acquire maximal functional or cosmetic results. After surgery splinting, exercise, and pressure may be indicated to achieve the best outcome.

---

*These can be ordered from Jobst Institute, Inc. in Toledo, Ohio or Bio-Concepts, Inc. in Phoenix, Arizona.

Sample treatment plan

Case Study

Mr. B. is a right-handed, 45-year-old automobile assembly worker who was burned in an automobile accident. He sustained deep second- and third-degree burns in the region of the left shoulder, left axilla, anterior surface of the left arm, and dorsum of the hand.

Mr. B. is considered a well-adjusted family man. He lives with his wife and two teenaged children in their own home. He is the sole support of his family. His leisure activities include spectator sports, card playing, gardening, golf, and home repairs.

He has been admitted to the burn unit of a rehabilitation center. Occupational therapy has been called on to treat Mr. B. through all phases of rehabilitation. The objectives are to maintain ROM; prevent contractures, deformity, and hypertrophic scars; restore maximal functional independence; and aid with adjustment to disability.

TREATMENT PLAN

A. Statistical data.

1. Name: Mr. B.
   Age: 45
   Diagnosis: 10% TBSA of deep second- and third- degree flame burns to the left upper extremity
   Disability: Potential axillary contracture, elbow flexion contracture, and clawhand deformity, and hypertrophic scars
   Surgery: Debridement and split thickness skin graft to left upper extremity
   Donor site: Left thigh
2. Treatment aims as stated in referral:
   Prevent contractures and deformity
   Maintain or increase ROM and strength
   Prevent hypertrophic scars
   Restore to maximal functional independence
   Aid with adjustment to disability
3. Precautions:
   Contraindications until dorsum of fingers are healed
   —No fist making
   —No passive PIP flexion
   —MP and IP joints are exercised separately
   Elastic bandages wrap lower left extremity when up after surgery

B. Other services.

Physician: Wound and medical assessment; prescribe medication; perform debridement or escharotomy as needed; supervise rehabilitation therapies; grafting
Nursing: Nursing care; positioning; administer medications; change dressings; carry out ADL
Physical therapy: Prevent contractures through ROM and strengthening exercises; hydrotherapy procedures
Psychologist: Evaluate psychological status; counsel; consultant to staff
Social worker: Explore financial problems; counsel patient and family
Family: Provide support, acceptance, encouragement, and assistance
Vocational counseling: Explore feasibility of return to same or similar job; explore job alternatives, if needed
Recreational therapy: Mental stimulation; activities for enjoyment and diversion; function of affected and nonaffected parts
Dietitian: Assess and monitor calorie and protein requirements and intake; provide supplemental diet as needed

C. OT evaluation.

Pregrafting.
Active and passive ROM: Observe
Muscle strength: Observe for function
ADL: Observe
Need for splints and positioning: Observe
Psychological status: Observe, interview, and consult with psychologist
Postgrafting.
Active and passive ROM: Measure
Muscle strength: Functional muscle test with precautions
Hand function: Test
ADL: Evaluate performance
Pressure garments: Assess need, measure, order, fit, and monitor
Psychological adjustment: Observe
Sensory modalities: Test for touch and thermal sensitivity; hypersensitivity
Vocational exploration: Evaluate simulated work skills
Assistive devices: Observe need

D. Results of evaluation.

1. Evaluation data.
   a. Physical resources.
      Pregrafting: Active ROM limited to 0° to 145° of shoulder flexion and abduction; full active flexion and extension of elbow and wrist; finger extension within normal limits; finger flexion limited by edema and pain as follows: MP joints (0° to 45°), PIP joints (0° to 30°), and DIP joints (0° to 5°); all remaining extremities are within normal limits
      Postgrafting: Shoulder flexion and abduction ROM increased to 0° to 150°, full motion possible at elbow and wrist; full finger extension possible; finger flexion increased as follows: MP (0° to 60°), PIP (0° to 45°), and DIP (0° to 10°); opposition only possible to tip of fourth finger; in fist making fingertips are 1 inch (2.5 cm) away from palm; strength in left arm rated good in all muscle groups; all remaining extremities are within normal limits
   b. Sensory-perceptual functions. Pregrafting: Not tested
      Postgrafting: Hypersensitivity to light touch and thermal stimuli; normal perceptual functions
   c. Cognitive functions. No cognitive deficits observed
   d. Psychosocial functions. Initial depression and withdrawal gradually being replaced by increasing motivation to recover and resume former life roles; active involvement and participation in the rehabilitation program increasing; patient realistic about injury, medical status, and future potential
   e. Prevocational potential. Since a good recovery is expected, patient will probably be able to return to former place of employment at a less demanding job on the line; physical endurance, work speed, and use of power tools will be evaluated during the stage of extended rehabilitation

Continued.

Sample treatment plan—cont'd

f. Functional skills.

Pregrafting: Patient able to do most hygiene and grooming, feeding, and dressing activities with uninvolved hand, using one-handed techniques, except for washing and combing hair

Postgrafting: Patient independent in all self-care activities and light home management activities and able to handle garden tools and do light gardening (raking and planting); he cannot play golf because of sudden stretching movements required; he can handle minor woodworking tools without difficulty and can hold cards with left hand, although it tires easily and he prefers to use a card holder

g. Hand function. Right hand is normal; left hand unable to perform gross grasp; maximal lateral pinch 3 pounds (1.4 kg) (below tenth percentile); maximal palmar prehension 2 pounds (0.9 kg) (below tenth percentile); performed below tenth percentile on all subtests of Jebsen-Taylor Hand Function Test

2. Problem identification

Pregrafting:

a. Potential contracture and deformity of left shoulder, elbow, wrist, and hand

b. Depression and withdrawal, initially

c. Anxiety about hospitalization and potential disability

Postgrafting:

d. Decreased physical endurance

e. Limitation of strength in left arm and hand

f. Limited ROM in left shoulder and hand

g Limited left hand function and coordination

h. Changed vocational and leisure roles

i. Potential hypertrophic scarring

j. Hypersensitivity of grafted areas

3. Assets/functions.

a. Normal right arm and lower extremities

b. Good coping skills

c. Supportive family

d. Good potential for reemployment

e. Severe deformity prevented in pregrafting and grafting stages of treatment

f. Intelligent, realistic outlook

g. Good motivation and cooperation with medical and rehabilitation efforts

E Problem	F Specific OT objectives	G Methods to meet objectives	H Gradation of treatment
Pregrafting stage a	Through splinting, positioning, and exercise, contracture and deformity will be prevented at shoulder, elbow, wrist, and fingers	Positioning and splinting the shoulder in 90° of abduction, elbow in 5° of flexion and hand with wrist extended, MPs flexed to 45°, PIP and DIP in complete extension, thumb abducted and extended	Revise splints as edema decreases to maintain maximal deformity positions
		Elevate arm above heart to reduce edema	
		Active ROM exercise, if possible for all joints, frequently for very short periods of time following precautions outlined on p. 287	Passive to active exercise if active ROM is not possible initially
b, c	Through a supportive and accepting approach and environment and appropriate activities, the patient's depression will subside, and he will participate more actively in the rehabilitation program	Therapist uses supportive, reassuring approach to patient	Increase interaction with staff and other patients
		Procedures are carefully explained and guided	
		Therapist explains potential disability and preventive measures to patient and family	
		Card and board games with other patients are used to enhance discussion of feelings, reactions to injury, anxieties about disfigurement, and acceptance; therapist acts as guide and facilitator	Increase independent decision making regarding activities and topics of discussion

E Problem	F Specific OT objectives	G Methods to meet objectives	H Gradation of treatment
Grafting stage a	Through appropriate splinting and positioning, grafted areas will be prevented from moving to promote healing	Axillary splint with shoulder abducted to 110°, hand elevated Elbow conformer splint to maintain full extension Antideformity splint for hand Splints worn 24 hours per day for 5 to 7 days	
a	Through active and resistive exercise during immobilization, muscle strength will be maintained at good grade in uninvolved areas	Active and resistive exercise to right upper extremity and both lower extremities	
Postgrafting stage a, d, e, f, g	Through exercise and functional activities, ROM, strength, and coordination in left arm will be maintained or increased	Gentle, active exercise to all joints of left arm against gravity Independent performance of self-care activities Board games or leather lacing positioned for maximal possible reach overhead, in front, and out to side of body	Increase to light resistive exercise as strength and tolerance improves Add gardening activities when well healed Add fine hand activities, such as peg games
a	Through positioning and splinting, ROM will be maintained	Left shoulder abducted at 90° at all times Left axillary and hand splints at night	Discontinue splinting when full ROM is gained
i	Through pressure garments, hypertrophic scarring will be minimized or prevented over grafted areas and donor site	Jobst vest with long left sleeve, left glove, and panty brief to be worn 23 hours per day for 9 to 12 months	Discontinue pressure garments when scars are no longer active
j	Through graded tactile stimulation, grafted areas will be desensitized so that touch, light rubbing, and pressure can be tolerated in everyday living	Self-application of touch and pressure stimuli and self-massage with lotion with caution for blistering and skin breakdown	Include fabric and brushes graded from soft to coarse Increase pressure during touch and massage

I. **Special equipment.**
   A. Ambulation aids.
      None required except elastic bandage wrap or pressure garments to lower left extremity when up
   B. Splints.
      Axillary splint: Maintain abduction at shoulder
      Elbow conformer: Maintain extension
      Antideformity splint: Prevent claw deformity for dorsal burn of the hand
   C. Assistive devices.
      None required

REVIEW QUESTIONS

1. What is the role of the occupational therapist in the pregrafting stage of treatment of the burn patient?
2. What is the purpose of splinting after burn injury?
3. Describe or demonstrate the anti-deformity position for bedrest in the supine position.
4. What types of exercise are commenced 7 days after grafting?
5. What is the precaution for exercising a hand with a dorsal burn? Why is this so?
6. What is the purpose of pressure garments?
7. In which position is the hand with palmar burn splinted?
8. Which important tendon can be ruptured when there is a dorsal burn? How can this be prevented?
9. How can the occupational therapist help the patient accept him or herself and prepare the patient for return to the community?
10. What are some of the social and psychological problems that the burn-injured patient may experience? Discuss how occupational therapy can help to prevent or minimize these problems during early phases of treatment and later during the extended rehabilitation program.
11. What are the precautions for lower extremity burns?
12. What are the indications to use pressure garments, and when are they discontinued?

REFERENCES

1. American Burn Association: Aims of the American Burn Association: prevention, care, teaching, research, New Orleans, American Burn Association. Mimeographed.
2. Dyer, C.: Burn care in the emergent period, J. Emerg. Nurs. **6**:9, 1980.
3. Gorham, J.A.: O.T. for the burn patient, lecture, San Jose, Calif., 1975, Department of Occupational Therapy, San Jose State University.
4. Gorham, J.A.: A mouth splint for burn microstomia, Am. J. Occup. Ther. **31**:2, 1977.
5. Krocker, C., Denor, B., and Nicoud, B.: Occupational therapy in the rehabilitation of burn patients, Milwaukee, 1977, St. Mary's Hospital.
6. Malick, M.H.: Burns. In Hopkins, H.L., and Smith, H.D., editors: Willard and Spackman's occupational therapy, ed. 6, Philadelphia, 1983, J.B. Lippincott Co.
7. Nolan, W.B.: Acute management of thermal injury, Ann. Plast. Surg. **7**:3, 1981.
8. O'Donnell, L.K.: Hand protocol: Bothin Burn Center rehabilitation therapy procedure manual, Saint Francis Memorial Hospital, San Francisco, Unpublished.
9. O'Donnell, L.K.: Hypertrophic scarring and contracture formation: Bothin Burn Center rehabilitation therapy procedure manual, Saint Francis Memorial Hospital, San Francisco, Unpublished.
10. Rivers, E.A., Strate, R.G., and Solem, L.D.: The transparent face mask, Am. J. Occup. Ther. **33**:2, 1979.
11. Schiff, W.: O.T. for the burn patient, lecture, San Jose, Calif., 1977, Department of Occupational Therapy, San Jose State University.
12. Tanigawa, M.C., O'Donnell, L.K., and Graham, P.L.: The burned hand: a physical therapy protocol, J. Phys. Ther. **54**:9, 1974.
13. Trombly, C.A., and Scott, A.D.: Occupational therapy for physical dysfunction, Baltimore, 1977, The Williams & Wilkins Co.
14. Von Prince, K., Curreri, W., and Pruitt, B.A.: Application of fingernail hooks in splinting burned hands, Am. J. Occup. Ther. **24**:556, 1970.
15. Von Prince, K., and Yaekel, M.: The splinting of burn patients, Springfield, Ill., 1974, Charles C. Thomas, Publisher.
16. Weil, R., et al.: Smoke inhalation injury, Ann. Plast. Surg. **4**:2, 1980.
17. Willis, B.A.: Burn scar hypertrophy: a treatment method, Galveston, Tex., 1973, Shriners Burn Institute.

CHAPTER **23**

Rheumatoid arthritis

LORRAINE WILLIAMS PEDRETTI
MARY C. KASCH

Rheumatoid arthritis is a chronic systemic disease that can affect the lungs, cardiovascular system, and eyes in some clients. However, joint involvement resulting from inflammatory disease of the synovium is the primary clinical feature.[7,16,18] The disease may range from mild to severe and can result in joint deformity and destruction of varying degrees.[16]

Although rheumatoid arthritis occurs most frequently between the ages of 20 and 40[7] and about three times more frequently in women than in men, it can occur from infancy to old age.[7,16,18]

The cause of the disease is unknown; however, it now appears that there are genetic factors that precipitate a continued immune reaction in the synovium. It has been documented that rheumatoid factor complex binding with synovial fluid complement precipitates the inflammatory reaction in a rheumatoid joint that results in its inflammation and pannus formation.[7,24] This can progress to erode the joint capsule, tendons, ligaments, and eventually cartilage and bone.[7,18]

DIAGNOSIS

The diagnosis is usually made by an analysis of the initial symptoms, the presence of rheumatoid nodules usually over bony prominences, radiological evidence of cartilage destruction or bony erosions, and presence of the rheumatoid factor in the blood serum.[18] Certain macroglobulins or antiglobulins constitute the rheumatoid factor.[7,24]

The number of clinical features present determines the classification of the disease. It can be designated as *possible, probable, definite,* or *classic* rheumatoid arthritis.[2,18]

COURSE

The onset of rheumatoid arthritis is usually gradual or insidious, although it may be abrupt. It is characterized by bilateral, symmetrical involvement of the small joints of the hands and feet.[2,18] The joints are typically painful, stiff, tender, hot, and occasionally, red. Muscles that act on the involved

joints may decrease in strength and size fairly early in the course of disease because of disuse. Range of motion (ROM) is limited because of edema and pain in the early stages and later may be due to destructive changes in the joint.[2]

The systemic manifestations should not be overlooked. Signs, which may be present in varying degrees, include fever, weight loss, weakness, fatigue, and generalized stiffness.[2] There may be an apparent depression and lack of motivation that may be related to the fatigue and organic symptoms and should be differentiated from the same symptoms that can be psychogenic.[18]

The course of the disease is unpredictable. Some individuals experience a single, brief episode, and others experience multiple episodes of varying severity. A small percentage of patients experience a gradual and continuous progression to severe joint deformity and dysfunction.[2]

The course is usually characterized by exacerbations and remissions. The client's level of function and independence can fluctuate from independent to completely dependent, varying with the stage and severity of the disease process.[16,18]

DRUG THERAPY

Drugs used include aspirin and aspirin-like analgesics, intraarticular steroids, gold salts, antimalarials, and cytotoxic agents.[11,18] Aspirin is the drug of choice because of its analgesic and antiinflammatory properties.[2,11,18] Nonsteroidal, antiinflammatory agents that can be used are indomethacin, phenylbutazone, ibuprofen, naproxen, and tolectin. Some of these have potentially serious side effects that are, fortunately, rare. They act to relieve inflammation but do not alter the course of the disease.[11,18]

Steroids are used as antiinflammatory agents, which usually are very effective. However, because of the multiplicity and potential seriousness of their side effects, they are reserved for patients who would become severely disabled without them.[18]

Gold salts also act as effective antiinflammatory agents. The mechanisms of their action unknown. Because of the close monitoring of the patient, which is required to identify potential toxicity, and the seriousness of the possible side effects, the use of gold salts is reserved for patients who are dependable, will comply with frequent visits for urinalysis and blood testing, are alert to side effects that must be reported immediately, and have failed to respond to more conservative forms of treatment.[2,18]

Antimalarial drugs, such as chloroquine and plaquenil sulfate, and cytotoxic agents, such as Cytoxan, Imuran, and penicillamine, are used infrequently and can benefit selected patients. Their undesirable side effects are serious considerations and may preclude their use.[11,18]

Surgical procedures that may be of benefit to patients with rheumatoid arthritis include synovectomy, tendon repair and transplant, tightening of ligaments, joint replacement, bone resection, and joint fusion.[2,11,18]

PSYCHOLOGICAL FACTORS

It has been suggested that rheumatoid arthritis is "psychosomatic," stress induced, or somehow related to specific personality variables. However, the research has not been adequate to produce definite associations between personality variables and the disease.[18,20]

Personality factors seen in patients with rheumatoid arthritis are found in persons with other chronic diseases and in the healthy population. The psychological factors are probably a response to chronic disease rather than a predisposing cause.[18] The patient may have suffered a serious change in physical function and life roles, and even appearance may be altered by deformity and drug side effects. These changes evoke an adjustment process akin to the grief process after a death. The patient may respond to the disability with depression, denial, a need to control the environment, and dependency.[18]

Some aspects of the illness that may

contribute to the psychological state include constant pain and fear of pain; changed body image and perception of self as a sick person; continuous uncertainty about the course and prognosis of the disease; sexual dysfunction because of pain or deformity; and altered social, family, vocational, and leisure roles.

Rehabilitation workers need to be aware of the client's response to disability and the adjustment that is in progress. All the factors and behaviors just cited will have an influence on rehabilitation. The interaction of personnel with the client can facilitate the development of healthy coping mechanisms and acceptance of disability. The reader is referred to Melvin[18] for a more detailed discussion of this subject.

SPECIFIC JOINT PROBLEMS AND DEFORMITIES*[12,15]
Pathogenesis of joint destruction

The initial event and prime cause of joint destruction is proliferation of the synovial membrane. The synovial membrane becomes so proliferated that it grows over and into cartilage, bone, and tendons and secretes enzymes that destroy them. The major microscopic fibers that hold the tissues of bone, cartilage, and tendons together are called collagen. The destruction of collagen is a major event, causing joint damage. This destruction is caused by the abnormal secretion of the enzymes collagenase and elastase by the abnormal synovium. The abnormal synovium also produces a thin, watery synovial fluid that is a poor lubricant and nutrient.

Polymorphonuclear white blood cells produced by the inflamed synovium bathe the joint by the millions, and when they break down, they release lysosomal enzymes and other enzymes that further alter the synovial fluid viscosity, cartilage, bone, and tendons to create a vicious cycle.

---

*Adapted primarily from Lages, W.: Pathogenesis of joint destruction, San Jose, Calif., 1976 and 1980, Santa Clara Valley Medical Center. Mimeographed.

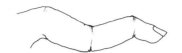

Fig. 23-1. Swan-neck deformity results in PIP hyperextension and DIP flexion.

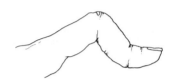

Fig. 23-2. Boutonnière deformity results in DIP hyperextension and PIP flexion.

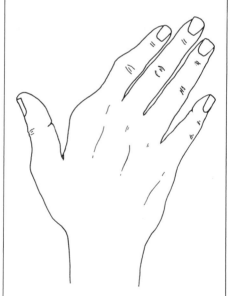

Fig. 23-3. MP joint ulnar drift.

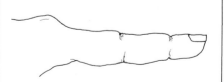

Fig. 23-4. MP palmar subluxation.

Specific joint problems

DIP AND PIP JOINTS OF SECOND TO FIFTH FINGERS

Swan-neck deformity. Swan-neck deformity results when synovitis weakens or destroys the lateral slips of the extensor tendon that insert into the base of the distal phalanx or weakens the intrinsic interossei and lumbrical muscles that insert into this tendon. The result is incomplete and weak to absent extension at the distal interphalangeal (DIP) joint with overbalanced contraction of the central slip of the extensor tendon that inserts at the base of the middle phalanx with hyperextension of the proximal interphalangeal (PIP) joint (Fig. 23-1).

The process can result in swan-neck deformity of the intrinsic plus type. If there is chronic, incomplete extension of the DIP, a contracture will ensue. Complete extension will be impossible, even passively. The overbalanced pull of the extensor central slip will result in more degrees of hyperextension of the PIP joint. The tendency toward resting hyperextension will result in gradual reduction of the range of flexion of the PIP joint.

Direct surgery involving the lateral slips of the extensor tendons is rarely done because of poor technical results. Sometimes synovectomy is indicated early to remove the invading synovium at the metacarpophalangeal (MP) joints. Daily passive ROM and gentle stretching are indicated for the DIPs. Active ROM should be done daily to the MPs, PIPs, and DIPs to prevent contractures. A small, short *dynamic* splint may be applied to the PIPs during daily activity to prevent progressive hyperextension. A three-point finger splint is sometimes used to maintain range of PIP flexion and relieve stress to the volar aspect of the PIP joint resulting from severe hyperextension.[18] Flexion contractures of the MPs, PIPs, and DIPs should be treated by active muscle contraction with stretch and not with passive or device stretch.

Isotonic and isometric resistive exercise to the finger extensors will not strengthen damaged tendons and may damage them further.

Boutonnière deformity. Boutonnière deformity can occur when synovitis at the wrist, MP, or PIP joints weakens or destroys the central slip of the extensor tendon that inserts into the base of the middle phalanx. There is often associated PIP joint arthritis. The result is incomplete and weak to absent extension at the PIP joint with overbalanced contraction of the lateral slips of the extensor tendon that insert into the base of the distal phalanx with hyperextension at the DIP joint (Fig. 23-2). The central slip of the extensor tendon is the major extensor of the finger, and if this problem is recent (days) and if *the physician does not know of it*, he or she should be informed immediately. Invariably a flexion contracture of the PIP joint and hyperextension of the DIP joint with loss of flexion range will ensue. Function of the finger will be seriously compromised.

Direct surgery of the central slips is often done if caught early enough, but there may be severe damage to the extensor tendon by the synovium, which may require a tendon graft from another site or may be irreparable. Because of this the fourth and fifth fingers are rarely operated on, whereas the second and third fingers often are operated on because of hand function priorities. Synovectomy will not restore tendon integrity but may be indicated to prevent the invasion of other tendons in proximity. Daily passive ROM is indicated for the MPs, PIPs, and DIPs to correct or prevent deformity. Active ROM exercises should be done daily to the MPs, PIPs, and DIPs to preserve joint ROM and muscle tone. *Dynamic* extension splints of the second and third fingers may be indicated to improve function and opposition.

Isotonic and isometric exercise or resistive exercise to the extensors will not help this deformity and may further damage tendons.

MP JOINTS OF SECOND TO FIFTH FINGERS

MP ulnar drift. Synovitis of the MP joints leads to weakness or destruction of the MP ligaments. The MP ligaments, particularly when the MPs are flexed at 45°, give medial and lateral stability. Both the extensor and flexor tendons to the fingers are bowed to produce an ulnar drift tendency of the tendons at the MP joints during normal

contractions. Forced contraction and especially forceful hand grip accentuate this force. With MP ligaments weakened the normal forces result in ulnar drift. The fifth MP joint buttresses the remainder of fingers from static, postural ulnar drift, but when the fifth MP ligament loses stability, ulnar drift can occur with gravity and posture even at rest (Fig. 23-3).

The result is that if the MP ligament damage is mild or if the stability of the fifth joint is preserved, the ulnar drift may occur only dynamically with finger extension-flexion. This gives weak pinch, which may result in thumb adduction and lateral pinch being substituted for true opposition. If the MP ligament damage is severe or if the stability of the fifth MP joint is lost, there will be ulnar drift even at rest, posturally, and the problem of opposition will be severe.

The dynamic and static ulnar drift plus lifting of the extensor hood by MP synovitis will result in dislocation of the extensor tendons from the extensor hood over the metacarpal heads into the space between the heads, leading to possible tendon injury and loss of ability to completely extend the MP joints. The lateral pinching of the thumb will result in radial subluxation and deformity of the IP joint of the thumb.

Treatment consists of early synovectomy, which may prevent progressive MP ligament damage. Extensor tendons dislocated ulnarly may be able to be replaced surgically with excision of MP synovial tissue. Severe problems may require replacement of the MP joints, since the MP ligaments cannot be successfully repaired surgically. Daily passive ROM exercises of the MP joints are indicated only if daily active ROM does not produce full flexion and extension. A joint protection program is strongly indicated to prevent forceful flexion and extension in activities of daily living (ADL). *Dynamic* ulnar deviation splints during the day coupled with *static* splints with the MPs in neutral deviation and 45° of flexion at night may halt progression of deformity and improve opposition.

Isotonic and isometric exercise or resistive exercise of the fingers will not help this deformity and may produce further MP ligament damage.

MP palmar subluxation-dislocation. Synovitis of the MPs results in MP ligament damage. Since finger flexors are much stronger and much more used than extensors, palmar dislocation will result. Palmar dislocation is often associated with ulnar drift but may occur by itself. Loss of effective MP extension and shortening and weakening of the intrinsic muscles are the usual isolated problems. Complete dislocation can occur (Fig. 23-4).

Early, complete surgical replacement or repair of the MP joints is the only effective treatment. Passive and active ROM exercises of the MPs to prevent loss of ROM are indicated. No exercises or splints are effective in correcting or treating this problem. A joint protection program is strongly indicated to prevent further progressive damage during ADL.

THUMB[15,18]

Flexion of MP joint with hyperextension of the IP joint (type I deformity). Chronic MP synovitis causes attenuation of the joint capsule, MP collateral ligaments, and the overlying extensor mechanism. Pain and distention of the joint capsule cause damage of the intrinsic muscles of the thumb. This may progress to MP palmar subluxation and ulnar-volar displacement of the extensor pollicis longus tendon. Once displaced this tendon acts as an MP flexor and with intrinsic muscle damage, causes hyperextension of the interphalangeal (IP) joint. The result is MP flexion and IP hyperextension.

Flexion of MP joint with IP hyperextension and CMC involvement (type II deformity). Type II deformity appears similar to type I deformity, but CMC joint damage and subluxation, a result of chronic synovitis of this joint, are the major factors. Once there is subluxation of the CMC joint, the adductor pollicis muscle pulls on the first metacarpal, which can result in a fixed adduction contracture with hyperextension of the *distal* phalanx.

MP hyperextension, IP flexion, and CMC joint involvement (type III deformity). The dynamics of type III deformity are initially the same as those described for type II deformity. However, type III deformity will result if there is a natural or pathological laxity of the MP joint with hyperextension of the proximal phalanx.

These problems may be treated surgically by extensor tendon repair, synovectomy, arthrodesis, or joint replacement. A joint protection program is indicated, and a CMC stabilization splint may be helpful to relieve pain and increase hand function.

WRIST JOINT

Wrist synovitis. Wrist synovitis can result in a variety of problems, which are discussed here.

CARPAL TUNNEL SYNDROME. The carpal tunnel under the transverse flexor carpal ligament is a tightly closed space, and inflammation can lead to high pressure on the median nerve, which runs in the carpal tunnel. This produces pain and sensory disturbances over the median nerve distribution in the hand and median nerve motor weakness and atrophy of the opponens pollicis, abductor pollicis brevis, and thenar atrophy. *If not already known by the physician, this should be promptly brought to his or her attention for treatment.* Sensory and motor deficits over the median nerve distribution and severe pain in the hand can result and can progress to permanent loss of feeling in the hand and weak to lost thumb opposition, which are serious impairments to hand use.

Until treatment heat and any exercises of the wrist other than active ROM are contraindicated. The hand should be kept elevated to reduce swelling, even at night. A cock-up splint to immobilize the wrist may also help and should be worn as much as possible during the day and all night. If splints, elevation, and corticosteroid injection fail to promptly resolve the problem, surgical release of the transverse carpal ligament is indicated.

SYNOVIAL INVASION OF THE EXTENSOR TENDONS. Dorsal swelling can be seen and felt in cases of invasion of the extensor tendon sheaths. This can lead to their weakness or rupture, resulting in weak to lost extension of the fingers at the MP, PIP, and DIP joints, flexion contractures, and loss of hand function, which is serious.

As soon as discovered, surgical synovectomy can correct and prevent further problems. Tendon repair may be done if caught promptly. Active ROM exercises at the wrist and night splints for the wrist can preserve function before surgery but are not substitutes for surgery. Passive and active ROM of the MP, PIP, and DIP are indicated to prevent flexion contracture.

Isotonic and isometric exercise or resistive exercise of the wrist extensors is of no value and may produce further damage.

SYNOVIAL INVASION OF THE CARPAL BONES. Synovial invasion of the carpal bone results in erosion and destruction of the intercarpal ligaments and joints. It can result in progressive loss of wrist motion, contracture of the wrist in a nonfunctional position, or in flexion subluxation-dislocation of the wrist (Fig. 23-5).

Loss of ROM can be minimized by active ROM exercise. Passive ROM should be gentle to avoid damaging ligaments. Using volar resting splints at night with the wrist in the position of function (neutral radioulnar position and slight wrist extension) can prevent contracture in nonfunctional positions. Surgery is not feasible except to fuse in more functional positions. Since surgery can only offer wrist fusion in the position of function, *static* wrist splints in the position of function produce the same end result. Splints causing loss of pronation-supination are contraindicated. Active pronation-supination ROM exercise and gentle passive ROM are indicated several times a day with the wrist out of the splint to prevent this. Joint protection of forceful flexion is strongly indicated. Isometric strengthening of wrist extensors is indicated.

Isotonic and isotonic resistive exercise may lead to subluxation-dislocation.

SYNOVITIS OF THE RADIOULNAR JOINT. Synovitis of the radioulnar joint, causing erosion of joint cartilage, usually results in progressive loss of pronation and supination at the wrist, particularly if there is associated elbow disease. It can result in partial to complete loss of pronation and supination of the wrist with severe functional impairment.

Surgical resection of the distal ulna can be done to restore lost pronation-supination. Active pronation-supination

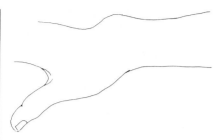

Fig. 23-5. Flexion subluxation of wrist.

ROM exercises and passive ROM are indicated daily to prevent loss. Pronation-supination in ADL is encouraged.

Isotonic or resistive exercises are contraindicated.

ELBOW JOINT

Elbow synovitis. The humeroulnar joint is a hinge joint, and synovitis results in loss of ROM. Disease of the radiohumeral joint can result in loss of pronation-supination at the elbow.

Loss of flexion can result in contracture that prevents feeding and many other ADL. Loss of extension can result in contracture that makes ADL and crutch use difficult and some tasks impossible. Loss of pronation-supination severely compromises the use of the hands and wrists in ADL. A dominant arm with severe loss of extension and pronation makes writing and other activities extremely difficult.

Flexion and extension contractures of the elbows are extremely difficult to improve surgically. Both elbows with severely limited flexion seriously impair ADL and functional activities; both elbows with severely limited extension make transfers and crutch use extremely difficult. The radial head can be resected to improve pronation-supination. With disease in the elbows splints and slings limiting movement are contraindicated unless daily ROM is preserved by a therapist or nurse. Active and passive ROM exercises are strongly indicated daily for the elbow. Isometric exercise is indicated for strengthening only if isotonic exercise is too painful. Isotonic exercise is best given through proper ADL instruction. Pain that may limit exercise can be reduced by corticosteroid injection. Loss of ROM is a greater concern than is joint damage, since the only surgical corrections for contractures are destructive of joints. Sometimes surgery is aimed toward improving extension at the expense of flexion in the dominant arm to permit crutch use and writing and improving flexion at the expense of extension in the nondominant extremity for feeding and personal grooming.

SHOULDER JOINT. The shoulder is a ball-and-socket joint that has some susceptibility to loss of motion.

Shoulder synovitis. The main result of synovitis is loss of some planes of ROM. A complication of shoulder synovitis is "frozen shoulder," which means very restricted ROM, and, unfortunately, is common. This results in major problems in ADL and in crutch ambulation. With shoulder contracture there is extremely severe restriction of ADL and other functions. Surgery is of little value in treating this problem. Corticosteroid injection early is very effective in reducing pain and restricted motion. Aggressive active and passive ROM and isotonic exercise are imperative, especially preceded by hot packs. A joint protection program is strongly indicated. Slings are a hazard and should be avoided.

Surgical intervention

Treatment of the patient with long-term rheumatoid arthritis will often include operative procedures to repair soft tissue or replace joints destroyed by the rheumatoid process.

Synovectomy, which is a surgical process of removing excessive synovium is an effort to control its proliferation, may be performed when the inflammation cannot be controlled by more conservative methods. It is most often delayed until soft tissue, such as finger extensors, appear to be jeopardized by the synovitis.

Resection implant arthroplasty is performed more successfully and more often since the development of high-grade Silastic spacers and joints. Early models of joints made out of metal and Silastic failed because of breakage of the implants from shearing forces applied during daily use. Current implant spacers are reinforced with Dacron and withstand normal hand usage more reliably than earlier models. Metal implants are generally no longer used in the fingers.

MP JOINT ARTHROPLASTY Although implants exist to replace almost any joint affected by arthritis, resection arthroplasty of the MP joints is the most common rheumatoid surgery in the hand. Guidelines given for timing of treatment vary with the surgeon, the patient, and the expertise of the treating therapist. The program described was developed for the Swanson-type Silastic implant, but the general principles would apply to other types of spacers as well.

Some joint replacements, such as in the total hip replacement, are designed to work like the joint they replace. However, the MP joint arthroplasty uses a joint spacer that is not a joint but acts as an interface between the metacarpal bone and the proximal phalanx. The stems of the Swanson spacer are not fixed within the intermedullary canal but move with a piston action within the bone. This allows adequate excursion of the implant for finger flexion and extension and reduces stress on the implant.

During the healing phase following the MP arthroplasty the implants go through an encapsulation period. During this time the tissue surrounding the Silastic forms a capsule that supports the stems of the spacer. Collagen fibers are present microscopically on the fourth or fifth day and gradually change from the cellular formation into collagen fibers.[17] This process appears to be complete by the end of the sixth week. During the encapsulation period it is extremely important that the joints be held in the desired position of extension and slight radial deviation.

During surgery the head of the metacarpal is resected and cleaned. The proximal phalanx is prepared but usually not resected. The bone canals are also prepared and the spacer carefully inserted. Soft tissue release of the ulnar intrinsic muscles, reconstruction of the radial intrinsic muscles, and reconstruction and alignment of the extensor hood may be performed during surgery.

The patient's hand is placed in a bulky dressing and immobilized for 3 to 6 days postoperatively. At that time a dynamic splint is applied, which places the fingers in slight radial deviation at the MP joints while lightly supporting the fingers into full extension and allowing active flexion to 70° (Fig. 23-6). A splint is worn 24 hours a day for the

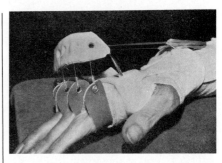

Fig. 23-6. Low profile dynamic splint is used to assist MP joints into extension while maintaining about 15° of radial deviation following implant arthroplasty of MP joints. MP joints should not be pulled into hyperextension by splint.

next 6 weeks. Some surgeons prefer a static splint, which maintains the fingers in the proper position while sleeping, and a dynamic splint during all waking hours. Frequent splint adjustments and goniometric measurements are necessary during this postoperative period to monitor joint position and excursion.

Starting with the application of the dynamic splint, passive ROM may be performed by the therapist on a daily basis to maintain 70° of pain-free passive flexion and full extension. Passive motion is applied gently with consideration to tissue reaction. The patient is instructed to perform active ROM and light ADL only in the splint for the first 6 weeks. This ensures that the fingers will not be used in an ulnarly deviated position. Heavy activities are restricted. During the 4 to 6 week period the patient may begin active flexion under the supervision of the therapist. Care is taken that flexion occurs at the MP joints and not primarily at the IP joints. A wide Velcro trapper may be placed on the fingers to prevent IP flexion during active MP flexion.[4] Also during this period flexion splinting may be begun if the patient has not regained a full 70° of flexion. The flexion cuff should allow for slight radial pull and should not be painful or cause swelling of the fingers.

Other exercises that should be stressed are "radial walking" of the fingers individually toward the thumb and active exercise of the extensors by placing the fingers in the intrinsic minus position (IP joints slightly flexed) while extending the MP joints.

Extension and flexion splints are adjusted for fit and wearing time based on goniometric measurements. Strength usually returns as the patient is allowed to use the hand for normal activities. Heavy resistive exercise is contraindicated.

Night splinting is continued for 12 to 14 weeks, although the patient may go without the splint during the day following the sixth week.

The principles of wound healing and encapsulation may be applied to joint implant arthroplasty of other joints. A balance of controlled splinting and active motion should be achieved following any joint arthroplasty.

PRINCIPLES OF REHABILITATION

Conservative management of rheumatoid arthritis is the preferred approach to its treatment. The long-term prognosis, using conservative methods, is usually as good as with more radical approaches. There is less risk of side effects using salicylates, appropriate rest, and rehabilitation measures than from drugs, such as gold salts, steroids, and cytotoxic agents.[7]

The goals of the basic treatment regime are to decrease inflammation and pain, preserve function, and prevent deformity. The treatment methods used include systemic, emotional, and joint rest; drug therapy; and appropriate exercise[7] and activity. In some instances surgery is required.[11]

Joint rest in non-weight-bearing positions and prone lying to prevent hip and knee flexion contractures are part of the program of rest. Splints to provide temporary rest of individual joints are used.[11]

The amount of rest required varies with the individual patient. In some instances complete bed rest will be necessary, whereas in others the patient may continue with normal daily living, incorporating 2 hours of rest into the daily schedule.[7]

It is of primary importance in the treatment program to preserve function of the hips, knees, elbows, and MP joints. Therefore exercise to other joints must not interfere with functions of these joints or be done at their expense. Complete joint rest is applicable to acutely involved joints only.

Self-care activities are permitted to pain tolerance, even in acute arthritis. Splinting should be maintained for as short a period as possible to prevent loss of ROM.[14]

Indications for splinting

Splinting is indicated for the wrist, MP and IP joints, and the ankle if it is acutely painful. Splinting is contraindicated at the shoulder and hip joints; at the elbow, except when weight bearing; and at the knee, unless there is joint instability.[14] Some of the splints commonly used in treatment of the arthritic hand are summarized from Melvin.[18] These include the volar resting, wrist stabilization, protective MP, combined, and ulnar drift positioning splints.

VOLAR RESTING SPLINT The volar resting splint is indicated when there is acute synovitis of the wrist, fingers, and thumb. Its purpose is to rest involved joints and thus decrease inflammation and pain. It is also used when multiple joint contractures are beginning to develop for the purpose of maintaining proper positioning during sleep.

WRIST STABILIZATION SPLINT. A wrist stabilization splint immobilizes the wrist but allows motion of the MP joints. It is used when hand function is limited by wrist pain to improve hand function and grip strength. It may be helpful when there is severe chronic wrist pain or inflammation to provide joint rest, decrease inflammation and pain, and protect extensor tendons from attenuation and rupture.

PROTECTIVE MP SPLINT. The protective MP splint maintains the MP joints in normal alignment, allowing 0° to 25° of MP flexion. It is used to protect the MP joints from ulnar deviation and the forces of volar subluxation.

COMBINED WRIST STABILIZATION AND PROTECTIVE MP SPLINT. A combined wrist stabilization and protective MP splint is used when both the wrist and MP joints are involved for the purposes just described.

ULNAR DRIFT POSITIONING SPLINT. An ulnar drift positioning splint prevents ulnar drift and maintains normal alignment of MP joints during pinch and grasp activities.

Splints and other orthoses must be removed regularly for ROM exercises to the involved joints.

The reader is referred to *Rheumatic Disease: Occupational Therapy and Rehabilitation* by J.L. Melvin for a full discussion and description of a wide variety of hand splints and their uses in the treatment of rheumatoid arthritis.

Indications for exercise

The concomitant use of the appropriate therapeutic exercise along with rest, in proper balance, is basic to the management of rheumatoid arthritis. The objectives of the exercise program are to preserve joint motion, muscle strength, and endurance. Active-assistive exercises are most useful and can be performed, within limits of pain tolerance, from the outset in the treatment program. As disease activity subsides and tolerance for exercise increases, gradation of the program may be increased to include active and resistive exercises.[7]

ACUTE STAGE. During the acute stage involved joints are inflamed and swollen. There may be systemic signs and symptoms, and bed rest may be required. Splints, braces, and positioning are used to provide joint rest and prevent deformity.

Active ROM exercise is started after 1 week and is gradually increased to active exercise to tolerance. Passive ROM exercise may be used only if the client is unable to complete the ROM with active motion. The purpose of these exercises is to improve or maintain joint mobility.

Isometric exercise without resistance (muscle setting) may be used to maintain muscle tone. Active exercise in water (hubbard tank or whirlpool) can be used to provide active exercise with minimal joint stress for maintenance of joint ROM and muscle tone.[1,14]

Active ROM exercises should be repeated 3 to 10 times once or twice daily. Isometric exercise should be repeated 3 to 10 times several times daily.[7] Active exercises should be performed in a manner to prevent active stretching and joint stress. Pain or discomfort that results from exercise and lasts more than 1 hour indicates that the exercise was too stressful and should be decreased.[18]

Active resistive exercise, isometric exercise against resistance, and stretching exercise are contraindicated during the acute stage of the disease.[14]

SUBACUTE STAGE. During the subacute stage of the disease a few joints are actively involved, and there may be mild systemic symptoms. Short periods of rest and splints for corrective or preventive purposes are used.

Gentle passive stretch and active isotonic exercise with minimal joint stress may be added to the passive or active ROM exercise program. Their purpose is to regain lost ROM in those joints that have become limited. Gradual isometric exercise twice daily for 5 to 10 minutes may be used to maintain or increase muscle strength and endurance.[1,14]

CHRONIC-ACTIVE AND CHRONIC-INACTIVE STAGES. During the chronic-active and chronic-inactive stages, stretch at the end of the ROM during exercise is recommended to increase ROM.[18] Active ROM, isometric, and isometric resistive exercises may also be continued.[14]

Isotonic resistive exercise should seldom be used.[7] It is thought to produce excessive and undesirable joint stress.[14] Melvin[18] outlines circumstances under which resistive exercises are used by some practitioners and describes specific exercise procedures.

A home exercise program that is designed for the particular client should be carried out. It is best for the therapist to write out the directions for exercises for the client to follow. The exercises should be done when the client is feeling best, often after a warm shower or bath and analgesic medication. Application of heat or cold for muscle relaxation and analgesic effect may be of benefit to some clients.[7,18]

Indications for activity

Treatment principles that apply to the therapeutic exercise just cited also apply to therapeutic activities. The activities that are selected should be nonresistive and provide opportunities for the maintenance or increase of ROM and strength. They should be meaningful and interesting to the client. Joint protection principles, to be discussed subsequently, should be employed during leisure and work activities and ADL.

Crafts and games as therapeutic modalities are not as frequently or effectively used as therapeutic exercise regimes. However, they can be of value and interest to some clients and should not be overlooked as a purposeful application of therapeutic exercise procedures. Activities that can be useful in the treatment of rheumatoid arthritis include weaving, Turkish knotting, macrame, and peg games.[18]

The use of crocheting, knitting, and similar traditional needlecrafts is controversial. In principle they are to be avoided because they involve the use of prolonged static contraction of hand muscles in the intrinsic plus position for holding tools and material. They also facilitate MP ulnar drift and MP volar subluxation through the forces in the hand during the performance of the activity. Melvin[18] points out that in general the only conditions in which knitting and crocheting can be harmful are when there are active MP synovitis, beginning swan-neck deformity caused in part by intrinsic tightness, and degenerative joint disease of the CMC joint of the thumb.

Adverse effects can be prevented by using an MP extension splint, performing intrinsic stretching exercises, and using a thumb CMC stabilization splint, depending on the specific potential problem. Frequent rest breaks during the activity or performing the activity for short, intermittent periods may also be helpful in preventing adverse effects. These are important considerations for those clients who would derive much pleasure and psychological benefit from these traditional and readily available avocational activities.[18]

ADL, including self-care and home management skills, is an important part of the rehabilitation program for the client with rheumatoid arthritis. Self-care activities to pain and fatigue tolerance should be performed even during early acute stages of the disease episode. The number and types of activities are gradually increased as the client's endurance and strength improve and pain and discomfort subside.[18]

These activities can be used to maintain or improve joint ROM, muscle strength, and physical endurance. Joint protection, work simplification, and energy conservation principles should be applied during the performance of these activities. The client, with the aid and direction of the therapist, needs to work out a daily schedule of intermittent rest and activity that is suitable for the stage of the disease, activity tolerance, and any special systemic or joint problems that affect performance.

These principles apply to work activities. Since there are more women than men affected by arthritis, there has been an emphasis in the literature on home management activities, and joint protection principles related to these focused on the traditional role of woman as homemaker. The therapist must not lose sight of the facts that men also perform homemaking tasks and that a substantial percentage of women are employed outside of their homes. Therefore job analysis and application of joint protection and energy conservation principles may be an important part of the rehabilitation program for both men and women. Prevocational evaluation may be necessary if a job change is necessitated by the disability.

For juvenile rheumatoid arthritis, school and leisure activities need to be considered and appropriate pacing of activities employed.

Assistive equipment

Assistive devices and equipment are used to reduce pain, decrease joint stress, and increase independence.[18]

In general the purposes of various devices are to (1) facilitate grasp (built-up soft handles on tools); (2) compensate for lost ROM (dressing sticks or reachers); (3) facilitate ease of performance (lightweight equipment or electrical appliances); (4) stabilize materials or equipment (nonskid mats or suction

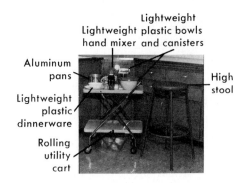

Fig. 23-7. Equipment designed to ease housework for client with arthritis.

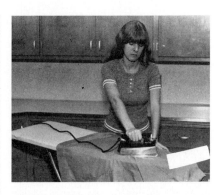

Fig. 23-8. During ironing full extension at elbow can be practiced.

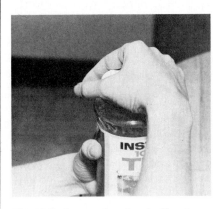

Fig. 23-9. Jar cap is twisted off, using palm of hand, and opened with right hand to prevent ulnar drift.

brushes); (5) prevent deforming stresses (extended faucet handles or adapted key holder); (6) prevent prolonged static contraction (book stand or bowl holder); (7) compensate for weak or absent motor function (universal cuffs or stocking devices); and (8) prevent accidents (bathtub grab bars and nonskid mats for shower or bathtub). Some suggestions to ease home management are shown in Fig. 23-7.

Principles of joint protection[6,18,21]

The purpose of joint protection training is to instruct the client in methods of reducing joint stress, decreasing pain, preserving joint structures, and conserving energy.[18]

The arthritic joint is predisposed to deterioration from abuse that can lead to reduced performance abilities.[6] Clients with rheumatoid arthritis need to employ joint protection principles in all of their daily activities to maintain maximal function and prevent joint damage and deformity.

MAINTAIN MUSCLE STRENGTH AND JOINT ROM.[6] During daily activities each joint should be used at its maximal ROM and strength consistent with the disease process. For example, long, sweeping, flowing strokes to maintain and increase ROM can be employed when ironing. The arms should be straightened as far as possible, especially on flat work (Fig. 23-8). When

vacuuming or mopping the floor, a long, forward stroke of the implement, then pulling it in close to the body so the arm is first fully straightened, then fully bent, will achieve full or nearly full range of elbow flexion and extension and shoulder motion. The use of dust mitts on both hands keeps fingers straight and prevents the static contraction and potentially deforming forces of holding a dust cloth. Light objects, such as cereal, oats, or sugar, can be kept on high shelves so that full ROM in the shoulder can be used with reaching.[21]

AVOID POSITIONS OF DEFORMITY AND DEFORMING STRESSES. Internal, that is, tight grasp around an object, and external, that is, propping up chin on side or back of fingers, forces in the direction of deformity should be avoided during daily activities. Some applications of this principle include always turning the fingers toward the thumb side, such as turning a doorknob toward the thumb or opening a door with the right hand and closing it with the left. Jars should be opened with the right hand and closed with the left (Fig. 23-9). When wringing out hand laundry, the object should be held steady with the left hand and twisted with the right in the direction of the thumb.[21]

Pressures along the thumb side of fingers should be avoided. These pressures contribute to ulnar deviation.

This position of ulnar deviation decreases the use of the hands. Pressure can be prevented by (1) avoiding leaning chin on fingers or palm of hand; (2) picking up coffee cup with two hands instead of with index, middle finger, and thumb; (3) twisting a jar cap off and on with the palm of the hand and not with the fingers (Fig. 23-9); (4) installing lever extensions on faucet handles to avoid use of fingers to run on and off; and (5) using electric can opener instead of hand-operated type, since this device requires sustained grasp of one hand and forced motion of the thumb and fingers of the other hand for operation.

Tight grasp should be avoided. This position increases the strength of the muscles that allow grasp and therefore, contributes to ulnar deviation and dislocation of joints. This happens in activities, such as carrying pails and baskets; using pliers, scissors, and screwdrivers; and holding spoons to stir or mix foods.

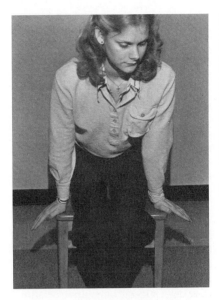

Fig. 23-10. Pushing off chair, using palms, helps prevent dislocation of finger joints.

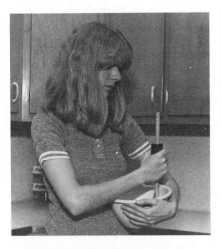

Fig. 23-11. Mixing bowl is stabilized with forearm. Spoon with soft, built-up handle is held so that pressure is toward radial side of hand.

When standing up, the client should be instructed to take the body weight through the wrist with fingers straight rather than on the fingers. "This will help reduce the pressure against the backs of the fingers. Excessive pressure in this area will contribute to dislocation of the knuckles"[21] (Fig. 23-10). The palm of the hand, rather than the fingers, should be used when taking down or hanging clothes in the closet. The palm can be used to lift the hanger at the exposed area in its apex. This method is most useful with heavy coats and jackets.

Excessive and constant pressure against the pad of the thumb should be avoided. For example, pressure against the pad of the thumb to open a car door, sew through thick fabric, and rise to a standing position all contribute to dislocation of the thumb joints.[21]

USE EACH JOINT IN ITS MOST STABLE, ANATOMICAL, AND FUNCTIONAL PLANE.[6] The client should be instructed to stand up straight from any sitting position. The client should stand or position self directly in front of a drawer to open it and not pull while standing to one side. In reaching for objects on a shelf the client should stand or position self directly in front of or under the shelf, not at the side. The wrist and fingers should always be used in good alignment.[21]

USE THE STRONGEST JOINTS AVAILABLE FOR THE ACTIVITY[6] Applications of using the strongest joints include using the hips and knees, not the back, when lifting and using the entire body to move heavy things. Carts and chairs should be pushed from behind; use straps for opening and closing heavy doors and drawers; and roll objects on counters and floors rather than lifting them. If any objects must be lifted, they should be scooped up in both hands, palms upward. This technique can be used when handling baking pans and casseroles if long oven mitts are used and in handling dishes, packages, books, and laundry.[21]

AVOID USING MUSCLES OR HOLDING JOINTS IN ONE POSITION FOR ANY UNDUE LENGTH OF TIME. Sustained muscle contraction is fatiguing and can contribute to joint subluxation and dislocation. Applications of this principle include (1) using a book stand instead of holding the book while reading; (2) when mixing, stabilizing the bowl with the palm of the hand and fingers against the body or a wall or in an open drawer to avoid holding the bowl with the fingers and thumb; (3) holding the mixing spoon with the thumb side pointing upward, not with the thumb pointing downward, and using a built-up handle to decrease the force of grasp (Fig. 23-11); (4) using the palm to scour pans, not the fingertips; (5) using the palm of the hand or the bend in the elbow instead of fingers in carrying handbags and coats; (6) using the side of the hand to push, as in shutting drawers, or using the little finger side of the hand in smoothing sheets on a bed; (7) squeezing the toothpaste tube with the palm of the hand, not between the thumb and fingers; and (8) holding objects, such as a vegetable peeler or knife, parallel to MP joints and not across the palms.[21]

NEVER BEGIN AN ACTIVITY THAT CANNOT BE STOPPED IMMEDIATELY IF IT PROVES TO BE TOO TAXING. In climbing up and down stairs, standing balance should be adequate to allow stopping and resting. In transferring from bed to wheelchair a sliding board should be used for less stress and to allow for stopping, if necessary. In getting in and out of a bathtub graded platforms to ascend and descend gradually at individual speed and tolerance can be used.

RESPECT PAIN. Some discomfort during treatment and activity may be tolerable and acceptable. If rest produces rapid relief, the level of activity need not necessarily be considered excessive.[6] However, pain lasting 1 or more hours after activity is a sign that the activity needs to be stopped or modified.[18,21] Pain can evoke protective muscle spasm and inhibit muscle contraction.[6]

Energy conservation and work simplification

Since prevention of fatigue is an important consideration in the management of rheumatoid arthritis, methods of simplifying work to save energy should be employed. One of the most important means to the end is to determine and carry out an appropriate balance between rest and play. The recommended amount of rest is 10 to 12 hours of rest per day, including a 1- to 2-hour nap in the afternoon.[18]

Short rest breaks of 5 to 10 minutes during daily activities can be very helpful in increasing overall endurance.[18] In general, 5 to 10 minutes of rest to 30 or 40 minutes[10] of activity is adequate. It may be difficult for the client to accept the notion of these short rest breaks, since it is often the desire to get work or housekeeping over with as quickly as possible. However, intermittent rest can actually save energy for more enjoyable tasks.[18] Work can be planned for an entire week and month. Light and heavy tasks can be alternated and work paced throughout the week, instead of doing a lot of work in 1 day. Work should be planned so that it is efficient, that is, not requiring getting up and down and moving to and fro repeatedly.

Time management needs to be explored if rushing is a tendency of the client. Rushing increases tension and fatigue. Most importantly the client should learn an energy-saving program and work schedule that prevent pushing to exhaustion.[21]

Other suggestions for conserving energy include (1) avoid bending and stooping by using long-handle reachers and flexible handle dust mops; (2) avoid long periods of standing during activities, such as ironing and food preparation; rather, use a high stool; (3) avoid extra trips by using a utility cart to convey as many items as needed at once; and (4) relax homemaking standards by using prepackaged foods and by air drying dishes, for example.

Work may be simplified by adjusting the work height for maximal comfort. The elbows should be flexed to 90°, and shoulders should be in a relaxed position. This can be accomplished without expensive home modification by using an adjustable ironing board as a work surface, placing a board over an open drawer, or using a high stool with a backrest to work at counters. A rack may be placed in the sink bottom to elevate the dishpan and thus prevent stooping during dish washing.

Work areas can be rearranged so that frequently used tools, equipment, and supplies are stored nearby and at easily reached levels. Counter tops may be used for convenient storage of small appliances. Commercial organizers, such as step shelves and revolving turntables, can make work easier.[21]

OCCUPATIONAL THERAPY FOR RHEUMATOID ARTHRITIS

The client with rheumatoid arthritis should be seen for occupational therapy services shortly after the diagnosis of arthritis is made. However, it is often the case that occupational therapy may not be initiated until many joints are involved, after surgery, or the disease is severe enough to cause hospitalization or moderate to severe performance limitations.[19]

Evaluation

OBSERVATION. The occupational therapist should observe the appearance of the hand for heat, redness, edema, deformity, deforming tendencies on motion, skin quality, and joint enlargement. In the early stages of the disease joints may appear puffy and soft. If the disease is active, joints may be red and hot. Later in the disease process enlarged joints may appear bony and hard.[10,19]

ROM. The occupational therapy evaluation includes active and passive ROM measurements. These may take a considerable amount of time if there is discomfort or pain in the joints. It may be necessary to perform the measurements gradually over two or three treatment sessions. The therapist should be aware of how the joints feel, that is, stiff, unstable, or crepitant. A major discrepancy between active and passive ROM may indicate significant muscle weakness.[19]

STRENGTH. Testing of muscle strength may be done by group or individual muscle testing. The usual procedures for manual muscle testing need to be adapted for the client who has arthritis. Resistance should be applied within the client's pain-free ROM rather than at the end of the ROM, as is usual in manual muscle testing. It is not unusual for clients with arthritis to have pain in the last 30° to 40° of joint motion. Therefore, if resistance is applied within the pain-free range, the inhibition of muscle strength by pain will be avoided.[18]

The use of the manual muscle test is controversial, since some physicians prohibit any resistance that can cause harm to diseased tissue and joints and place deforming forces on the joint.[25] Functional muscle or motion testing may be used if resistance is prohibited.

In both the ROM assessment and the muscle strength test the therapist should make note of the time of day and the amount of antiinflammatory or analgesic medication taken. These medications can affect results of the evaluation.[18]

HAND FUNCTION. Hand function testing is important. Pinch and grip strength testing with instruments is controversial for the reasons just stated.[25] Grip and pinch can be tested with an adapted blood pressure cuff and measured in millimeters of mercury.[10,18] A test of hand function that evaluates grasp and prehension patterns, such as the Jebsen Test of Hand Function[9] or the Quantitative Test of Upper Extremity Function,[3] should be administered.

SPECIFIC JOINT DEFORMITIES AND PROBLEMS. Tests for specific deformities or potential deformities of the hand should be administered as appropriate. The therapist might evaluate for possible carpal tunnel syndrome, swan-neck deformities, boutonniére deformities, flexor tendon nodules, ulnar drift, MP and wrist subluxation, intrinsic and extrinsic muscle tightness, ruptured tendons, extensor tendon displacement, and laxity of the MP collateral ligaments.[10]

Extrinsic muscle tightness. To test for tightness (contracture) or adherence of the extensor digitorum communis (EDC) tendon, the wrist is positioned at neutral. Then the MP joint is passively flexed to different positions, and simultaneously the PIP and DIP joints are flexed. The test is positive if the position of the proximal joint (MP) influences the degree of flexion possible at the distal joints (IPs). For example, when the MP joint is fully flexed, the PIP joint will lack full active or passive flexion. When the PIP joint is fully flexed, it will not be possible to fully flex the MP joint because the tendon does not have sufficient length to go over all the joints it crosses when they are all flexed.[11,18]

Swan-neck deformity. Swan-neck deformity results in hyperextension of the PIP joint and incomplete extension or slight flexion of the DIP joint. There are several causes of swan-neck deformity. Three types are discussed here. It is important for the therapist and physician to know the underlying cause if appropriate treatment is to be instituted.

One type of swan-neck deformity is caused by initial involvement at the MP joint[18] and results in intrinsic muscle tightness. To test for this type the test for extrinsic muscle tightness is applied first to prove that the extensor tendons do not have adhesions.[11] Then the MP joint is passively moved into full extension, and the PIP joint is flexed. Resistance to PIP flexion indicates intrinsic tightness. The PIP joint will not flex fully in this position if the intrinsic muscles are shortened. The reason for this is that the lumbricales act to extend the IP joints during MP flexion. By extending MP joints and flexing PIP joints these muscles are fully stretched. If they have become shortened, there will be insufficient elasticity or length to achieve the test position. Intrinsic muscles become weak, scarred, and shortened when they are invaded by pannus during the rheumatoid disease process.[11,18]

Another type of swan-neck deformity is a result of initial involvement at the DIP joints[18] and rupture of the lateral slips of the extensor tendons (Fig. 23-12). To test for this type the test for extrinsic tightness is applied first to prove that there is no adherence of the extensor tendon.[11] Then the MP joint is moved into extension, and the PIP joint is flexed to prove that there is no intrinsic tightness. Then the client should extend the finger actively. If there is a rupture of the lateral slips of the extensor tendon, the DIP joint will drop into flexion because ruptured lateral slips of the EDC cannot function to extend the joint. The middle slip of the EDC, acting on the PIP joint, pulls too hard and hyperextends the joint when active extension is attempted, resulting in the swan-neck appearance. This type of swan-neck deformity is caused by tendon ruptures resulting from inflammatory infiltration of pannus and attrition from bony spurs.[11]

A swan-neck deformity with initial involvement at the PIP joint[18] is caused by rupture of the flexor digitorum sublimis (FDS) tendon (Fig. 23-13). To test for this the test for extrinsic tightness is applied as before. The MP joint is moved into hyperextension, and the PIP joint is flexed to rule out intrinsic tightness. The client is then asked to flex the finger into the palm actively. If the FDS tendon is ruptured, it will not be possible to flex the PIP joint. The tendon rupture is a result of synovitis of the PIP joint with infiltration of the FDS

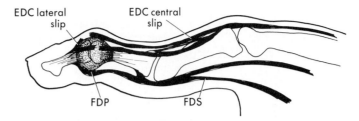

Fig. 23-12. Swan-neck deformity resulting from rupture of lateral slips of EDC tendon.

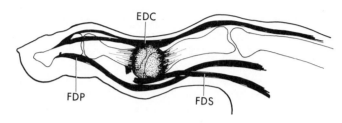

Fig. 23-13. Swan-neck deformity as a result of rupture of FDS tendon.

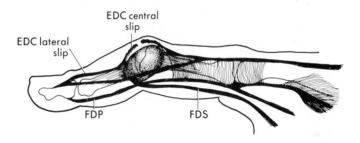

Fig. 23-14. Boutonnière deformity caused by rupture or lengthening of central slip of EDC tendon.

tendon, causing its rupture, or to bony spurs producing tendon erosion.[11,18]

Boutonnière deformity. Another deformity of the fingers in rheumatoid arthritis is the boutonnière deformity. This appears as flexion at the PIP joint and hyperextension at the DIP joint. The boutonnière deformity is caused by a rupture or lengthening of the central slip of the EDC tendon (Fig. 23-14). To test for this the client should actively extend the finger. Loss of active PIP extension is indicative of the rupture. The deformity is described as mild if the loss is 5° to 10°, as moderate if the loss is 10° to 30°, and as severe if 30° or more is lost.[18] The central slip of the extensor tendon is ruptured as a result of inflammatory infiltration or bony

spurs. Therefore it cannot function to extend the PIP joint on which it acts. The lateral slips slide volarly below the normal angle of pull and act to flex the PIP joint and hyperextend the DIP joint, resulting in the typical boutonnière appearance.[11,18]

Trigger finger. Trigger finger deformity is caused by a nodule or thickening of the FDS tendon at the entrance to the flexor tunnel (tendon sheath). This is caused by a rheumatoid nodule on the FDS tendon that blocks or makes difficult the slipping of the tendon through its sheath, preventing full extension of the PIP joint.[11,18] To test for this problem the examiner should ask the client if the fingers ever catch or stay closed when attempts are made to open the hand. If the client reports that this is the case, the examiner should determine if it occurs rarely, occasionally, or consistently; if there is any pain associated with it; and if it inhibits function. The therapist should palpate for a nodule over the flexor pulleys.[18] A click or crepitation may be palpated at the point where the nodule is pulled through the sheath. The palpation point is in the palm distal to the palmar creases at the base of the involved finger. The deformity is described as mild if there is inconsistent, painless triggering during active motion; as moderate if there is constant triggering during active motion or if it is intermittent but painful; and as severe if it prevents full active motion and is severely painful.[18]

Ulnar drift (see Fig. 23-3). Ulnar drift at the MP joints is another common deformity of rheumatoid arthritis. The therapist may test for the deformity by measuring the angle between the proximal phalanx and the MP joints during active extension. This measurement should be compared with the normal ROM. The index finger normally has 10° to 20° of ulnar deviation during active extension. The severity of the ulnar drift is described as follows:

Severity	Index finger	Fingers 3 to 5
Mild	20° to 30°	0° to 10°
Moderate	30° to 50°	10° to 30°
Severe	50° or more	30° or more[18]

MP subluxation (see Fig. 23-4). MP subluxation is also seen in the rheumatoid hand. It is the volar subluxation of the proximal phalanx on the metacarpal head. The therapist can test for this deformity by palpating over the dorsum of the joint when it is at the 0° neutral position. If there is subluxation, a "step" can be felt between the metacarpal and the first phalanx. The deformity is described as mild if the step is palpable, but full extension is possible; as moderate if the step is visible, palpable, and there is a slight limitation of extension; and as severe if there is gross malalignment and definite limitation of ROM.[18]

Wrist subluxation (see Fig. 23-5). Subluxation of the wrist is a volar slippage of the carpal bones on the radius. It is caused by weakness of the supporting ligaments caused by chronic synovitis. To test for wrist subluxation the thera-

pist should palpate from the distal radius to the carpals on the dorsal side of the forearm. If there is subluxation, there will be a step. It may be merely palpable if mild, visible if moderate, and grossly malaligned if severe.[18]

Sensation. Sensory evaluation is indicated if there is potential nerve compression caused by swelling. Modalities that should be tested are senses of touch, pain, temperature, and position. Paresthesias should be noted.

Endurance. The client's physical endurance should be evaluated by observation and an assessment of the daily or weekly schedule. Specific lower extremity evaluation may be carried out by the occupational or physical therapist. The occupational therapist should observe the gait pattern and mode of rising and sitting and the client's posture during ambulation and when sitting. The therapist should observe for any obvious joint limitations and weakness in the lower extremities and have data from specific evaluation of ROM, strength, and deforming tendencies in the legs. These factors are important considerations in planning treatment, presenting joint protection and energy conservation techniques, and positioning to prevent loss of ROM in the lower extremities.

Performance. Assessment of performance is a very important part of the occupational therapy program. Evaluation of ADL, including self-care, child care, home management, and work activities, should be carried out by interview and observation. A home evaluation should be carried out to assist the client in learning new methods and in making modifications to simplify work, save energy, and protect joints from undue stress. Job performance may be evaluated by observation in a real or simulated situation. The job tasks can be analyzed, and joint protection principles can be applied, if possible. Pacing of work responsibilities may be a consideration to incorporate the required rest periods into the working day.

Treatment objectives

The general objectives of treatment for clients with rheumatoid arthritis are to (1) maintain or increase joint mobility; (2) maintain or increase muscle strength; (3) increase physical endurance; (4) prevent or correct deformities,

if feasible; (5) minimize the effect of deformities; (6) maintain or increase ability to perform daily life tasks; (7) increase knowledge about the disease and the best methods of dealing with physical performance and psychosocial effects; and (8) aid with stress management and adjustment to physical disability.

Treatment methods

Methods used by occupational therapists to minimize the dysfunction that can result from rheumatoid arthritis include a variety of exercises, just described, tailored to the client's needs and stage of the disease. For clients not in the acute stage of the disease, exercise should be incorporated into daily activity as much as possible to reduce the need for a formal and rigid program of daily exercise.[19]

Training in ADL is an important aspect of the occupational therapy program for many clients. This includes training in joint protection, energy conservation techniques, and use of assistive devices and special equipment. Self-care, child care, home management, and work activities may be included in the ADL training program. Joint protection principles and energy-saving techniques should be introduced gradually, and the number and complexity of procedures should be increased as the client incorporates previously learned skills into daily life. For some clients arts and crafts or games, as described earlier, can be a meaningful part of the treatment program. This will depend on the client's needs, interests, and life-style and should be explored with the client and not overlooked.

Splints to protect joints and prevent or retard the development of deformity are usually made by the occupational therapist. The therapist may recognize the need for splints and recommend them to the physician in some instances. Some splints that may be of benefit in the treatment of rheumatoid arthritis include the resting, cock-up, ulnar drift, MP extensor assist, flexor assist, CMC stabilization, and three-point finger extension splints.[18]

Psychosocial factors may be treated by exploring the client's attitude toward the disability, the client's goals, how the client deals with pain and fear, and performance priorities and objectives. Activity groups, such as movement or exercise classes, home management classes, or arthritis education classes, can serve as mutual support and problem-solving groups. Occupational therapists may lead or participate with other rehabilitation specialists in such activity groups. Sexual counseling may be necessary to teach joint protection techniques during sexual activity and explore attitudes about body image, self-acceptance, and acceptance by the partner as a sexual being. Several excellent treatments of this subject are available.[58,22,23]

Education of the client and family about the disease, potential disability, treatment, and home program to achieve maximal function is essential. Such education can be provided through classes and literature available from the Arthritis Foundation. Family roles may need to be changed or modified as a result of one member's physical dysfunction. Therefore it is important for families to understand and support the disabled member and lend aid for tasks the client cannot or should not do.[19]

The occupational therapist should assist in designing a home program for the client. This should include a suitable work and rest schedule, activities, and exercises that will maximize function and minimize deformity and dysfunction. The home program should be outlined for the client in writing.

Treatment precautions

Fatigue should be avoided, and pain should be respected. It may be difficult for the client to do things in the morning because of stiffness of joints. A warm shower may be helpful to begin moving. Static, stressful, or resistive activities should be avoided. The use of a ball, putty, or clay for squeezing should be avoided, since these involve forceful flexion of the fingers, which can produce ulnar deviation, MP subluxation, and extensor tendon displacement.[10] If sensation is impaired, techniques to prevent injury to the desensitized part must be taught and observed by client and therapist.[19] If warmth is used to relax muscles and increase mobility, it should be limited to 20 minutes. Longer periods of warmth can increase inflammation and, later, produce increased swelling and pain. Resistive exercises for strengthening muscles do *not* improve joint stability and should not be used with this as an objective. Joint instability is usually due to ligamentous laxity, and resistive exercises can make this worse.[11]

Sample treatment plan

Case study

Mrs. J. is a 36-year-old woman with a diagnosis of rheumatoid arthritis. The onset was 3 years ago. She is a wife and the mother of an 8-year-old girl. She lives with her husband and daughter in a three-bedroom, single-level tract home. Mrs. J.'s primary role is that of homemaker. However, she has held a part-time job at a florist shop doing wreath design and construction and flower arranging. She both enjoys this work and sees her salary as a necessary adjunct to the family income.

Mrs. J. experiences intermittent acute disease episodes that have primarily involved the elbows, wrists, MP, and PIP joints bilaterally. There are slight losses of ROM and strength at all involved joints.

To date there is no permanent deformity, but ulnar deviation, MP subluxation, boutonnière deformity, wrist subluxation, and further limitation of ROM at all involved joints are possible deformities.

Medical management has been through rest and salicylates. Medical precautions are no strenuous activity, no resistive exercise or activity, and avoidance of fatigue.

She was referred to occupational therapy during the acute phase of her most recent episode for prevention of deformity and loss of ROM and maintenance of maximal function. She continued with occupational therapy services during the subacute period with the same goals.

TREATMENT PLAN

A. Statistical data.
 1. Name: Mrs. J.
    Age: 36
    Diagnosis: Rheumatoid arthritis
    Disability: Limited ROM, strength, and potential deformity of elbows, wrists, MP, and IP joints bilaterally
 2. Treatment aims as stated in referral:
    Prevent deformity
    Prevent loss of ROM
    Maintain maximal function

B. Other services.
 Medical services: Supervise medical management and rehabilitation therapies
 Physical therapy: May be used for specific exercise program
 Social services: Client and family counseling, if needed; financial arrangements, if appropriate
 Vocational counseling: Explore feasibility of return to same or modified occupation in floral work.

C. OT evaluation.
 Active and passive ROM: Test
 Muscle strength: Observe, test
 Sensation: Test
 Carpal tunnel syndrome: Test
 Boutonnière deformity: Test
 MP stability: Test
 Ulnar drift: Measure
 Wrist subluxation: Observe
 MP subluxation: Observe
 Hand function: Test
 ADL: Interview, observe
 Endurance: Interview, observe
 Prevocational skills: Observe
 Adjustment to disability: Observe
 Interpersonal and coping skills: Observe

D. Results of evaluation.
 1. Evaluation data.
    a. Physical resources. ROM measurements are equal for active and passive motion and bilaterally.
       Joint measurements
          Elbows: 10° to 130°
          Wrists
             Extension: 0° to 40°
             Flexion: 0° to 70°
          MP joints: 10° to 80°
          PIP joints: 10° to 110°
       Strength
          Elbow flexors: G
          Elbow extensors: F+
          Wrist extensors: F+
          Wrist flexors: G
          Grasp: G
          Finger extensors: F+
          Thumb muscles: N

Continued.

Sample treatment plan—cont'd

All other joint motions and muscle groups are within normal limits. MP joints are slightly unstable with 10° of ulnar drift on active motion. There is no evidence of wrist or MP subluxation, boutonniére deformity, or carpal tunnel syndrome at this time. Hand function testing reveals difficulty with fingertip prehension, and pinch and grip are good but not normal in strength. Forceful use of the thumb in opposition enhances ulnar drift and produces MP discomfort.

b. Sensory-perceptual functions. Sensory modalities of touch, pain, temperature, and position are intact. Perceptual functions are normal.

c. Cognitive functions. Cognition is normal. Client appears alert, intelligent, and interested in her progress.

d. Psychosocial functions. Client interacts comfortably with staff and other clients. She is cooperative and helpful. Her husband reported that she withdrew from social situations somewhat after her last

disease episode. She interacts comfortably with him and with her daughter, although her patience is very limited when she is fatigued or in pain. Her daughter has some understanding of her mother's problems and is usually willing to help with light chores.

e. Prevocational potential. Observation of the job performance of another worker by the occupational therapist and observation of Mrs. J. in simulated job tasks revealed that some aspects of the job would contribute to development of deformity. Cutting and twisting floral wire, forcing stems and stem support into Styrofoam, and binding wreaths were thought to be likely to enhance ulnar drift and MP subluxation because of the resistance and direction of joint forces. However, wreath design and layout and fresh flower arrangement are possible alternatives. Mrs. J.'s employer is willing to retain her on a part-time basis to perform these duties.

f. Functional skills. During

acute episodes Mrs. J. is severely limited in ADL. She leaves all home management to her husband and daughter during these periods and is not able to work. She only manages to do light self-care activities independently. During inactive periods, Mrs. J. is independent in light housekeeping, self-care, and work activities. She fatigues after 2 hours of light to moderate activity and requires a 20-minute rest period.

2. Problem identification.
   a. Muscle weakness
   b. Limited ROM
   c. Potential deformity
   d. Fluctuating vocational role
   e. Limited ADL independence
   f. Fluctuating role as wife and mother
   g. Tendency to social withdrawal
   h. Limited endurance
3. Assets-functions.
   a. No lower extremity involvement
   b. Good preservation of function
   c. Supportive and intact family unit
   d. Potential job skills, flexible employer
   e. Intelligence, motivation

E Problem	F Specific OT objectives	G Methods used to meet objectives	H Gradation of treatment
Acute stage a	Through appropriate exercise to elbows and wrists, muscle strength will be maintained	Isometric exercise without resistance to biceps, triceps, and flexors and extensors, carpi radialis and ulnaris, 3 to 10 repetitions 3 times daily Active ROM exercises; self-care to tolerance	Increase number of exercise sessions
b	Through appropriate exercise, ROM of affected joints will be preserved at present level	Active or active-assisted ROM exercises to elbow, MP and PIP flexion and extension, wrist flexion and extension, radial and ulnar deviation; active ROM exercise may be carried out in warm whirlpool bath coordinated with physical therapy	Grade to active exercise and add gentle active and passive stretching during subacute stage
b, c	Through splinting, joints will be rested to prevent damage and potential deformity	Hand resting splints in the position of function for night wear and use during periods of inactivity; short cock-up splint to protect the wrist may be useful when hands are active or being exercised	Decrease use of splint; remove splint for exercise and during self-care activities
e	Given instruction in joint protection, client will perform self-care to tolerance during acute episode	Self-feeding, using built-up, soft handle utensils; oral hygiene with electric toothbrush or built-up toothbrush; sponge and tub bathing, using wash mitt; self-dressing, using loose, slipover garments	Increase number of activities as disease activity subsides

E Problem	F Specific OT objectives	G Methods used to meet objectives	H Gradation of treatment
Subacute or inactive stage			
a	Through exercise and daily activities, muscle strength of affected joints will increase to one-half grade higher than initial evaluation	Light ironing, dust mopping, and dish washing Isometric exercise with resistance to elbow and wrist flexors and extensors, MP and PIP extensors, 3 to 10 repetitions 5 times daily; manual resistance is applied	Increase amount of activity, within physical tolerance Maintain at light resistance; increase number of exercise periods, if tolerated
b	Through appropriate exercise and activity, ROM of affected joints will be increased or maintained	Active ROM exercise to elbow, wrist, MP and PIP motions; gentle passive stretching to elbow flexion and extension, MP flexion and extension, and PIP extension Light dust mopping, dusting, table setting, diswashing with wash mitt	
c	Given instruction in joint protection techniques, deformity will be prevented or retarded in development	Individual and group instruction in techniques of joint protection applied to home management and work activities Avoid positions of deformity; always turn fingers to thumb side when opening and closing doors, jars, and make-up containers; place foam rubber tubing on handles of flower clippers; use strongest joints available; lift vases and bowls between palms of both hands; lift wreaths on forearm; spread sheets with forearm rather than fingertips; avoid long periods of holding or positioning; use stabilizers for bowls and vases; place foam curler on pencil for light grasp; stand up and move about from time to time while working	Increase number of techniques as each is mastered and applied in daily life
d	Explore potential for return to same or modified job in floral wreath design and construction	Client describes all steps of the involved tasks Therapist observes normal worker performing tasks; analyzes activity for potential deforming forces; determines need for job modification and application of joint protection and energy conservation principles in the workplace; modifies job to floral design and fresh flower arrangement; provides built-up pencil and protective ulnar deviation splint to be used during drawing, writing, and handling of flowers and clippers	Begin with one or two simple job tasks to be performed at home; job trial for 2 to 4 hours a day with 10 minutes of rest for every 40 minutes worked

I. **Special equipment.**
  1. Ambulation aids.
    None required
  2. Splints.
    Hand resting splints: For joint rest and maintenance of optimal position during acute episodes
    Short cock-up splint: For rest and protection of wrist when hand is in use during acute and possibly subacute stages

Protective ulnar deviation splint: To prevent ulnar drift during housekeeping and work activities
  3. Assistive devices.
    a. Electric mixer, can opener, toaster oven
    b. Lightweight dust mop with flexible handle
    c. Lever handles on faucets
    d. Fabric loops on oven doors so they may be opened with arm movement and not fingertips

  e. Utility cart
  f. High stools with backrest for kitchen and for work place
  g. Adapted key holders
  h. Wash mitts
  i. Dust mitts
  j. Foam rubber tubing to build handles on utensils and pencils

REVIEW QUESTIONS

1. What is the outstanding clinical feature that produces joint limitation and deformity in arthritis?
2. What sex and age groups are most frequently affected by arthritis?
3. What is meant by "rheumatoid factor"?
4. List four systemic signs of rheumatoid arthritis.
5. What is the characteristic course of the disease?
6. Describe the appearance and mechanics of two common finger deformities that may affect the DIP and PIP joints in rheumatoid arthritis.
7. What are the deformities that can result at the MP joints? How are they treated or prevented?
8. What are the major problems at the elbow and shoulder in arthritis? How can they be prevented?
9. What kinds of exercises are appropriate for arthritis clients in the acute stage of disease?
10. When is stretching exercise indicated?
11. When is joint rest indicated in treatment of arthritis?
12. Which joints should not be splinted in treatment of arthritis?
13. Which joints are frequently splinted in treatment of arthritis?
14. What is the role of the occupational therapist in splinting for arthritis?
15. List appropriate occupational therapy evaluation procedures for rheumatoid arthritis.
16. What are the general objectives of occupational therapy in treatment of arthritis?
17. What kinds of activities are contraindicated for the arthritis client during the acute stage of disease?
18. What kinds of activities are appropriate during the acute stage?
19. When the acute stage of the disease has abated, how can the client's activity be graded?
20. Discuss some of the ways work can be simplified for the arthritic client.
21. List some of the principles of joint protection directed toward maintaining ROM of the elbow and shoulder joints. Give some practical examples of methods of application of the principles to household tasks.
22. List five assistive devices for self-care or home management that could be useful to an arthritic client, and give the rationale for each.

REFERENCES

1. Arthritis Foundation: Guidelines for treatment of adult rheumatoid arthritis: exercise guide for physicians. Adapted by Dr. William Lages, San Jose, Calif., 1972, Santa Clara Valley Medical Center. Mimeographed.
2. Arthritis Foundation: Arthritis manual for allied health professionals, The Professional Manual Subcommittee of the Education Committee, Allied Health Professions Section, New York, 1973, The Arthritis Foundation.
3. Carroll, D.: A quantitative test of upper extremity function, J. Chronic Dis. **18:** 479, 1965.
4. Carter, M.S., and Wilson, R.L.: Postsurgical management in rheumatoid arthritis. In Hunter, J.M., and others: Rehabilitation of the hand, St. Louis, 1978, The C.V. Mosby Co.
5. Comfort, A.: Sexual consequences of disability, Philadelphia, 1978, George F. Stickley Co.
6. Cordery, J.C.: Joint protection: a responsibility of the occupational therapist, Am. J. Occup. Ther. **19:**285, 1965.
7. Engleman, E., and Shearn, M.: Arthritis and allied rheumatic disorders. In Krupp, M., and Chatton, M., editors: Current medical diagnosis and treatment, Los Altos, Calif., 1980, Lange Medical Publications.
8. Fries, J.F.: Arthritis, a comprehensive guide, Reading, Mass., 1979, Addison-Wesley Publishing Co., Inc.
9. Jebsen, R.H., et al.: An objective and standardized test of hand function, Arch. Phys. Med. Rehabil. **50:**311, 1969.
10. Kasch, M.: O.T. for rheumatoid arthritis, lecture, San Jose, Calif., 1975, Department of Occupational Therapy, San Jose State University.
11. Lages, W.: Arthritis and connective tissue diseases, lectures, San Jose, Calif., 1974 to 1978, Department of Occupational Therapy, San Jose State University.
12. Lages, W.: Pathogenesis of joint destruction. San Jose, Calif., 1976 and 1980, Santa Clara Valley Medical Center. Mimeographed.
13. Lages, W.: Principles of treatment program for rheumatoid arthritis, San Jose, Calif., 1976, Santa Clara Valley Medical Center. Mimeographed.
14. Lages, W.: Rheumatoid arthritis: indications for exercise, San Jose, Calif., 1976, Santa Clara Valley Medical Center. Mimeographed.
15. Lages, W.: Specific joint problems in rheumatoid arthritis, San Jose, Calif., 1976 and 1980, Santa Clara Valley Medical Center. Mimeographed.
16. Larson, C.B., and Gould, M.: Orthopedic nursing, ed. 8, St. Louis, 1974, The C.V. Mosby Co.
17. Madden, J.W., DeVore, G., and Arem, A.J.: A rational postoperative management program or metacarpophalangeal joint implant arthroplasty, J. Hand Surg. **2:**326, 1977.
18. Melvin, J.L.: Rheumatic disease: occupational therapy and rehabilitation, Philadelphia, 1982, F.A. Davis Co.
19. Paterson, M.: O.T. for rheumatoid arthritis, lectures, San Jose, Calif., 1977, Department of Occupational Therapy, San Jose State University.
20. Pelletier, K.R.: Mind as healer: mind as slayer, New York, 1977, Dell Publishing Co., Inc.
21. Quan, P.E., and English, C.: Principles of joint protection and energy conservation, San Jose, Calif., Department of Occupational Therapy, Santa Clara Valley Medical Center. Mimeographed. (Adapted from Cordery, J.C.: The conservation of physical resources as applied to the activities of patients with arthritis and connective tissue diseases. In Rothenberg, E., editor, and Kandel, D., editorial chairman: Dynamic living for the long-term patient, World Federation of Occupational Therapists, study course III, 1962, Dubuque, Iowa, 1964, Wm. C. Brown Co., Publishers.)
22. Richards, J.S.: Sex and arthritis: sexuality and disability, **3:**97, 1980.
23. Sidman, J.M.: Sexual functioning and the physically disabled adult, Am. J. Occup. Ther. **31:**81, 1977.
24. Swezey, R.L.: Rehabilitation in arthritis and related conditions. In Kottke, F.J., Stillwell, G.K., and Lehmann, J.F., editors: Krusen's handbook of physical medicine and rehabilitation, Philadelphia, 1982, W.B. Saunders Co.
25. Trombly, C.A., and Scott, A.D.: Occupational therapy for physical dysfunction, Baltimore, 1977, Williams & Wilkins.

CHAPTER 24

Acute hand injuries

MARY C. KASCH

Treatment of the upper extremity is important to all occupational therapists who work with physically disabled persons. The incidence of upper extremity injuries is significant and accounts for about one third of all injuries. The nearly 16 million upper extremity injuries that occur annually in the United States result in 90 million days of restricted activity and 12 million visits to physicians. The upper extremities are involved in about one third of work-related farm injuries and one third of disabling industrial injuries. In addition, disease and congenital anomalies contribute to upper extremity dysfunction, and it is estimated that only about 15% of those suffering from severe cerebral vascular accident recover hand function.[30]

The hand is vital to human function and appearance. It flexes, extends, opposes, and grasps thousands of times daily, allowing the performance of necessary daily activities. The hand's sensibility allows feeling without looking and provides protection from injury. The hand touches, gives comfort, and expresses emotions. Loss of hand function through injury or disease thus affects much more than the mechanical tasks that the hand performs. Hand injury may jeopardize a family's livelihood and at the least affects every daily activity. The occupational therapist with training in physical and psychological assessment, prosthetic evaluation, fabrication of orthoses, and assessment and training in the activities of daily living (ADL), and in functional restoration is uniquely qualified to treat upper extremity disorders.

Hand rehabilitation, or hand therapy, has grown as a specialty area of both physical and occupational therapy, and some of the treatment techniques used with hand patients have emerged from both specialties to be used by the hand therapist. It is not the purpose of this chapter to instruct the occupational therapy student in physical modalities. Rather, treatment techniques that have been found to be beneficial to hand injury patients are presented. It is assumed that these techniques will be provided by the therapist best trained to provide them. Hand rehabilitation requires advanced and specialized training by both physical and occupational therapists.

Treatment techniques, whether thermal modalities or specifically designed exercises, are used as a bridge to reach a further goal of returning to functional performance. Thus some modalities may be used as "enabling modalities" in preparation for functional use. It is within this context that treatment techniques will be presented in this chapter.

Treatment of the injured hand is a matter of timing and judgment. Following trauma or surgery a healing phase must occur in which the body performs its physiological function of wound healing. Following the initial healing phase when cellular restoration has been accomplished, the wound enters its restorative phase. It is in this phase that hand therapy is most beneficial. Early treatment that occurs in this restorative phase is ideal and in some cases essential for optimal results. Although sample timetables may be presented, the therapist should always coordinate the application of any treatment with the hand surgeon. Surgical techniques may vary, and inappropriate treatment of the hand patient can result in failure of a surgical procedure. Communication between the surgeon, therapist, and patient is especially vital in this setting. A comfortable environment in which group interaction is possible may increase patient motivation and cooperation. The presence of the therapist as an instructor and evaluator is essential, but without the patient's cooperation limited gains will be achieved. Treating the psychological loss suffered by the patient with a hand injury is an integral part of the rehabilitative therapy as well.

EXAMINATION AND EVALUATION

When approaching a patient who has a hand injury, the therapist must be able to evaluate the nature of the injury and the limitations it has produced. First the injured structures must be identified by consulting with the hand surgeon, reviewing operative reports and x-ray films, and discussing the injury with the patient. Evaluation of bone, tendon, and nerve function must be ascertained using standardized evaluation techniques whenever possible.

The patient's age, occupation, and hand dominance should be taken into account in the initial evaluation. The type and extent of medical and surgical treatment that has been received and the length of time since such treatment are important in determining a treatment plan. Any further surgery or conservative treatment that is planned should also be noted. The treatment plan should have the written approval of the referring physician.

The purposes of hand evaluation are to identify (1) physical limitations, such as loss of range of motion (ROM), (2) functional limitations, such as inability to perform daily tasks, (3) substitution patterns to compensate for loss of sensibility or motor function, and (4) established deformities, such as joint contracture.

Arm and hand function are mutually dependent and have an intimate relationship in effective function.[14] Some upper extremity movements are more valuable for function than others. The wrist is the key joint in the position of function.[11] Wrist stability is necessary for finger performance. Skilled hand performance depends on wrist stability, mobility, and ability to make fine adjustments in position. It also depends on arm and shoulder stability and mobility for fixing or positioning the hand for functional use. The thumb is of greater importance than any other finger. Effective pinch is almost impossible without a thumb, and attempts will always be made to salvage or reconstruct an injured thumb. Proximal interphalangeal (PIP) joint motion is important for finger function.[11]

Physical evaluation

The effect of trauma or dysfunction on anatomical structures is the first consideration in evaluating hand function. The joints must be assessed for active and passive mobility, fixed deformities, and any tendency to assume a position of deformity. The ligaments must be evaluated for laxity or contracture and their ability to maintain joint stability. Tendons must be examined for integrity, contracture, or overstretching; muscles are tested for strength and function. The degree of mobility, elasticity, adherence, and trophic changes in the skin should be observed. The vascular system is assessed by observing the skin color and temperature of the hand and evaluating for presence of edema.

SOFT TISSUE TIGHTNESS. Joints may develop intrinsic dysfunction following trauma. Mennell describes joint dysfunction as loss of joint play or intrinsic play of the joint associated with pain and functional impairment. Joint dysfunction may result from (1) intrinsic trauma, (2) immobilization, or (3) resolution of some more serious pathological condition.[45] It is necessary to restore accessory motions before the joint can be moved through passive ROM by the therapist.[44]

It is important to assess if limited motion is caused by joint tightness or tightness of the extrinsic or intrinsic muscles.

To test for extrinsic extensor tightness the metacarpophalangeal (MP) joint is passively held in extension and the PIP joint is moved passively into flexion. Then the MP joint is flexed, and the PIP joint is again passively flexed. If the PIP joint can be flexed easily when the MP joint is extended but not when the MP joint is flexed, the extrinsic extensors are adherent.[1]

Intrinsic tightness is tested by passively holding the MP joint in extension and applying pressure just distal to the PIP joint. This is repeated with the MP joint in flexion. If there is more resistance when the MP joint is extended, intrinsic tightness is indicated.[1]

If there is no difference in passive motion of the PIP joint when the MP joint is held in extension or flexion and there is limitation of PIP joint flexion in any position, tightness of the joint capsule is indicated, and treatment techniques to reduce joint stiffness should be initiated.

GRIP AND PINCH STRENGTH. Upper extremity strength evaluation is usually performed following the healing phase of trauma. Strength testing is *not* indicated following recent trauma or surgery.

A standard adjustable handle dynamometer is recommended for assessing grip strength. Although variables, such as age, will affect the strength measurements, maximal readings will usually be obtained at the second or third position and either the first or second attempt at gripping[24] (Fig. 24-1).

The subject should be seated with the shoulder adducted, the elbow at 90° of flexion, and the forearm held in neutral position. The dynamometer should be lightly held by the examiner to prevent accidental dropping of the instrument. The subject then forcefully grips the dynamometer three successive times, alternating the two hands if possible. The noninjured hand is used for comparison. Normal tables can be found in the literature listed in the references.[29]

Pinch strength should also be tested on a standard pinch dynamometer. Palmer pinch (thumb tip to index fingertip), lateral or key pinch (thumb pulp to lateral aspect of the middle phalanx of the index finger), and three-point pinch (thumb tip to tips of index and long fingers) should be evaluated. As with the grip dynamometer, three successive trials should be obtained and compared bilaterally[24] (Fig. 24-2).

Grip and pinch strength can be expressed in pounds or kilograms. The metric system is more commonly used

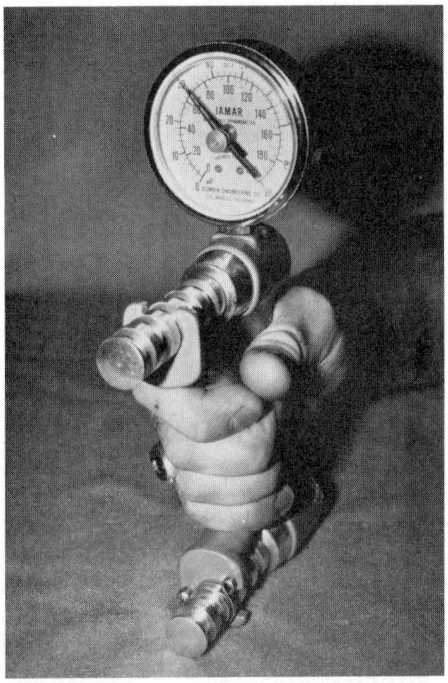

Fig. 24-1. Jamar dynamometer is used to evaluate grip strength in both hands.

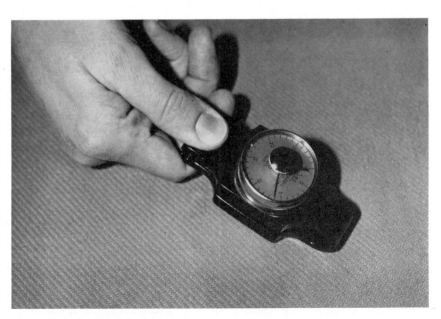

Fig. 24-2. Pinch guage is used to evaluate pinch strength in variety of prehension patterns of pinch.

in medicine, and many surgeons prefer measurements in kilograms. For accurate comparison consistency is important in describing test results.

Manual muscle testing is also used to evaluate upper extremity function. Accurate assessment is especially important when preparing the patient for tendon transfers or other reconstructive surgery. The student who wishes to study muscle testing of the hand is referred especially to J.V. Basmajian's work.[5]

EDEMA ASSESSMENT. Hand volume is measured to assess the presence of extra- or intracellular edema. It is generally used to determine the effect of treatment and activities. By measuring volume at different times of the day the effects of rest versus activity may be measured as well as the effects of splinting or treatment designed to reduce edema.

A commercially available volumeter[17] may be used to assess hand edema. The volumeter has been shown to be accurate to 10 ml[62] when used in the prescribed manner. Variables that have been shown to decrease the accuracy of the volumeter include (1) the use of a faucet or hose that introduces air into the tank during filling, (2) movement of the arm within the tank, (3) inconsistent pressure on the stop rod, and (4) the use of a volumeter in a variety of places. The same level surface should always be used.[24] The evaluation is performed as follows (Fig. 24-3):

1. A plastic volumeter is filled and allowed to empty into a 500 ml graduated cylinder until the water reaches spout level. The cylinder is then emptied and dried thoroughly.
2. The patient is instructed to immerse the hand in the plastic volumeter, being careful to keep the hand supinated.
3. The hand is lowered until it rests gently between the middle and ring fingers on the dowel rod. It is important that the hand does not press onto the rod.
4. The hand remains still until no more water drips into the cylinder.
5. The hand is removed, the cylinder is placed on a level surface, and a reading is made.

A method of assessing edema of an individual finger or joint is circumferential measurement using either a circumference tape[34] or jeweler's ring size standards. Measurements should be made before and after treatment and especially following the application of thermal modalities or splinting. Patients will often note swelling but objective data will help the therapist to determine the benefits of treatment. Edema control techniques will be discussed later in this chapter.

SENSIBILITY. Sensibility of the hand must be assessed following nerve trauma and repair. Tests, such as Tinel's sign,[33] may be used to plot the regeneration of a nerve. The tests of nerve function, such as two-point discrimination, are always performed at the fingertips.

Recovery of sympathetic response (sweating, pain, and temperature discrimination) may occur early but does not correlate with functional recovery.[19] O'Rain[49] observed that denervated skin does not wrinkle. Therefore nerve function may be tested by immersing the hand in water for 5 minutes and noting

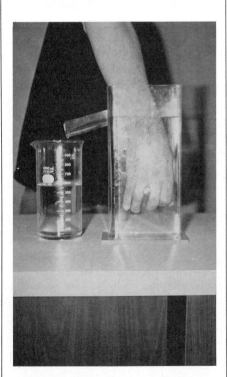

Fig. 24-3. Volumeter is used to measure volume of both hands for comparison. Increased volume indicates presence of edema.

the presence or absence of skin wrinkling. This test may be especially helpful in diagnosing a nerve lesion in young children. The ability to sweat is also lost with a nerve lesion. A ninhydrin test[47] evaluates sweating of the finger.

The wrinkle test and the ninhydrin test will objectively measure return of sympathetic function. Recovery of sweating has been shown to correlate with the recovery of protective sensation.

During the first 2 to 4 months following nerve suture, axons will regenerate and travel through the hand at a rate of about 1 mm per day or 1 inch per month. Tinel's sign may be used to follow this regeneration.[33] The test is performed by tapping gently along the course of the nerve, starting approximately at the nerve suture, moving distally to elicit a tingling sensation in the fingertip. The point at which tapping no longer elicits this tingling is noted and indicates the extent of nerve growth. As regeneration occurs, paresthesias will develop. Although this hypersensitivity may be uncomfortable to the patient, it is a positive sign of nerve growth.

At this point the therapist can begin to evaluate 30 cps vibration, 256 cps vibration, moving touch, and constant touch. These tests will be repeated until 6 months after repair or until each is present at the fingertip.[19]

Vibration is tested first with a 30 cps tuning fork. The fork should be at room temperature. The patient faces the therapist with the former's hand resting lightly in the therapist's hand so that feedback will not come from the table. As with other sensibility tests, the uninvolved hand is tested first for reference. After the patient understands what is being asked, the therapist starts the tuning fork and rests it lightly on the proximal palm. It is moved distally until the patient is no longer able to identify the vibration. It should be stressed that the patient must distinguish between pressure and vibration. After the patient has recovered the ability to detect moving touch and constant touch to the tip of the finger, vibration of 256 cps may be tested. Testing is performed in the same manner.[20]

Moving touch is tested using the eraser end of a pencil. The eraser is placed in an area of normal sensibility and, pressing lightly, is moved to the distal fingertip. The patient notes when the perception of the stimulus changes. Light and heavy stimuli may be applied and noted.[42]

Constant touch is tested by pressing with the eraser end of a pencil, first in an area with normal sensibility and then moving distally. The patient responds when the stimulus is altered again; light and heavy stimuli may be applied.[42]

Discrimination, the second level of sensibility assessment, requires the subject to distinguish between two direct stimuli. The two-point discrimination test, first described by Weber in 1853, was developed and further modified by Moberg[46] to assess the functional level of sensation. Two-point discrimination is not tested until constant touch is perceived at the fingertip.[19]

The test is performed as follows:[33]

1. The patient's vision is occluded.
2. An area of normal sensation is tested as a reference, using a blunt caliper or bent paper clip.
3. The calipers are set 10 mm apart and are randomly applied longitudinally in line with the digital nerves, with one or two points touching. The skin should not be blanched by the caliper. The distance is decreased until the patient no longer feels two distinct points, and that distance is measured. From 3 to 4 seconds should be allowed between applications, and the patient should have four out of five correct responses.[8] Because this test indicates sensory function, it is usually administered at the tips of the fingers. It may be used proximally to test nerve regeneration. Normal two-point discrimination at the fingertip is 6 mm or less.[1]

Moving two-point discrimination has been proposed as a method to measure the innervation density of a quickly adapting fiber and receptor system, which would be more valid than the Weber test that only evaluates the slowly adapting fiber and receptor system. Moving two-point discrimination

is not tested until moving touch is perceived at the fingertip. The test is performed as follows:[19]

1. The patient's vision is occluded.
2. An area of normal sensation is tested as a reference, using a blunt caliper or bent paper clip.
3. The fingertip is supported by the examining table or the examiner's hand.
4. The caliper, separated 5 to 8 mm, is moved longitudinally from proximal to distal along the surface of the fingertip. One and two points are randomly alternated. The patient must correctly identify the stimulus in seven out of eight responses before proceeding to a smaller value. The test is repeated down to a separation of 2 mm.

The Semmes-Weinstein monofilaments measure cutaneous pressure thresholds. The test is composed of 20 nylon monofilaments that are graded by thickness and stiffness between a range of 1.65 and 6.65. These numbers represent a formula that can convert the force applied into grams of pressure. The monofilaments are held perpendicular to the finger and gently bounced off the skin just until the fiber bends. With the heavier monofilaments, only one motion is used. The Semmes-Weinstein monofilaments do not correlate accurately with the measurement of two-point discrimination. Thus application of the monofilaments may be clinically objective but interpretation of the results may be much more complex because of variations in the instrument.[19]

Recognition of common objects is the final level of sensory function. Moberg popularized the phrase "tactile gnosis"[46] to describe the ability of the hand to see by feeling to perform complex functions. Moberg later stated that normal tactile gnosis requires a two-point discrimination of 3.5 mm.[47] Other authors have asserted that the test for two-point discrimination does not clearly correlate with function but rather with the regeneration of slowly adapting fiber and receptors.[19] Moberg suggested the use of the "picking-up test."[46] Subjects were asked to pick up a number of objects and place them in a small box. Trials were made with each hand, first with the aid of vision, then blindfolded.

Each trial was timed, and the test was repeated at intervals. Observation of hand use during the blindfolded phase was also important. Dellon[19] suggests a modified picking-up test in which the patient is asked to identify the object he or she is picking up while blindfolded. The modified picking-up test is felt to correlate most directly with tactile gnosis.

Functional evaluation

Evaluation of hand function or performance is important because the physical evaluation does not measure the patient's ingenuity and ability to compensate for loss of strength, ROM, sensation, or presence of deformities.[14]

The physical evaluation should precede the functional evaluation because awareness of physical dysfunction can result in a critical analysis of functional impairment and an understanding of why the client functions as he or she does.[43]

The effect of the hand dysfunction of the use of the hand in ADL should be observed by the occupational therapist. In addition some type of a standardized performance evaluation, such as the Jebsen Test of Hand Function[27] or the Carroll Quantitative Test of Upper Extremity Function,[14] should be administered.

The Jebsen Test of Hand Function[27] was developed to provide objective measurements of standardized tasks with norms for client comparison. It is a short test that is easy to administer, is inexpensive, and is put together by the person administering the test. The test consists of seven subtests, comprising (1) writing a short sentence, (2) turning over 3 × 5-inch cards, (3) picking up small objects and placing them in a container, (4) stacking checkers, (5) eating (simulated), (6) moving empty large cans, and (7) moving weighted large cans. Norms are provided for dominant and nondominant hands for each subtest and also are divided by sex and age. Instructions for fabricating the test, as well as specific instructions for administering the test, are provided by the authors.[27] This has been found to be a good test for overall hand function.

The Quantitative Test of Upper Extremity Function described by Carroll[14] was designed to measure ability to perform general arm and hand activities used in daily living. It is based on the assumption that complex upper extremity movements used to perform ordinary ADL can be reduced to specific patterns of grasp and prehension of the hand, supination and pronation of the forearm, flexion and extension of the elbow, and elevation of the arm.

The test consists of six parts, comprising (1) grasping and lifting four blocks of graduated sizes to assess grasp; (2) grasping and lifting two pipes of graduated sizes from a peg to test cylindrical grip; (3) grasping and placing a ball to test spherical grasp; (4) picking up and placing four marbles of graduated sizes to test fingertip prehension or pinch; (5) putting a small washer over a nail and putting an iron on a shelf to test placing; and (6) pouring water from pitcher to glass and glass to glass, placing hand on top of head, behind head, and to mouth, and writing the name to assess pronation, supination, and elevation of the arm. The test uses simple, inexpensive, and easily acquired materials. Details of materials and their arrangement, test procedures, and scoring can be found in the original source.

Other tests that have been found to be useful in the evaluation of hand dexterity are the Crawford Small Parts Test,[16] the Bennett Hand Tool Dexterity Test,[9] and the Purdue Pegboard Test.[56] All of these tests include comparison with normal subjects working in a variety of industrial settings. These tests are especially useful when administering a work capacity evaluation. Tests may be purchased and come with instructions for administering the test and the standardized norms. Melvin lists a variety of additional hand function tests.[43]

Observation

The occupational therapist should observe the appearance of the hand and arm. The position of the hand and arm at rest and the carrying posture can yield valuable information about the dysfunction. How the patient "treats"

the disease or injury should be observed. Is it overprotected and carefully guarded or ignored? The skin condition of the hand and arm should be noted. Are there lacerations, sutures, or evidence of recent surgery? Is the skin dry or moist? Are there scales or crusts? Does the hand appear swollen? Does the hand have an odor? Is the skin normally mobile? Palmar skin is less mobile than dorsal skin normally. Are there contractures of the web spaces? The therapist should observe the relationship between hand and arm function as the patient moves about and performs test items or tasks. If the patient has difficulty assuming the functional position, the therapist may assist by stabilizing the patient's wrist and placing the thumb in opposition.

The therapist should ask the patient to perform some simple bilateral ADL, such as buttoning a button, putting on a shirt, opening a jar, and threading a needle, and observe the amount of spontaneous movement and use of the affected hand and arm. Is it relatively or completely static or slightly to completely dynamic when required for function?

Clinical tests for specific dysfunction

PERIPHERAL NEUROPATHY. Several quick clinical observations to detect dysfunction of peripheral nerves are available, based on the sensory and motor function of the individual nerve.

The ulnar nerve may be tested by asking the patient to make a cone with the fingers or abduct and adduct the fingers. The radial nerve may be tested by asking the patient to extend the wrist and fingers. Median nerve function is tested by asking the patient to oppose the thumb to the fingers and flex the fingers.[15] The median nerve may be affected by carpal tunnel compression in conditions such as rheumatoid arthritis. Early signs of median nerve compression are sensory in nature and may be tested in two ways. First, to elicit Tinel's sign of median nerve compression, the examiner taps over the volar aspect of the wrist at the base of the thumb metacarpal. A positive response of paresthesias along the median distribution in the thumb is indicative of compression. Phalen's test involves

complete passive flexion or extension of the wrist to elicit the same response described for Tinel's sign. The complete passive flexion or extension increases the nerve compression and results in the abnormal sensory response.

It is important to test for median nerve compression periodically in clients with rheumatoid arthritis involving the wrist, since synovial proliferation under the transverse carpal ligament can cause compression on the median nerve. It is important to correct this problem before it progresses to include motor dysfunction of the muscles innervated, which are so critical to hand function.

TREATMENT
Fractures

In treating a hand or wrist fracture the surgeon will attempt to achieve good anatomical position through either a closed (nonoperative) or open (operative) reduction. Internal fixation with Kirschner wires, metallic plates, and/or screws may be used to maintain the desired position. The hand is usually immobilized in wrist extension and MP joint flexion with extension of the distal joints whenever the injury allows this position.[64] Trauma to bone may also involve trauma to tendons and nerves in the adjacent area. Treatment must be geared toward the recovery of all injured structures, and this fact may influence treatment of the fracture.

Occupational therapy may be initiated during the period of immobilization, which is usually 3 to 5 weeks. Uninvolved fingers of the hand must be kept mobile through the use of active motion. Edema should be carefully monitored, and elevation is required whenever edema is present.

As soon as there is sufficient bone stability, the surgeon will allow mobilization of the injured part. The surgeon should provide guidelines for the amount of resistance or force that may be applied to the fracture site. Activities that correct poor motor patterns and encourage use of the injured hand should be started as soon as the hand is pain free. Early motion will prevent the adherence of tendons and reduce edema through massage of the lymphatic and blood vessels.

Closed functional treatment of fractures, or fracture bracing, is a technique described by Sarmiento[51] in which the fracture is treated with rigid immobilization for a brief period of time until the pain subsides. Immobilization is then discontinued, and the fracture is placed in a fracture brace that stabilizes the fracture while allowing function.

"Fracture bracing is predicated on the belief that bone contact, end to end or otherwise, is not required for bony union; and that rigid immobilization of joints above and below a fracture, as well as prolonged rest, are detrimental to fracture healing. Closed functional bracing of fractures calls for functional activity in order to obtain greater osteogenesis."[51]

Occupational therapists may participate in the fabrication of fracture braces and may supervise a program of progressive functional activity for the patient who is treated with closed functional bracing. Ferraro[23] documents the success of closed functional bracing of metacarpal fractures with minimal interference in the ADL and work activities of the patients.

As soon as the brace or cast is removed, the patient's hand must be evaluated. If edema remains present, edema control techniques can be initiated using techniques described later in this chapter. A baseline ROM should be established, and the application of appropriate splints may begin. A splint may be used to correct a deformity that has resulted from immobilization or it may be used to protect the finger from additional trauma to the fracture site. An example of this type of splinting would be the application of a Velcro "buddy" splint (Fig. 24-4) or a Bedford finger stall[38] (Fig. 24-5). A dorsal block splint that limits full extension of the finger may be used following a fracture or dislocation of the PIP joint. A dynamic splint may be used to achieve full ROM or prevent the development of further deformity.

Intraarticular fractures may result in injury to the cartilage of the joint, resulting in additional pain and stiffness. An x-ray examination will indicate if there has been damage to the joint surface that might limit the treatment of the joint. Joint pain and stiffness following fracture without the presence of

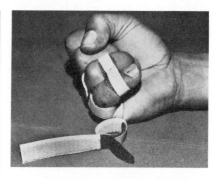

Fig. 24-4. Velcro "buddy" splint may be used to protect finger following fracture or encourage movement of stiff finger. (Available from Smalley and Bates, Inc., 85 Park Avenue, Nutley, N.J.)

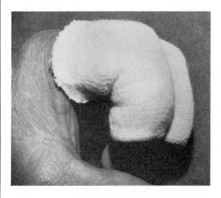

Fig. 24-5. Bedford finger stall may be used as "fellow traveler" to protect injured finger. Slight compression applied by stretch gauze may reduce edema, and pressure may alleviate pain. Finger stall can be worn for prolonged periods of time.

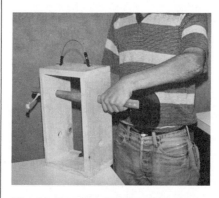

Fig. 24-6. Weight well is used for strengthening upper extremity with progressive resistance applied to weakened musculature. It is also useful in retraining prehension patterns of pinch and grip.

joint damage should be alleviated by a combination of thermal modalities, restoration of joint play, or joint mobilization and corrective and dynamic splinting followed by active use. Resistive exercise can be started when bony healing has been achieved.

Wrist fractures are common and may present special problems for the surgeon and therapist. Colles' fractures of the distal radius are the most common injury to the wrist[11] and may result in limitations in wrist flexion and extension, as well as pronation and supination resulting from the involvement of the radioulnar joint. Use of splints, active motion that emphasizes wrist movement, and joint mobilization may be beneficial. The weight well[3] (Fig. 24-6) may be used to provide resistance to wrist motions.

The carpal scaphoid is the second most commonly injured bone in the wrist[11] and is often fractured when the hand is dorsiflexed at the time of injury. Fractures to the proximal portion of the scaphoid may result in nonunion because of poor blood supply to this area. Scaphoid fractures will require a prolonged period of immobilization, sometimes up to several months in a cast, with resulting stiffness and pain. Care should be taken to mobilize noninvolved joints early.

Trauma to the carpal lunate may result in avascular necrosis of the lunate or Kienböck's disease.[11] This may result from a one-time accident or may be caused by repetitive trauma. Lunate fractures are usually immobilized for 6 weeks. Kienböck's disease may be treated with a bone graft, Silastic implant, or partial wrist fusion.

Stiffness and pain are common complications of fractures, but the control of edema coupled with early motion and good patient instruction and support will minimize these complications.

Nerve injuries

Nerve injury may be classified into the following three categories:

1. Neurapraxia is contusion of the nerve without wallerian degeneration. The nerve recovers function without treatment within a few days or weeks.

2. Axonotmesis is an injury in which nerve fibers distal to the site of injury degenerate, but the internal organization of the nerve remains intact. No surgical treatment is necessary, and recovery usually occurs within 6 months. The length of time may vary, depending on the level of injury.

3. Neurotmesis is a complete laceration of both nerve and fibrous tissues. Surgical treatment is required. Microsurgical repair of the fascicles is common. Nerve grafting may be necessary in situations where there is a gap between nerve endings.[10]

Peripheral nerve injuries may occur as a result of disruption of the nerve by a fractured bone, laceration, or crush injury. Symptoms of nerve injuries will include weakness or paralysis of muscles that are innervated by motor branches of the injured nerve and sensory loss to areas that are innervated by sensory branches of the injured nerve. Before evaluating the patient for nerve loss the therapist must be familiar with the muscles and areas that are innervated by the three major forearm nerves.

RADIAL NERVE. The radial nerve innervates the extensor-supinator group of muscles of the forearm, including the brachioradialis, extensor carpi radialis longus, extensor carpi radialis brevis, extensor digitorum communis, extensor digiti minimi, extensor indicis, extensor carpi ulnaris, supinator, abductor pollicis longus, extensor pollicis brevis, and extensor pollicis longus. The sensory distribution of the radial nerve is a strip of the posterior upper arm and the forearm; dorsum of the thumb; and index and middle fingers and radial half of the ring finger to the PIP joints. Sensory loss of the radial nerve does not usually result in dysfunction.

Clinical signs of a high-level radial nerve injury (above the supinator) are pronation of the forearm, wrist flexion, and the thumb held in palmar abduction resulting from the unopposed action of the flexor pollicis brevis and the abductor pollicis brevis.[66] Injury to the posterior interosseous nerve will spare the extensor carpi radialis longus, and an inexperienced examiner may miss the nerve lesion. Clinical signs of a low-level radial nerve injury include incomplete extension of the MP joints of the

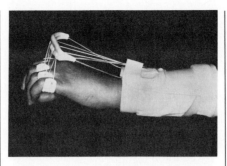

Fig. 24-7. Low-profile radial nerve splint is carefully balanced to pull MP joints into extension when wrist is flexed and allows the MP joints to fall into slight flexion when wrist is extended, thus preserving normal balance between two joints and preventing joint contracture. (Splint courtesy of Judy C. Colditz, O.T.R., Raleigh Hand Rehabilitation Center.)

fingers and thumb. The interossei will extend the interphalangeal (IP) joints of the fingers but the MP joints will rest in about 30° of flexion.

A dorsal splint that provides wrist extension, MP extension, and thumb extension should be provided to protect the extensor tendons from overstretching during the healing phase and to position the hand for functional use (Fig. 24-7). A dynamic splint is commonly provided. A less obvious splint may increase patient acceptance.

ULNAR NERVE. The ulnar nerve in the forearm innervates only the flexor carpi ulnaris and the median half of the flexor digitorum profundus. It travels down the volar forearm through the canal of Guyon, innervating the intrinsic muscles of the hand, including the palmaris brevis, abductor digiti minimi, opponens digiti minimi, flexor digiti minimi, dorsal and volar interossei, third and fourth lumbricales, and medial head of the flexor pollicis brevis.

The sensory distribution of the ulnar nerve is the dorsal and volar surfaces of the little finger ray and the ulnar half of the dorsal and volar surface of the ring finger ray.

A high-level ulnar nerve injury results in hyperextension of the MP joints of the ring and small fingers (also called "clawing") resulting from overaction of the extensor digitorum communis that is not held in check by the third and fourth lumbricales.[66] The IP joints of

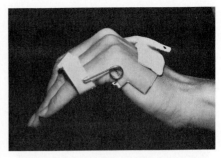

Fig. 24-8. Dynamic ulnar nerve splint blocks hyperextension of MP joints that occurs with paralysis of ulnar intrinsic muscles. It allows MP flexion, which maintains normal ROM of MP joints. (Splint courtesy of Mary Dimick, O.T.R., University of California-San Diego Hand Rehabilitation Center.)

the ring and small fingers will not demonstrate a great flexion deformity because of the paralysis of the flexor digitorum profundus. The hypothenar muscles and interossei will be absent. The wrist will assume a position of radial extension caused by the loss of the flexor carpi ulnaris. In a low-level ulnar nerve injury the ring and small fingers will claw at the MP joints and the IP joints will exhibit a greater tendency toward flexion because the flexor digitorum profundus will be present. Wrist extension will be normal.

Clinical signs of a high-level ulnar nerve injury may include clawhand with a loss of the hypothenar and the interosseous muscles. In a low-level ulnar nerve injury the flexor digitorum profundus and flexor carpi ulnaris will be present and unopposed by the intrinsic muscles. When attempting lateral or key pinch the IP joint of the thumb will flex instead of extend because of paralysis of the intrinsic muscles. This is also known as Froment's sign. Long-standing compression of the ulnar nerve in the canal of Guyon will result in a flattening of the hypothenar area and conspicuous atrophy of the first dorsal interosseous muscle.[11]

With a low-level ulnar nerve injury a small splint may be provided to prevent hyperextension of the small and ring fingers without limiting full flexion at the MP joints. Stabilization of the MP joints will allow the extensor digitorum communis to fully extend the IP joints (Fig. 24-8).

Sensory loss of the ulnar nerve results in frequent injury to the ulnar side of the hand, especially burns. Patients must be instructed in visual protection of the anesthetic area.

MEDIAN NERVE. The median nerve innervates the flexors of the forearm and hand and is often called the "eyes" of the hands because of its importance in sensory innervation of the volar surface of the hands. Median nerve loss may result from lacerations as well as compression syndromes of the wrist, such as the carpal tunnel syndrome.

Motor distribution of the median nerve is to the pronator teres, palmaris longus, flexor carpi radialis, flexor digitorum to the index and long fingers, flexor digitorum sublimis, flexor pollicis longus, pronator quadratus, abductor pollicis brevis, opponens pollicis, superficial head of the flexor pollicis brevis, and first and second lumbricales.

Sensory distribution of the median nerve is to the volar surface of the thumb, index and middle fingers, and radial half of the ring finger and dorsal surface of the index and middle fingers and radial half of the ring finger distal to the PIP joints.

Clinical signs of a high-level median nerve injury are ulnar flexion of the wrist caused by loss of the flexor carpi radialis, lack of palmar abduction, and opposition of the thumb. Active pronation will be absent, but the patient may appear to pronate with the assistance of gravity. In a wrist-level median nerve injury the thenar eminence will appear flat, and there will be a loss of thumb flexion, palmar abduction, and opposition.[66]

The sensory loss associated with median nerve injury is particularly disabling because there will be no sensation to the volar aspects of the thumb and index and long fingers. The patient when blindfolded will substitute pinch to the ring and small fingers to compensate for this loss. An injury in the forearm that involves the anterior interosseous nerve will not result in sensory loss.

Splints that position the thumb in palmar abduction and slight opposition will increase functional use of the hand (Fig. 24-9). If clawing of the index and long fingers is present, a splint should be fabricated to prevent hyperextension

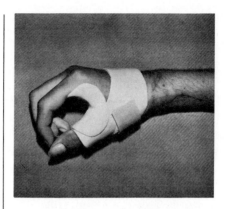

Fig. 24-9. Thumb stabilization splint may be used with median nerve injury to protect thumb and to improve function by placing thumb in position of pinch. Normal pinch cannot be achieved with median nerve injury because of paralysis of thumb musculature.

of the MP joints. Patients report that they avoid use of the hand with a median nerve injury because of lack of sensation rather than because of muscle paralysis. Despite this, the weakened or paralyzed muscles should be protected.

POSTOPERATIVE MANAGEMENT FOLLOWING NERVE REPAIR. Following nerve repair the hand is placed in a position that will minimize tension on the nerve. For example, following repair of the median nerve, the wrist will be immobilized in a flexed position. Immobilization usually lasts for 2 to 3 weeks, after which protective stretching of the joints may begin. The therapist must exercise great care not to put excessive traction on the newly repaired nerve.

Correction of a contracture may take 4 to 6 weeks. Active exercise is the preferred method of gaining full extension, although a light dynamic splint may be applied with the surgeon's supervision. Splinting to assist or substitute for weakened musculature may be necessary for an extended period during nerve regeneration. Splints should be removed as soon as possible to allow for active exercise of the weakened muscles. However, it is important to instruct the patient in correct patterns of motion so that substitution does not occur.

Initially treatment is directed toward

the prevention of deformity and correction of poor positioning during the acute and regenerative stages. Patients must be instructed in visual protection of the anesthetic area. ADL should be evaluated, and new methods or devices may be needed for independence. Use of the hand in the patient's work should be evaluated, and the patient should be returned to employment with any necessary modifications of his or her job or adaptations of equipment as soon as possible.

Careful muscle, sensory, and functional testing should be done frequently. As the nerve regenerates, splints may be changed or eliminated. Exercises and activities should be revised to reflect the patient's new gains, and adapted equipment should be discarded as soon as possible.

As motor function begins to return to the paralyzed muscles, a careful program of specific exercises should be devised to facilitate the return. Proprioceptive neuromuscular facilitation techniques, such as hold-relax, contract-relax, quick stretch, and icing may assist a fair strength muscle and increase ROM. Functional electrical stimulation[2] will also provide an external stimulus to help strengthen the newly innervated muscle. When the muscle has reached a good rating, functional activities should be used to complete the return to normal strength.

SENSORY REEDUCATION. Evaluation of sensibility has been described in some detail earlier in this chapter. This information should be used to prepare a program of sensory re-education following nerve repair.

Sensory reeducation[20,42] was described as early as 1926 but was not popularized until 1974. Dellon has used the 30 cps tuning fork, moving touch, constant touch, and 256 cps tuning fork to evaluate for introduction of the early phase of sensory reeducation. When each submodality has reached the proximal phalanx, exercises of constant or moving-touch may be initiated by stroking or pressing the eraser end of a pencil proximally to distally. The patient first watches as the stimuli is applied, then closes his or her eyes and tries to perceive the stimulus, then may watch again. This process is repeated four times per day for about 5 minutes.

Late phase sensory reeducation may begin when the patient perceives constant touch and moving touch at the fingertip. This may be as early as 6 months postrepair but can be done anytime the criteria have been met, even several years following nerve suture. Late-phase exercises are designed to regain tactile gnosis, and they are graded, starting with large, familiar objects. The patient again watches while manipulating the objects, then shuts his or her eyes, concentrating on the perception of the object, then again open the eyes. Gradations in size, shape, and texture are used, and responses may be timed to help the patient gauge progress. Stimulation of the area through massage with different textures and locating objects buried in a texture box may also be effective for sensory reeducation. Some patients carry a pocketful of loose change, and they manipulate the coins several times a day, trying to identify them without looking.

It must be emphasized that sensory reeducation requires use of the hand to achieve full sensibility and tactile gnosis. Microsurgical techniques have made this more possible from a technical standpoint but cannot replace the need for thorough evaluation and instruction by the therapist.

TENDON TRANSFERS. If, following a minimal period of 1 year after nerve repair, a motor nerve has not reinnervated its muscle, the surgeon may consider tendon transfers to restore a needed motion. The rules of tendon transfer are to evaluate (1) what is absent, (2) what is needed for function, and (3) what is available to transfer.[25] Some muscles, such as the extensor carpi radialis longus and the sublimis to the ring finger, are commonly used for transfers because their motions are easily substituted by the extensor carpi radialis brevis and flexor digitorum profundus to the ring finger, respectively. The surgeon may request assistance in evaluating motor status from the therapist to determine the best motor transfer.

Therapy before tendon transfer is essential if the motor being used is not of normal strength. A muscle will lose a grade of strength when transferred, and a strengthening program of progressive resistive exercises, functional electrical

stimulation, and isolated motion will help ensure success of the transfer.

Following transfer, many patients require instruction to perceive the correct muscle during active use of the transfer. Use of biofeedback, careful instruction, and supervised activity to note any substitution patterns during active use will usually help the patient to use the transfer correctly. Therapy must be initiated before the patient has time to develop incorrect use patterns. Functional electrical stimulation may be used to isolate the muscle and to strengthen it postoperatively.

Tendon injuries

FLEXOR TENDONS. Injuries to tendons may be isolated or may occur in conjunction with other injuries, especially fractures or crushes. Flexor tendons injured in the area between the distal palmar crease and the insertion of the flexor digitorum superficialis are considered to be the most difficult to treat, because the tendons lie in their sheaths in this area beneath the fibrous pulley system, and any scarring will cause adhesions. This area is often referred to as "no-man's-land" or "zone 2."

Primary repair of the flexor tendons within zone 2 is most frequently attempted following a clean laceration. Several methods of postoperative management have been proposed with the common goal to promote gliding of the tendons and to minimize the formation of scar adhesions.

Kleinert[31] was an early advocate of primary repair of flexor tendons using rubber band traction of the injured finger postoperatively. The wrist is positioned in 30° to 45° of flexion, and a rubber band is attached from a fingernail suture to the wrist where it is held in place by a safety pin (Fig. 24-10). This method allows full passive flexion and active extension against the rubber band. The patient is instructed not to attempt active flexion. The MP joints must be held in 70° to 90° of flexion for the PIP joints to move through their full ROM. The splint is removed after 21 days, and the patient begins a program of active and passive flexion and extension.

Duran and Houser[21] suggested the use of controlled passive motion to

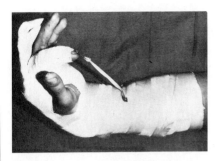

Fig. 24-10. Following flexor tendon repair wrist is placed in 30° of flexion with rubber band from fingernail to wrist, allowing full passive IP joint flexion and active extension. Note that MP joints maintain full flexion in dressing.

achieve optimal results following primary repair, since 3 to 5 mm of tendon excursion is sufficient to prevent adherence of the repaired tendons. On the third postoperative day the patient begins a twice daily exercise regimen of passive flexion and extension of six to eight motions for each tendon. Care is taken to keep the wrist flexed and the MPs in 70° of flexion during passive exercise. Between exercise periods the hand is wrapped in a stockinette. At 4½ weeks the protective dorsal splint is removed and the rubber band traction is attached to a wrist band. Active extension and gentle active flexion are done for 1 week and gradually increased over the next several weeks.

A third postoperative program is complete immobilization for 3½ weeks following tendon repair. Immobilization has not resulted in consistently good results and may lead to a greater incidence of tendon rupture following repair because a tendon gains tensile strength when submitted to gentle tension at the repair site.[54]

When active flexion is begun, it should be directed at the IP joints with the MP joint blocked. This may be accomplished using a blocking splint,[22] a small wooden block known as a Bunnell block (Fig. 24-11), or the opposite hand (Fig. 24-12). The MP joints should be held in extension during blocking so the intrinsic muscles that act on it cannot overcome the power of the repaired flexor tendons. Care should be taken not to hyperextend the PIP joint and overstretch the repaired tendons.

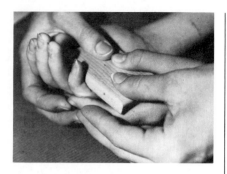

Fig. 24-11. Bunnell block is used to exercise each joint individually, allowing full tendon excursion, following surgical repair.

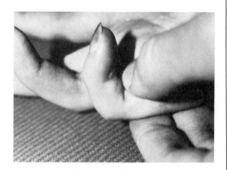

Fig. 24-12. Manual blocking of MP joint during flexion of PIP joint.

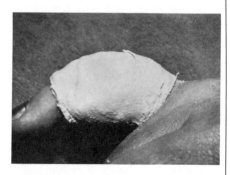

Fig. 24-13. Plaster cylindrical splint is used to apply static stretch of PIP joint contracture. It is not removed by patient and must be replaced frequently by therapist with careful monitoring of skin condition.

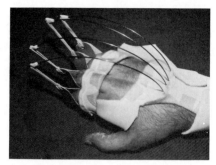

Fig. 24-14. Dynamic outrigger splint using spring steel outriggers with a lumbrical block can be used to assist PIP joint extension, stretch against scar adhesions of extrinsic flexors, or reduce PIP joint contractures. Proper fit and tension of rubber bands must be frequently assessed by therapist.

After 6 weeks passive extension may be started and splinting may be necessary to correct a flexion contracture at the PIP joint. A cylindrical plaster splint may be fabricated to apply constant static pressure on the contracture as described by Bell[7] (Fig. 24-13). Static splinting may be especially effective with a flexion contracture greater than 25°. Gentle dynamic traction may be applied using a commercial splint or one that is fabricated by the therapist (Fig. 24-14).

If a persistent flexion contracture is present after 8 weeks, a splint with greater tension, such as a Joint-Jack, may be applied. Night splinting in extension is often necessary to maintain extension gains made during the day. Dynamic flexion splinting may be necessary if the patient has difficulty regaining passive flexion.

At about 8 weeks the patient begins light resistive exercises and activities. The hand should now be used for light ADL, but the patient should continue to avoid heavy lifting with or excessive resistance to the affected hand. Sports activities should be discouraged. However, activities such as clay work, woodworking, and macrame are excellent.

When evaluating a hand that has sustained a tendon injury, passive versus active limitations of joint motion must be evaluated. Limitations in active motion may indicate joint stiffness, muscle weakness, or scar adhesions. If passive motion is greater than active motion, the therapist should consider that tendons may be caught in the scar tissue. The therapist should be able to determine if a tendon is adhering and causing a flexion contracture or if the tendon is free, but the joint itself is stiff. Treatment should be based on this type of evaluation.

ROM, strength, function, and sensibility testing (if digital nerves were also injured) should be performed frequently with splints and activities geared to progress. Although performance of ADL is generally not a problem, the therapist should ask the patient about any problems he or she may have or anticipate. Disuse and neglect of a finger, especially the index finger, are common and should be prevented.

Gains in flexion and extension may continue to be recorded for 3 to 4 months postoperatively. A finger with limber joints and minimal scarring preoperatively will function better after repair than one that is stiff and scarred and has trophic skin changes.[12] It is important therefore that all joints, skin, and scars be supple and movable before reconstructive surgery is attempted. A "functional" to "excellent" result is obtained if the combined loss of extension is less than 40° in the PIP and distal interphalangeal (DIP) joints of the index and middle fingers and is less than 60° in the ring and little fingers[50] and if the finger can flex to the palm.[12]

If the tendon is damaged as a result of a crush injury or the laceration cannot be cleaned up enough to allow for a primary repair, staged flexor tendon reconstruction may be done. At the first operation a Silastic rod is inserted beneath the pulley system and attached to the distal phalanx. Other reconstructive procedures, such as pulley reconstruction, are performed at the same time. A mesothelial cell–lined pseudosheath is formed about the rod and a fluid similar to synovial fluid is formed in the recovery phase.[32] The second stage is performed about 4 months later when the digit can be moved passively to the palm. A tendon graft is inserted and the Silastic rod removed. The postoperative program is carried out in the same manner as for a primary tendon repair.

Following a two-stage tendon reconstruction or primary repair, a tenolysis may be performed if there is a significant difference between the active and passive motion. Tenolysis is usually not performed for 6 months to 1 year after tendon repair. At the time of tenolysis surgery scar adhesions are removed from the tendon, and gliding of the tendons is assessed. Patients are often asked to move their fingers in the operating room at the time of lysis to determine the extent of scar removal. Active motion is begun within the first 24 hours using bipuvacaine hydrochloride (Marcaine) blocks[52] or transcutaneous electrical nerve stimulation (TENS)[13] to control pain. Tenolysis may significantly improve the final results of surgery.[32]

EXTENSOR TENDONS. Dorsal scar adherence is the most difficult problem following injury to the extensor tendons because of the tendency of the dorsal extensor hood to become adherent to the underlying structures and thus limit its normal excursion during flexion and extension.

Injuries to extensor tendons proximal to the MP joint may be immobilized for 3 weeks. After this the finger may be placed in a removable volar splint that is worn between exercise periods for an additional 2 weeks. Progressive ROM is begun at 3 weeks, and if full flexion is not regained rapidly, dynamic flexion may be started at 6 weeks.

Extensor tendon injuries that occur distal to the MP joint require a longer period of immobilization, usually 6 weeks. A progressive exercise program is then initiated with dynamic splinting during the day and a static night splint to maintain extension.

Dynamic splints may include a PIP-DIP splint first described by Hollis and now available commercially[34] (Fig. 24-15), a web strap made of lamp wick or elastic, a fingernail hook with rubber band traction, a traction glove, or another splint.

If a lysis of scar tissue is required because of persistent scar adhesion, the surgeon may place a thin sheet of Silastic between the tendon and bone at the time of surgery to reduce further scar

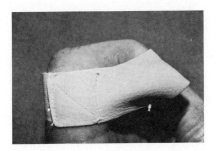

Fig. 24-15. PIP-DIP splint may be used to increase flexion of both PIP and DIP joints. Tension can be adjusted with Velcro closure. Wearing time should be determined by therapist.

adherence. The patient begins exercising within the first 24 hours, and splints are applied as needed. Active exercise is essential, and the patient must be carefully instructed in a home program. The patient is encouraged to use the hand for all activities except those requiring heavy resistance. After 4 to 6 weeks the Silastic sheet is removed and ROM should be maintained.

TOTAL ACTIVE MOTION AND TOTAL PASSIVE MOTION. Total active motion (TAM) and total passive motion (TPM) is a method of recording joint ROM that is used to compare tendon excursion (active) and joint mobility (passive). It is the measure of flexion minus extensor lag of three joints. TAM and TPM have been recommended for use in reporting joint motion by the American Society for Surgery of the Hand.[1]

TAM is computed by adding the sum of the angles formed by the MP, PIP, and DIP joints in flexion minus incomplete active extension at each of the three joints. For example, MP joint flexion is 85° with full extension; PIP is 100° and lacks 15° extension; and DIP is 65° with full extension; therefore

$$TAM = 85 + 100 + 65 - 15 = 235°$$

TAM should be measured while making a fist. It is used for a single digit and should be compared with the same digit of the opposite hand or subsequent measurements of the same digit. It should not be used to compute a percentage of loss or impairment.

TPM is calculated in the same manner but measures only passive motion.

Edema

Edema is a normal consequence of trauma but must be quickly and aggressively treated to prevent permanent stiffness and disability. Within hours of trauma vasodilation and local edema occur with an increase in white blood cells to the damaged area.[37] The inflammatory response to the injury results in a decrease in bacteria.

The patient is instructed at the time of injury to keep the hand elevated, and a compressive dressing is used to reduce early swelling. Pitting edema is present early and can be recognized as a bloated swelling that "pits" when pressed. This may be more pronounced on the dorsal surface where the venous and lymphatic systems provide return of fluid to the heart. Active motion is especially important to produce retrograde venous and lymphatic flow.

If the swelling continues, a serofibrinous exudate invades the area. Fibrin is deposited in the spaces surrounding the joints, tendons, and ligaments, resulting in reduced mobility, flattening of the arches of the hand, tissue atrophy, and further disuse.[37] Normal gliding of the tissues is eliminated and a stiff, often painful hand will be the result. Scar adhesions will form and further limit tissue mobility. If untreated, these losses may become permanent.

Early recognition of persistent edema through volume and circumference measurement is important. It may be necessary to use several of the suggested edema control techniques.

ELEVATION. Early elevation with the hand above the heart is essential. Slings tend to reduce blood flow and should be avoided. Resting the hand on pillows while seated or lying down is effective. Resting the hand on top of the head or using devices that elevate the hand with the elbow in extension have been suggested. Suspension slings may be purchased or fabricated.

ACTIVE ROM. Normal blood flow is dependent on muscle activity. Active motion does not mean wiggling the fingers but rather complete ROM done firmly. Casts and splints must allow mobility of uninjured parts while protecting newly injured structures. The shoulder and elbow should be moved several times a day.

The patient should use the hand for ADL within the limitations of resistance prescribed by the physician. Light ADL that can be accomplished while in the dressing are permitted.

CONTRAST BATHS. Alternating soaks of cold and warm water that is 66° and 96° F (18.9° and 35.6° C) has been recommended as a method preferred over warm water soaks or whirlpool baths. The contrast baths can be done for 20 minutes, alternating the hand between cool water for 30 seconds and warm water for 3 minutes. Start and end with cool water. A sponge can be placed in each tub so that the hand is moved during the soaking period. The tubs should be placed as high as possible to provide elevation of the extremity. The alternating warm and cool water will cause vasodilation and vasoconstriction, resulting in a pumping action on the edema. Combined with elevation and active motion edema may be reduced and pain is often alleviated by this technique.

RETROGRADE MASSAGE. A retrograde massage may be done by the therapist, but it should be taught to the patient so that it can be done frequently through the day. The massage assists in blood and lymph flow. It should be started distally and stroked proximally with the extremity in elevation. Active motion should follow the massage until the muscles are fatigued.

PRESSURE WRAPS. Wrapping with soft string[36] or Coban elastic wrap may be employed to reduce edema (Fig. 24-16). Starting distally, the finger is wrapped snugly with Coban or string. Each involved finger should be wrapped distally to proximally until the wrap is proximal to the edema. The wrap remains in place for 5 minutes and then is removed. Active exercise may be done while the finger is wrapped or immediately following. Measurements should be taken before and after treatment to document an increase in ROM and a decrease in edema. The wrapping may be repeated three times a day.

Light compression may be applied throughout the day with a light Coban wrap, an Isotoner glove, or a Jobst garment. The compression should not be constricting and should be discontinued if ischemia results. Isotoner gloves may be purchased through a retailer. Jobst Institute, Inc. markets a standard glove that comes in several sizes and may be used in the same manner as an Isotoner glove. Jobst garments may be specially fitted and fabricated for the individual (Fig. 24-17).

A variety of pressure wraps, such as the temperfoam edema mitt, are used by hand centers. Tubular gauze, a surgical glove, and Bedford finger stalls provide compression to a specific finger. No one method is superior to the other, but a combination of techniques may be used at different stages of healing and according to patient comfort. The basic treatment of goals of elevation, compression, massage, and above all, active motion, should be followed to achieve early control of edema.

Scar remodeling

A scar is the result of wound healing and is a dynamic rather than static function of wound physiology. Fibroblasts begin to synthesize collagen on the third day following trauma or surgery. Collagen continues to synthesize rapidly for the first 4 week and remains metabolically active for a prolonged period. Scar architecture is altered by an early gliding motion that allows reweaving of the early random fibers into tissue that resembles preinjury tissue. This process is called scar remodeling, and it appears to be augmented by a carefully planned treatment regimen.

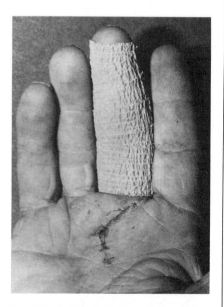

Fig. 24-16. One-inch Coban is wrapped with minimal pressure from distal end to proximal crease of digit. Patient is instructed to be aware of vascular compression or "tingling." Coban may be worn several hours a day to reduce edema. (Available from Medical Products Division/3M, St. Paul, Minn.)

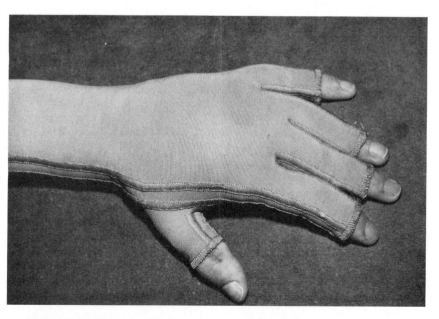

Fig. 24-17. Custom-fit Jobst garment may be used to reduce edema or to reduce and prevent hypertrophic scar formation following burns or trauma. Inserts may be used in conjunction with garment to increase pressure over natural curves, such as dorsum of wrist.

PRESSURE. A hypertrophic scar or a scar that is randomly laid down and thickened is reduced by the application of pressure. Jobst garments are effective in providing pressure. Use of an insert or neoprene fabric, Elastomer (382 Medical Grade Elastomer made by Dow-Corning), or Otoform[63] under the pressure garment will increase the efficacy of the treatment. Pressure should be applied for most of the 24-hour period, and with a hypertrophic burn scar this treatment should continue for a period of 6 months to 1 year following the injury. Other forms of pressure outlined in the section on edema control may also be used.

MASSAGE. Gentle to firm pressure of the scarred area using a thick ointment, such as lanolin, will rapidly soften scar tissue and should be followed immediately with active hand use so that tendons will glide against the softened scar. Vibration to the area with a small, low intensity vibrator will have the same effect. Active exercise using facilitation techniques and against resistance or functional activity should follow vibration.

Thermal heat in the form of paraffin dips, hot packs, or Fluidotherapy immediately followed by stretching while the tissue cools will provide stretch to the scar tissue. Wrapping the scarred or stiff digit into flexion during the application of heat will often increase mobility in the area.

ACTIVE ROM AND ELECTRICAL STIMULATION. Active ROM provides an internal stretch against resistant scar, and its use cannot be overemphasized. If the patient is unable to achieve active motion because of scar adhesions or weakness, use of a battery-operated electrical stimulator may augment the motion. Functional electrical stimulation may be done by the patient for several hours at home and has been shown to increase ROM and tendon excursion.[2]

A high-voltage, pulsating, direct current is used by many physical therapists as a treatment to increase motor activity and may be used for scar remodeling. Ultrasound treatments are often prescribed but may be more effective if done within the first few months following trauma.

Pain syndromes

Pain is the subjective manifestation of trauma transmitted by the sympathetic nervous system, which may interfere with normal functioning. Because pain leads to overprotection of the affected part and disuse of the extremity, it should be treated early.

DESENSITIZATION. Stimulation of the large afferent A nerve fibers will lead to a reduction of pain by decreasing summation in the slowly-adapting, small, unmyelineated C fibers, which carry pain sensation. The A axons can be stimulated mechanically with pressure, rubbing, vibration, TENS, percussion, and active motion. Desensitization techniques are based on the amplification of inhibitory mechanisms.

Yerxa has described a desensitization program that "employs short periods of contact with three sensory modalities: dowel textures, immersion or contact particles, and vibration."[67] This program allows the patient to rank 10 dowel textures and 10 immersion textures on the degree of irritation produced by the stimulus. Treatment begins with a stimulus that is irritating but tolerable. The stimulus is applied for 10 minutes 3 or 4 times a day. The vibration hierarchy is predetermined and is based on cps of vibration, the placement of the vibrator, and the duration of the treatment. Complete instructions for assembling the Downey Hand Center desensitization kit can be found in the literature in the references.[4] The recently developed Downey Hand Center Hand Sensitivity Test can be used to establish a desensitization treatment program and to measure progress in decreasing hypersensitivity.[67]

NEUROMAS. Neuromas are a complication of nerve suture or amputation. A traumatic neuroma is an unorganized mass of nerve fibers that results from accidental or surgical cutting of the nerve. A neuroma in continuity occurs on a nerve that is intact.[55] They may be clinically identified by a specific, sharp pain. Stimulation of a neuroma will usually cause the patient to quickly pull the hand away; many patients report a burning pain that radiates up the forearm. Neuromas are disabling because any stimulation will cause intense pain and the patient avoids the sensitive area.

A generalized desensitization program may not work because the patient never develops a tolerance for stimulation of the neuroma. Injection of cortisone acetate may help break up the neuroma, making desensitization techniques more effective. Surgical excision of the neuroma or burying the nerve endings deeper may be necessary.

REFLEX SYMPATHETIC DYSTROPHY. Reflex sympathetic dystrophy (RSD) is a term used to describe a disabling reaction to pain that appears to be triggered by vasospasm following an injury. The sympathetic nervous system plays a major role in the process.[48] The degree of trauma does not correlate with the severity of the pain and may occur following an injury. Abnormal edema and constrictive dressings may be a factor in initiating the vasospasm. A vasospasm "causes tissue anoxia and edema and therefore more pain, which continues the abnormal cycle."[48] Circulation is decreased, which causes the extremity to become cool and pale. Fibrosis following tissue anoxia and protein-rich exudates results in joint stiffness. The patient may cradle the hand and prefers to keep it wrapped. There may be an exaggerated reaction to touch, especially light touch. Osteoporosis may be apparent on x-ray films by 8 weeks after trauma following active use of the hand. Burning pain, associated with causalgia, is a symptom of RSD. RSD is alleviated by interruption of the sympathetic nerve pathways.

The first goal of treatment is reduction of the pain and hypersensitivity to light touch. This may be accomplished with application of warm (not hot) moist heat, Fluidotherapy, gentle handling of the hand, and TENS. Narcotics may become addictive and should be avoided in favor of physical techniques that inhibit the perception of pain. Pain that cannot be controlled may be treated with the injection of stellate ganglion blocks by the surgeon. Stellate ganglion blocks may be beneficial in treating sympathetic symptoms but are usually a late treatment if other conservative measures fail to help.

As soon as pain is controlled, active motion and functional activities should be begun. Patients may benefit from several treatment sessions per week. Therapy should be coordinated with stellate ganglion blocks to take advantage of the pain-free period. Splints that reduce joint stiffness should be used.

A tendency to develop RSD should be suspected in any patient who seems to complain excessively about pain, appears anxious, and complains of profuse sweating and temperature changes in the hand. Patients will tend to overprotect the hand. Early intervention with a structured therapy program of functional activities, group interaction, and exercises that include the hand and shoulder may prevent the occurrence of a fully developed RSD. This is a problem that is best recognized early and treated aggressively but with empathy.

TRANSCUTANEOUS ELECTRICAL NERVE STIMULATION. TENS is a treatment technique that is thought to stimulate the afferent A nerve fibers in the high-frequency mode and stimulate the release of neural hormones, the enkephalins, in the low-frequency mode. Its efficacy as a treatment for pain control is well developed in medical literature. As with other electrical modalities that may be used by hand therapists, TENS should be correlated with functional use of the hand.

Current literature[28] indicates that TENS should be used for treatment periods not to exceed 60 minutes to achieve pain control. A TENS diary should be used to record level of pain on a scale of 0 to 10 before and after treatment, as well as activities that exacerbate the pain. Use of TENS may be tapered down as the pain-free periods increase to avoid overuse. Treatment can be continued as long as necessary to provide pain control.

Joint stiffness

Joint stiffness has been discussed in other sections of this chapter because it is seen following almost any hand trauma or disease. In the acute phase it may also result from "internal splinting" done unconsciously by the patient to avoid pain. It may be prevented by early mobilization, reduction of edema, active and passive ROM, and appropriate splinting techniques.

Treatment of established joint stiffness is more difficult. Thermal modalities, joint mobilization, ultrasound and electrical stimulation, dynamic splinting, serial casting, and active and passive motion in preparation for functional use should all be included in the treatment regimen.

Inflammatory problems

Tendinitis may be the result of overuse of a muscle group, incorrect positioning for use, or trauma. It may be insidious or related to a specific injury. It is often the result of repetitive motions. Examples of soft tissue inflammatory problems are carpal tunnel syndrome, lateral epicondylitis (tennis elbow), de Quervain's disease, and trigger fingers. Treatment varies by the specific disorder but general guidelines may be followed.[61]

Acute phase treatment is geared toward decreasing the inflammation through "dynamic rest." Splints are used for immobilization but removed three times per day for exercise. Painful activities are avoided. Inflammation is decreased by the application of icing techniques or contrast baths. Antiinflammatory medications may be prescribed, and ultrasound phonophoresis has been beneficial to many patients. High-voltage electrical stimulation may also be used. Vibration is contraindicated, since vibration may contribute to inflammatory problems.

When the inflammation has been controlled, the patient begins the exercise phase of treatment. After warming up the muscles by slow stretching, controlled progressive exercise is begun. Resistance should be given at the end of range when doing progressive resistive exercise. A tennis elbow armband can be worn over the extensor muscle bellies and will limit full excursion of the muscle during active use of the arm. Resistance should be increased slowly and should not cause an increase in pain. Patients are instructed to resume icing and stretching techniques if symptoms exacerbate.

An evaluation of the job site, tools used, and hand position during work activities may be indicated with the patient whose symptoms are related to job demands. Modification of the equipment used and strengthening of the dominant muscle groups and their an-

tagonist muscles may permit continued employment while controlling the inflammatory problem.

Carpal tunnel syndrome is an example of a frequently seen inflammatory problem. Symptoms of this syndrome are caused by pressure on the median nerve as it travels beneath the transverse carpal ligament at the volar surface of the wrist. It may be associated with trauma, edema, retention of fluids as a result of pregnancy, flexor tenosynovitis, repetitive wrist motions, or static loading of the wrist.

Symptoms are night pain that is severe enough to waken the patient; tingling in the thumb and index and long fingers; and, if advanced, wasting of the thenar musculature caused by pressure on the motor branch of the nerve. Early carpal tunnel syndrome may be recognized by a thorough nerve evaluation.

Conservative treatment is usually attempted first and includes splinting the wrist in 20° to 30° extension, contrast baths to reduce edema, wearing Isotoner gloves, and activity analysis. Ultrasound may be used to reduce inflammation, and icing techniques are often beneficial. Specific strengthening exercises should be given when the pain and inflammation have been controlled.

Diagnosis of carpal tunnel syndrome has increased,[35] and it is thought to occur more frequently in industrial settings with highly repetitive technical jobs that require the wrist to be held in dorsiflexion or palmar flexion while manipulating small objects. A direct cause and effect relationship has not been documented but is suspected. Occupational therapists may be asked to visit the job site and make recommendations for adaptation of the workplace to reduce the incidence of this syndrome.

Surgical correction of carpal tunnel syndrome is done by releasing the transverse carpal ligament.

Strengthening activities

Acute care is followed by a gradual return of motion, sensibility, and preparation to return to normal ADL. Strengthening the injured and neglected extremity is usually not accomplished by the patient at home, since he or she is often fearful of further injury and pain. Every hand clinic has its own armamentarium of strengthening exercises and media, and a few suggestions are provided here.

WEIGHT WELL. The weight well[3] was developed at the Downey Community Hospital Hand Center in Downey, California and is available commercially.[34] It is an open box that is secured to the table with a clamp. Dowel rods with a variety of handle shapes are placed through holes in the box and weights are suspended from the rods. The rods are turned against resistance throughout the ROM to encourage full grasp and release of the injured hand, wrist flexion and extension, pinch, and pronation and supination patterns. The weight well can be graded for resistance and repetitions and is an excellent tool for progressive resistive exercise.

THERABAND. Theraband is a 6-inch (15.2 cm) wide rubber sheet that is available by the yard and is color coded by degrees of resistance. It can be cut into any length required and used for resistive exercise for the upper extremity. Use of Theraband is limited only by the therapist's imagination, and it can be adapted to diagonal patterns of motion, wrist exercises, following treatment of tennis elbow, and other uses. The theraband can be combined with dowel rods and other equipment to provide resistance throughout the ROM. It is inexpensive and easy to incorporate into a home treatment program.

HAND STRENGTHENING EQUIPMENT. Hand grips of graded resistance are available from rehabilitation supply companies and sporting goods stores. Big Grips can be purchased in 10-, 15-, 30-, and 60-pound sizes and are recommended because they easily conform to the shape of the hand. They can be used for progressive resistive hand exercises. The Hand Helper is also used, and resistance is varied by the addition of rubber bands. Small, hand-shaped rubber grippers are available and may be used for blocking exercises.

The therapist is cautioned against using overly resistive spring-loaded grippers often sold in sporting good stores. These devices may be beneficial to the seasoned athlete but are usually too resistive for the recently injured.

Therapy putty can be purchased in bulk, and the amount given to the patient is geared to hand size and strength. Putty is also available in grades of resistance. It can be adapted to most finger motions and is easily incorporated into a home program.

Household items, such as spring-type clothes pins and a toy called the Obie Doll, have been used to increase strength of grasp and pinch. Imaginative use of common objects should present a challenge to the hand therapist.

Functional activities

Functional activities are an integral part of rehabilitation of the hand. Functional activities may include crafts, games, dexterity activities, ADL, and work samples. Many of the treatment techniques described to this point are employed to condition the hand for normal use.

Activities should be started as soon as possible at whatever level the patient can perform them with adaptations to compensate for limited ROM and strength. They should be used as an adjunct to other treatments. The occupational therapist must continually assess the patient's functional capacities and initiate changes in the treatment program to incorporate activities as soon as possible in the restorative phase.

Vocational and avocational goals should be established at the time of initial evaluation and taken into account when planning treatment. The needs of a brick mason may be quite different from those of a mother with small children, and the environmental needs of the patient must not be neglected.

Crafts should be graded from light resistance to heavy resistance and from gross dexterity to fine dexterity. Crafts that have been found to work extremely well with hand injuries include macrame, turkish knot weaving, clay, leather, and woodworking.

All of these crafts can be adapted and graded to the patient's capabilities and have been found to have a high level of patient acceptance. When integrated into a program of total hand rehabilitation, they are viewed as another milestone of achievement and not as a diversion to fill up empty hours. For example, the pride of accomplishment for a patient who sustained a Volkmann's contracture caused by ischemia and who completed her first project in nearly 4 years is evidence that crafts belong in hand rehabilitation.

Activities that do not have an end product but provide practice in dexterity and ADL skills also fit into the category of functional activities. Developmental games and activities that require pinch or grasp and release may be graded and timed to increase difficulty. ADL boards that have a variety of opening and closing devices provide practice for use of the hand at home and increase self-confidence. String and finger games are challenging coordination activities that can be done in pairs and are fun to do.

Many times a hobby can be adapted for use in the clinic. Fly-tying is a difficult dexterity activity but one that will be enjoyed by an avid fisherman. Golf clubs and fishing poles can be adapted in the clinic to allow early return to a favorite form of relaxation.

Humor and patient interaction with the therapists and the other patients are factors that are vital but intangible benefits of treatment. Treatment should be planned to promote both.

Physical capacity evaluation

EVALUATION PHASE. The ultimate goal of therapy for an injured worker is to return to full employment. Many weeks or months may have elapsed between the time of the injury and the point at which the physician feels a return to work is appropriate from a medical standpoint. Despite the fact that x-ray examinations may show full healing and restored ROM, many patients do not feel they have the strength, dexterity, or endurance to return to their former job. Pain may continue to be a limiting factor, especially with heavy activities. Light duty or part-time positions may not be available, and the physician, therapist, industrial insurance carrier, and most of all, the patient are frustrated by the lack of an objective method of evaluating an individual's physical capacity for work. Occupational therapists with training in evaluation, kinesiology, and adaptation of environmental factors coupled with a functional approach to the patient may play a key role in physical capacity evaluation.

A renewed interest in evaluation of prevocational factors has brought the profession of occupational therapy full circle. As one of the cornerstones of the profession in its early years, "prevocational evaluation" has been neglected in many centers during the last two decades. Occupational therapists in the 1980s have rediscovered a need that the profession is in a unique position to provide. The term "prevocational evaluation" ambiguously implied that occupational therapists were involved in assessing the vocational needs of patients they treated. However, the development of the term "physical capacity evaluation" (PCE) more clearly describes the process of measuring an individual's ability to perform the physical demands of work. The results of this evaluation allow the therapist, worker, physician, and vocational counselor to establish a specific attainable employment goal using reliable data. This relieves the physician of the responsibility of returning the patient to work without objective information about the patient's ability to do a job. It also allows the patient to test his or her abilities for him or herself and may result in increased self-confidence about returning to work.

Many techniques for performing a physical capacity evaluation have been proposed.[6,26,40,41] Some basic steps may be followed regardless of the specific technique adopted. The patient should be evaluated for grip and pinch strength, sensation, and ROM. Edema and pain must also be assessed and reassessed during the course of the evaluation. The GULHEMP (general physique, upper extremity, lower extremity, hearing, eye sight, mentality, and personality) Work Capacity Evaluation Worksheet[40] may be used as a general method of determining functional abilities. The GULHEMP Physical Demands Analysis Worksheet[40] may be used to evaluate the job.

Job analysis may also be provided by a rehabilitation counselor and through information provided by the patient. The therapist should consult the *Dictionary of Occupational Titles* (DOT)[58] to obtain information about the worker traits required for the expected job.

This dictionary contains 12,900 job descriptions and 20,000 job titles. If sufficient information about the job is not available through these methods, an on-site job analysis by the therapist may be necessary.

Once the physical demand characteristics of work have been documented, it is possible to evaluate the patient's ability to perform them.

Baxter[6] has described a physical capacity evaluation adapted for upper extremity injuries[7] based on the physical capacity requirements found in the *Dictionary of Occupational Titles*. Following evaluation the therapist may recommend a work therapy program. Work therapy can include simulated job tasks to increase job performance.

Matheson[40,41] has written several manuals and articles that describe Work Capacity Evaluation (WCE). This test includes evaluation of the patient's feasibility for employment (worker characteristics, such as safety and dependability), employability, work tolerances (such as strength, endurance, and the effect of pain on work performance), the physical demand characteristics of the job, and the worker's ability to "dependably sustain performance in response to broadly defined work demands".[40]

Tests with well-accepted reliability, such as the Purdue Pegboard Test,[56] the Crawford Small Parts Dexterity Test,[16] the Minnesota Rate of Manipulation,[57] and the Jebsen Hand Dexterity Test,[57] may be administered as a screening process. These tests will give the therapist valuable information through observation whether or not the normal tables are used or the test is adapted to an individual worker.

Many evaluation tests and job simulation devices are available and should be reviewed before establishing a physical capacity evaluation program. To choose appropriate work samples, the job market in a specific area should be determined. This can be done by consulting with vocational schools, rehabilitation counselors, and employment agencies in the area.

Work samples, available through Jewish Employment and Vocational Service,[60] Singer,[53] Valpar,[59] and Work Evaluation Systems Technology (W.E.S.T.)[65] may be used to test specific skills. Job samples may also be developed by the therapist using information on jobs in the local area. Discarded electronic assembly boards, a lawn mower motor, automobile engine, or other items from the local hardware store may provide valuable information about the worker's ability.

Curtis and Engalitcheff[18] have developed an electromechanical work simulator that may be used for both work evaluation and upper extremity rehabilitation. It is available from Baltimore Therapeutic Equipment (BTE) in Baltimore. Use of the BTE-work simulator is enjoying increasing popularity in hand rehabilitation centers and allows the therapist to evaluate a wide range of job tasks with a minimal amount of space. It is equipped with interchangeable handles that simulate a variety of tools and job situations, and it can be adjusted for various work heights and ROM. Resistance and monitoring the time over which a task is performed can be electronically programmed.

A combination of "normed" tests, job samples, job simulation, and work capacity evaluation devices may provide the therapist with the best information about a worker's physical capacity. For more information about vocational evaluation and rehabilitation, the therapist should write to the Materials Development Center at the University of Wisconsin-Stout in Menomie, Wis.[39]

WORK HARDENING. Work hardening is the progressive use of simulated work samples to increase endurance, strength, productivity, and often feasibility. Work hardening may be performed for a period of weeks, and the progressive ongoing nature of the work usually results in improvements in physical capacity. It is an important contribution to vocational rehabilitation.

Since PCE is also performed over time, it may be difficult to identify the difference between PCE and work hardening. A PCE is generally done when the patient has stopped improving with traditional therapy methods and may have been released from acute medical care. The patient may be unable to return to his or her former employment or it is questionable if the patient would be able to do his or her former work. A PCE may be initiated by a physician, rehabilitation counselor, insurance adjustor, or lawyer.

Work hardening may be initiated earlier in the rehabilitation process, perhaps by the treating physician or therapist who recognizes that an individual may have difficulty returning to his or her former employment. It is performed before the end of medical care and may serve as a final "checkout" before discontinuing treatment.

It is important to stress that PCE and work hardening are adjuncts to the vocational rehabilitation process. Occupational therapists are trained to observe behavior and have the skills necessary to translate that observation into useful data. PCE and work hardening should not be a process that is in competition with the work of rehabilitation or vocational counselors but provides badly needed information about a worker's physical functioning and may serve as a program to foster reentry into the job market.

Sample Treatment Plan

Case Study

Bob is a 32-year-old right-handed male who works for the state in a mid-level management position. His right hand was crushed in a log splitter when his hand got lodged between the end of the log and the metal plate while operating the machine. The injury resulted in avulsion of the adductor pollicis and an intercarpal dislocation between the third and fourth metacarpals between the capitate, the hamate, the lunate, and the triquetrum. He also sustained a chip fracture of the right radius with no displacement. The patient was referred to occupational therapy to (1) increase passive and active ROM of the right hand, (2) increase ROM of the right wrist, (3) increase strength of the right hand, (4) decrease edema in the right hand, and (5) assess functional capabilities.

TREATMENT PLAN

A. **Statistical data.**
   1. Name: Bob
      Age: 32
      Diagnosis: Intercarpal dislocation of right wrist and compounded soft tissue injury in first right web space
      Disability: Intermetacarpal dislocation resulting in flattened transverse metacarpal arch and malalignment of ring and little fingers relative to radial side of the hand; ulnar symptomatology because of compression of ulnar nerve and canal of Guyon; avulsion of the adductor pollicis resulting in inability to bring thumb into the second metacarpal; pain, edema, and limitation of motion resulting in inability to use right hand at time of referral

   2. Treatment aims as stated in referral:
      Increase passive and active ROM of the right hand
      Increase ROM of the right wrist
      Increase strength of the right hand
      Decrease edema in the right hand
      Assess functional capabilities

B. **Other services.**
   At the time of injury the patient underwent soft tissue debridement and repair. His hand was placed in a large bulky dressing, and he was discharged from the hospital to await delayed repair of the remainder of his injuries because of the unusual degree of swelling immediately following his injury. Ten days after injury the edema had subsided significantly, and he returned to the hospital for reduction and internal fixation of the intercarpal dislocation with decompression of the ulnar nerve at the wrist and delayed primary closure of the first web space.

C. **OT evaluation.**
   The patient was referred to therapy 3 weeks after injury and 10 days after surgical repair. The bulky dressing was removed on the date of referral, and the occupational therapist was instructed to construct a stabilizing wrist splint to protect and repair the fractured radius. Pins remained in place at that time
      Hand volume measurement: Test
      Active and passive ROM of fingers and thumb and active ROM of the wrist: Test
      Sensory modalities: Test
      ADL: Observe
      Jebsen Test of Hand Function: Test

D. **Results of evaluation.**
   1. Evaluation data.
      a. Physical resources.
         (1) The right-hand volume was 607 ml on the right and 492 ml on the left.
         (2) Active and passive ROM are reported in Table 24-1;[1] Note the loss of ROM in all fingers with an increasing loss moving radially to ulnarly. Because of pain and swelling in the hand, individual measurements of each joint were not made passively, but passive measurements were made of the MP joints because they were the most markedly stiff. Passive measurements to the distal palmar crease were recorded to allow comparison at subsequent visits. Passive ROM was noted to be greater than active ROM, and it was thought that the flexor tendons were adhering in scar tissue at the wrist level. The patient also noted that he could not "feel the muscles pulling." The thumb web space was noted to be contracted, which would be expected with the type of injury that he sustained. There was scar tissue in this area and a volar scar that was similar to the incision made for a carpal tunnel release. Early contractures of the PIP joints of the ring and small finger were noted and were thought to be caused again by adhesions of the flexor tendons in the palmar scar.

Continued.

Sample Treatment Plan—cont'd

(3) Sensation was normal in all fingers but the small finger, which had limited light touch sensation and two-point discrimination greater than 10 mm. This was to be expected with compression of the ulnar nerve at the time of the injury and was expected to resolve over the next 6 to 8 weeks.

(4) The patient had been unable to perform any ADL with the right hand since the time of his injury as a result of immobilization of the hand. At the time of his initial therapy visit the patient's hand was placed in a protective wrist splint, and he was instructed to begin doing light ADL within his pain tolerance.

(5) The Jebsen Hand Function test was deferred initially. It was administered toward the end of treatment.

b. Psychosocial functions. The patient and his wife were seen for the initial evaluation and the early treatment phase. The patient's family was extremely supportive in carrying out his treatment program with him at home and in making sure that the patient was not overly dependent for his self-care needs. The patient and his family seemed to understand the importance of increasing his activity level as early as possible. The patient also had an extremely positive attitude toward his rehabilitation and followed through with the treatment that was outlined in his home program. He was

---

Table 24-1
Bob's ROM

Affected hand	Active ROM						Passive ROM			
	Extension flexion				Tips from palm (cm)		Extension flexion		Tips to palm (cm)	
	Initial		Final		Initial	Final	Initial	Final	Initial	Final
Thumb										
MP	0/40	40	0/50	50						
IP	0/55	55	0/90	90						
TAM		95		140						
Index finger										
MP	0/30	30	0/86	86			0/40			
PIP	0/75	75	0/105	105			★			
DIP	0/15	15	0/55	55			★			
TAM		120		246	5.0	0				3.0
Long finger										
MP	0/30	30	0/92	92			0/42			
PIP	0/58	58	0/105	105			★	Full ROM		
DIP	0/30	30	0/77	77			★			
TAM		118		274	7.0	0				3.0
Ring finger										
MP	0/15	15	0/85	85			0/30			
PIP	10/62	52	0/100	100			★			Full ROM
DIP	0/20	20	0/75	75			★			
TAM		87		260	7.0	0				3.5
Small finger										
MP	0/15	15	0/85	85			0/20			
PIP	20/42	22	0/95	95			★			
DIP	0/37	37	0/85	85			★			
TAM		74		265	6.0	0				3.0
Wrist										
Extension	−2		47							
Flexion	27		67							
Pronation	50		85							
Supination	46		90							

Final strength measurements
Grip: 68 lb, 70 lb, 75 lb (right)
     84 lb, 80 lb, 86 lb (left)
Palmar pinch: 4 lb, 2 lb, 2 lb (right)
     11 lb, 12 lb, 11 lb (left)
Lateral pinch: 2 lb, 1½ lb, 2 lb (right)
     15 lb, 17 lb, 16 lb (left)

Initial hand volume
607 ml right
492 ml left

Final hand volume
515 ml right
510 ml right

★Not tested

Sample Treatment Plan—cont'd

highly motivated to return to all his former activities and stated that the supportive atmosphere he experienced in his therapy program enabled him to perform many activities he would have been afraid to attempt on his own, and he credited the therapy he received with helping him restore normal hand function long before he would have been able to do it independently.

c. Prevocational potential. Because Bob held a management position, he was able to return to work within 1 week after his injury with his hand in a bulky dressing. He was unable to write at that time but did learn to use his left hand for necessary writing. His staff assisted him in any activities that he was unable to perform, such as lifting or bilateral activities.

2. Problem identification.
   a. Presence of edema
   b. Loss of passive motion of all finger joints, especially MP joints
   c. Decreased active motion, especially in ring and little fingers
   d. Contraction of thumb web space because of scar tissue
   e. Scar adhesions of flexor tendons and palmar scar
   f. Loss of ROM of wrist
   g. Loss of abduction of fingers
   h. Loss of adduction of thumb
   i. Decreased grip and pinch strength of right hand
   j. Decreased functional use of right hand
   k. Demineralization of small bones of hand following immobilization

E Problem	F Specific OT objectives	G Methods used to meet objectives	H Gradation of treatment
a	Decrease edema	Elevation except during use (may use Gardner Arm Elevator or Zimmer Orthopedic Products) Contrast baths Flex and extend to maximal position in each bath (use sponge) Active motion through full range Isotoner glove worn constantly Retrograde massage Jobst Compression Unit used in conjunction with physical therapy For edema localized to one finger, nonrestrictive wrapping with Coban or lamp wick for several hours will reduce edema String wrapping or tight compression wrap for 5 minutes several times a day Custom-fit Jobst glove	Methods are graded, for example, if elevation and active motion do not reduce edema, attempt contrast baths, then pressure wrapping; all may not be needed
b	Increase joint mobility	Thermal modalities combined with stretching for tissue softening Gentle, passive ROM to all affected joints; immediately follow with active ROM or isolated active motion of affected joints and muscles Dynamic flexion splint with wrist protected to increase joint flexion especially of the MP joints Individual joints splinted with variety of commercial and custom-made splints, including lamp wick or web straps, flexion outriggers, fingernail hooks attached to rubber bands that pull the fingers into passive flexion, and commercially available splints Use of a continuous passive motion device*	Increase time of activity Increase dynamic forces and length of time worn

*Under development by Sutter Biomedical, Inc. 3940 Ruttin Road, San Diego, Calif. 92123

Continued.

Sample Treatment Plan—cont'd

E Problem	F Specific OT objectives	G Methods used to meet objectives	H Gradation of treatment
c	Increase excursion and strength of affected tendons and muscles	Full controlled active range of each finger; observe hand to note any neglect or substitution of any muscles; allow active muscle pull to stretch soft tissue and remodel scar	Increase repetition
		Allow isolated pull through of any tendons that appear to be stuck in scar tissue, that is, block MP and PIP flexion in ring finger and use full DIP (flexor digitorum profundus) motion to pull free of scar	Hold-relax or contract-relax techniques to facilitate motion desired
		Light resistance in grasping with Play doh, temper-foam blocks, or foam sponges; working against resistance helps the patient to feel active motion through pressure and proprioceptive feedback and increases muscle strength	Active assist of exercise compensates for lack of strength while allowing full tendon excursion; as more resistance is allowed to the wrist, begin exercise with graduated dowel rods, "Exertwist" device, or weight well to allow full grasp with flexion and extension of the wrist
		Work with Bunnell block to isolate PIP and DIP joints	Increase repetition
		Place ruler perpendicularly to palm; have patient attempt to get closer to palm each exercise session; patient measures and records best measurement; for extension, patient can attempt to touch a ruler projecting distally from dorsal surface of hand	Always attempt to decrease measurement
		Exercise with graduated dowel rods or rolling pin for grasp and release and pronation-supination, twisting with other hand	Decrease dowel size
		Weight well exercise to increase finger grasp, pinch, extension, and flexion of the wrist and pronation and supination of forearm	Progressive resistive exercise with weights applied to the weight well
		Functional activities that promote pinch, grasp, release, and wrist motions	Increase difficulty of activity or strength required; gross to fine prehension (grasp and pinch)
		Functional electrical stimulation (FES) to be used in home program	Start with 20 minutes of FES twice a day; progress gradually to 2 hours three times a day
		Use activities that promote needed motions, always positioning properly	Increase amplitude and length of on-time duty cycle
d	Stretch web space; soften scar	Splint that applies constant, uniform pressure to scar and places thumb in maximal abduction (wear 23 hours a day)	As web stretches, new splints are made always to maximal abduction (serial splinting)
		Massage scar with lanolin or tacky ointment if patient is allergic to wool (lanolin is made from sheep fat and will cause a rash in patients with wool allergy); gentle massage with low-intensity vibrator combined with stretching	
		Active motion four times a day for 15 minutes each	

Sample Treatment Plan—cont'd

E Problem	F Specific OT objectives	G Methods used to meet objectives	H Gradation of treatment
e	Pull tendons free of adhesions	Friction massage with no ointment, using Dycem pad between thumb and skin, for friction may also be used to break up scar adhesions (combine with active motion) Dynamic extension splinting Isolated DIP (flexor digitorum profundus) and PIP (flexor digitorum superficialis) active motion Pressure wrapping with Coban or compressive cloth using insert of Silastic, neoprene sheet, or Otoform mold placed beneath the compressive wrap Low-intensity vibration over scar combined with stretching techniques Friction massage to scar combined with stretching of active motion FES	Increase force of traction; work against resistance Frequently replace mold as scar decreases
f	Increase mobility of soft tissue	Dynamic flexion splint (a variety might be necessary as gains are made) Active motion to maintain gains made by splinting	Increase traction; increase time spent in splint
g	Increase MP mobility (MP tightness limits abduction); increase strength of interossei and long extensors (assists in abduction)	Passive stretching of joints into abduction with fingers extended Lay hand flat and draw around fingers (have patient try to go beyond pattern) Isolate abduction combined with MP joint extension with palm supported and IP joints in a relaxed, slightly flexed position, concentrating joint motion at MP joint Resist abduction and adduction with therapy putty, splint, or other device; resist MP extension using opposite hand Contract-relax or hold-relax exercises to facilitate abduction and adduction	Increase force (limit by pain and swelling); make new patterns Increase repetitions Increase resistance
h	Increase grip strength	Exercises and activities that provide resistance, allow full active ROM, and hand use as needed in vocation (may also use avocation interests if appropriate); as strength increases, evaluate need for forearm and shoulder strength; evaluate and treat the entire extremity (see also methods for problem c)	Increase resistance; increase time of activity; increase variety of activities

Continued.

Sample Treatment Plan—cont'd

Discharge summary

Bob was seen for a period of 5 months in therapy, daily for the first 6 weeks, then with decreasing frequency. Subjectively he felt that his hand was normal, except for activities that required fine pinch and dexterity. He did not feel limited as a result of his hand injury, and had learned to adapt to any difficulty in pinching.

Final volume, strength, and ROM measurements may be found in Table 24-1. Sensibility was normal. There appeared to be atrophy in his median nerve innervated thumb muscles, and it was thought by the surgeon that a portion of the motor branch of the median nerve was damaged by the avulsion of the adductor pollicis at the time of injury. This accounted for his lack of dexterity and strength in the thumb. Because of the nature of the injury, it was not thought that this could be repaired surgically.

Test results on the Jebsen Test of Hand Function were within the norms listed for the test. The Purdue Pegboard Test was also administered, and scores indicated poor fine dexterity. The right hand tested alone fell in the lower 25th percentile. This points out the need to use more than one test in evaluating hand function, since somewhat different functions are evaluated by each test.

Bob was encouraged to continue to exercise at home, use his hand as much and as normally as possible, and return if any further problems developed.

REVIEW QUESTIONS

1. Discuss three approaches to postoperative care of flexor tendon injuries. What would be the significance of each method in initiating occupational therapy?
2. To what does "joint dysfunction" refer? What are its causes?
3. List three treatment techniques that might be used in treatment of a pain syndrome.
4. Explain the three classifications of nerve injury.
5. Define the area referred to as "no-man's land." What is the significance of injury to this area?
6. What techniques would be employed to evaluate the physical demand characteristics of work?
7. List three methods of applying pressure to a hypertrophic scar.
8. What functional activities could be used for restoration of hand function following laceration and repair of the extrinsic finger flexors?
9. How does physical capacity evaluation differ from prevocational evaluation and vocational assessment?
10. List five components of hand evaluation.
11. List three objectives of splinting as they relate to injury of the radial, median, and ulnar nerves.
12. Describe the test for intrinsic and extrinsic tightness.
13. What are the characteristics of a reflex sympathetic dystrophy? What are the treatment goals?
14. List four commonly used dexterity tests.
15. Define "work hardening." How can work hardening be incorporated into occupational therapy?
16. How is the presence of edema evaluated? List three methods used to reduce edema.
17. Explain the difference between acute phase and restorative phase treatment for an inflammatory problem. How would these factors influence occupational therapy?
18. What is the goal of sensory reeducation following nerve repair? List the hierarchy of nerve function return as it relates to sensory reeducation.

REFERENCES

1. American Society for Surgery of the Hand: The hand examination and diagnosis, ed. 2, New York, 1983, Churchill Livingstone, Inc.
2. Baker, L.L.: Functional electrical stimulation: a practical clinical guide, ed. 2, Downey, Calif., 1981, Rancho Los Amigos Hospital.
3. Barber, L.M.: Occupational therapy for the treatment of reflex sympathetic dystrophy and posttraumatic hypersensitivity of the injured hand. In Fredericks, S., and Brody, G. S., editors: Symposium on the neurologic aspects of plastic surgery, St. Louis, 1978, The C.V. Mosby Co.
4. Barber, L.M.: Desensitization of the traumatized hand. In Hunter, J.M., et al.: editors: Rehabilitation of the hand, ed. 2, St. Louis, 1984, The C.V. Mosby Co.
5. Basmajian, J.V.: Practical functional anatomy. In Hunter, J.M., et al., editors: Rehabilitation of the hand, ed. 2, St. Louis, 1984, The C.V. Mosby Co.
6. Baxter, P.L.: Physical capacity evaluation and work therapy. In Hunter, J.M., et al.: editors: Rehabilitation of the hand, ed. 1, St. Louis, 1978, The C.V. Mosby Co.
7. Bell, J.A.: Plaster cylinder casting for contractures of the interphalangeal joints. In Hunter, J.M., et al., editors: Rehabilitation of the hand, ed. 2, St. Louis, 1984, The C.V. Mosby Co.
8. Bell, J.A.: Sensibility testing: state of the art. In Hunter, J.M., et al., editors: Rehabilitation of the hand, ed. 2, St. Louis, 1984, The C.V. Mosby Co.
9. Bennett, G.K.: Hand-tool dexterity test, New York, 1981, Harcourt Brace Jovanovich, Inc.
10. Bora, F.W.: Nerve response to injury and repair. In Hunter, J.M., et al., editors: Rehabilitation of the hand, ed. 1, St. Louis, 1978, The C.V. Mosby Co.
11. Boyes, J.H.: Bunnell's surgery of the hand, ed. 5, Philadelphia, 1970, J.B. Lippincott Co.
12. Boyes, J.H., and Stark, H.H.: Flexor-tendon grafts in the fingers and thumb, J. Bone Joint Surg. 53A:1332, 1971.
13. Cannon, N.M., et al.: Control of immediate postoperative pain following tenolysis and capsulectomies of the hand with TENS, J. Hand Surg. 8:625, 1983.
14. Carroll, D.: A quantitative test of upper extremity function, J. Chronic Dis. 18:479, 1965.
15. Chusid, J.G.: Correlative neuroanatomy and functional neurology, ed. 15, Los Altos, Calif., 1973, Lange Medical Publications.
16. Crawford, J.E., and Crawford, D.M.: Crawford small parts dexterity test manual, New York, 1981, Harcourt Brace Jovanovich, Inc.
17. Creelman, G.: Volumeters unlimited, Idyllwild, Calif.
18. Curtis, R.M., and Engalitcheff, J.: A work simulator for rehabilitating the upper extremity: preliminary report, J. Hand Surg. 6:499, 1981.
19. Dellon, A.L.: Evaluation of sensibility and reeducation of sensation in the hand, Baltimore, 1981, Williams & Wilkins.
20. Dellon, A.L., Curtis, R.M., and Edgerton, M.T.: Reeducation of sensation in the hand after nerve

injury and repair, Plast. Reconstr. Surg. **53**:297, 1974.

21. Duran, R.J., and Houser, R.G.: Controlled passive motion following flexor tendon repair. In A.A.O.S.: Symposium on tendon surgery in the hand, St. Louis, 1975, The C.V. Mosby Co.

22. English, C.B., Rehm, R.A., and Petzoldt, R.L.: Blocking splints to assist finger exercise, Am. J. Occup. Ther. **36**:259, 1983.

23. Ferraro, M.C., et al.: Closed functional bracing of metacarpal fractures, Orth. Rev. **12**:49, 1983.

24. Fess, E.E., and Moran, C.A.: Clinical assessment recommendations, Indianapolis, 1981, American Society of Hand Therapists.

25. Fields, J.: Anatomy and kinesiology of the upper extremity, lecture presented at San Jose State University, San Jose, Calif., 1976.

26. Harrand, G.: The Harrand guide for developing physical capacity evaluations, Menomonie, Wis., 1982, Stout Vocational Rehabilitation Institute.

27. Jebsen, R.H., et al.: An objective and standardized test of hand function, Arch. Phys. Med. Rehabil. **50**:311, 1969.

28. Kasch, M.C., and Hester, L.A.: Low-frequency TENS and the release of endorphins, J. Hand Surg. **8**:626, 1983.

29. Kellor, M., et al.: Technical manual of hand strength and dexterity test, Minneapolis, 1971, Sister Kenney Rehabilitation Institute.

30. Kelsey, J.L., et al.: Upper extremity disorders: a survey of their frequency and cost in the United States, St. Louis, 1980, The C.V. Mosby Co.

31. Kleinert, H.E., Kutz, J.E., and Cohen, M.J.: Primary repair of zone 2 flexor tendon lacerations. In A.A.O.S.: Symposium on tendon surgery in the hand, St. Louis, 1975, The C.V. Mosby Co.

32. LaSalle, W.B., and Strickland, J.W.: An evaluation of the two-stage flexor tendon reconstruction technique, J. Hand Surg. **8**:263, 1983.

33. Lister, G.L.: The hand: diagnosis and indications, London, 1977, Churchill Livingstone.

34. LMB Hand Rehabilitation Products, Inc., San Luis Obispo, Calif.

35. Lublin, J.S.: Unions and firms focus on hand disorder that can be caused by repetitive tasks, The Wall Street Journal, January 14, 1983.

36. Mackin, E.J., and Maiorano, L.: Postoperative therapy following staged flexor tendon reconstruction. In Hunter, J.M., et al., editors: Rehabilitation of the hand, ed. 1, St. Louis, 1978, The C.V. Mosby Co.

37. Madden, J.W.: Wound healing: the biological basis of hand surgery. In Hunter, J.M., et al., editors: Rehabilitation of the hand, ed. 2, St. Louis, 1984, The C.V. Mosby Co.

38. Mark One Health Care Products, Inc., Philadelphia, Pa.

39. Materials Development Center, Stout Vocational Rehabilitation Institute, University of Wisconsin-Stout, Menomonie, Wis.

40. Matheson, L.N.: Work capacity evaluation: a training manual for occupational therapists, Trabuco Canyon, Calif., 1982, Rehabilitation Institute of Southern California.

41. Matheson, L.N., and Ogden, L.D.: Work tolerance screening, Trabuco Canyon, Calif., 1983, Rehabilitation Institute of Southern California.

42. Maynard, C.J.: Sensory reeducation following peripheral nerve injury. In Hunter, J.M., et al., editors: Rehabilitation of the hand, ed. 1, St. Louis, 1978, The C.V. Mosby Co.

43. Melvin, J.L.: Rheumatic disease occupational therapy and rehabilitation, ed. 2, Philadelphia, 1982, F.A. Davis Co.

44. Mennell, J.M.: Joint pain, Boston, 1964, Little, Brown & Co.

45. Mennell, J.M., and Zohn, D.A. Musculoskeletal pain diagnosis and physical treatment, Boston, 1976, Little, Brown & Co.

46. Moberg, E.: Objective methods of determining functional value of sensibility in the hand, J. Bone Joint Surg. **40A**:454, 1958.

47. Moberg, E.: Aspects of the sensation in reconstructive surgery of the upper extremity, J. Bone Joint Surg. **46A**:817, 1964.

48. Omer, G.: Management of pain syndromes in the upper extremity. In Hunter, J.M., et al., editors: Rehabilitation of the hand, ed. 2, St. Louis, 1984, The C.V. Mosby Co.

49. O'Rain, S.: New and simple test of nerve function in the hand, Br. Med. J. **3**:615, 1973.

50. Peacock, E.E., Madden, J.W., and Trier, W.C.: Postoperative recovery of flexor tendon function, Am. J. Surg. **122**:686, 1971.

51. Sarmiento, A., and Latta, L.L.: Closed functional treatment of fractures, New York, 1981, Springer-Verlag, Inc.

52. Schneider, L.H., and Hunter, J.M.: Flexor tenolysis. In A.A.O.S.: Symposium on tendon surgery in the hand, St. Louis, 1975, The C.V. Mosby Co.

53. Singer Education Division, Career Systems, Rochester, N.Y.

54. Strickland, J.W., and Glogovac, S.V.: Digital function following flexor tendon repair in zone II: a comparison of immobilization and controlled passive motion techniques, J. Hand Surg. **5**:537, 1980.

55. Thomas, C.L., editor: Taber's cyclopedic medical dictionary, ed. 14, Philadelphia, 1981, F.A. Davis Co.

56. Tiffin, J.: Purdue pegboard examiner manual, Chicago, 1968, Science Research Associates, Inc.

57. Trombly, C.A., editor: Occupational therapy for physical dysfunction, ed. 2, Baltimore, 1983, Williams & Wilkins.

58. U.S. Department of Labor, Employment, and Training Administration: Dictionary of occupational titles, ed. 4, Washington, D.C., 1977, U.S. Government Printing Office.

59. Valpar Corporation, Tucson, Ariz.

60. Vocational Research Institute, Jewish Employment and Vocational Service (JEVS), Philadelphia, Pa.

61. Walker, S.W.: Treatment of soft tissue inflammatory problems of the forearm and hand (mimeographed), San Jose, Calif., 1983.

62. Waylett, J., and Seibly, D.: A study to determine the average deviation accuracy of a commercially available volumeter, J. Hand Surg. **6**:300, 1981.

63. WFR Corp., Ramsey, N.J.

64. Wilson, R.E., and Carter, M.S.: Management of hand fractures. In Hunter, J.M., et al., editors: Rehabilitation of the hand, ed. 2, St. Louis, 1984, The C.V. Mosby Co.

65. Work Evaluation Systems Technology (W.E.S.T.), Huntington Beach, Calif.

66. Wynn Parry, C.B.: Rehabilitation of the hand, ed. 4, London, 1981, Butterworth & Co.

67. Yerxa, E.J., et al.: Development of a hand sensitivity test for the hypersensitive hand, Am. J. Occup. Ther. **37**:176, 1983.

CHAPTER 25

Cardiac dysfunction

DENISE FODERARO

In 1980 over 1 million American deaths were attributed to cardiovascular disease. According to the National Center for Health Statistics that is more deaths than were recorded as a result of cancer, accidents, pneumonia, and influenza combined.[6]

This powerful message from the American Heart Association has inspired many preventive and public awareness programs. The medical community attempts to control risk factors and strives to develop better technological advances in critical care monitoring and medical or surgical intervention. The results of these efforts are enabling Americans with cardiovascular diseases to survive with little residual disability.

Societal trends combined with these advances in cardiovascular technology have affected cardiac mortality in a manner similar to trends noted with accident victims in the 1960s. As society became more safety conscious with new laws concerning national speed limits and seat belts and roadside and emergency techniuqes became more advanced, more persons were surviving once fatal spinal cord and head injuries. This created a genesis of specialty rehabilitation centers to care for their specialized needs. Similarly, trends toward better cardiac emergency care, surgical advances making transplants possible and bypass surgery almost routine and extensive clinical research commending early mobilization programs[61] have inspired the genesis of specialty cardiac rehabilitation programs.

There is one striking difference. Whereas accident victims need not fear recurrence of injury, patients with cardiac disease must attend to the continuing process of arteriosclerosis, which in many cases caused their injury. Increased research in this area suggests that participation in cardiac rehabilitation exercise programs halts and at times reverses the arteriosclerotic disease process.[44]

Judy Padé, O.T.R., and Barbara Baum Zoltan, M.S., O.T.R., are gratefully acknowledged for their support and assistance.

Arteriosclerosis does not only affect the coronary circulation but often is manifest in the cerebral and peripheral circulation as well. It is not uncommon that a 65-year-old victim of a stroke also has a significant cardiac disease or that following a coronary episode a patient cannot engage in an aggressive conditioning program because of extensive peripheral vascular disease. These are the types of patients in general rehabilitation clinics who require special program modifications to accommodate their cardiovascular conditions and complications.

All occupational therapists working in the field of physical dysfunction must have a working knowledge of the cardiovascular system to provide safe, effective rehabilitation programs to all patients.

This chapter provides a basic review of cardiovascular anatomy, physiology, and pathophysiology. Its purpose is (1) to enable the therapist to obtain the necessary medical information through chart review and patient interview and (2) to identify and understand the appropriate precautions when treating both the less serious or "uncomplicated" cardiac problems and the more involved or "complicated" cardiac conditions. With this background knowledge the therapist can plan an appropriate activity progression guided by accurate and continuous vital sign monitoring. In this way the patient may attain a maximal yet safe level of independent function.

THE CARDIOVASCULAR SYSTEM
Normal cardiovascular function[8,28,31,50]

Although many anatomy and physiology courses in occupational therapy curricula adequately review cardiac anatomy, coronary circulation, the conduction system, and the basics of muscle physiology, little time is devoted to integrating these systems in an attempt to understand "the cardiac cycle."[15,21,28] This intricate interplay of events within the heart is responsible for coordinating the direction and volume of blood flow.

By this process the heart (1) systematically delivers oxygen to vital organs and tissues of the body, (2) removes carbon dioxide and other metabolic by-products, and (3) regulates body core temperature to maintain effective hemostasis for continued and optimal occurrence of the cellular events responsible for the heart's function as an efficient pump.

ANATOMY AND CIRCULATION. The right side of the heart (right atrium and right ventricle) collects blood (venous return) and delivers it to the lungs where it can be reoxygenated, whereas the left side of the heart (left atrium and left ventricle) collects blood from the lungs and delivers it to the systemic circulation. Four heart valves assist in the paced passage and direction of blood flow within the heart (Fig. 25-1). The opening and closing of the valves depends on volume and pressure changes within the heart and on the papillary muscles, which are connected to the inner myocardium and innervated by the conduction system. Although the heart muscle is always filled with blood, it receives its blood supply from the coronary circulation (Fig. 25-2).

The left main coronary artery and the right coronary artery are the major arteries that supply the outer layer of the heart muscle called the epicardium. These arteries divide further and extend into the myocardial wall called the endocardium. The small structure of these arteries predisposes them to arteriosclerotic disease, often referred to as coronary artery disease or CAD.

Cardiologists universally refer to these coronary arteries by abbreviations, such as LAD or left anterior descending coronary artery. The name of the artery describes the portion of the heart it supplies. CAD, which causes a blockage in the LAD vessel, interferes with blood supply to the left anterior aspect of the heart or the left ventricle. Since the left ventricle is responsible for pumping blood into the systemic circulation and to the brain, the consequences of LAD disease are often serious.

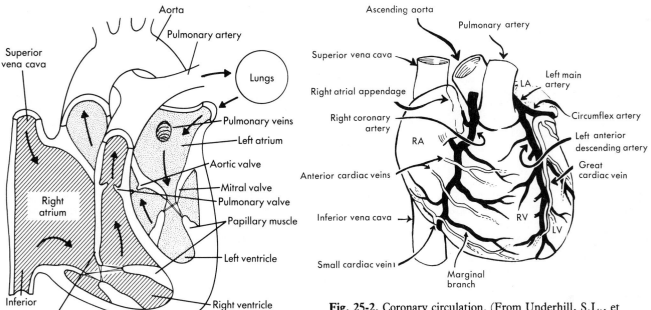

Fig. 25-1. Anatomy of the heart. (From Andreoli, K.G., et al.: Comprehensive cardiac care: a text for nurses, physicians, and other health practitioners, St. Louis, 1983, The C.V. Mosby Co.)

Fig. 25-2. Coronary circulation. (From Underhill, S.L., et al., editors: Cardiac nursing, Philadelphia, 1982, J.B. Lippincott Co.)

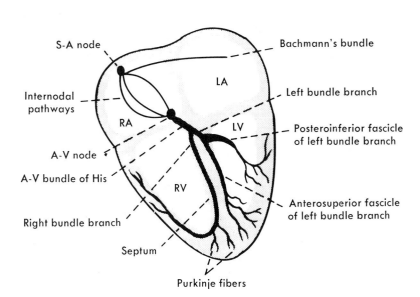

Fig. 25-3. Cardiac conduction. (From Andreoli, K.G., et al.: Comprehensive cardiac care: a text for nurses, physicians, and other health practitioners, St. Louis, 1983, The C.V. Mosby Co.)

INNERVATION. Heart muscle, like skeletal muscle, requires nervous innervation to contract. A specialized nervous conduction network (Fig. 25-3) is responsible for systematically depolarizing the muscle and eliciting myocardial contraction. This timed and coordinated sequence of depolarization and contraction is initiated by the sinoatrial (SA) node or pacemaker of the heart. From the SA node the impulse makes its way to the ventricles through the atrioventricular (AV) node, bundle branches, and Purkinje fibers.

Because depolarization is the result of electrical cellular changes, this process can be studied and recorded graphically by the electrocardiogram (ECG, EKG).[23] Surface electrodes are placed on the limbs and chest to monitor the sequence, timing, and magnitude of the impulse as it travels through the conduction system (Fig. 25-4). Each graphic segment (P, QRS, and T waves) corresponds to the wave of depolarization as it travels through the various chambers of the heart. For instance, the P wave represents electrical

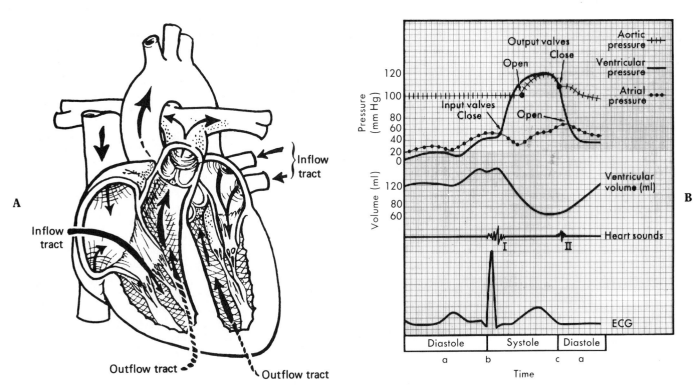

Fig. 25-4. Electrocardiography. (Adapted from Andreoli, K.G., et al.: Comprehensive cardiac care: a text for nurses, physicians, and other health practitioners, St Louis, 1983, The C.V. Mosby Co.)

stimulation arising from and creating depolarization in the atria. The QRS complex corresponds to the wave of depolarization as it travels through the bundle of His to the ventricles. The timing of depolarization can be studied by counting the blocks on ECG paper. If the PR interval or QRS complex is widened or longer than normal, a conduction abnormality or "block" in the system can be suspected.

The SA node adjusts its rate to meet the demands of the body and working muscle. It is sensitive to vagal and sympathetic nervous input.[8] This explains why heart rate increases during anxiety or in response to circulating catecholamines, such as epinepherine and norepinepherine, as produced with exercise. This mechanism also explains why heart rate decreases with deep breathing, meditation, or other relaxation techniques.

THE CARDIAC CYCLE.[15,21,28] The cardiac cycle is the timed interplay of events occurring within the heart to systematically maintain and adjust cardiac output. Understanding this normal cardiac physiology and a synthesis of

cardiac anatomy, hemodynamics, and conduction is the basis for understanding cardiac pathophysiology and associated symptoms in patients with cardiac disease. It is only through this understanding that a therapist can safely evaluate and formulate a progressive treatment plan.

The cardiac cycle occurs in two phases, input (diastole) and output (systole) (Fig. 25-5, *A*). The following discussion is a review of the cardiac cycle.

Input (diastole). The time interval from *a* to *b* in Fig. 25-5, *B*, represents the phase of ventricular filling. This is referred to as diastole or resting phase, since it requires no active contraction from the ventricle. Some texts subdivide this phase into periods of quick and slow filling. More simply, during diastole the input valves (mitral and tricuspid) are open, and the output valves (aortic and pulmonary) are closed. This allows blood from the systemic pulmonary and coronary circulation to passively fill the ventricles. As ventricular volume increases, the pressure within the ventricles increases (Fig. 25-5, *B*).

Fig. 25-5. A, Input and output. **B,** The cardiac cycle. (Adapted from Underhill, S.L., et al., editors: Cardiac nursing, Philadelphia, 1982, J.B. Lippincott Co.)

At this time the SA node spontaneously initiates a wave of depolarization (P wave) that stimulates the atrial muscles to contract and "kick" their contents into the ventricle. This creates a greater ventricular volume and pressure. Once the ventricular pressure exceeds the atrial pressure, the input valves close, and the first heart sound is heard.

The wave of depolarization (QRS wave) then stimulates the ventricles to contract. The ventricles begin their contraction isometrically because both the input and output valves are closed. This contraction generates an even greater ventricular pressure. Once this ventricular pressure exceeds the pressure across the output valves, the valves open, allowing blood flow into the systemic and pulmonary circulation. The numerical value assigned to the pressure required to open the output valves is the diastolic pressure or lower number of a blood pressure reading. High diastolic pressure (greater than 90 mm Hg) makes this isometric contraction phase longer, taxes the heart muscle, and requires medical attention.

Output (systole). Once the aortic and pulmonary valves are open, the ventricles continue to contract isotonically (Fig. 25-5, *B, b* to *c*). The maximal peak pressure generated by the ventricles to eject blood is called the systolic blood pressure and is the upper number of the blood pressure reading. Once the ventricles empty their contents, their volume and corresponding pressures decrease. When ventricular pressure falls below the pressure in the output vessels (aorta and pulmonary artery), the output valves close and create the second heart sound. The total amount of blood ejected during one contraction is called stroke volume. The amount of blood ejected per minute is called cardiac output. The reader is referred to the references for a more detailed understanding of the factors influencing the cardiac cycle and ultimate cardiac output; some of these factors are concepts of preload and afterload, Starling's law, length tension velocity relationships of cardiac muscles, and valve and rhythm dysfunction.

Pathophysiology

ISCHEMIC HEART DISEASE. The coronary circulation supplies oxygen to the myocardium so that it may continue myocardial metabolism to meet the demands of working muscle. An imbalance of oxygen supply and demand created by arteriosclerotic narrowing of the coronary arteries results in myocardial injury or myocardial infarction (death of tissue).

The immediate consequences of ischemia include an excess accumulation in the myocardium of metabolic byproducts, such as potassium, hydrogen ions, lactate production, and lysosomal enzymes.[56] The presence of these metabolites adversely affects further metabolism and may result in a decreased myocardial contractility, which can then decrease stroke volume.[32] Since the ST and T waves on the ECG correspond to the status of the myocardium following ventricular contraction or "systole," ischemia often manifests as a change in these ECG segments.[50] An ST segment depression indicates ischemia whereas an elevation indicates myocardial injury (Fig. 25-6).[50]

In addition, these circulating byproducts predispose the myocardium to an increased occurrence of "ectopic beats" or irregular heart beats arising from irritable portions of the heart muscle. Depending on the origin and frequency of these ectopic beats, overall cardiac output may decrease further and life-threatening cardiac rhythms may develop.

$$\text{Cardiac output} = \text{Stroke volume} \times \text{Heart rate}^{50}$$

$$CO = SV \times HR$$

Once stroke volume is decreased as a result of altered myocardial contractility, the heart attempts to maintain cardiac output by increasing heart rate.

Faster heart rates increase the myocardial oxygen demand and further predispose the heart to ischemia. Furthermore, if heart rates are greater than 110 beats per minute, the diastolic filling phase of the cardiac cycle is reduced, which further impinges on cardiac output.[35]

Ischemia clinically manifests as "angina pectoris," literally interpreted as chest pain. However, since the afferent neural network in cardiac muscle is very different from skeletal muscle, this "pain" is often vague; is experienced as a pressure sensation; and is interpreted by the brain by association with more common sensations, such as arm, neck, back, and/or jaw discomfort.[56]

Myocardial ischemia significant enough to cause angina usually results in temporary ventricular failure, particularly left ventricular failure.[43] If the left ventricle is not able to handle preload or afterload, the system will back up, causing pulmonary venous congestion with associated shortness of breath. This congestive heart failure[43] (CHF) is indicative of ventricular failure and can manifest by shortness of breath, angina with associated ECG changes, a drop in blood pressure reflecting inability to handle preload or afterload, fatigue, and/or peripheral edema. Once cardiac output is significantly diminished, the kidneys perceive a hypovolemic state, and they in turn retain water. This creates an even greater preload on an already failing heart. If uncontrolled, CHF can result in death.

Myocardial infarction (MI) occurs when severe ischemia lasts longer than 20 to 30 minutes. The extent and secondary complications of MI depend on the site of infarct, degree of atherosclerosis, influence of collateral circulation, and oxygen requirements of the myocardium.[56]

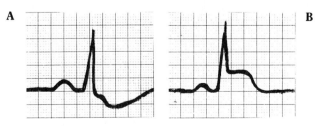

Fig. 25-6. Changes in ST segments. **A,** ST segment depression. **B,** ST segment elevation.

MIs can be either "transmural," in which the whole thickness of the myocardium is involved, or "nontransmural," in which a lesion is usually confined to the subendocardial layer of the myocardium. This subendocardial layer is particularly susceptible to ischemia, and patients with this diagnosis require close medial surveillance during rehabilitation to prevent its progression to a full thickness infarct.[56] MIs are described by their location and size. An anterolateral MI affects both the anterior and lateral walls. Other types include septal, inferior, posterior, or any combination of these.

Nausea and vomiting are often associated with an acute MI. Other symptoms depend on the severity of MI (site and size) and the development of complications (CHF, arrhythmias, or cardiogenic shock). Those patients who develop complications are placed in a high-risk category, need close medical surveillance, and require slower progression in rehabilitation.

VALVULAR DISEASE.[55,58] With age or in response to recurrent bacterial endocarditis the valve leaflets may become fibrous and prevent the valves from closing. A backward flow or "regurgitation" occurs, creating a valve "insufficiency." Clinically, this regurgitation can be heard as a murmur. In mitral insufficiency this backward flow creates an excessive blood volume that dilates the left atria and ventricle. This causes a congestion in the pulmonary circulation with resultant shortness of breath. This stretched atrium also becomes susceptible to erratic heart rates, such as atrial fibrillation. Such heart rates interfere with ventricular filling and complete emptying. Blood tends to stagnate, and emboli are common complications. Valvular disease with resultant emboli is a common cause of cerebral vascular accident (CVA).

Aortic insufficiency and regurgitation similarly dilate and hypertrophy the left ventricle. This volume overload may result in CHF. Furthermore, hypertrophied muscles require an increased myocardial oxygen consumption. If the coronary circulation is unable to supply the oxygen, ischemia results. Aortic stenosis, if severe, will affect cardiac output. Symptoms caused by a decreased cardiac output include arrhythmias as a result of decreased coronary circulation perfusion, cerebral insufficiency or confusion, syncope, or "blacking out" when exerting effort, and dizziness related to a drop in blood pressure. Aortic stenosis warrants close medical management. Depending on severity, exercise may be contraindicated, and patients may require surgery, since these patients are at high risk for sudden death.

CARDIOMYOPATHY.[50,57] Cardiomyopathy simply means disease of the heart muscle. Although coronary arteries and valves may be intact, the cellular mechanics (actin and myosin) responsible for muscle contraction have been altered. This is usually the result of toxic substances, like alcohol, in the blood stream, which accounts for the high incidence of cardiomyopathy among chronic alcoholics. Other systemic diseases, such as muscular dystrophy, may also affect heart function in this manner.[42] The symptoms produced by myopathic states of the myocardium are related to a decreased ability to achieve muscle contraction, as previously discussed. Severe cases of cardiomyopathy, which cannot be controlled medically, produce a severely limited individual who is a prime candidate for occupational therapy intervention with energy conservation and equipment, such as an electric wheelchair. These patients, if lucky, may go onto receive heart transplants.

RISK FACTORS. The Framingham study[21] has correlated the presence of several risk factors to the accelerated progression of the arteriosclerotic process. The American Heart Association[3] divides them into: (1) controllable risk factors: hypertension, smoking, obesity, sedentary or stressful life-style, diabetes, and other metabolic conditions (gout, hyperthyroidism, and lipidemia) that can be controlled through medication, diet, and life-style modification; and (2) uncontrollable factors: age, male sex, and heredity.

The Framingham study, a landmark study, inspired much research in an effort to understand the physiological and metabolic mechanisms responsible for arteriosclerosis. Medical science is now beginning to understand which factors control the development of arteriosclerosis. Much emphasis has been on prevention through exercise and diet. Consequently, much research has been performed on the cardiovascular benefits of aerobic conditioning at a target heart rate for a sustained 30- to 45-minute period.[9,22,26] Research shows that such conditioning alters glucose and lipid metabolism and affects intrinsic cardiac and skeletal muscle mechanisms of oxygen transport and use, thus making the entire cardiovascular system a more efficient one. This efficiency explains why resting heart rate goes down after a 6-week period of retraining.

Heart disease however is not solely the effect of arteriosclerosis. There are medical conditions and disabilities that have associated and secondary cardiac involvement. Some of these are as follows[42,55]:

Alcoholism
Anemia
Ankylosing spondylitis
Arteriosclerosis
Cerebralvascular disease
Diabetes
Friedreich's ataxia
Gout
Hypertension
Marfan's syndrome
Obesity
Peripheral vascular disease
Progressive muscular dystrophy
Progressive systemic sclerosis
  (scleroderma)
Rheumatoid arthritis
Systemic lupus erythematosus

Patients in general rehabilitation clinics may require program modification and close surveillance of vital signs because of these secondary diagnoses.

PATIENT MANAGEMENT
Medical and surgical management

The cardiologist's immediate concern is to preserve viable myocardium by controlling complications that may jeopardize healing and overall cardiac function. This is accomplished by a necessary period of bed rest during which hemodynamics are stabilized by medications that control arrhythmias, afterload, and preload and augment muscular contractility.

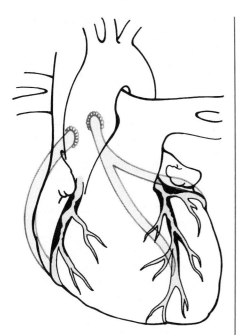

Fig. 25-7. Coronary artery bypass. (From Heart facts, 1983. © Reproduced with permission. American Heart Association.)

Once the patient is stabilized at rest, medical surveillance continues through the cardiac program to assure medical stability during activity. Both patients with complicated conditions who have difficulty achieving stability and patients with uncomplicated conditions who are progressing toward discharge are studied further to examine the precipitous cause of the event. If patients demonstrate significant CAD and are appropriate surgical candidates, coronary bypass surgery is performed. In this procedure a vein from another location (usually a leg) is placed in the heart to reroute blood around the occluded area and perfuse the myocardium (Fig. 25-7).

Other surgeries include valve replacement, aneurysm repairs, pacemaker inserts, and complete transplants. New techniques, like the percutaneous transluminal arterioplasty, float a balloon-tipped catheter to the point of occlusion. The balloon is inflated and the occlusion is compressed against the arterial wall.[61] This technique avoids costly open-heart surgery, and its long-term effectiveness is currently being examined.

Psychosocial aspects

As with any physical disability, patients who experience an MI progress through various stages of psychosocial reaction and adjustment. Anxiety produced by discomfort and imminent fear of death is often overwhelming. While the emergency health care team rapidly attempts to meet the physiological demands of the patient in an effort to avert life-threatening conditions, the patient's psychological needs are often of secondary concern.[13]

Anxiety places an increased physiological demand on the heart muscle at a time when it needs rest. It is most often noted during the first 48 hours of a patient's admission and at times of changing environments, such as transfers to step down units and at discharge. Sedation may be used to alleviate anxiety; however, excessive sedation may produce medical problems and interfere with integrating the realities of the event, which is a necessary step toward successful rehabilitation.[13]

Anxiety is best alleviated through supportive and educational communication.[27] Once a patient verbalizes his or her feelings and learns of the nature of the condition and ways to control it, anxiety usually diminishes.

Denial is a mechanism used when an individual cannot cope with the surrounding events. Denial is common in coronary disease because of the vague characteristics of symptoms and the hidden nature of the disability. At times denial is considered a healthy response,[51] and health professionals must be careful not to strip the patient of this coping mechanism by forcing the patient to face reality too quickly.[13]

Depression is most commonly seen from the third to sixth day after MI.[13] A patient's fears and feelings of inadequacy may be based on a misconception that may be reinforced from equally fearful and often noninformed family members.[11]

Although initial efforts are made to alleviate stress, patients must eventually be educated to handle it, not circumvent it.[13] Relaxation programs,[1] assisted therapeutic introspection and examination of coping patterns, changes in life expectations and beliefs, and self-help groups[41] are methods to effectively deal with stress. "It is only when the patient has confronted stress successfully that he can resume a fully functioning way of life."[13]

The entire health team has the responsibility to prepare the cardiac patient to deal with a new life. The medical and psychological training of occupational therapists enables them to be an integral part of the rehabilitation team.

CARDIAC REHABILITATION

Early mobilization of patients after coronary incidence is now standard cardiological practice. This current philosophy of treatment considerably differs from management of the patient with cardiac disease in the 1950s and 1960s. At that time strict bed rest was prescribed for 6 to 8 weeks, since pathological studies quoted "6 weeks" as required for the transformation of necrotic myocardium to form scar tissue.[60] Physicians did not want to interfere with this delicate healing process, and recommendations for bed rest often continued 3 to 4 months after discharge. Stair climbing was often restricted for a 1-year period.

The 1960s marked the advent of coronary care units with better monitoring techniques for the patient with acute coronary distress. At this time Wenger implemented her hallmark 14-step, early mobilization, activity program at Grady Memorial Hospital.[14] The implementation of such programs across the country demonstrated that progressive activity under supervised conditions prevented the effects of bed rest, shortened hospital stays, facilitated earlier return to work, and reduced the anxiety and depression that often led to the "cardiac cripple" mind set.[60]

Following a "coronary event," current medical management of patients includes an acute recovery phase (1 to 3 days) to stabilize cardiac hemodynamic conditions. This is followed by a subacute recovery phase called phase 1 of cardiac rehabilitation during which a course of progressive, low-energy expenditure hospital activity is prescribed.[51] Such a program decreases the ill effects of bed rest and increases a patient's functional capacity in anticipation of a safe, early hospital discharge.[60]

Following the subacute recovery phase, patients usually undergo a predischarge graded exercise test (GXT), as appropriate, to better assess prognosis and to quantify their maximal functional capacity. By administering a symptom-limited GXT, a safe target heart rate (THR) is identified and can be used as a guideline during home, vocational, and exercise activity programs. Patients continue this cardiac-conditioning exercise program in phase 2, the outpatient phase of their convalescence. After a six-week program, the true benefits of cardiovascular conditioning occur.[22] The majority of patient education, risk factor modification, and lifestyle changes takes place during this phase of rehabilitation.[52]

Individuals continue to advance to greater exercise intensities in phase 3 and 4 programs. They further develop their own knowledge and self-monitoring techniques so that medical surveillance only needs to occur on an intermittent basis.

Optimally, as the rehabilitative process of recovery is completed, phase 1 through phases 3 and 4, the once anxious and functionally limited patient becomes an educated individual who continues risk factor modification and exercise as a way of life. The patient consequently attains maximal functional capacity and can resume an active role in society.

Program objectives[51]

PHASE 1—INPATIENT REHABILITATION

1. To decrease the effects of prolonged bed rest; such as thromboembolism, atelectasis, orthostatic hypotension, hypovolemia, muscle atrophy, osteoporosis, and negative nitrogen and protein balance
2. To increase maximal functional capacity by providing a monitored, low-level activity program that includes exercise and activities of daily living (ADL)
3. To identify medical problems during increased activity and to monitor the effectiveness of various therapeutic regimes
4. To decrease patient anxiety and depression related to coronary heart disease, hospitalization, and eventual return to work and leisure roles

5. To provide an educational program so that patients may understand their medical condition and begin to learn effective life-style and risk factor modification
6. To provide diet education to the patient and family so that they may incorporate diet modifications into the patient's life
7. To minimize the need for home care services through early mobilization, early assessment of equipment needs, and coordinated discharge planning and family training, as indicated
8. To establish an appropriate exercise prescription and activity guidelines by performing a predischarge GXT
9. To identify the method for continued patient follow-up with referral, as appropriate, to phase 2, outpatient rehabilitation program

PHASE 2—OUTPATIENT REHABILITATION

1. To increase physical work capacity through a cardiovascular conditioning program by which the patient ultimately progresses to a diversified exercise program for 20 to 30 minutes at THR
2. To achieve patient compliance and independence in self-monitoring and home program performance so that exercise becomes a part of daily life
3. To support and encourage diet and risk factor modification as a permanent life-style change
4. To continue to decrease patient anxiety and depression by restoring confidence with increased activity, providing educational support groups for both patients and families, and promoting the development of constructive coping mechanisms used to deal with temporary or permanent disability
5. To promote an early, safe return to work and leisure skills by providing simulated task evaluations, specific guidelines for job modification, and retraining, as appropriate
6. To increase functional capacity of the severely limited patient (such as class III or IV in the boxed material on p. 345) to maximal capacity by offering comprehensive patient and family training in work efficiency and energy conservation techniques with the use of durable medical equipment, as appropriate

PHASE 3—COMMUNITY-BASED OUTPATIENT REHABILITATION.

1. To promote the transition from a medically supervised program to a community-based group or independent program with medical follow-up and exercise prescriptions, updated on an intermittent basis

• • •

[In summary,] cardiac rehabilitation is the process concerned with the full development of each cardiac patient's physical, mental, social and vocational potential. It is designed to restore the patient to an optimally productive, active and satisfying life as soon as possible after the recognition of heart disease.[14]

Team approach

Achieving such program objectives is a colossal endeavor and is not the sole responsibility of a single health profession.[18] In small community hospitals the cardiac rehabilitation team includes a physician and a nurse. In larger and more formalized rehabilitation programs other health professionals may be involved, including dietitians, exercise physiologists, occupational therapists, pharmacists, physical educators, physical therapists, psychologists, respiratory therapists, social workers, and vocational counselors.

The degree of the health professionals' involvement is largely dependent on (1) their availability, (2) their role as defined within the rehabilitation facility, (3) their specialty skills and experience in treating patients with cardiac disease, and (4) the financial resources available for the delivery of professional services.

Comoss et al.[18] used a schematic representation (Fig. 25-8) to describe the roles of varied health professionals in cardiac rehabilitation.

Whichever health professionals are involved, the most important members of the cardiac team are the patient and family.

Patient population

Following is a list of patients most often referred to medically supervised and "monitored" rehabilitation programs[51]:
I. Patient population for cardiac rehabilitation
   A. Myocardial infarction
   B. Angina pectoris

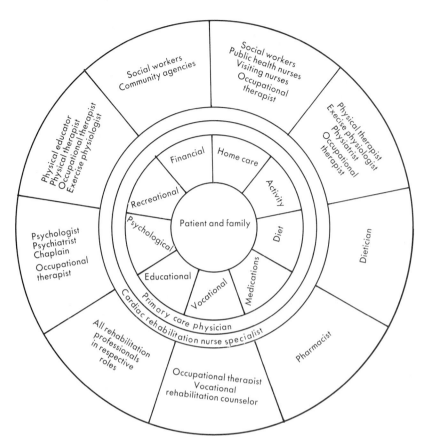

Fig. 25-8. The cardiac team. (Adapted from Comoss, P., Burke, E., and Swails, S.: Cardiac rehabilitation: a comprehensive nursing approach, Philadelphia, 1979, J.B. Lippincott Co.)

various cardiac conditions are urged to consult these references. *All* patients with the diagnoses just mentioned may not need occupational therapy intervention. Cost-effectiveness is of prime importance in today's health care environment. Therapists must be able to support their proposed rehabilitation programs and goals with sound physiological principles as documented in the literature discussing cardiac rehabilitation.

Program guidelines

Although graded activity is beneficial in minimizing the ill effects of bed rest and maximizing functional capacity, there are several conditions for which exercise is absolutely contraindicated[29,31]:

1. Acute illness—includes evolving MI; unstable angina; primary active pericarditis; respiratory, gastrointestinal, febrile illness with fever greater than 100° F (37.78° C); and thrombophlebitis and/or recent systemic or pulmonary embolism
2. Active, chronic, systemic disease (uncontrolled)—includes thyroid, renal, hepatic, gout, and rheumatic diseases
3. Anatomical abnormalities—includes dissecting aneurysm; uncompensated valvular heart disease, such as severe aortic stenosis; and gross cardiomegaly
4. Functional abnormalities—includes uncontrolled atrial or ventricular arrhythmias, second- or third-degree heart block, resting diastolic blood pressure of 120 mm Hg, resting systolic blood pressure of 200 mm Hg, orthostatic systolic blood pressure drop of 20 mm Hg or more, and uncompensated heart failure

Patients must be medically stable before initiating or continuing with any progressive activity program. Special considerations, however, do exist when a patient may be "relatively" stable on an optimal medical regime. These specific conditions require a modified rehabilitation program with close medical supervision[27,30]:

1. Resting diastolic blood pressure over 100 mm Hg or resting systolic blood pressure over 180 mm Hg
2. Hypotension
3. Sinus tachycardia greater than 120 beats per minute at rest

C. Cardiac surgery
D. Controlled congestive heart failure
E. Cardiomyopathy
F. Patients at high risk for potential heart disease
II. Patient population for general rehabilitation
   A. The 65-year-old paraplegic, amputee, and/or CVA patient with significant CAD and/or previous MI
   B. The 70-year-old patient with a fractured hip and a history of CHF and chronic atrial fibrillation
   C. The patient with muscular dystrophy or alcoholism and documented cardiac involvement
   D. The patient with a head injury resulting from suspected arrhythmia

E. General rehabilitation patients at high risk for coronary incidence

A monitored, graded activity progression is prescribed for all these patients: however, each condition varies, and activity progressions and modalities must reflect this. Too often therapists use a "cookbook," protocol approach. Although general guidelines apply to each of them, specific precautions and rates of progression will vary according to the patient's current condition, prognosis, and individualized rehabilitation goals.

The American Heart Association's Committee on Exercise has published guidelines for exercising individuals with various forms of heart disease.[30,31] Therapists wishing to increase their understanding of the physiological rationale for rehabilitation of patients with

4. Fixed rate pacemaker
5. Cardiomyopathy
6. Intermittent claudication
7. Any neuromuscular, musculoskeletal, or arthritic disorders that could prevent activity

THE ROLE OF OCCUPATIONAL THERAPY

During phase 1 of a cardiac rehabilitation program, the occupational therapist is primarily responsible for encouraging the patient's self-care activity to achieve a safe yet maximal level of independent self-care. The process involves a great deal of patient and family education and instruction in energy conservation techniques to avoid stress to a healing myocardium. This monitored progression of activity gives the therapist an opportunity to evaluate the effectiveness of the patient's current medical regime and assists the patient in avoiding the ill effects of prolonged bed rest.

Similarly, in phases 2 and 3 of cardiac rehabilitation the therapist advances the patient to high-energy activities geared to return the patient to more demanding vocational and leisure pursuits. Some patients never advance to high-energy activities because of serious cardiac disease. For these patients the occupational therapist's role is essential. These patients with end-stage cardiac disease may be on a maximal medical regime and still have difficulty performing simple self-care activities. The occupational therapist's role is to evaluate the patient's technique of ADL performance and to identify ways to decrease the energy used so the patient can begin to perform the task without symptoms. Adaptive aids and durable medical equipment are often necessary for these patients. Patient success with these simple activities, although using a varied technique, is of tremendous psychological benefit. Continued participation in their ADL gives them a sense of control and independence and thus alleviates the patient's and family member's fear and anxiety.

As with any other patient evaluation and treatment there are special evaluation tools and techniques pertinent to patients with cardiac disease.

Evaluation procedures

CHART REVIEW. A thorough chart review is advised before meeting the patient. This implies that the therapist must be familiar with cardiac terminology and have a basic understanding of how a patient's clinical course and various test results affect program progression and ultimate treatment goals.

Work sheets are helpful in expediting the chart review process and in organizing the information gained from the medical chart and patient interview. A sample work sheet as used at Santa Clara Valley Medical Center is included in Fig. 25-9. Other work sheets are included in Ogden's *Initial Evaluation of the Cardiac Patient*.[47] Readers wishing to further their understanding of cardiac terminology and medical information gathered from the charts are referred to *Cardiac Nursing* by Underhill et al.[58] and *Comprehensive Cardiac Care* by Andreoli et al.[8]

PATIENT INTERVIEW. Once a thorough chart review is complete, the therapist conducts an initial patient interview to obtain an activity history. Social, financial, architectural, psychological, cognitive-behavioral, vocational and/or avocational factors, and how they influence treatment planning may be further assessed.

The initial patient interview is frequently the patient's first contact with a member of the cardiac rehabilitation team. Moreover, it often occurs at a significantly anxious time; for instance, the patient has just been informed of the MI, has just been weaned from the ventilator, or has just been moved to the transitional care unit. Although the patient may not engage in significant physical activity during the first visit, the cardiac rehabilitation process begins. The patient-therapist relationship is established. The therapist must outline the terms and expectations of the relationship so that the patient (1) understands the importance of gradually increasing activity: (2) understands the logistics of the cardiac rehabilitation program (scheduling and activity modalities); (3) begins to feel comfortable asking personal or repeated questions; and (4) begins to take an active part in the rehabilitation process, including reporting signs and symptoms experienced during activity.

Various questionnaires may be used as an adjunct to direct patient interview to fully assess a patient's activity history. Most questionnaires have had significant shortcomings. The value of only a few of them has been documented empirically; a few have been validated against objective outcome measures.[20] The ADAPT© Quality-of-Life-Scale,[20] on the other hand, is a brief questionnaire designed to assess a patient's activity level. Among pulmonary patients it significantly correlates with maximal oxygen consumption achieved during exercise testing. ADAPT© can potentially be used with varied patient populations, including those with cardiac diagnoses.

Cost efficiency issues have inspired methods of completing such questionnaires in group and/or on an independent basis. Some questions may provoke an anxiety response. Although this may not be of major concern with patients in phase 2 or phase 3 of the recovery process, administering such a questionnaire to patients in phase 1 without immediate or simultaneous discussion may produce undue anxiety.

MONITORED SELF-CARE EVALUATIONS. Self-care evaluations are most often performed in phase 1 of cardiac rehabilitation. They consist of ADL that require very little energy expenditure and may include hygiene, grooming, simple bathing, dressing, and functional mobility tasks.[48]

The therapist chooses a combination of low-level self-care activities to both mobilize and evaluate the patient. The therapist's choice of activities is based on the patient's past medical and functional history, the patient's current clinical status and course of recovery, the therapist's knowledge of cardiovascular dynamics, and the metabolic energy costs of increasing activity.

For instance, a 74-year-old man is admitted to the hospital with a recurrent bout of CHF. Before his admission to the hospital his activities were limited to independent bathing and dressing (on a chair) and walking for two blocks before experiencing shortness of breath. His hospital course is complicated with kidney problems and CHF that has been difficult to control. He has been resting in bed for 1 week, and his current hospital activity includes

```
                    Santa Clara Valley Medical Center
                         Occupational Therapy

            CHART REVIEW WORKSHEET FOR PATIENTS WITH CARDIAC DISEASE

   I.  THIS ADMISSION                    II.  ACTIVITY HISTORY

       Admission date and symptoms:           Social situation (assistance available,
                                               stairs, bathrooms):


       Workup (vital signs, laboratory, ECG,  Vocational and avocational activities:
       and examinations):



       DIAGNOSIS:

       Complications:                          Preadmission activities and limitations:

                                                 General mobility:

       Current hospital activity:               Ambulation:

       PRECAUTIONS:                             Self-care:

                                                Homemaking:

                                                Community:

       Significant medical history:            Patient goals (appropriate?):


       Risk factors:                           Discharge status plans:
       _____Obesity or sedentary life-style
       _____Family history, age, sex predispose
               to cardiac disease
       _____Smoking history,_____ pkg/yr_____
       _____HTN_____  yr _____
       _____Diabetes (adult onset)
       _____Lipid abnormality
       _____High cholesterol
       _____Type A personality, stress
       Medications:
```

Fig. 25-9. Chart review worksheet for cardiac patients.

out-of-bed activity with assistance for short periods to use the commode.

The initial self-care evaluation for this patient may consist of a 30-minute treatment session during which the patient will learn energy efficient ways of moving in bed and performing bed-to-commode transfers with minimal use of isometrics or Valsalva maneuver (straining and holding breath). Within the 30-minute treatment session, the patient may be asked to tolerate sitting on the edge of the bed unsupported for a sustained 15- to 20-minute period while performing intermittent upper and lower extremity tasks so the therapist can assess basic range, strength, coordination, and balance. The therapist encourages the patient to perform rhythmic ankle pumping to avoid venous pooling in the lower extremities and resultant dizziness. A significant drop in blood pressure related to sitting or standing up is called orthostatic hypotension. Slow transitional movements, support stockings, and rhythmical extremity movements help to prevent it. This patient may then be asked to stand for a 1- to 2-minute period while gently swaying side to side for augmented venous return so that the patient may begin to tolerate short periods of standing to better care for his toileting needs.

On the other hand, if this patient had an uncomplicated clinical course and was admitted for a 3-day hospitalization to adjust his medication regime for his long-standing CHF, the activities in his initial self-care evaluation would differ. The therapist may quickly assess this patient's basic mobility status (bed mobility, transfers, and standing balance) and then have the patient proceed with washing and dressing himself while seated on a chair in the bathroom.

Such decisions concerning the graduation and progression of activities involve an understanding of the energy costs of activity and the multiple factors that influence it, as discussed under "Treatment progressions."

SIMULATED TASKS EVALUATION. Monitored task evaluations measure the cardiovascular response to a combination of lower and upper extremity work and variations in body position.[48] The tasks that are monitored

simulate what the patient will actually be doing at home or at work to determine if this level of activity is safe to resume under nonmonitored circumstances. These tasks typically require more energy than that required during selfcare and are therefore performed when the patient progresses to phase 2 or 3 of the cardiac rehabilitation program. Treadmill exercise tests are routinely used to evaluate a patient's functional capacity; however, the information obtained is based solely on lower extremity performance. Since upper extremity work elicits a different and more pronounced cardiovascular response,[9] simulated task evaluations can better evaluate a patient's response to specific vocational and leisure tasks.

A numerical scoring system of task analysis has been developed by Ogden.[46] She analyzes tasks by six variables: rate, resistance, muscle groups used, involvement of trunk muscles, arm position, and isometric work (straining). This system of analysis assists the therapist in evaluating which tasks demand the highest energy demand from the heart. Perhaps the application of this system is more useful to cardiac teaching and work simplification. Here the therapist reduces the energy demands of a task by altering the aforementioned variables. Other factors, such as environmental temperature, emotional stress related to the task, and length of time (sustained versus intermittent) the patient performs the task, must be considered.

The need for a simulated task evaluation most often arises when the patient is ready to return to a blue-collar job. For instance, Mr. J., a 53-year-old cafeteria dishwasher, had a coronary artery bypass following his MI 2 months ago. He has been involved in an aggressive cardiac rehabilitation program consisting of walking, bicycling, and arm ergometry (arm crank) at a target heart rate of 120 beats per minute. He can now tolerate sustained, 30 minute activities that are 4½ times the amount of energy he requires at rest. His treadmill test produced fatigue and a suboptimal blood pressure response. The question arises whether Mr. J.'s current activity tolerance is sufficient for a safe return to work as a dishwasher. The therapist

performs a chart review, patient interview, and job analysis that includes an interview with the patient's employer and an on-site observation to determine the energy demands of the job. The therapist finds that the job is full-time employment performed in three parts daily:

1. Dish tray assembly for 2 hours (sustained standing and light upper extremity activity)
2. General cleaning of work stations for 2 hours (intermittent activity with frequent bending and reaching)
3. Dishwashing for 3 hours (sustained standing with frequent stacking and lifting 5 to 10 pounds at once on an assembly line)

These tasks take place in a warm environment; the patient has no control over pace or rest period because of the fixed-rate assembly line and union regulations concerning breaks. The therapist designs a simulated task evaluation that takes place over 3 hours. The therapist evaluates cardiovascular responses to (1) sustained standing and light upper extremity activity, (2) intermittent activity with frequent bending and reaching, and (3) sustained standing with moderate upper extremity work at a fixed, moderate pace. The therapist finds that the patient has significant difficulty and demonstrates abnormal cardiovascular responses. The therapist discusses this with the cardiologist who implements a medication change and suggests a change in the patient's physical conditioning program so it is geared toward those tasks the patient must perform at work. In this case the simulated task evaluation gave the cardiologist crucial information of functional performance that could not be obtained from a routine treadmill test. Occupational therapists are becoming more involved with simulated work evaluations for patients with cardiac disease. Further methods, studies, and applications of such evaluations should be developed.

Evaluation tools

Therapists assess a patient's cardiovascular response to activity by monitoring five parameters: heart rate, blood pressure, ECG readings, signs and symptoms of cardiac dysfunction, and heart sounds. In some facilities therapists are not required to monitor ECG and heart sounds. This author believes that, if treating a cardiac population, therapists should develop skills in basic ECG interpretation[23] and in recognition of abnormal heart sounds.[37] Instruction in these skills is beyond the scope of this text.

Monitoring skills and techniques should be objective, expedient, and accurate. Furthermore, therapists must be able to assess these parameters in relation to cardiovascular hemodynamics and adverse cardiac symptoms.

HEART RATE. "Normal" heart rates vary with age, sex, activity, attitude, temperature, health status, emotion, amount of coffee or tobacco intake, and electrolyte and fluid imbalances.[22] Basically, normal adult heart rate is 60 to 100 beats per minute. Abnormal heart rates are either too slow (called bradycardia; less than 60 beats per minute), too fast (called tachycardia; greater than 100 beats per minute), or irregular (called arrhythmias).

If the heart rate is bradycardic, the cardiac output may not be sufficient to meet the energy demands of the brain, systemic circulation, and working muscles. This results in fatigue; and if bradycardia is severe, dizziness, confusion, or syncope (loss of consciousness) can result. In highly trained athletes bradycardia is normal and reflects a highly efficient cardiovascular system. In other cases bradycardia that is symptom free at 50 to 60 beats per minute may be desired to decrease the work of the myocardium. This is often the result of medications, like propranolol (Inderal), in the beta blocker category. A sudden development of bradycardia, however, especially if associated with symptoms, warrants further medical workup and could be indicative of severe cardiac conduction dysfunction, that is, heart blocks that may necessitate inserting a cardiac pacemaker.

Tachycardic heart rates (HR) may be caused by general deconditioning or conditions that alter stroke volume (SV), the amount of blood ejected with each heart beat. Tachycardia may be the heart's attempt to maintain cardiac output (CO) since CO = SV × HR. Heart rates greater than 110 do not allow adequate filling time in diastole, which further impinges on stroke volume. Furthermore, tachycardic heart

rates increase myocardial oxygen demand. The increase may exceed available supply and cause myocardial ischemia.

Heart rate can be monitored by several methods: palpation, (feeling), auscultation (listening), and ECG monitoring (skin electrodes). Pulses can be palpated and counted at the radial, brachial, carotid, and temporal sites. Therapists must exercise caution if monitoring carotid pulse, since this site is close to the carotid sinus that if overstimulated, can cause bradycardia. If the pulse is regular, it is counted for 10 seconds and multiplied by 6, giving total beats per minute.

Auscultation, or listening to the heart with a stethoscope to monitor heart rate, is recommended for patients with poor peripheral pulses or irregular heart beats. The stethoscope is placed over the apex of the heart (the fifth intercostal space at or just medial to the left midclavicular line).[10] This is the point of maximal impulse refered to as PMI. Apical pulses, if irregular, should be counted for a full 60-second period for accuracy. The ECG method of monitoring heart rate is a simple technique of reading heart rate from an accurate digital display. Heart rate can also be measured from ECG strips by counting blocks on the paper as they correlate to assigned heart rates[23] or by using a special rate ruler. Appropriate documentation of heart rate includes the number of beats per minute and a comment on regularity, such as "72 beats per minute and irregular."

BLOOD PRESSURE.[15,43,55] Blood pressure is simply the pressure of blood against the arteries created by the pumping of the heart and the peripheral resistance of flow. This pressure is responsible for driving the blood through the circulatory system to perfuse vital organs, tissues, and working muscle. The reader is referred to the cardiac cycle (Fig. 25-5). The diastolic blood pressure (lower number) is the amount of pressure generated by ventricular contraction that is responsible for opening the aortic and pulmonary valves. Systolic blood pressure (upper number) is the peak pressure that the ventricles continue to generate over and above the point at which the valves open. For instance, if 80 mm Hg is

necessary to open the aortic and pulmonary valves and the ventricle continues to contract to a maximal force of 120 mm Hg, then the blood pressure is 120/80 mm Hg. The numerical difference (40 mm Hg) or the amount of pressure generated from the time the valves open to peak pressure is the pressure available to propagate blood along the systemic circulation. This is called pulse pressure. If this pulse pressure becomes less than 20 mm Hg (90/80), profusion to the distal tissues may not be sufficient. In severe cases circulatory shock or collapse may occur with permanent damage related to the amount of time the vital organs and tissues do not receive oxygen.

Normal blood pressures increase with age.[22] Since arteriosclerosis and a decrease in the distensibility of the arteries is often associated with age, more pressure is required to propel blood through the system. Pressures become hypertensive if they are between 160/90 to 200/110 mm Hg or greater. A particularly high systolic blood pressure may generate too much pressure in the arteries and could result in an aneurysm or CVA. In addition, diastolic hypertensive states require that the ventricles perform increased and often sustained contractions that may result in myocardial hypertrophy. In this case the heart needs even more oxygen as a result of the increase in muscle fibers. If the oxygen cannot be supplied to meet this demand, ischemia may result.

If systolic blood pressure is less than 90 mm Hg, hypotension or low blood pressure exists. Similarly, low blood pressure affects perfusion and the delivery of blood to vital organs and peripheral tissues. Hypotension may be associated with dizziness and lightheadedness. In severe cases of hypotension caused by circulatory inadequacy hands and feet may become cold, the patient's color may be dusky or pale, lips may be cyanotic or bluish, and the patient may become confused, indicating degrees of cerebral anoxia.

When patients are admitted to a medical service, physicians will usually indicate vital sign precautions in the nursing orders; these may differ according to the patient's condition, medications, and past medical history. They are usually written as, "Call H.O.

(house officer or on-call physician) if SBP > 150 < 90; DBP > 90 < 50; HR > 120 < 50" (Systolic blood pressure greater than 150 or less than 90; diastolic blood pressure greater than 90 or less than 50; heart rate greater than 120 or less than 50).

Blood pressure is monitored by two methods, invasive and noninvasive. Invasive techniques require that an arterial line be placed into the artery for direct blood pressure monitoring. Although this is the most accurate and the most often used in acute care for the hemodynamically unstable patient, it is not feasible in a rehabilitation setting. If a patient is receiving therapy with a central arterial line in place, therapists can record blood pressures from the digital readout on the monitor. Most often therapists will record blood pressure from noninvasive techniques by use of a sphygmomanometer or blood pressure cuff. Because this method is indirect, it is subject to many sources of error that the therapist must attempt to minimize.

An indirect measurement is one that uses and examines associated factors (cuff pressure) to derive and define the desired measurement (blood pressure).[55] More simply, if a given blood pressure is 120/80 mm Hg and the therapist pumps the cuff to 200 mm Hg, the brachial artery will be completely occluded, since cuff pressure (200) exceeds peak arterial pressure (120). If a stethoscope is placed over the artery at this time, no sounds will be heard, since there is no blood flow. Once the therapist gradually releases the cuff pressure to 120 mm Hg, the artery's peak pressure may be able to squeeze some blood through a now partially occluded artery, and pulse sounds will be heard under the stethoscope. The point at which the first two sounds are heard corresponds to the point where the arterial pressure now exceeds the cuff pressure.[55] The therapist then reads the number on the dial to quantify this point of pressure as the systolic blood pressure. The systolic blood pressure is *not* the point where the needle or column of mercury visually bounces. Systolic blood pressure measurements are associated with auscultation or listening, not vision. As the therapist continues to release pressure, the artery be-

comes less occluded, enabling greater blood flow and louder sounds under the stethoscope. Once the artery is not occluded and full blood flow is established, the sounds will disappear (for example, 80 mm Hg). This point corresponds to diastolic blood pressure. There are some instances where these sounds (called Korotkoff sounds)[36] will continue all the way to zero. Here the therapist notes the number at which the sounds change in quality. The American Heart Association has established guidelines for a universal method of recording blood pressure. They recommend that systolic blood pressure be recorded at the point where the first two consecutive sounds are heard and diastolic blood pressure be recorded when the sounds change or become muffled.[5]

Sources of error can arise from faulty tools and techniques and errors in measurement.[36] Blood pressure cuffs have many components,[15] and each of these must be in good repair. The most common problems are noncalibrated meters and cracked or kinked tubing because of placement. Aneroid (dial) meters should be calibrated every 6 months, whereas mercury (column) meters only require calibration once per year.[36] All systems require calibration if the dial or column meniscus does not return to zero.

The relationship between the size of the cuff and circumference of the arm must be considered when choosing which cuff to use.[36] If a standard cuff is used on a very thin arm, the therapist will obtain a false, low pressure reading, whereas a standard cuff applied to an obese arm will result in a false, high reading. Blood pressures measured when cuff/arm size relationships are not considered will be erroneous. Alternate cuffs, for instance, pediatric or "large" adult cuffs, should be available in the clinic.

Additional sources of error may include placing the stethoscope underneath the cuff to hold it in place, varying the position of the arm during serial blood pressure monitoring, repeating inflation of the cuff to make sure measurement is correct, and deflating cuff too rapidly or slowly.[36]

Interpretation of blood pressure responses is based on accurate and expedient measurement. To ensure accuracy

therapists are urged to use the same arm, position, evaluator, and equipment when measuring responses. In addition, therapists must be able to obtain a blood pressure response in 30 to 40 seconds. Once activity is stopped, blood pressure begins to recover, and peak response will be missed.

Most therapists are not confident in blood pressure monitoring techniques; if blood pressure is difficult to take, they immediately identify their technique as the source of error. Therapists must remember that most patients referred for cardiac rehabilitation have abnormal cardiovascular systems and a difficult blood pressure may be indicative of an inappropriate cardiovascular response to activity. There are additional techniques that can be used to augment blood pressure sounds. In fact, if auscultation with a stethoscope cannot determine a blood pressure, the palpation method can be used.[15] With this method no stethoscope is needed. The therapist deflates the cuff; the moment the arterial pulse returns, systolic blood pressure is recorded. Blood pressure monitored in this manner is recorded as 120/P (palpated).[6]

ECG. Patients with cardiovascular disease are prone to arrhythmias, which, if frequent, can decrease cardiac output, cause symptoms, and affect overall cardiac function. If severe, they could be life threatening. All therapists must be trained in cardiopulmonary resuscitation as a basic life-support measure. Therapists working with patients who have known or suspected heart disease must be able to recognize signs and symptoms related to cardiac dysfunction. For therapists not trained in ECG interpretation this includes noting how irregular a pulse becomes (10 irregular beats per minute) during or after activity. Therapists using ECG during therapy should be familiar with monitoring equipment, including problems and artifacts (monitor interference). "They also should be capable of recognizing, at a minimum, the following EKG dysrhythmias: 1) sinus tachycardia, 2) sinus bradycardia, 3) premature atrial complexes, 4) atrial tachycardia, 5) atrial flutter, 6) atrial fibrillation, 7) junctional rhythms, 8) atrioventricular blocks of all degrees, 9) premature ventricular complexes, 10) ventricular tachycardia, 11) ventricular fibrillation and 12) cardiac standstill or asystole."[4] Changes in ST segments on the ECG should also be recognized, since these changes parallel cardiac ischemia and cardiac dysfunction. Because ECG interpretation is beyond the scope of this text, the reader is referred to Dubin's *Rapid Interpretion of EKG*.[23] Sample strips are shown in Fig. 25-10 so that the reader may gain an understanding that any arrhythmia either too fast, too slow, or two irregular interferes with cardiac output and function.

SIGNS AND SYMPTOMS OF CARDIAC DYSFUNCTION. Whenever patients become symptomatic or display signs of intolerance to an activity, the therapist should evaluate and record the event by noting the following[53]:

1. Exact complaint
2. Body location
3. Quality
4. Quantity
5. Chronology
6. Setting
7. Aggravating or alleviating factors
8. Associated symptoms

Angina. Many chest pains are not associated with ischemia. Angina pectoris induced by ischemia has specific hallmark characteristics. Typically, it is felt substernally with or without radiation to the shoulders, arms, back, throat, and/or jaw. Its quality is often described as a "heaviness, pressure, squeezing and/or tightness."[10] Some patients experience indigestion, and have difficulty describing this discomfort. "Sticking, stabbing, throbbing or needle-like pain is seldom angina."[10] Patients who have difficulty describing this vague discomfort may gesture with a clenched fist to their chest. Angina typically lasts less than 15 minutes; and if longer, it may indicate further damage as a result of infarction. Patients should be asked to quantify the severity of the pain on an angina rating scale[10] with 10 being the worst pain felt. The surrounding activities that induce angina should be examined. Angina typically occurs during ambulation, shaving, bowel movement, stair climbing, observation of athletic events, or arguing, or after a meal. Once these exacerbating factors are stopped, angina dissipates; prompt relief (3 minutes) may

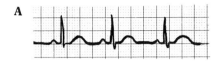

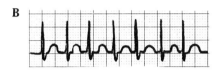

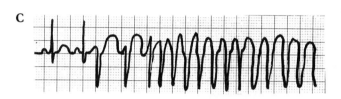

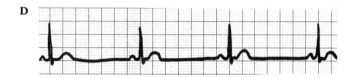

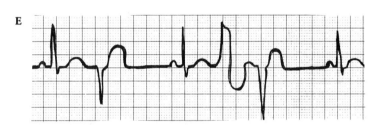

Fig. 25-10. Sample ECG readings of cardiac arrythmias. **A,** Regular sinus rhythm. **B,** Sinus tachycardia (too fast). **C,** Ventricular tachycardia (too fast). **D,** Sinus bradycardia (too slow). **E,** Multifocal premature ventricular contractions (too irregular).

occur with sublingual nitroglycerin tablets, a quick-acting vasodilator. Associated symptoms may include nausea, palpitations, and dizziness. Angina is not the only indication of ischemia. Some patients never experience angina with MI. Instead, weakness or dyspnea (shortness of breath) may be a symptom.

Dyspnea.[10,53] Dyspnea, difficulty breathing, is a common symptom in heart disease and may be indicative of left ventricular failure. When dyspnea is noted on exertion, the therapist must note the quantity of activity that produces this. This functional method of recording dyspnea is preferred over the "numerical values" often used to describe dyspnea (for instance, +2 dyspnea). Orthopnea, is shortness of breath created by resting in the supine position. Since this position creates a greater venous return, stroke volume increases in accordance with Starling's Law,[10] thus demanding more work from the myocardium. Often a diseased myocardium is not capable of handling the demand, and shortness of breath or orthopnea will result. "Two pillow orthopnea" describes the propped-up position necessary to relieve this symptom.

Fatigue. Fatigue is often an initial sign of heart disease. When patients report fatigue, therapists must determine whether it is localized or generalized. Asking which muscles are fatigued will assist the patient in localizing it. If the patient has difficulty localizing the symptom and uses words like exhausted and drained and appears fatigued, the cause may be centralized, as in heart disease. One objective method of rating fatigue is Borg's rate of perceived exertion (RPE) scale[12] (see boxed material at right). Patients experiencing centralized fatigue are asked to assign a number to their fatigue based on their perception of the difficulty of activity. Myocardial oxygen consumption studies have correlated RPE scores of greater than 15 RPE to 75% of maximal myocardial oxygen consumption.[12] RPE scores have been used during graded exercise tests and exercise training sessions to guide the clinician in grading or stopping the activity.[51] RPE has been successfully used during monitored self-care and simulated task evaluations. Such an objective rating scale

Rate of perceived exertion	
6	
7	Very, very light
8	
9	Very light
10	
11	Fairly light
12	
13	Somewhat hard
14	
15	Hard
16	
17	Very hard
18	
19	Very, very hard
20	

From Borg, G., et al.: Med. Sci. Sports Exerc. **14:**376, 1982.

warrants further examination and application to other physical disabilities, such as arthritis and multiple sclerosis.

• • •

In summary, whenever any sign or symptom is noted with activity, the therapist must accurately note its characteristics and associated factors for proper interpretation.

Assessment

If a patient has tolerated rehabilitation activities well, it implies that no adverse signs or symptoms were noted and that heart rate, blood pressure, and ECG responses were appropriate. Monitoring and assessing a *response* implies measuring and quantifying a change. Therefore therapists record each of these parameters before activity (resting phase), during activity (peak phase), and 4 to 5 minutes after the activity has stopped (recovery phase). To isolate the response to activity the therapist must monitor and record vital signs in the position of peak activity. For instance, if peak activity is performed while standing at the sink, baseline and recovery vital signs should be noted in the standing position.

Postural responses should also be noted, particularly since orthostatic hypotension is a common occurrence after immobility and is often a side effect of diuretic and antianginal medication regimes. Therapists must be able to assess patient responses so they may establish appropriate treatment progressions for patients. The boxed material below lists appropriate (desired) and inappropriate cardiovascular responses to activity.[51]

Cardiovascular responses to activity

Appropriate	Inappropriate
Heart rate: Increases with activity to a maximum of approximately 20 beats above resting rate	Heart rate: Excessive heart rate response to activity ($>$20 beats above resting rate); resting tachycardia ($>$120); bradycardic response to activity (pulse drops or fails to rise with increased work loads)
Blood pressure: Peak systolic blood pressure increases as work load increases	Blood pressure: Hypertensive responses (220/110 mm Hg maximum); postural hypotensive responses ($>$10 to 20 mm Hg systolic blood pressure decrease); any drop in systolic blood pressure with activity; failure of systolic blood pressure to rise with activity
ECG readings: Absence of arrhythmias and segment changes	ECG readings: Any rapid arrhythmias or increase in ectopic activity; development of 2 or 3 degree heart blocks; ST segment depression ($>$3 to 4 mm); any ST segment elevation
Symptoms: Absence of adverse symptoms	Symptoms: Excessive shortness of breath; angina and/or associated symptoms of nausea, sweating, and extreme fatigue (RPE $>$15); cerebral symptoms (confusion or ataxia)

From Santa Clara Valley Medical Center: Cardiac rehabilitation program protocol, San Jose, Calif., 1983. Unpublished.

In instances where significant maladaptive responses are noted, communication lines to the referring physician must be expedient. Emergency precautions and procedures[23] must be established in any program before placing any demand on patients with documented heart disease.

Treatment progressions

GRADED ACTIVITIES. Program progressions are guided by the patient's current clinical status, prognosis, and tolerance of current activities with appropriate cardiovascular responses. The rate of progression is further guided by the patient's past functional history and severity of coronary event. The physician synthesizes this information and ultimately categorizes the patient into one of four functional categories (see boxed material at right).[42] Patients in class I will obviously progress the most rapidly, depending on their continued demonstration to tolerate activities appropriately. Patients in classes III and IV will progress slowly and may never achieve total independence in self-care.

Progressions are further guided by the energy costs of activities and the factors that influence them. Energy expenditure is measured by the amount of oxygen that is consumed. Years ago this was expressed in calories but has been refined recently to METs. One MET (basal metabolic equivalent) is equal to the energy consumed when a patient is at rest in a semi-Fowler position (semireclined with extremities supported). This is equal to 3.5 ml O_2 per minute per kilogram of body weight. As soon as one sits up, walks, or performs activities, this metabolic demand and oxygen consumption increases. For instance, dressing requires 2 METs or twice the amount of energy required at rest. Several MET lists establish a comprehensive catalog of a variety of activities that require 1 to 9 METs. Table 25-1 is an example of such an energy cost list. The references cited in the table can be found at the end of the chapter.

This method of grading activity, however, is a general guideline. Caution must be exercised when extrapolating the results of a treadmill test to apply to vocational and leisure tasks. For instance, if a patient achieves 5 METs on the treadmill, this does not necessarily

---

Functional classification of cardiac disease

Class I: Patients with cardiac disease but without resulting limitations of physical activity. Ordinary physical activity does not cause undue fatigue, palpitation, dyspnea, or anginal pain.

Class II: Patients with cardiac disease resulting in slight limitation of physical activity. They are comfortable at rest. Ordinary physical activity results in fatigue, palpitation, dyspnea, or anginal pain.

Class III: Patients with cardiac disease resulting in marked limitation of physical activity. They are comfortable at rest. Less than ordinary physical activity causes fatigue, palpitation, dyspnea, or anginal pain.

Class IV: Patients with cardiac disease resulting in inability to carry on any physical activity without discomfort. Symptoms of cardiac insufficiency or of the anginal syndrome may be present even at rest. If any physical activity is undertaken, discomfort is increased.

From New York Heart Association, Inc.: Nomenclature and criteria for diagnosis of diseases of the heart and great vessels, ed. 8, Boston, 1979, Little, Brown & Co.

---

mean that the patient can resume all activities listed at 5 METs on the energy cost list. Various factors, such as pace, position, muscles used, isometrics, techniques, and environmental factors, influence the energy cost of an activity.

Choosing "very light-light"[41] activities for a patient just recovering from an acute MI or cardiac surgery is essential. During a patient's acute recovery (phase 1) physicians wish to promote healing of the myocardium but also wish to avoid the deconditioning effects of inactivity. Physicians do not wish any activity to produce tachycardia or a heart rate response greater than 20 beats per minute above rest, since such myocardial work would interfere with healing. Patients in phase 1 rehabilitation should not be permitted to perform tasks greater than 3.5 METs. Most self-care can be achieved within this very light-light work category.

Note that sexual activity is listed at 5 METs. Patients just recovering from heart attacks often have questions concerning safe sexual activity. Since sexual activity is "intermittent" and does not require prolonged, sustained high levels of rhythmical physical activity, physicians advise return to sexual activity if patients can tolerate walking up and down two flights of stairs without symptoms.[52] Therefore patients may be able to perform 5-MET–level activity as long as performance is intermittent and can perform a lower level or 3.5-MET–level activity if performance is continu-

ous or sustained. To ensure that patients gradually resume daily activities a step-by-step program similar to the one used at Santa Clara Valley Medical Center is advised (Table 25-2).

In phase 1 the therapist gradually progresses the patient from simple bed mobility and commode transfers to independent dressing and showering, listed at 3.5 METs, under controlled environmental conditions.

Myocardial healing and musculoskeletal and cardiac conditioning have occurred by 6 to 8 weeks after coronary event. At this time most patients can tolerate increased MET-level activities greater than 3.5 METs and are ready for simulated task evaluations.

Energy conservation

As mentioned throughout the chapter, a balance of low-level activity and rest is essential to the healing myocardium, especially during phase 1 rehabilitation. Knowledge of how various activities evoke differing cardiovascular responses is the basis of energy conservation and work simplification principles.[7] Ogden[45] prefers to use the term *work efficiency* to describe such principles because it is a more positive and "less restrictive" term and because such principles are based on how activities affect the actual efficiency of cardiovascular function.

Such exercise physiology principles are included in many physiology texts,[9,22] but little is written concerning

Text continued on p. 351.

Table 25-1
Santa Clara Valley Medical Center's MET levels of ADL and vocational and recreational activities

1 MET	METs	Ref	2 METs	METs	Ref	3 METs	METs	Ref	4 METs	METs	Ref
Daily activities											
Resting supine	1	(17)	Walking 1 mph	2	—	Walking 2 mph	3	—	Hot shower	4.2	(34)
Supported sitting in arm chair, full support semireclined 45° with knees up	1	(34)	Walking 1.5 mph	2.5	—	Walking 2.5 mph			Bowel movement on bed pan	4.7	(34)
			Wheelchair propulsion 1.2 mph	2	(17,38)	Using bedside commode	3	—	Walking downstairs	4.5	(17)
			Washes hands, face and brushes hair	2	(17,38)	Bowel movement (toilet)	3.6	(17)			
Unsupported sitting on bed edge, at ease	1.3	(19,38)	Dressing, undressing	2.5	(34)	Warm shower	3.5	(34)			
Self-feeding (sitting supported)	1.2	(19,38)	Washing, dressing, undressing	2.7	(34)	Stairs (slowly at 24 ft/min)	3.5	(17)			
Standing relaxed	1.5	(2)									
Transfers bed to chair	1.65	(34)									
Homemaking skills											
Hand sewing	1	(17)	Polishing furniture	2	(17)	Cleaning windows	3-4	(17,25)	Bed making (stripping)	4.4	(19,38)
Light machine sewing	1.5	(17)	Dusting	2.5	(19,38)	Light bed making	3.9	(34)	Washing floor (kneeling)	4.3	(19,38)
			Electric vacuuming	2.6	(19,38)	Ironing (standing)	3.5	(17)	Polishing floor	4.1	(19,38)
Sweeping floor	1.5	(17)	Manual vacuuming	2.9	(19,38)	Mopping	3.5	(17)	Pushing power mower	3-4	(54)
			Scrubbing (standing)	2.5	(17)	Waxing floor	3.4	(19,38)			
			Peeling potatoes	2.5	(17)	Hanging wash	3.5	(17)			
			Kneading dough	2.5	(17)	Wringing by hand	3.5	(17)			
			Washing small clothes	2.5	(17)	Preparing meals	3	(34)			
			Misc. carrying	2.9	(19,38)						
Vocational tasks											
Clerical			*Tradesmen*								
Desk work	1.8-2.2	(54)	Shoe repair	2.2	(19,38)	Light janitorial work	3	(25)	Welding (moderate load)	3-4	(25)
			Fixing soles	1.9	(19,38)	Bartending	3	(25)			
Operating electric office machinery	2.2	(54)	Industrial machine sewing	2.5	(17)	Locksmith work (filing)	3	(19,34)	Chiseling	4.6	(19,38)
			Tailoring, cutting	2.2	(19,38)				Wheelbarrow 115 lb/2.5 mph	4	(17)
Manual typing	1.2	(19,38)	Radio, bench assembly	2.5	(17,34)	Tailoring (pressing)	3.6	(19,34)			
Electric typing	1.1	(19,38)				Auto repair	3	(25)			
						Tractor plowing	3.5	(17)			

5 METs			6 METs			7 METs			8 METs			9 METs		
	METs	Ref		METs	Ref		METs	Ref		METs	Ref		METs	Ref
Walking 3.5 mph Up/down stairs	5.5	(17)	Ambulation with braces and crutches	6.5	(17)	Ascending stairs with 17 lb load (27 ft/min)	7.5	(17)				Ascending stairs with 25 lb load (54 ft/min)	13.5	(17)
30 ft/min	5	—												
36 ft/min	5.5	—												
Marital sexual relations	5	—												
Carrying bags, groceries	4-5	(54)	Manual lawn mowing	6.5	(17,54)				Tending furnace	8.5	(17)			
Shoveling light earth, digging garden	5-6	(25)	Splitting wood	6.5	(17,54)									
Sawing soft wood	5.1	(19,38)	Planing soft wood	6.1	(19,38)	Heavy hammering	7.4	(17,19,38)	Shoveling 14 lb (10/min)	8-9	(25)	Shoveling 16 lb (10/min)	>10	(25)
Sawing hard wood	5.9	(19,38)	Planing hard wood	6.6	(19,38)	Shoveling 10 lb (10/min)	6-7	(25)						
Drilling hard wood	5.7	(19,38)				Digging ditches	7-8	(25)						
Light carpentry	4-5	(25)				Carrying 30 lb	7-8	(25)						
Paper hanging	4-5	(25)												
Painting, masonry	4-5	(25)												

Continued.

Table 25-1—cont'd

Santa Clara Valley Medical Center's MET levels of ADL and vocational and recreational activities

1 MET			2 METs			3 METs			4 METs		
	METs	Ref		METs	Ref		METs	Ref		METs	Ref
Engineering			*Building*								
Watch repair	101.5	(17)	Measuring,	2.8	(19,38)	Bricklaying	3.5	(17)			
Light assembly line	1.5	(19,38)	sawing			Plastering	3.5	(17)			
Draftsman	1.5	(19,38)	Light stone brick work	2.7	(19,38)	Mixing cement	3.8	(19,34)			
Printing	1.8	(19,38)	Hacksawing (standing)	2.5	(34)	Joining floor boards	3.6	(19,34)			
Setting type (standing)	1.6	(34)	Metal work (hammering)	2.1	(34)	Driving trailer truck in traffic	3-4	(54)			
Recreational tasks											
Watching TV, conversation	1	(17)	Playing piano	2	(17,34)	Golfing, power cart	3	(25)	Energetic musician	3-4	(25)
			Driving car	2	(19,38)						
Knitting, crocheting	1	(17)	Bimanual activity sanding 50 strokes/min	2	(34)	Cycling, 5 mph level	3	(25)	Archery	3-4	(25)
Rug hooking	1.1	(19,38)				Bowling	3.5	(17)	Sailing small boat	3-4	(25)
Writing (sitting)	1.6	(19,38)	Flying, motorcycling	2	(25)	Playing with children	3.5	(19,38)	Fly fishing (standing in water)	3-4	(25)
Painting (sitting)	1.5	(17)	Weight lifting 10 lb 15/45 min	2.8	(34)	Power boat driving	3	(25)	Horseshoe pitching	3-4	(25)
Drawing (standing)	1.9	(19,38)	Canoeing 2.5 mph	2.5	(17)	Billiards, shuffleboard	3	(25)	Gardening (raking, hoeing, weeding)	4.5	(17,54)
Playing cards (sitting)	1.6	(19,38)	Slow horseback riding	2.5	(17)	Playing most musical instruments	3	(25)	Dancing	4.5	(17)
Leather tooling (sitting)	1.4	(34)							Swimming (20 yd/min)	4	(17)
Lacing	1.5	(34)							Golfing	4	(17)
Carving	1.7	(34)							Volleyball (6 man noncompetitive)	3-4	(25)
Weaving floor loom	1.6	(19,38)							Badminton (social doubles)	3-4	(25)

5 METs			6 METs			7 METs			8 METs			9 METs		
	METs	Ref		METs	Ref		METs	Ref		METs	Ref		METs	Ref
Horse ploughing	5	(17)	Shoveling light earth	5-6	(25)									
Haying	5.9	(19,38)												
Many calisthenics	4-5	(25)	Push-ups	6.5	—	Water skiing	6-7	(25)	Squash (social)	8.5	(17,25)	Squash (competitive)	>10	(25)
Deep knee bends	5.5	(17)	Weight lifting 10-20 lb lifted 36/15 min	6.5	(34)	Spading	7	(17)	Running (5.5 mph)	8-9	(25)	Running 6 mph	10.0	(25)
Canoeing (4 mph)	5-6	(25)				Jogging (5 mph)	7-8	(25)	Cycling (13 mph)	8-9	(25)	7 mph	11.5	
Stream fishing	5-6	(54)	Cycling (10 mph)	5-6	(25)	Cycling (12 mph)	7-8	(25)	Cross country skiing (4 mph)	8-9	(25)	8 mph	13.5	
Cycling (8 mph)	4-5	(25)	Trotting on horseback	6.5	(17)	Vigorous downhill skiing	7-8	(17,25)				9 mph	15.0	
Roller, ice skating (9 mph)	5	(38,54)	Dancing (folk and square dancing)	6-7	(25)	Horseback (galloping)	7-8	(25)				10 mph	17.0	
Dancing (Foxtrot)	4-5	(25)				Mountain climbing	7-8	(25)				Cross country skiing (> 5 mph)	>10	(25)
Golfing, carrying clubs	4-5	(25)	Light downhill skiing	6-7	(25)	Ice hockey	7-8	(25)	Handball (social)	8-9	(25)	Handball (competitive)	>10.0	(25)
Table tennis	4-5	(25)	Tennis (singles)	6-7	(17,54)	Touch football	7-8	(25)	Vigorous basketball	8-9	(25)			
Tennis (doubles)	4-5	(25)	Badminton (competitive)	6-7	(25)	Basket, paddleball	7-8	(25)						
Badminton (singles)	4-5	(25)				Canoeing (5 mph)	7-8	(25)						

Table 25-2

Santa Clara Valley Medical Center's post MI and post open-heart surgery rehabilitation program*

Stage	Physical therapy	Occupational therapy	Dietary	Nursing
Phase 1—inpatient program				
1 in ICU or on ward 1.5 METs	Check and record heart rate, blood pressure, and ECG readings in supine, sitting, and standing positions In semi-Fowler position: 5-10 times active assistive exercise Ambulate 50-100 ft, with assistance, as tolerated Teach breathing patterns with exercises Postoperative: deep breathing exercises Chest: physical therapy as indicated	General mobility (bed mobility transfers to commode and position changes) with energy conservation techniques (environmental set-ups, equipment, and pacing) Sedentary leisure tasks, with arms supported (reading, writing, and cards)	Interview patient and review chart for pertinent medical history Note: Diet history Usual eating patterns Height, weight, and pertinent laboratory values Calculate basal metabolic equivalent Assess nutritional status	Psychological and emotional support to patient and family (preoperative education as indicated) Supported sitting (15 min-1 hr) Self-feedings, arms supported Dependent: assisted bed bathing Reinforcement of mobility, energy conservation, ADL techniques, and ambulation as per occupational therapy and physical therapy
2 in ICU or on ward 1.5 METs	Same as stage 1 except exercises are active	Stage 1 continued with focus on: Unsupported sitting (5-30 min) Standing tasks (seconds to 2 min) Simple hygiene, semifowler sitting position	Same as above	Progression of ADLs and ambulation as per individualized activity sheets above patient's bed
3 On ward 1.5-2 METs	In sitting position: 5-10 times active upper extremity (UE) and lower extremity (LE) exercise with coordinated breathing Ambulate 100-200 ft, with monitoring (2-3 min)	Unsupported sitting ½-1 hr Standing tasks (3-5 min) Bedside bathing (assist with feet and back) Bathroom privileges Light leisure tasks	**After MI** Begin diet education; explain basic principles of diet prescription Include family members in diet education process Reinforce and review diet principles frequently Continue diet education with outpatient dietitian after discharge	Same as above
4 2 METs	In standing position; 5-10 times active UE and LE exercise with coordinated breathing Ambulate 300 ft with monitoring (3-5 min)	Standing tasks (5-8 min) UE sustained activity (2-5 min) Total body bathing at sink	**After surgery** Monitor intake Allow patient to participate in menu selection but offer alternative foods within diet limitations to achieve optimal intake Initiate diet education and involve family members just before discharge Continue diet education with outpatient dietitian	Continued reinforcement and progression of ward activities as per ADL and exercise sheets above patient's bed
5 2 METs	Same as stage 4 except ambulate 400-600 ft with monitoring (5-10 min)	Standing tasks (8-12 min) UE sustained activity (5-7 min) Total hygiene, bathing, and dressing at sink		
6 2 METs	Same as stage 4 except ambulate 400-600 ft with monitoring (5-10 min) Stair climbing 1 flight monitored A predischarge graded exercise test (GXT) is recommended at this time	Standing tasks (12-15 min) with intermittent UE activity UE sustained activity (7-10 min) Total body mobility: bending for small object retrieval and reaching Moderate leisure tasks		

From Santa Clara Valley Medical Center: Cardiac rehabilitation program protocol, San Jose, Calif., 1983. Unpublished.
*Education program to be performed by all team members as per SCVMC *Cardiac Rehabilitation Education Manual*.

Table 25-2—cont'd

Santa Clara Valley Medical Center's post MI and post open-heart surgery rehabilitation program*

Stage	Physical therapy	Occupational therapy	Dietary	Nursing
7 3-3.5 METs	Home program outlined with warm-up exercises and timed walks 3-4 times daily	Tub transfers Total showering task (hair washing, total body washing, drying, and dressing) Simple homemaking tasks Energy conservation techniques with activity 3.5 METs (or greater as indicated by GXT) Home program with ADL guidelines and recommendations for equipment, as appropriate		Discharge education: Medications Wound care Follow-up medical appointments
Phase 2—outpatient program	Exercise program under continuous telemetry ECG monitoring; combination of calisthenics, walking, bicycle ergometry, and resisted arm exercises Frequency: 2-3 times/week for 6-8 weeks supplemented with home exercise 2-3 days/week Duration: 30-60 min/session Intensity: varies from 2-10 METs, depending on the patient target heart rate (THR) derived from entry GXT; usually 70% of maximal heart rate attained on GXT or at RPE of 11-15 Progression: Patients are progressed according to heart rate, systolic blood pressure, and symptomatic RPE responses to exercise; the duration of exercise is generally increased before the intensity of exercise in patients with low-level physical work capacities	Patients not yet independent with full self-care maximal functional capacity <3.5 METs) will be followed to provide home program guidelines for self-care and/or homemaking; such guidelines may include specific energy conservation techniques and/or the use of durable medical equipment All home programs are designed by simulating these specific activities under monitored conditions to evaluate safe performance Work tasks are similarly assessed and referral to a vocational rehabilitation counselor is pursued as indicated	Patients are followed by the outpatient dietitian as needed	

how these are applied to ADL, especially for the individual with severe cardiac disease. For instance, upper extremity work elicits a greater cardiovascular response than lower extremity activity. Also standing requires a greater cardiovascular positional adjustment and more energy than sitting. Any isometric muscular activity interferes with easy blood flow through the muscle and impinges a demand on the cardiovascular system and Valsalva maneuvers (straining and breath holding) interfere with blood return to the heart and elicit large increases in blood pressure. In warm environments (for example, a hot shower) the body has the added task of maintaining its core temperature and must direct blood to the periphery for cooling, which demands cardiovascular work and increased heart rate. Similarly, blood is shunted away from the muscles and to the stomach immediately after meals, and any activity immediately after a meal will elicit a higher heart rate and a higher myocardial oxygen demand.

Santa Clara Valley Medical Center
Occupational Therapy
Self-Care Activity Guide

Name: _____

Therapist: _____

Key:

☐ Contraindicated at this time. Dependent on total nursing assistance.

☐ Supervision or assistance needed. *0*, Verbal or set-up assistance. *1*, Minimal assistance. *2*, Moderate assistance. *3*, Maximal assistance.

☐ Let patient go ahead. The patient can proceed safely and independently.

	METs					
Date						
Feeding	METs					
In bed, legs up, arms supported	1.0					
On bed edge, legs dangling	—					
In chair	1.2					
Mobility						
Sitting	1.3					
Standing relaxed	1.4					
Turning in bed	—					
Repositioning and scooting	—					
Supine to sit	—					
Bedpan	4.0					
Transfering to commode	3.0					
Walking to bathroom (1 mph)	2.0					
Retrieving objects from drawer	—					
Retrieving objects from floor	2.9					
Total body mobility and tub transfers	—					
Bathing and hygiene						
Set up: Gathering all supplies	—					
Proceeding in bed, back supported, legs up	—					
Proceeding on bed edge	—					
Proceeding on chair in bathroom	—					
Standing in bathroom	2.0					
Washing face and hands, combing hair	2.0					
Washing face, chest, arms, and legs above knees	2.0					
Washing perianal area	2.0+					
Washing feet	2.0+					
Washing back	2.0+					
Sitting shower	—					
Standing shower	3.5					
Showering, drying, and dressing	3.5+					
Washing hair	—					
Dressing						
Set up: Gathering all supplies						
Sitting on chair	—					
Standing and sitting ad lib	—					
Donning blouse or shirt	2.0					
Donning pants or trousers	2.0					
Donning shoes and socks	2.0+					

Fig. 25-11. ADL flow sheet. (Reproduced with permission. Occupational Therapy Department, Santa Clara Valley Medical Center, San Jose, Calif.)

The therapist must analyze how these principles affect the patient's function. For instance, putting on shoes and socks is an intermittent activity listed at 2.5 METs. It is puzzling to find that on a treadmill test Mrs. M. can tolerate 4 METs of activity but experiences shortness of breath and fatigue with putting on shoes and socks. Close observation of this task reveals that because of the patient's arthritis she strains and holds her breath to reach her feet. When this doesn't work, she stands and hops on one foot to twist and reach to put on her sock. In this case putting on shoes and socks is no longer 2.5 METs. The therapist discovering this may instruct the patient in the use of adaptive dressing aids.

Energy conservation also addresses patterns of activities. For instance, Mrs. R. can perform a standing shower (3.5 METs) with good cardiovascular responses and no symptoms. However, as she dries herself and then attempts to redress, she experiences increased heart rates and fatigue. Therefore a shower chair may be necessary, and a system of work and rest (such as work 5 minutes and rest 2 minutes) can be introduced.

Patients need much guidance and education in this area. Once a patient understands the principles of work efficiency, anxiety is reduced, and the patient feels in control of the events. For instance, Mr. J. was extremely depressed because last evening he had chest pain during his shower; he now feels his cardiac condition is worse because this never happened before. On further examination the therapist discovers that Mr. J. had to run up and down the steps twice to get the phone before taking a shower. It is understandable that if he starts at a high heart rate, activity will certainly increase the rate further; in this case it was increased beyond Mr. J.'s angina threshold. Therapeutic intervention is to educate Mr. J. in environmental and activity factors that increase heart rate and to instruct him in pulse monitoring. If Mr. J.'s pulse is greater than 90, he should wait to take a shower. Meditation or progressive relaxation 10 minutes before showering may be necessary so that showering begins at a heart rate of 70 beats per minute.

Patient education sheets can be used to instruct the patient in such principles. Furthermore a method of work simplification can be used to instruct patients in analyzing new tasks to be simplified at home or in their work environment.

PATIENT AND FAMILY EDUCATION. Patient and family education is of prime importance in cardiac rehabilitation. Topics covered include basic cardiac anatomy, basic exercise physiology, medications, pulse monitoring, diet and risk factor modification, energy conservation, and energy cost of activities.[41,52] The occupational therapist may be involved with instruction in several of these topics. Some occupational therapists coordinate cooking classes with the dietitian to address diet education and assess a patient's performance and use of energy conservation with kitchen tasks.

One useful tool for patients to see their own progress and refer to the energy costs of daily activities is the use of a color-coded ADL sheet. The therapist explains the progression of activities in cardiac rehabilitation on the sheet and color codes activities that patients can perform independently. Activities that are contraindicated are in red, and activities requiring some assistance or supervision are coded yellow (caution) (Fig. 25-11).

Patient and family education can be performed creatively in a variety of ways, such as direct instruction, experiential performance, demonstration, reinforcement, problem solving, and repeated practice. The reader is referred to the references that have evaluated the effectiveness of various presentation techniques geared toward patient education.[16,39]

Sample treatment plan

Case study

D.D. is a 64-year-old man admitted 4 days ago with a 5-hour history of bilateral arm pain and tightness in his throat associated with fatigue and shortness of breath.

Diagnostic workup disclosed an acute anterolateral MI with subsequent complications of CHF and arrhythmias.

This patient is divorced and lives alone. He is a retired plumber and enjoys doing odd maintenance jobs around the house.

He was referred to occupational therapy for ADL evaluation and activity progression per cardiac protocol.

He was transferred out of the ICU and onto a general medicine floor today.

TREATMENT PLAN

A Statistical data.
1. Name: D.D.
   Age: 64
   Diagnosis: Acute anterolateral MI (post day 4) with complications
   Disability: Altered functional capacity
2. Treatment aims as stated in referral:
   Achieve maximal, functional level of ADL without adverse cardiovascular signs of symptoms

B. Other services.
Medical service: Continued medical surveillance of patient's progress and effectiveness of current medical regime with increasing activity and program adjustments as indicated
Nursing: Provision of nursing and supportive care: reinforcement of ADL and ambulation programs in accordance with rehabilitation progress; provision of educational program with nursing emphasis on anatomy and physiology, medications, tests, and wound care
Social service: Assistance in family and social adjustment; exploration of financial resources for follow-up services and arrangement for equip-

Continued.

Sample Treatment Plan—cont'd

ment; outpatient and home health and/or homemaker services as needed
Physical therapy: Graded exercise program with focus on musculoskeletal conditioning progressing to cardiovascular conditioning program with various use of modalities (such as ambulation, arm ergometer, and calisthenics); formulation of home program; ordering of exercise equipment for program as necessary
Dietary service: Diet evaluation and modification with follow-up patient and family education as needed

C. **OT evaluation.**
Chart review
Activity history and interview
Family interview
Monitored ADL
  Basic mobility
  Self-care
Cognitive and behavioral assessment

D. **Results of evaluation.**
1. Evaluation data.
   a. Chart review.
      (1) Tests. *Echocardiogram* identifies abnormal dyskinetic motion of left ventricle. *Catheterization* shows diffuse coronary artery disease; patient is not a surgical candidate. *ECG readings* record rapid atrial fibrillation successfully cardioverted. *Chest x-ray* examination finds cardiomegaly (enlargement) and lung infiltration. *Laboratory tests* show abnormal enzymes (CPK: 1000, MB% 18% = large MI.)
      (2) Complications. CHF is now controlled on furosemide (Lasix), recurrent angina after infarct is now stabilized on nifedipine. Initial arrhythmia complications of atrial fibrillation are now converted to regular sinus rhythm with occasional irregular beats (PVCs).
      (3) Medical history. Positive risk factors include a 50-pack-a-year smoking history, an old MI 3 years ago with recurrent bouts of CHF as a result of poor compliance with medications, and a positive family history for

cardiac disease and borderline diabetes. D.D. also has degenerative joint disease and an old injury in right hip from car accident.
   b. Activity history/interview.
      (1) Mobility. D.D. has some problems bending because of his hip problem and shortness of breath; transfers to the tub bottom are difficult, but he "manages."
      (2) Self-care. D.D. reports independent self-care but difficulty with socks and shoe ties because of shortness of breath and "strain on hip."
      (3) Ambulation. D.D. walks with a cane a maximal distance of 2 to 3 blocks. He makes frequent stops because of shortness of breath and fatigue.
      (4) Community activities. D.D. doesn't drive but uses buses. Sometimes he tires with grocery bags.
      (5) Homemaking. D.D. reports that he is independent with all homemaking; however, he must have "arthritis because neck pain limits laundry and vacuuming tasks." He eats out for most meals.
      (6) Vocational and leisure activities. D.D. enjoys fix-it maintenance and attends senior citizen socials.
   c. Monitored ADL.
      (1) Basic mobility.
         (a) Bed mobility. He cannot lie flat because of shortness of breath, so bed is elevated at 30° at head. In rolling and supine-to-sit positions he is independent, but he uses many Valsalva maneuvers and isometrics.
         (b) ROM. Upper extremity is intact. In the lower extremity D.D. cannot cross his legs. Internal and external rotation is limited at right hip. Hip flexion is 0° to 100°.

         (c) Sit-stand mobility. D.D. is independent from bed height (20 inches) and from toilet, but he uses isometrics and Valsalva maneuvers to get up from a 16-inch surface.
         (d) Sitting tolerance. D.D. sits unsupported for 15 minutes without orthostatic responses. He can tolerate supported sitting for 1 hour by his report.
         (e) Standing tolerance. He manages 2 minutes without orthostatic responses, which is adequate for toileting.
      (2) Self-care.
         (a) Meals: D.D. is independent with supported sitting.
         (b) Bathing: He is independent in simple hygiene.
         (c) Body bathing: He experiences neck pain and blood pressure drop with dizziness while washing arms at 1.5 MET level. All other self-care is not appropriate at this level and will be performed by nursing personnel.
   d. Cognitive and behavioral data. D.D. talks profusely, often boasting of his excellent physical condition for a man of his age. A week before his heart attack he showed some friends how he could do 10 push-ups. He listens to some energy conservation suggestions but seems to have difficulty accepting guidance from others, insisting that he has a better way. He belittles cardiovascular symptoms. He doesn't seem to have any understanding of how shortness of breath, fatigue, or neck pain are related to the heart. He believes that people should work through their pain, just like "in the army." Overall, he is pleasant and cooperative. At the end of

the session he quietly and somewhat out of character asked, "Did I do OK?"

2. Problem identification.
   a. Complicated course and poor left ventricular function indicates high-risk status, slow rehabilitation progression, and probable limited functional prognosis.
   b. "Diffuse coronary artery disease/not a surgical candidate" means that compliance with an optimal medical regime and work efficiency approach to ADL is the only means of returning to near independent function.
   c. Symptoms noted with low-level self-care means poor functional capacity and a possibility for further medication change.
   d. D.D. lives alone so he has little family support.
   e. He has a history of poor compliance with medications.
   f. ROM is decreased in lower extremities. D.D. uses many isometrics and Valsalva maneuvers to compensate for decreased motion.
   g. He has little knowledge of current condition and associated signs and symptoms.
   h. D.D. is somewhat resistive to energy conservation suggestions.

3. Assets.
   a. D.D. has financial security.
   b. He enjoys social contact and activities.
   c. He is invested in his physical condition and seeks reaffirmation of his condition.
   d. D.D. is beginning to communicate underlying fears of his condition ("Did I do OK?").

E Problem	F Specific OT objectives	G Methods used to meet objectives	H Gradation of treatment
a, b, c	Given training and practice performance of self-care skills will be independent at a modified MET level without symptoms	Daily practice in ADL with slow progression and close monitoring of blood pressure, heart rate, signs and symptoms, and ECG Use of energy conservation techniques and equipment as necessary: sit-down bathing with shower chair, limited standing, and slow and rhythmical pace with intermittent rests Limited bending and reaching: use of long-handled bath brush, easy to reach set-ups (shower-caddy), and extra long bath towel. Control of temperature: lukewarm water only and good exhaust fan or door slightly open to prevent buildup of humidity Limited upper extremity activity above heart level: washing hair slowly with intermittent rests; easy-care hair cut; avoiding straining to reach back of hair with brush	Gradual progression if all signs are appropriate; if adverse signs develop, consultation with medical team Progression according to MET level: Bathing: full support in bed; independent for hands and face only; increase to include arms and chest Full support in bedside chair: independent for all body parts except feet and back; use of long bath brush for legs; standing for short periods for independent perianal care No support chair in bathroom: independent for all body parts; use of brush for back and feet; use of extra long towels and sit-down shower
c, f	Given training and assistive devices patient will be independent in lower extremity dressing with minimal use of Valsalva maneuvers and isometrics caused by compensating for decreased hip motion	Dressing: sit-down method, intermittent standing Pace: slow and rhythmical with rests between upper and lower extremity dressing and after each lower extremity item; controlled by verbal cues (working to music or to a metronome), by regulating schedule and extending uninterrupted time set aside for ADL, or by prefacing activity with relaxation techniques or breathing exercises or guided imagery Limited bending and reaching: use of cross-legged technique, reachers, long-handled shoe horn, slip-on shoes, sock aid, and/or No-Bows	Similar gradation as for problems a, b, and c, progression with upper extremity then lower extremity dressing Establishment of effective pacing followed by decreasing external cues so patient develops intrinsic pacing skills Establishment of rest periods; rest period after bathing; gradual increase of the number of activities that can be safely done before a rest period Time rest and activity periods: gradual decrease in rest phases and increase in time spent in activity longer

Continued.

Sample treatment plan—cont'd

E Problem	F Specific OT objectives	G Methods used to meet objectives	H Gradation of treatment
b, c, d	Given training and daily practice patient will be independent in functional mobility without symptoms	Daily practice with bed mobility techniques using proper body mechanics to minimize isometrics and Valsalva maneuvers Task analysis of bed mobility: Begin with rolling, legs out of bed, gravity assisted, and side to sit while exhaling No use of bedrails Seek medical clearance to lie flat; if shortness of breath interferes, pursue equipment set-up: electric bed, pillow props, and wedged cushion	Physical assistance with scooting, repositioning, and coming to sit Performance of all unresisted motions: rolling and feet out of bed Use of bed controls for up to sit Performance of all antigravity motions: up to sit and feet into bed; no straining or exhaling on effort; no equipment
g, h	Given demonstration and practice patient will be independent in energy conservation and pacing techniques and will carry them over to ADL consistently	Demonstration of energy-efficient transfer techniques with daily practice Demonstration of use of larger muscle groups (legs) for transfers; Discourage straining, pulling, and gripping with arms Body mechanics technique: coming to standing by moving to edge of chair, stable foot placement, lean forward, breath out, and stand Training in energy efficient "sit first" technique for car and tub transfers	Initially, transfers from higher surfaces; progression to transfers to and from lower surfaces (standard toilet and household furniture) Initially, with firm surfaces; progression to cushions; If still straining with proper breathing and body mechanics, use equipment and have patient avoid difficult surfaces unless assistance is available
e, g, h	Given instruction patient will demonstrate a working knowledge of activity guidelines, restrictions, and symptoms so he can explain them to other patients	Educational presentations (multisensory) and individual and group methods Structured problem-solving exercises: discussion and/or experiential trial and error techniques; patient is given criteria to judge what makes up an energy efficient technique: no symptoms (blood pressure, heart rate, ECG appropriate; RPE score less than 11-13); Patient judges and is led to decision Patient is informed of all vital sign monitoring and interpretation and is involved in assessing his own vital signs; he can take his own pulse, read ECG strip, and listen to heart beat Written guidelines for home use Program questionnaire (quiz) Patient is responsible for explaining general guidelines to new patients Arrangements with home health agency for homemaking services and medication and dietary compliance	Instruction Experiential Demonstration Reinforcement Problem solving Practice Follow up: Activities up to 2.5 METs are permitted Energy conservation to be used with all self-care activities from 2.5 to 3.5 METs Following guidelines for 6 weeks; after course of conditioning, reassessment of home program No activities over 3.5 METs

I. Special equipment.
1. Shower chair.
2. Long-handled bath brush.
3. Long-handled dressing aids.
4. Shoe adaptations (No-Bows or elastic laces).
5. Reacher.
6. Raised toilet seat.

REVIEW QUESTIONS

1. Describe the sequence of events (cardiac cycle) responsible for the heart's function as a systematic pump.
2. Name the symptoms and consequences encountered with prolonged cardiac ischemia.
3. Name the cardiac risk factors that can be contolled by medical and therapeutic intervention.
4. Which patients in general rehabilitation clinics may require special program modification as a result of secondary cardiac involvement?
5. Under what circumstances is exercise and activity absolutely contraindicated?
6. List the signs and symptoms of cardiac intolerance to activity.
7. Demonstrate and describe the method of taking an accurate blood pressure.
8. What are "METs," and how are they used in cardiac rehabilitation?
9. Design a cardiac rehabilitation activity program to be performed over 1 week for a 53-year-old man with cardiomyopathy. He has been described as a class III cardiac case.

REFERENCES

1. Aiken, L.H., and Henrichs, T.F.: Systematic relaxation as a nursing intervention technique with open heart surgery patients, Nurs. Res. **20:**212, 1971.
2. American Heart Association: Exercise testing and training of apparently healthy individuals: a handbook for physicians, New York, 1972, American Heart Association.
3. American Heart Association: Coronary risk handbook, Dallas, 1973, American Heart Association.
4. American Heart Association: Cardio-pulmonary resuscitation: advanced life support, JAMA Suppl. Aug. 1980.
5. American Heart Association: Recommendations for human blood pressure determination by sphygmomanometers, Dallas, 1980, American Heart Association Communications Division.
6. American Heart Association: Heart facts: 1983, Dallas, 1983, American Heart Association.
7. American Heart Association: The heart of the home, Dallas, American Heart Association.
8. Andreoli, K.G., et al.: Comprehensive cardiac care: a text for nurses, physicians, and other health practitioners, St. Louis, 1983, The C.V. Mosby Co.
9. Astrand, P.O., and Rodahl, K.: Textbook of work physiology, New York, 1970, McGraw-Hill, Inc.
10. Bates, B.: A guide to physical examination, ed. 2, Philadelphia, 1979, J.B. Lippincott Co.
11. Bedsworth, J.A., and Molen, M.T.: Psychological stress in spouses of patients with myocardial infarction, Heart Lung **11:**450, 1982.
12. Borg, G., et al.: RPE collection of papers presented at ACSM Annual Meeting, 1981, Med. Sci. Sports Exerc. **14:**376, 1982.
13. Bragg, T.L.: Psychological response to myocardial infarction, Nurs. Forum **14:**383, 1975.
14. Brock, L.L., et al.: Cardiac rehabilitation unit program guide, Dallas, 1977, American Heart Association.
15. Burch, G.E., and De Pasquale, N.P.: Primer of clinical measurement of blood pressure, St. Louis, 1962, The C.V. Mosby Co.
16. Chatham, M., and Knapp, B.: Patient education handbook, Bowie, Md., 1982, Robert J. Brady Co.
17. Colorado Heart Association: Exercise equivalents, Denver, 1970, Cardiac Reconditioning and Work Evaluation Unit, Spalding Rehabilitation Center. Pamphlet.
18. Comoss, P., Burke, E., and Swails, S.: Cardiac rehabilitation: a comprehensive nursing approach, Philadelphia, 1979, J.B. Lippincott Co.
19. Coronary Heart Disease Rehabilitation/Cardiac Rehabilitation Unit, Denver, 1971, University of Colorado Medical Center, Department of Physical Medicine and Rehabilitation. Pamphlet.
20. Daughton, D.M., et al.: Maximum oxygen consumption and the ADAPT© Quality-of-Life Scale, Arch. Phys. Med. Rehabil. **63:**620, 1982.
21. Dawber, T.R.: The Framingham study: the epidemiology of arteriosclerotic disease, Cambridge, Mass., 1980, Harvard University Press.
22. de Vries, H.A.: Physiology of exercise, Dubuque, Iowa, 1978, Wm. C. Brown Co., Publishers.
23. Dubin, D.: Rapid interpretation of EKGs, Tampa, Florida, 1974, C.O.V.E.R, Inc.
24. Ellestad, M.H., et al.: The exercise standards book, Dallas, 1979, American Heart Association.
25. Fox, S.M., Naughton, J.P., and Gorman, P.A.: Physical activity and cardiovascular health: the exercise prescription, frequency and type of activity, Mod. Concepts Cardiovasc. Dis. **41:**6, 1972
26. Froelicher, V.F.: Exercise in the prevention of atherosclerotic heart disease. In Wenger, N., editor: Exercise and the heart, Philadelphia, 1978, F.A. Davis Co.
27. Gentry, W.D., and Haney, T.: Emotional and behavioral reaction to acute myocardial infarction, Heart Lung **4:**738, 1975.
28. Halpenny, C.J.: The cardiac cycle. In Underhill, S.L., et al., editors: Cardiac nursing, Philadelphia, 1982, J.B. Lippincott Co.
29. Haskell, W.L.: Design of a cardiac conditioning program. In Wenger, N., editor: Exercise and the heart, Philadelphia, 1978, F.A. Davis Co.
30. Kattus, A.A., et al.: Exercise testing and training of apparently healthy individuals: a handbook for physicians, Dallas, 1972, American Heart Association.
31. Kattus, A.A., et al.: Exercise testing and training of individuals with heart disease or at high risk for its development: a handbook for physicians, Dallas, 1975, American Heart Association.
32. Katz, A.: Effects of ischemia and hypoxia upon the myocardium. In Russak, H., and Zohman, B., editors: Coronary heart disease, Philadelphia, 1971, J.B. Lippincott Co.
33. Katz, A.M.: Physiology of the heart, New York, 1977, Raven Press.
34. Kottke, F.J.: Common cardiovascular problems in rehabilitation. In Krusen, F.H., Kottke, F.J., and Ellwood, P.M., editors: Handbook of physical medicine and rehabilitation, Philadelphia, 1971, W.B. Saunders Co.
35. Kruida, H.: Fundamental principles of circulation physiology for physicians, New York, 1979, Elsevier North-Holland, Inc.
36. Lancour, J.: How to avoid pitfalls in measuring blood pressure, Am. J. Nurs. **76:**773, 1976.
37. Lehmann, J.: Auscultation of heart sounds, Am. J. Nurs. **72:**1242, 1972.

38. Maloney, F.P., and Moss, K.: Energy requirements for selected activities, Denver, 1974, Department of Physical Medicine, National Jewish Hospital. Unpublished.

39. Megenity, J., and Magenity, J.: Patient teaching: theories, techniques and strategies, Bowie, Md., 1982, Robert J. Brady Co.

40. Milnor, W.R.: The heart as a pump. In Mountcastle, V.B., editor: Medical physiology, vol. II, ed. 14, St. Louis, 1979, The C.V. Mosby Co.

41. Newton, K., and Sivaraian, E.: Cardiac rehabilitation: life style adjustments. In Underhill, S.L., et al., editors: Cardiac nursing, Philadelphia, 1982, J.B. Lippincott Co.

42. New York Heart Association, Inc.: Nomenclature and criteria for diagnosis of diseases of the heart and great vessels, ed. 8, Boston, 1979, Little, Brown and Co.

43. Niles, N., and Wills, R.: Heart failure. In Underhill, S.L., et al., editors: Cardiac nursing, Philadelphia, 1982, J.B. Lippincott Co.

44. Oberman, A., and Kouchoukos, N.: Role of exercise after coronary artery bypass surgery. In Wenger, N., editor: Exercise and the heart, Philadelphia, 1978, F.A. Davis Co.

45. Ogden, L.D.: Cardiac rehabilitation program design: occupational therapy, Downey, Calif., 1981, Cardiac Rehabilitation Resources.

46 Ogden, L.D.: Guidelines for analysis and testing of activities of daily living with cardiac patients, Downey, Calif., 1981, Cardiac Rehabilitation Resources.

47. Ogden, L.D.: Initial evaluation of the cardiac patient: occupational therapy, Downey, Calif., 1981, Cardiac Rehabilitation Resources.

48. Ogden, L.D.: Procedure guidelines for monitored self-care evaluation and monitored task evaluation, Downey, Calif., 1981, Cardiac Rehabilitation Resources.

49. Passmore, R., and Durnen, J.V.: Human energy expenditure, Physiol. Rev. **35**:801, 1955.

50. Rushmer, R.F.: Cardiovascular dynamics, Philadelphia, 1976, W.B. Saunders Co.

51. Santa Clara Valley Medical Center: Cardiac rehabilitation program protocol, San Jose, Calif., 1983. Unpublished.

52. Scalzi, C., and Burke, L.: Myocardial infarction: behavioral responses of patient and spouses. In Underhill, S.L., et al., editors: Cardiac nursing, Philadelphia, 1982, J.B. Lippincott Co.

53. Silverman, M.: Examination of the heart: the clinical history, Dallas, 1978, American Heart Association.

54. Sivarajan, S.E.: Cardiac rehabilitation: activity and exercise programs. In Underhill, S.L., et al., editors: Cardiac Nursing, Philadelphia, 1982, J.B. Lippincott Co.

55. Sokolow, M., and McIlroy, M.B.: Clinical cardiology, Los Altos, Calif., 1977, Lange Medical Publications.

56. Solack, S.: Pathophysiology of myocardial ischemia and infarction. In Underhill, S.L., et al., editors: Cardiac nursing, Philadelphia, 1982, J.B. Lippincott Co.

57. Trobaugh, G.: Cardiomyopathies. In Underhill, S.L., et al., editors: Cardiac nursing, Philadelphia, 1982, J.B. Lippincott Co.

58. Underhill, S.L.: Valvular disorders. In Underhill, S.L., et al., editors: Cardiac nursing, Philadelphia, 1982, J.B. Lippincott Co.

59. Vander Werf, T.: Cardiovascular pathophysiology, New York, 1980, Oxford University Press.

60. Wenger, N.: The physiological basis of early ambulation after myocardial infarction. In Wenger, N., editor: Exercise and the heart, Philadelphia, 1978, F.A. Davis Co.

61. Wulff, K., and Hong, P.: Surgical intervention for coronary artery disease. In Underhill, S.L., et al., editors: Cardiac nursing, Philadelphia, 1982, J.B. Lippincott Co.

CHAPTER 26

Low back pain

SALLY ABELE ROOZEE

Low back pain has probably plagued human beings since they stood upright.[7] Today low back pain has become a national health problem. In 1980 statistics from *Time*[7] predicted that 8 out of every 10 Americans will have a back problem some time in their lives. Anderson[1] states that more people miss work because of back pain than because of any other disease or injury. In a study done by Frymoyer[4] it is estimated that 217 million work days are lost annually because of back pain. In dollars and cents it is estimated that Americans spend more than $50 billion each year on low back pain. This amount includes expenses of hospital and medical services, as well as loss of work productivity, compensation payments, and litigation.[6]

With statistics as staggering as these, it can be easily recognized that low back pain is a surmounting economic and health concern. Because of this fact, occupational therapists will become increasingly involved in the treatment and prevention of low back pain. The skills and knowledge that an occupational therapist possesses lend themselves well to the treatment of low back pain, and as the occupational therapist's involvement increases, he or she will find it to be an exciting and challenging field in which to work.

Why do individuals have back aches? Health care professionals cite many reasons that may be responsible for the prevalence of low back pain in America. The evolutionary predicament of human beings going from a quadruped to a biped stance with the back taking the abuse may be one of the causes for the prevalence of low back pain. Other causes or risk factors may be attributed to an ever increasing sedentary lifestyle. Because of the conveniences of modern technology, Americans are physically not as active as their grandparents. Americans tend to be overweight, which contributes to extra stress on the spine. The back is further abused by the practice of bad habits, such as poor posture and the use of poor body mechanics in activities of daily living (ADL). Prolonged postures and certain repetitive motions can also contribute stress to the spine. Last but not least is the unavoidable accident or the trauma-induced injury to the back. Any or all of these factors contribute to the wear and tear of the structures of the spine that may result in low back pain or an injury to the back.

Low back pain is a complex and multifaceted problem. The patient that experiences low back pain may be affected physically, psychologically, economically, socially, and recreationally. As a result, this disability requires medical professionals who are knowledgeable, sensitive, and versatile for successful treatment.

MEDICAL MANAGEMENT
Anatomy of the spine

To understand the medical and therapeutic management of low back pain, a brief review of anatomy and anatomical terms is necessary.

The spine is comprised of 33 vertebrae: 7 cervical, 12 thoracic, 5 lumbar, 5 sacral, and 4 coccygeal stacked on top of each other. The cervical, thoracic, and lumbar vertebrae remain distinct and separate from each other throughout life. The adult sacral and coccygeal vertebrae are fused or united with each other to form two bones, the sacrum and the coccyx.[3] Intervertebral disks separate the vertebrae, and a system of muscles and ligaments helps to provide alignment and mobility to the spine. The function of the vertebral column is to support human beings in an upright position that is mechanically balanced to conform to the stress of gravity.[2]

The vertebrae in the cervical, thoracic, and lumbar areas are all slightly different in size and shape, but they each have the same basic components. The vertebral body is the large portion of the vertebra and the area that is the weight-bearing surface. The transverse processes are located on both sides of the vertebral body. These processes serve as points of attachments for muscles. Slightly above and below the transverse processes are the facets. These articulations determine the direction of movement between two adjacent vertebrae. By their directional planes the facets prevent or restrict movement in a direction contrary to the planes of articulations.[2]

Two other areas on the vertebrae are the pedicles and the laminae, which are bony arches that help form the protective spinal foramen. The spinous process is the posterior portion of the vertebrae, which one feels as the "bumps" along the spine. These processes also serve as attachment sites for muscles.

In between the vertebrae are the intervertebral disks. The disks separate the vertebrae, act as shock absorbers, and serve as cushions on which the vertebrae may move. The disk is much like a jelly doughnut with a fibrous outer ring, the anulus, and the center, a colloidal gelatin, known as the nucleus pulposus. The mechanism by which a disk functions is similar to a water balloon between two hands. As compressive forces push evenly down on the vertebral body, the distribution of the nucleus is equal in all directions. If the force is exerted more on one side than another, however, the nucleus is forced predominately in the opposite direction of the force. This mechanism exists with the various movements of the spine, such as forward flexion, extension, and lateral flexion.

As an individual ages the disk loses some of its water and elastic properties. This results in the intervertebral disk space becoming narrower. The facets are closer and in some instances may touch each other, the mechanism of the disk becomes more sluggish, and the anulus is more brittle. All of these changes, which occur as a part of the natural aging process, make human beings more susceptible to back problems as they become older.

The most important factor to remember about a disk is that it is constantly under pressure. The pressure is increased every time an individual bends forward slightly. The repetiveness with which one flexes forward every day continues to exert pressure on one area of the disk. Little tears gradually begin to appear in the anulus, and then one day a movement as simple as bending over to pick up a newspaper may result in a herniated disk. This process is insidious, painless, and there are no warning signs. However, it is a situation that can be prevented.

The ligaments of the spine run longitudinally along the vertebral column. They restrict movement in some directions and prevent any significant shearing action by their points of attachment.[2] The intervertebral disks are surrounded by ligaments anteriorly and posteriorly. The anterior longitudinal ligament runs anterior to the vertebral bodies and is broad and strong with intimate attachment to each vertebral body. In contrast the posterior longitudinal ligament is situated along the posterior surface of the vertebral bodies, which also forms the anterior surface of the spinal canal.[5] This ligament is intact throughout the entire length of the vertebral column until it reaches the lumbar region, which is of functional and potential pathological significance. At the first lumbar level it begins to progressively narrow so that on reaching the last lumbar, first sacral interspace, the ligament is half of its original width. This ultimate narrow posterior ligamentous reinforcement contributes to an inherent structural weakness at the level where there is the greatest static stress and the greatest spinal movement producing the greatest kinetic strain.[2]

The muscles of the low back are numerous and interrelate and function together in many instances. For the purpose of this chapter, muscles will be grouped together according to their action on the spine. The muscles that extend the spine include the quadratus lumborum; the sacrospinalis, also known as the erector spinae; the multifidus; the intertransversarii; and the interspinales.[3] These muscles work together to maintain an individual in an upright posture and to actively extend the lumbar spine. The primary flexors of the lumbar spine are the abdominal muscles that include the obliquus externus abdominis, the obliquus internus abdominis, the transversalis abdominis, and the rectus abdominis. Along with the abdominal muscles, the psoas major and minor are also considered flexors of the lumbar spine.[3] To classify a muscle as either a flexor or extensor of the

lumbar spine implies bilateral simultaneous muscle action. However, unilateral action of some muscles will result in lateral bending or lumbar abduction. Therefore the abductors of the lumbar spine are the quadratus lumborum, psoas major and minor, musculi abdominis, and the intertransversarii.[3] In summary the muscles of the lumbar spine function to allow motion to occur and help to maintain the upright posture.

The spinal cord is encased by the vertebrae and supporting structures. As the nerve roots descend the spinal canal, they cross the disk immediately above the intervertebral foramen.[2] As they emerge from the foramen, the nerves divide into the anterior and posterior primary divisions, and one branch goes immediately to the facets.[2] Because of this close relationship of the nerves to the structures of the spine, the nerve roots are susceptible to impingement and entrapment.

In summary the spine is comprised of a network of structures, the vertebrae, disks, ligaments, and muscles, all working together to keep a person upright, to allow movement to occur, and to provide stability. The lumbar spine withstands the greatest kinetic strain, and it is also the area that is most vulnerable to trauma and injury.

Diagnosis

Medical diagnosis of a low back problem involves a multifaceted evaluation. Initially the physician will obtain a thorough history from the patient, which includes the following questions. When did the symptoms occur? What brought on the symptoms? Describe the pain. How often does the pain occur? What relieves the symptoms? What aggravates the symptoms? How does this limit functioning?

The physical examination, according to Finneson,[3] should consist of 12 steps.

1. Inspection, that is, observing the patient as he or she moves, walks, and sits as well as observing the spine and buttocks is the first part of the examination.
2. The patient's gait is observed for a short distance, and then the physician may ask the patient to walk on his or her heels and then on the

toes to detect any muscle weakness.
3. Mobility of the spine is examined next by having the patient go through the motions of trunk flexion, extension, lateral flexion, and rotation. Range of motion (ROM) or mobility of the spine is generally not recorded in degrees, but rather as "normal," "slightly" limited (moves through three-fourths ROM), "moderately" limited (moves through one-half ROM), or "severely" limited (moves through one-fourth or less ROM).
4. The patient squats with complete flexion of the knees and hips. Any pain produced in the low back, knees, or hips is noted.
5. Reflex testing of the deep tendon reflexes of the ankle and patella is conducted on the patient to determine if there is any nerve root problems.
6. Leg length is measured to determine that the low back pain is not produced by a discrepancy in the length of the patient's two legs.
7. Sensation testing for light touch and pain is performed on the individual with back pain symptoms.
8. Motor strength is evaluated by testing the muscles in the lower extremities. Measurement of the circumference of the thigh and the calf of both legs may also be done to determine if there is any significant difference in the size of the two extremities.
9. Straight leg raising is done on both lower extremities to determine if there is sciatic nerve involvement. This test will also indicate the tightness of the hamstring muscles.
10. Internal and external rotation of the hip is performed as part of the evaluation process to eliminate any hip disease. Pain with internal rotation of the hip indicates a sacroiliac dysfunction.
11. Spinal pressure is examined, which involves applying pressure over the spinous processes of the lumbar spine to determine areas of local tenderness or reproduction of sciatic pain.
12. Arterial pulses of the inguinal, popliteal, and dorsalis pedis sites are carefully checked.[3]

As an adjunct to the physical examination, a physician may order other diagnostic tests to assist in the determination of the cause of the low back symptoms. An x-ray examination may be ordered to detect fractures, dislocation, infections, tumors, and other metabolic diseases. Common abnormalities seen on an x-ray film may include transitional vertebrae (either a sacralized lumbar vertebra or a lumbarized sacral vertebra), spina bifida, increased lumbar lordosis, scoliosis, intervertebral disk narrowing, asymmetrical lumbosacral facets, osteoarthritis, and spondylolisthesis.[3] In the majority of low back pain patients, however, a specific cause of the symptomatology is not clearly demonstrated by x-ray examinations. Therefore further testing may be necessary. Contrast x-ray studies, such as myelograms and diskograms, may be done to determine the condition of the spinal canal and the disks.

In recent years a computerized tomography (CT) scan has been developed that has many advantages over conventional x-ray films. The CT scan is noninvasive and permits visualization of fine anatomical detail by providing displays of thin slices of various planes. Furthermore, it permits discrimination of more differing tissue densities than conventional x-ray film techniques. Soft tissue organs, muscle, bone, fat, blood, metal, and iodinated contrast material all can be clearly distinguished on a CT scan.[3] Traditionally the lumbar myelogram has served as the primary diagnostic imaging method of the lumbosacral spine in the low back pain syndrome. However, a CT body scan of the lumbar spine has significant advantages over the earlier procedure in terms of accuracy, risk, accessibility, availability, and an ease of performance and is fast becoming one of the primary diagnostic tools in low back pain.[3]

Other diagnostic tests may be done to determine motor or sensory disorders. Electromyography and nerve conduction velocity studies are among the additional tests that the physician may order. Lumbar epidural or facet blocks may be done as a diagnostic procedure or as a method of treatment. These procedures generally involve injecting a peripheral nerve or facet with an anesthetic agent and sometimes a corticosteroid.

Nonsurgical management of low back pain

In the management of low back pain the physician's objectives are alleviating pain, restoring motion and mobility, minimizing residual impairment, preventing recurrence, and preventing entry into a chronic pain cycle.[2] One of the most important treatments in low back pain is rest. Patients who have low back discomfort from any cause will generally instinctively attempt to avoid activity and will rest. The method and extent of rest largely depend on the severity and nature of the symptoms. For example, an individual suffering from mild low back discomfort may only be restricted from heavy lifting, prolonged standing and flexion postures, excessive stooping, and long automobile trips.[3] In other cases, however, strict bed rest at home or in a hospital may be necessary. In strict bed rest all meals are to be taken in bed and the patient is not allowed to get up except for toilet activities. Generally the preferred position in bed is lying supine with the knees and hips slightly flexed or lying on one side with the knees flexed. However, this may vary according to the patient's condition and the physician's preference. It must be recognized that in prolonged bed rest a certain degree of muscle atrophy will occur as a result of lack of activity and muscle disuse. Additionally there may be loss of calcium from the bones, loss of protein, and certain circulatory changes may cause light-headedness in some cases.[3] Once bed rest is discontinued, a program of strengthening and improving endurance will be necessary.

Traction is a time-honored procedure used in the conservative treatment of low back dysfunction. It has gained the reputation of being "specific" treatment for the herniated lumbar disk. However, traction in the manner and force usually applied does not distract the vertebrae but decreases the lordosis, thus separating the facets and opening the foramina. It also gradually overcomes the spasm of the erector spinae.[2]

Recently medical literature has advocated total body weight traction applied in the hospital environment in a mechanical circular bed. This uses the concept that 30% of the total body weight is found below the third lumbar vertebra. If the patient is suspended at the thoracic cage, this amount of weight is applied as lumbar traction.[2]

Modalities used in the conservative treatment of low back pain may include therapeutic cold, superficial heat, ultrasound, or transcutaneous electrical nerve stimulation. According to Finneson,[3] therapeutic cold is the most effective modality in the treatment of acute low back pain. He stated that physiological cooling is associated with a decrease in the tissue metabolic rate and a vasoconstriction of the arterial system. The vasoconstriction leads to an effect that penetrates tissues deeper than does heat. Superficial heat can be effective in low back pain problems. However, it produces a vasodilation that can promote swelling. Therefore an individual with low back pain following trauma who may have tissue disruption has a tendency to produce swelling, and this treatment would be contraindicated.[3] Ultrasound is another method of providing heat to deeper tissues. This modality is generally not indicated in the acute phase of low back pain as a result of the tendency of heat to produce swelling.

Transcutaneous electrical nerve stimulation (TENS) is a modality that uses a mild electrical current to modulate the sensation of pain. TENS does not cure any of the symptoms causing the pain, but it can help reduce the severity and duration of the pain and may be used instead of medication. The device consists of a small pocket-size, battery-operated pulse generator that can be worn clipped to the clothing. Electrodes are adhered to the skin at or near the site of pain or over a nerve trunk representative of the painful area. Cables or leads attached to the electrodes run to the pulse generator where they are connected. TENS can only be used with the prescription of a physician.

Medications may be prescribed for individuals suffering from acute low back pain and may include analgesics, muscle relaxants, antiinflammatory drugs, and antidepressant drugs. Medications for the alleviation of pain are best used on a specified basis of every 4 to 6 hours depending on the life of the drug, rather than as requested by the patient. For patients susceptible to addiction or dependency drugs become a reward for pain and are difficult in later periods of illness to decrease or discontinue.[2]

Most muscle relaxants are sedatives and are capable also of being depressants. It is recommended that they be given in limited doses and eliminated before too much depression occurs. Oral antiinflammatory medication is valuable when administered for a limited time. It, as other drugs, has side effects that must be carefully explained to the patients. Antidepressant drugs may be prescribed and are valuable in patients who have been premorbidly depressed or who react to their acute impairment with depression.[2]

Once a person has recovered from the painful acute stages of low back pain, bed rest has been discontinued, and the patient is on limited activity, exercise becomes an important treatment in low back pain. As cited previously, bed rest is a common treatment for the patient with low back pain, but even with bed rest the side effects of decreased strength and endurance are encountered. An exercise program may include specific exercises for the low back, strengthening exercises for supporting structures, and endurance exercises. Education of the patient with low back pain is another important facet in the treatment phase. The educational phase should include principles of body mechanics, energy conservation, simple anatomy of the spine, and principles of injury prevention.

The combination of rest, modalities, exercise, and education should help most patients suffering from low back pain. However, there will be a small percentage of patients who will have to undergo surgical intervention to alleviate the problem. Today most physicians are trying the conservative methods of treatment before recommending surgery. If a patient does undergo surgery, a recovery stage similiar to that stated previously will be instituted as well. Immediately after surgery the patient will be ordered to rest in bed, progressing to limited activity, and later to an exercise and maintenance program, which will include the same components described earlier.

Acute versus chronic pain

Acute, symptomatic pain serves the useful purpose of warning an individual that something is wrong and serves as a diagnostic aid to the physician. Yet when the sudden, jabbing sharpness of acute pain persists and results in a chronic condition, pain then becomes a complex malady and a menace to the individual, his or her family, and ultimately to society. The point at which acute low back pain becomes chronic is a debatable issue. Finneson[3] stated that chronic low back pain can be defined as that which is present for more than 3 days. Cailliet[2] stated that low back pain considered to have existed less than 2 months can be termed acute. Since there is disagreement as to the exact timing when acute pain becomes chronic, perhaps it is better to state that chronic intractable low back pain is more of an attitude on the part of the patient.[8] Acute pain demands a need for immediate relief. Medication, rest, modalities, and often surgery will accomplish this goal. Chronic pain may have mechanical irritating factors, such as structural defects, disk herniations, and congenital or disease problems. Contributing nonmechanical factors include anxiety, depression, frustration, and paranoia.[8] No matter when acute low back pain becomes chronic, the individual with chronic pain has a complex condition.

The patient with chronic low back pain may have some of the same symptoms and restrictions as the individual with acute pain. For example, the patient is suffering from pain, which restricts his or her ADL, such as tying shoes, driving a car, and performing yard activities and household tasks. The pain further restricts the patient's social and recreational events because he or she is unable to sit through a movie or church, for example. The patient cannot play ball with his or her children and is unable to work because the pain restricts the activities required for the job. However, once the pain persists for a length of time, unlike the patient with acute low back pain, the person suffering from chronic pain soon may undergo a change in income status because he or she can no longer work. The spouse may have to take a job or increase the number of hours working, and there may be a reversal of roles in the family. The patient continues to make trips to physicians only to have more of the same tests, more medication, and possibly to have initial or recurrent surgery only to end up feeling the same. The patient becomes frustrated, feels hopeless, and develops a mistrust of the medical profession. The constant pain makes him or her irritable. The inability to work and function as previously makes him or her depressed, despondent, and angry. The increasing isolation from activities, friends, and even family members makes the patient fearful. The pain is ever present, serving as a reminder of all of his or her inabilities and slowly eroding self-esteem, motivation, and courage. It is obvious then that the patient suffering from chronic low back pain presents a picture of physical, psychological, economic, and social limitations.

REHABILITATION

Since the patient with low back pain, and especially chronic low back pain, has a myriad of symptoms and disabilities and because the syndrome is such a complex one, it is best dealt with by a variety of professionals. A team approach to treating low back pain is the best and preferred method of handling this syndrome. The team might include a physician, physiatrist, neurologist, orthopedist, psychiatrist or pscyhologist, physical therapist, occupational therapist, recreational therapist, social worker, and a vocational counselor.

Role of occupational therapy

The goal of an occupational therapist in the treatment of any patient is to help the patient achieve the maximal level of functional independence. In treating patients the occupational therapist makes an assessment of the person's limitations and problems, and a treatment program is designed around these facts to help alleviate or at least improve the existing conditions. No matter what problem or diagnosis exists or what methods of treatment are used, the occupational therapist's role is to provide the patient with the best opportunity to achieve maximal functional independence.

As noted previously, the patient with chronic low back pain has physical, psychological, social, and economic limitations. The occupational therapist has the skills to work with people who are depressed, angry, or have low self-esteem; the skills to assess joint restrictions, muscle weakness, and nerve involvement; and the skills to help people accomplish their daily activities with minimal effort and as independently as possible. With these skills the occupational therapist is a vital and important member of the health care team in the treatment of low back pain.

Assessment

The assessment of a patient with low back pain should include a four-part evaluation. If the occupational therapist is working as a member of a team, part of the assessment process may be done by another team member, such as the physical therapist. The entire assessment process is described here, but it can be adapted according to the division of responsibilities and the facilities available in the treatment environment (Fig. 26-1).

SUBJECTIVE ASSESSMENT. The first part of the evaluation consists of the "subjective assessment." This involves obtaining information from the patient through an interview and reading the medical records. First the therapist should obtain a pain history from the patient. A blank chart with the outline of a person with front and back views may be given to the patient with the instructions to draw in the areas of pain. Many times the manner in which the patient marks in his or her pain on the chart provides the evaluator with insight as to how the patient perceives the pain. For example, some patients merely mark the chart with a light line or "X" to represent where the pain is located. Other people will mark in the painful area heavily, practically coloring in the entire back or extremity. Although having the patient mark on the pain chart is not meant as an interpretative measure, the evalutor can surmise that when the patient colors in the area of pain marking in most of the chart that the patient views the pain as all-encompassing.

After the patient has marked the pain on the chart, the evaluator should follow through by asking the patient some additional questions. When did the pain occur? What caused the pain? Next, a description of the pain is obtained to include the quality of the pain, such as sharp, burning, or jabbing; the frequency of the pain, such as constant or intermittent; and the intensity of the pain, such as excruciating, moderate, or mild. Next, a series of questions can be asked to determine when the pain is worse, what exacerbates the condition, and what alleviates the pain. The evaluator will also want to know how the patient perceives that his or her ADL are interrupted or limited because of the low back pain. Furthermore, the therapist will want to know if this condition has existed in the past, and if so, what treatments seemed to help and which aggravated the condition. Finally, the evaluator needs to ascertain if the patient is taking any medication, what kind, and how often it is used. It is also important to ask the patient if he or she is using any orthotic or bracing devices.

Once the pain history has been obtained, it is important to ascertain what a typical day for the patient entails. This can be done by using the daily schedule described in Chapter 4. The patient is asked to describe in detail a typical day. Another method is to present the patient with a chart that breaks the day into small increments on which he or she can complete a daily schedule.

Finally, the evaluator should determine what the home and work situations entail. If the patient is still working or hopes to return to work, the evaluator should ask for a job description. Detail is necessary. Does the patient sit, stand, walk, or climb? Does the patient have to lift or carry objects, and if so, how much weight is he or she required to lift or carry, for how long, and for what distances? The evaluator should ask the patient to describe any problem tasks that he or she is involved with now or that he or she expects as problem tasks once the patient returns to work. It is also important to determine what the home atmosphere is like. Does the spouse work? Are there small children at home? What household or

yard tasks does the patient typically engage in on a routine basis?

PHYSICAL ASSESSMENT. The second phase of the evaluation is the physical assessment. In this category if the therapist is working as a member of a team, it should be determined definitely which discipline will undertake which parts of the evaluation. It is not fair to the patient for two disciplines to perform the same tests or procedures, especially if both services charge for the evaluation. Furthermore, it is a waste of time to duplicate certain procedures. If two or more disciplines work closely together to determine what the evaluation should include and what procedures will be followed, cooperation can be achieved and redundancy can be avoided.

ROM is the first part of the physical assessment. Even though a patient is suffering from low back pain, a quick assessment of the upper extremities is indicated. Certain motions do put a strain on the lower back, and the evaluator will want to know this. For example, shoulder flexion exceeding 90° causes a shift in the center of gravity, resulting in increased lordosis, which may aggravate a patient's symptoms. The upper extremity ROM test can be done actively with the patient standing and mimicking the evaluator's motions. Any limitations in ROM are noted in degrees, and any exacerbation of pain is recorded. ROM of the lower extremities should be done with more exactness than the upper extremities. Hip flexion, hip extension, straight leg raise, and hip internal and external rotation, which are key motions, should be tested passively, noting any limitations in degrees and any pain on execution of the test. Hip flexion should be tested with the patient lying supine, knee flexed, and then the hip flexed through the available ROM. Hip internal and external rotation are also done with the patient lying supine. The straight leg raise test should be done with the patient lying supine and both legs extended. When the lower extremity is to be tested the knee should remain fully extended with movement occurring at the hip through the patient's available ROM. A sitting straight leg raise test

Name: _____

Room number: _____

Physician: _____

O.T. AND P.T. LOW BACK EVALUATION

Subjective assessment

Age: _____   Date of onset: _____

Mechanism of injury: _____

_____

Description of pain: _____

_____

What aggravates pain? _____

What eases pain? _____

What time of day is pain worse? _____

Is pain better or worse when:

Lying _____   Position _____ Lying to sit _____
Sitting _____   Sitting time _____ Sit to stand _____
Standing _____   Standing time _____

Description of daily routine: _____

_____

Which tasks can or cannot be done?

Sleeping _____   Household tasks _____
Dressing _____   Yard tasks _____
Sink activities _____ Driving _____
Sitting _____   Working _____
Lifting _____   Reaching _____

Previous history

Back injuries or problems: _____

Hospitalizations: _____

Physical therapy: _____

Chiropractor: _____

Surgeries or procedures: _____

What treatments increased pain? _____

What treatments decreased pain? _____

Present medications: _____ Frequency: _____

Fig. 26-1. Low back evaluation.

Physical assessment

Range of motion

    Upper extremities (gross): _____

    Lower extremities:

	Left	Pain	Right	Pain
Hip flexion				
Hip extension				
Straight leg raise test in lying position				
Straight leg raise test in sitting position				
Hip external rotation				
Hip internal rotation				

    Trunk:

        Trunk flexion (standing) _____

        Trunk flexion (supine) _____

        Trunk extension (standing) _____

        Trunk extension (supine) _____

        Trunk hyperextension _____

        Lateral flexion (right) _____ (left) _____

        Trunk rotation (to right) _____ (to left) _____

Sensation (sharp to dull): _____
_____

Strength:

    Upper extremity (gross) _____
_____

    Trunk (functional) _____

    Lower extremity:

	Left	Pain	Right	Pain
Hip flexion (L2)				
Knee extension (L3)				
Dorsiflexion (L4)				
Extensor hallucis longus (L5)				
Plantar flexion (S1)				
Quad set (functional)				

Fig. 26-1, cont'd. Low back evaluation.

Functional assessment

ADL assessment:

	Level	Body mechanics	Pain
Lying			
Sitting			
Standing			
Supine lying to sitting			
Sitting to standing			
Tying shoes			
Sink activities			
Sweeping and vacuuming			
Reaching overhead			

Level code: IE = Independent
IG = Independent but movements guarded
A = Assisted
U = Unable
ND = Not done

Lifting:

0-36 inches _____

36-72 inches _____

0-72 inches _____

Endurance walk:

Time _____

Distance _____

Treadmill incline:

Minutes _____

mph _____

Upper extremity weights:

Bench press _____

Elbow flexion _____

Shoulder flexion _____

right _____

left _____

Lower extremity weights:

Leg press _____

Static quad _____

Posture (standing): _____

Sitting tolerance: _____ Standing tolerance: _____

Low back exercises: _____

Carrying:

Weight _____

Time _____

Distance _____

Treadmill level:

Minutes _____

mph _____

Bicycle:

Resistance _____

Time _____

Distance _____

Abduction:

right _____

left _____

_____

Fig. 26-1, cont'd. Low back evaluation.

Psychological assessment

Cooperative: _____ Motivated: _____

Hostile: _____ Withdrawn: _____

Outgoing: _____

Remarks: _____

Treatment goals

_____   _____

_____   _____

_____   _____

_____   _____

_____   _____

Plan _____

_____

_____

_____

_____

_____

_____

_____

_____ OTR

_____ RPT

_____ DATE

Fig. 26-1, cont'd. Low back evaluation.

may be done to observe any inconsistencies in the patient's performance. For a sitting straight leg raise test the patient should be sitting on the edge of a firm surface. The evaluator asks the patient to sit up straight so 90° hip flexion is present, then asks the patient to straighten out the knee and lift the leg as high as he or she can without tilting backward. The evaluator will watch that the patient does not compensate by leaning backward, thus decreasing the angle at the hip joint. If the patient can achieve only 40° straight leg raise in a supine position and 90° in a sitting position, this indicates a discrepancy and should be noted and investigated. Active ROM should be evaluated for trunk flexion, trunk extension, trunk hyperextension, lateral bending, and trunk rotation. The results for trunk extension, rotation, and hyperextension

should be recorded in degrees. Results from trunk flexion and lateral bending can be recorded either in degrees or in inches from a set landmark. For example, on trunk flexion the distance from the patient's fingertips to the floor can be measured and recorded. Lateral bending can be measured as inches above or below the knee joint. For all the previously mentioned motions any complaints of pain expressed during the testing should be recorded according to location and motion that evoked the pain.

Sensation testing is another part of the physical assessment. Generally sharp and dull sensation is tested. Using a pin wheel the examiner tests the patient's lower extremities in the dermatomal distributions. Any sensory abnormalities may help to indicate any possible nerve problems.

Evaluating the patient's strength is another important part of the assessment. Generally specific muscle testing of the trunk and lower extremities is performed, and a quick muscle test of the upper extremities should be done. Instead of testing the individual muscles in the entire trunk and lower extremities, the evaluator selects muscle groups that represent each nerve root in the lower extremity. Muscle testing is typically done on trunk flexion, hip flexion, knee extension, dorsiflexion and plantar flexion of the ankle, and extension of the great toe. Dorsiflexion and plantar flexion of the ankle may also be done by asking the patient to walk on the toes and the heels.

FUNCTIONAL ASSESSMENT. In the functional assessment as in the physical assessment, if the therapist is working with other team members, it must be determined who will be doing each part of the evaluation. The functional assessment can be thought of as the current status of the patient. What can the patient do now? What are the patient's capabilities and shortcomings?

To start, a functional assessment of the patient's capabilities of ADL is necessary. Some of this can be done through observation, and part of the assessment data may be obtained by interviewing and performing simulated tasks. It is not uncommon for patients with low back pain to complain or demonstrate difficulty in tying shoes, putting on shoes and socks, standing at a sink to shave or apply make-up, standing to wash dishes, sweeping, vacuuming, washing windows, and mowing the lawn. It is best for the evaluator to ask the patient to actually try these tasks or to simulate them as closely as possible.

As the evaluator is having the patient try certain tasks, he or she must always be observant of the manner in which the patient attempts the tasks. Does the patient use proper body mechanics? Does the patient do the task with ease, guardedly, with much effort, or is he or she unable to attempt the task at all? Is there any facial grimacing visible or sound of effort audible? All these factors should be noted. Even during the initial interview and physical assessment, the evaluator should observe the patient's movements. How does the patient get in and out of a chair? What sitting posture does the patient assume? How long can the patient sit before he or she must adjust his or her posture? In the physical assessment how does the patient get up from and down to the supine position?

In evaluating the use of body mechanics the evaluator should have the patient lift a box or object weighing no more than 5 pounds (2.3 kg) from the floor to a tabletop and then from a tabletop to a position 72 inches (182.9 cm) overhead. Again the way the task is accomplished should be observed and recorded. After instructing the patient in proper lifting techniques, the evaluator should gradually increase the amount of weight the patient is handling to obtain a maximal weight that the patient can lift to and from the three different heights (floor, tabletop, and overhead).

The patient's carrying capacity needs to be assessed. This can be done by asking the patient to carry the amount of weight he or she was able to lift to the tabletop. The evaluator asks the patient to walk a measured course until he or she becomes tired or starts to feel the pain becoming aggravated. This task is timed. The distance the patient was able to travel with the weight, the amount of weight carried, and the time are recorded.

The patient's posture should be evaluated. This can be accomplished by asking the patient to stand next to a plumb line. If a plumb line is not available, the evaluator asks the patient to stand erect and observes the patient's posture, noting any increases or decreases in the normal curves of the spine. The sitting posture can also be observed and noted. The patient's sitting and standing tolerances should be determined. If the evaluator has the opportunity to have the patient sit for a class, workshop, or interview, the therapist can document the amount of time the patient was able to sit. If the evaluator is unable to observe the patient in such a situation, then the evaluator asks the patient how long he or she thinks he or she can sit but compares it to something with a time frame, such as "Can you sit through a 30 minute television program?" The evaluator will want to determine the tolerance for standing as well, and the same techniques or questioning can be used.

PSYCHOLOGICAL ASSESSMENT. During the evaluation process the evaluator has an opportunity to talk with and become acquainted with the patient. From this contact with the patient, the evaluator will be able to obtain an idea of the client's psychological state. The patient throughout the evaluation process may express anger, frustration, hostility, or depression, and these attitudes should be noted as part of the evaluation. If there is a psychiatrist or psychologist on the rehabilitation team, however, a specific psychological assessment should be carried out by that professional.

On completion of the assessment treatment goals and a treatment program need to be established. The overall goal in treating the individual with low back pain is to help the patient reach the maximal level of independence. Of course the goals established for each individual may differ according to the findings of the assessment. However, there are a few general goals that will apply to most patients suffering from low back pain. The goals are to improve and maintain ROM and flexibility; to improve endurance; to develop proper ways of using the body (body mechanics); to understand the structures of the spine, how they work, and what the adverse forces are that should be avoided; and to improve functional capabilities.

Treatment

EDUCATION. One of the most important phases of the treatment program for a patient with low back pain is education. The person who has injured his or her back, is 10 times more likely to reinjure the back again within 1 year following the initial injury. Therefore teaching the patient how the back works, how to use proper body mechanics, and how to avoid unnecessary stresses are all important in preventing reinjury. The educational phase of a treatment program should include five areas of concentration. The first area is back anatomy, that is, teaching the patient the simple anatomy of the spine and the interrelationship of the structures and how they work together. Body mechanics, or how to use the body to obtain the most from it with the least amount of physical stress to the spine, is a vital part of the educational program. This includes discussion about the correct ways to stand, sit, sleep, lift, carry, stoop, climb, reach, sweep, vacuum, and rake.

Since psychological and emotional stresses can aggravate pain, sessions on stress management should be offered to the patient with low back pain. This can be done by using biofeedback, relaxation techniques, and classes on how to cope and reduce the everyday stresses of daily life.

Sessions about time management can be offered to the patient as a way of helping the patient learn how to pace his or her day and work tasks to avoid fatigue and overexertion. This is especially important for the patient who is just beginning to resume regular activities. This person may have the impulse or desire to immediately step back into a regular routine before he or she is physically ready to take on the stresses following surgery, a period of prolonged bed rest, or a period of limited activity. Besides helping the patient manage his or her time, discussion of realistic goal planning is imperative and complements the sessions of time management.

The last area of the educational phase should include a session on energy conservation. These sessions can help the person learn to reorganize home and office space to reduce the stresses placed on the back. For example, the individual should minimize the amount of reaching, bending, and twisting that is done in the daily activities while at work. Many times by simply reorganizing a cupboard or desk much of the reaching, bending, or twisting is eliminated.

The educational part of the patient's treatment program can be taught by any of several professionals. If the therapist is working in a team environment, the anatomy, time management, and stress management classes can be shared or presented by the individual most qualified and comfortable with the material, such as the occupational therapist or the physical therapist. The body mechanics and energy conservation sessions are generally instructed by the occupational therapist, but the physical therapist may also instruct patients in these areas. Again it is important to accomplish the goals set forth without conflict or duplication of services.

EXERCISE. In a setting in which a team approach to the treatment of low back pain is being used, the endurance training and lower extremity strengthening is customarily done by the physical therapist, whereas the upper extremity strengthening and functional training is done by the occupational therapist.

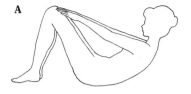

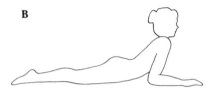

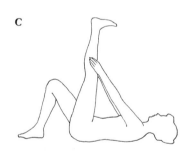

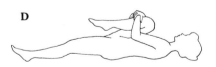

Fig. 26-2. Low back exercise. **A,** Partial sit-up. **B,** Back extension exercise. **C,** Straight leg raise exercise. **D,** Single knee to chest exercise.

Treatment programs for patients with low back pain usually involve instructing patients in specific exercises. The primary physician usually prescribes the type and frequency of exercises to be given to the patient. Depending on the diagnosis and condition of the patient's back the physician may prescribe flexion or extension exercises or even a combination of the two. Flexion and extension exercises refer to the action of the trunk and back. Flexion exercises generally involve trunk flexion exercises, such as sit-ups and single and double knee to chest exercises. Extension exercises refer to extension of the spine and include trunk hyperextension and hip extension exercises (Fig. 26-2). If any of the exercises aggravates a patient's pain beyond normal stretching or pulling sensation, the patient should stop, and the physician should be consulted.

In addition to specific exercises for the low back, exercises to improve the patient's upper and lower extremity strength may be a part of the treatment plan. Strengthening both the upper and lower extremities helps the patient lift, carry, and manage weighted objects better, and because the stronger muscles are doing the work, it eliminates stress that otherwise might be exerted to the back. Strengthening of the upper extremities can be done by using weight equipment or by merely using barbells or cuff weights. Generally the areas to strengthen are the elbow flexors, shoulder depressors, scapular stabilizers, and pectoralis major and minor. Strengthening of the lower extremities should be done by using specific equipment, such as a leg press. Static setting of the quadriceps muscles (quad sets) can be used as part of the strengthening program for the lower extremities.

Since many patients with low back pain have been on limited activity during their convalescence, there is usually a need to improve endurance. Endurance training can be done with a variety of activities, such as walking, riding a stationary bicycle, walking on a treadmill, or climbing stairs. The important factor in endurance training is that the patient should be started slowly and progressed at a steady, slow rate to allow him or her to build up tolerance and to prevent the creation of more pain and discomfort.

FUNCTIONAL PRACTICE. Another important phase of any treatment program is to provide the patient with the opportunity to practice many of the body mechanics techniques he or she has been taught. Standing, sitting, and lying posture should be practiced. If there is a video camera and monitor available, videotaping the patient's posture in various positions can be a valuable adjunct to therapy. Even taking a picture with an instant print camera can be beneficial and provide immediate feedback to the patient.

Functional practice of lifting, reaching, and carrying techniques is necessary in the treatment of low back pain. Not only does this practice help teach the patient the correct way to handle objects safely, but the activity can be graded so the patient gradually increases the amount of weight lifted and learns what he or she can and cannot handle. In the functional practice different size objects should be used, such as a box, suitcase, laundry basket, and grocery bag. Differing amounts of weight can be added or subtracted according to the patient's tolerance for the particular activity. For any patients who were injured on the job the carrying and lifting practice results are important information for the employer or the insurance agency. The information in many cases may determine whether the patient may return to the former occupation or not.

Functional practice of body mechanics can also be carried out in a "par course." This is a set of activities put together in an orderly sequence that the therapist asks the patient to perform. Many times this activity lends itself to videotaping and can be used for comparative testing before and after treatment. Depending on the purpose of the par course activity, a sequence of tasks are combined that requires a variety of body mechanic techniques. For example, the par course may start with the patient going to a cupboard or shelf and reaching for a few items, putting them into a box or sack, carrying it to a table, and setting it down. Then the patient may be asked to sweep paper shreds and pick the debris up in a dustpan. Any combination of activities can be put together. Generally patients like this type of activity because it is not repetitive, it stimulates real situations, and it sparks some interest. Functional practice activities are usually designed and administered by the occupational therapist, especially since so many of the activities are actual or simulations of ADL.

To include job simulation as part of the treatment program, special equipment and space may be needed. If the occupational therapy department serves a large number of worker's compensation cases, the work simulation may be an integral part of the program. Providing accurate, relevant, and well-documented data to an employer or insurance carrier is important in helping to determine the feasibility of return to employment. Simple job simulations can be devised for some people. For example, for a secretary, it would be easy to set up a situation in which the patient can type, file, and answer phones. However, some of the manual, heavy labor occupations entail more sophisticated equipment and space than is available in many facilities. Since work simulation in some cases is vital, the patient may have to be referred to another agency for a thorough work evaluation assessment.

PSYCHOLOGICAL SUPPORT. The approach that a therapist takes with low back pain patients will set the atmosphere for the entire treatment environment. A direct, honest, and sincere approach is always best. A therapist should strive to always inform the patient about any procedure in which the patient is about to become involved. Sharing with the patient why a certain task or procedure is about to be undertaken and relating it specifically to his or her condition will help alleviate the patient's apprehension, fear, or mistrust. This is especially true with those patients experiencing chronic low back pain. A therapist should not make promises of eliminating a patient's pain. A better approach to take is one that acknowledges the presence of the pain but focuses more on the functional goals and improvements. In dealing with patients with chronic pain a therapist may have to discourage the patient's "pain behavior," such as talking incessantly about the pain, holding the back with every movement, or moaning and grimacing. Generally if the therapist is sincere and honest, the patients will respond with cooperation and trust.

In the treatment plan for a patient with low back pain psychological support is vital. Many times patients will exhibit anger, frustration, depression, and low self-esteem. Depending on the extent of these symptoms, a psychologist or psychiatrist may be dealing with the patient. Engaging the person in leisure time activities or crafts, however, can do much to improve the outlook and feelings about him or herself. The occupational therapist can structure activities for the patient that are at a level that he or she can handle and that will provide him or her with a challenge so the patient has a feeling of accomplishment and self-worth. If a department has a workshop or craft area available, this is an ideal setting to allow patients with low back pain to participate in crafts. It is especially beneficial if more than one patient can work together while making crafts because interaction and socialization will occur.

Recreational therapy through the use of leisure activities can play an equally important part in the psychological support of individuals. Socialization, interaction, and accomplishment of a project all contribute to a patient's feelings of self-worth.

Group or individual counseling sessions may be conducted with patients who are experiencing chronic low back pain and who are exhibiting anger, frustration, and depression. However, trained personnel, such as a psychiatrist or psychologist, should be involved in these sessions. Family members may be encouraged to attend these or similar sessions to help them cope with the changes the patient and the family are experiencing.

Family members may also become involved in the educational process if time, circumstances, and situations allow this or if special sessions for family education can be established. Helping the family understand the anatomy and mechanisms of the spine will enhance their understanding of what a loved one might be encountering and may prevent another back problem in the family.

PAIN MODULATION. Pain modulation or pain reduction may be another part of the treatment program for the patient with low back pain. Any increase, decrease, or elimination of medications is handled by the physician, but it is important for other team members to be aware of this so they can be alerted to any changes in behavior that might indicate a drug reaction. With proper training and preparation therapists may become involved in pain reduction or modulation through the modalities of biofeedback, TENS, and relaxation. These can all be used in conjunction with other phases of the treatment program.

Progression of treatment

When to start a patient on certain phases of the treatment program and when to progress the patient in his or her activities once he or she is on a full treatment program are decisions based on the physician's recommendations, the therapist's knowledge, and the individual's performance. When a patient is in the acute stages of low back disability, the activities are limited and often the patient is resting in bed and in so much pain that even the educational phase of treatment will be of no benefit. At this stage rest and control of the pain are the primary objectives of the treatment program. The patient with chronic pain has different treatment goals. This person generally is not resting in bed but has been on limited activities for an extended period of time and to start the patient on a full treatment program may be detrimental. Once a physician has permitted the patient to participate in activities, the therapist must pay close attention and progress the patient at a slow, steady pace. Many of the therapist's clues to treatment progression will be given by the patient, and an alert, observant therapist will watch for the clues and grade the activities accordingly. For example, if a therapist is asking the patient to walk a certain distance and the first day the patient completes the task he or she is flushed, out of breath, and

complaining of increased pain, the program should not be progressed, and perhaps the activity level should be reduced. If on the third or fourth day, however, the patient completes the task with no increased symptoms and does not appear flushed or breathless, then perhaps the patient is ready to progress. When using weights in strengthening activities, progressive resistive exercise programs (PRE) are the safest for patients with low back pain. When a patient has successfully completed a maximal amount of weight on the PRE method, the therapist can ask the patient to try a few more repetitions at the maximal amount of weight. If the patient succeeds in completing 10 more repetitions at his or her maximal amount of weight, then it is time for the patient to progress to a higher weight limit. This type of progression can apply to any activity, even if it does not involve weight lifting. For example, if the patient has been riding on a stationary bicycle at 1 speed for 5 minutes with no difficulty and has even been increasing the mileage, the therapist can grade the program by increasing one of the parameters. In this case the therapist would probably increase the time and later the amount of resistance.

In any activities that are done with the patient it will be helpful to record and obtain as much objective data as possible because the data give an accurate picture of the patient's performance. For example, with an endurance walk activity the course should be measured for distance, and the patient and therapist should keep account of the number of laps the former does in a specified amount of time. On a stationary bicycle resistance, time, and mileage can all be recorded. On a treadmill incline, speed, and time are the available parameters.

By carefully progressing patients in their programs there should be no aggravation of pain and little muscle soreness. By meticulously progressing patients the therapist will instill confidence while allowing good habits and techniques to become ingrained.

Body mechanic techniques

Posture is the basic foundation of all good body mechanics. As stated earlier, the spine is composed of a column of

vertebrae, which is a curved column rather than a straight one. The curves serve a purpose and provide strength to the column. Therefore for proper alignment of the spine and good posture, it is important that these curves be maintained. Since the purpose of this chapter is to discuss low back pain, the focus of attention will be on the lumbar spine.

The lumbar spine withstands the most stresses. It supports the weight of the body and allows several motions to occur. The lumbar spine is also the most vulnerable area because it does not have the same ligamentous support as the other areas of the spine. Therefore it is especially important to be aware of the curves in the lumbar area. Any exaggeration of the curve contributes additional stresses to the structures of the lumbar area.

For proper posture one must be aware of the curves in the spine and the factors that influence these curves. The position of the pelvis plays an important role in the curves of the low back. By rotating the pelvis forward and backward, the lumbar curve is increased and decreased. Flexibility of the muscles in the lumbar, pelvic, and lower extremities is another factor that influences the curve of the lumbar spine. For example, tight hamstring muscles exert a pull on the pelvis that results in a flattening of the lumbar curve. The amount of weight an individual carries and the condition of the abdominal muscles are still other factors that can influence the lumbar curve. Finally it is important to remember that the body is a system of interrelated and connecting parts and that movement or position of one structure is likely to influence the position of another structure. This holds true in the back and extremities. For example, by flexing the knees and hip joints, the pelvis is influenced, which affects the low back. Likewise raising the arms above shoulder level changes the center of gravity and changes the curve in the low back. Even the height of the heel on a shoe can affect the lumbar curve. Keeping these facts in mind, Figures 26-3 to 26-8 and the boxed material on p. 373 demonstrate basic principles for posture and body mechanics.

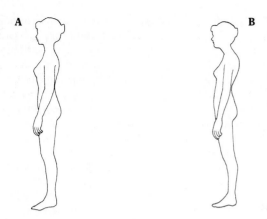

Fig. 26-3. Standing. **A,** Correct. **B,** Incorrect.

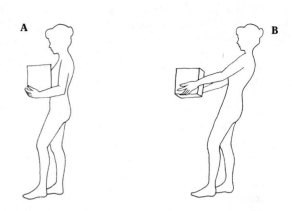

Fig. 26-6. Carrying. **A,** Correct. **B,** Incorrect.

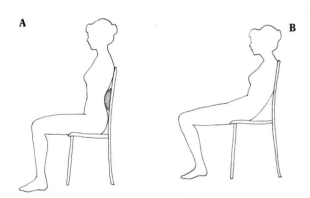

Fig. 26-4. Sitting. **A,** Correct. **B,** Incorrect.

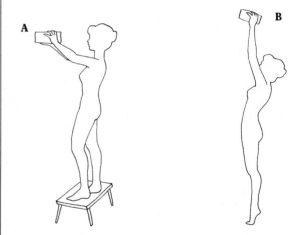

Fig. 26-7. Reaching. **A,** Correct. **B,** Incorrect.

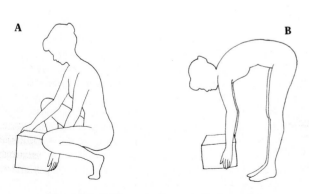

Fig. 26-5. Lifting. **A,** Correct. **B,** Incorrect.

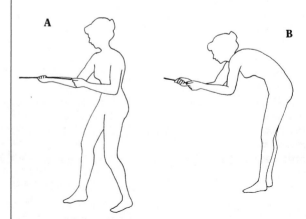

Fig. 26-8. Pulling. **A,** Correct. **B,** Incorrect.

Correct posture for body mechanic techniques

Standing posture (Fig. 26-3)	Stomach should be flat.
	With a plumb line dropped all curves must transect the line to be gravity balanced.
	Observe the spine and check that the curves are not exaggerated.
Prolonged standing posture	Avoid prolonged standing, especially in shoes with a high heel.
	Move about and stretch whenever possible.
	Use a footstool to prop one foot on from time to time.
Sitting posture (Fig. 26-4)	Avoid prolonged sitting.
	Get up every 45 minutes to stretch in the opposite direction.
	Use a lumbar support in the chair to maintain the lumbar curve.
	Use a footstool as an alternative to lumbar support.
Lying posture	Lie on one side.
	When lying on the back, put pillows under the knees.
Principles for lifting (Fig. 26-5)	Feet should have a wide base of support.
	Squat and bend the knees, not the back.
	Lift with the legs.
	Tighten the abdominal muscles.
	Avoid twisting.
	Keep object close.
	Be sure the lumbar curve is present.
Carrying (Fig. 26-6)	Carry the object close to you.
	Use the arms and carry at waist level.
	Avoid torquing or twisting movements.
	Check to be sure lumbar curve is present.
Reaching (Fig. 26-7)	Avoid reaching above the shoulders without taking precautions.
	Use a footstool or ladder when possible.
	Rearrange an area so you do not have to reach across a desk or cabinet for commonly used items.
Pushing	Push instead of pulling when possible.
	Use mechanical devices to help push heavy or large items.
	Push with the legs or entire body to break the inertia.
Pulling (Fig. 26-8)	Avoid pulling an object if possible.
	Keep the knees partially bent.
	Maintain a wide base of support.
	Shift the body weight to give extra pull.
	Do not pull with the back muscles.
	Try to keep the lumbar curve present.

Sample treatment plan

Case study

Mr. M. is a 29-year-old single man who was injured on the job 2 years ago. When he was lifting a 50-pound box, he lost his balance and felt a pull in his low back. Subsequently he underwent two lumbar laminectomies, one 3 months following his injury and the other one 6 months ago. Currently he continues to complain of pain in his right lower back and complains that he is unable to function and be as active as he was before his injury. His diagnosis is low back strain.

Mr. M is a picture framer and would like to return to work. He enjoys fishing, skiing, and basketball, and he wants to be able to engage in these sports again.

He was referred to an inpatient back rehabilitation program. The goals were to improve ROM, flexibility, strength, endurance, and body mechanics, and restore him to his maximal level of independence so that he can resume his former work and leisure roles.

TREATMENT PLAN

A. Statistical data.
  1. Name: Mr. M.
     Age: 29
     Diagnosis: Low back strain
     Disability: Constant pain in lower right back; decreased functional capabilities
  2. Treatment aims as stated in referral:
     Improve ROM and flexibility
     Improve strength and endurance
     Improve body mechanics
     Restore to maximal functional independence

B. Other services.
  Physician: Prescribe treatment, modalities, and any medication if necessary; supervise rehabilitation services
  Nursing: Assist in patient's orientation to nursing floor; administer medications; reinforce and follow through with body mechanic techniques in patient's ADL
  Psychiatrist: Evaluate patient's psychological status; recommend any medication

Physical therapy: Evaluate physical potential of patient; strengthen lower extremities; increase endurance in conjunction with occupational therapy
Social worker: Explore financial problems; help family and patient adjust to hospital setting; provide support, education, and encouragement to family members
Family: Provide support and encouragement to the patient
Recreational therapy: Provide leisure time activities to help improve patient's self-esteem and decrease depression
Vocational rehabilitation: Explore feasibility of return to present occupation or explore new job possibilities and retraining

C. OT Evaluation.
  1. Evaluation data.
     a. Subjective findings.
        The patient complains of constant and burning pain in his right lower back. The pain is aggravated by prolonged standing and is relieved somewhat by lying down. The patient intermittently wears a back brace. He attempts to return to work but has to take time off or quit because of pain. He lives by himself; when not working he does daily chores and watches television
     b. Physical resources.
        (1) ROM: Patient demonstrates limited ROM in trunk flexion, trunk extension, and lateral flexion; all are limited to within one-half of normal range on the right and three fourths normal range on the left. Trunk rotation is limited to one half normal range on the right and three fourths normal range on the left. He experiences an increase of pain with these motions. Lower extremities limitations include straight right leg raise of 0° to 45°, straight left leg raise of 0° to 90°, right hip flexion of 0° to 100°, and right hip abduction of 0° to 50°.

        (2) Strength: Strength was normal throughout except for right ankle dorsiflexion and right extensor hallucis longus; both were graded as fair plus (F+).
        (3) Functional skills: Patient is independent but guarded in dressing and sink activities. He complains of pain when putting on shoes and socks and demonstrated poor body mechanics with these activities. He has difficulty with sweeping, vacuuming, and mopping and used poor body mechanics. Outdoor tasks and driving are not attempted, since in the past they have aggravated his pain. He further demonstrates improper body mechanics when sitting and when moving from a sitting to standing position. His standing posture demonstrates increased lordosis with head jutting forward.
        Lifting: Patient is able to lift 10 pounds (4.5 kg) from 0 to 36 inches (0 cm to 91.4 cm) and 36 inches to 72 inches (91.4 cm to 182.8 cm) with only a "pulling" sensation.
        Carrying: Patient is able to carry 10 pounds (4.5 kg) for 5 minutes for 323 feet (98.4 meters) with no complaints of pain.
        Lower extremity weights: Patient is able to extend leg with 75-pound (34 kg) weights and hold a 90° static quad for 12 seconds.
        Upper extremity weights: Patient is able to flex elbow with 15-pound (6.8 kg) weights, depress scapula with 20-pound (9.1 kg) weights, and flex shoulder with 45-pound (20.4 kg) weights.

Sample treatment plan—cont'd

Treadmill: Patient able to run 1.5 mph for 10 minutes with no aggravation of pain.

Stationary bicycle: Patient is able to resist with 3.3 pounds (1.5 kg) for 2 miles in 15 minutes but experienced right leg pain.

Endurance walk: Patient is able to walk 947 feet (328 meters) in 30 minutes with some stopping because of pain.

Psychological status: Patient expresses some anger at his insurance company. He is pleasant but withdrawn and has lost social contact with many of his friends.

2. Problem identification.
   a. Constant pain in right low back
   b. Some limitations in ROM
   c. Slight decrease in strength
   d. Low lifting and carrying capabilities
   e. Poor endurance
   f. Improper body mechanics
   g. Some display of anger, withdrawal, low self-esteem
   h. Change or loss in vocational role
3. Assets.
   a. Expresses desire to get better
   b. Expresses desire to return to work
   c. No exhibition of muscle atrophy or gross loss of strength
   d. Limitations in ROM because of inactivity; no bony problems
   e. Young
   f. Cooperative, appears motivated to follow treatment program

The following treatment plan is modeled after the program at Saint Francis Memorial Hospital in San Francisco, in which back rehabilitation is a team effort between occupational and physical therapies. This treatment plan is merely an example and would not be suitable for any and every patient with low back pain. Each patient needs to be evaluated and then have a treatment plan designed specifically to meet his or her needs.

E Problem	F Specific OT objectives	G Methods used to meet objectives	H Gradation of treatment
a	Given appropriate modalities, pain will be modulated or reduced so that patient can increase functional activities and return to work	TENS Biofeedback to aid the patient's ability to relax Teach patient several relaxation methods; may include progressive relaxation, visualization techniques, or a form of meditation Stress reduction techniques, such as energy conservation and time management	Start and use TENS as needed for pain relief; may wean off of device as pain decreases Daily biofeedback training until patient can maintain a relaxed state for 5 minutes; increase time to 20 minutes Daily trials and practice of various relaxation techniques until find one that is effective and can maintain a state of relaxation for 5 minutes; increase time to 20 minutes
a, b	Given exercise and muscle flexibility, ROM will increase and pain will be reduced so that normal ROM is attained in the lower extremities	Occupational or physical therapist to instruct patient in low back exercises for trunk mobility, hamstring stretching, and hip flexibility; exercises are as follow: 1. Lumbar rotation: Patient supine, both knees bent, head and shoulders on mat; bring both knees to the right by rotating the pelvis; repeat on left side 2. Double knee to chest: Patient supine with both knees bent; bring right knee to chest, hold with right hand; bring left knee to chest, hold with left hand; lift head up toward knees, hold for 5 seconds; lower head and legs one at a time to mat	Start with 5 repetitions for each exercise unless exercise aggravates pain; repetitions increased 1 per day until a total of 10 is reached; progression holds for all of the following five exercises If pain at certain level, decrease number of repetitions and maintain at lower level for several days

Continued.

Sample treatment plan—cont'd

E Problem	F Specific OT objectives	G Methods used to meet objectives	H Gradation of treatment
		3. Straight leg stretch: Patient supine, one leg bent, one leg straight out on mat; bend straight leg toward chest, straighten and lift as high as possible without bending knee; tilt toes toward nose, hold for 5 seconds and return; repeat with other leg 4. Pelvic roll: Patient supine, one leg bent, one leg straight, head and shoulders on mat; bring bent knee toward straight leg by rotating pelvis (keep foot on mat); hold for 5 seconds, return to starting position; repeat with other leg 5. Back extension: Patient prone, elbows bent, hands by shoulders; slowly push up with arms to a position that can be tolerated; hold for 5 seconds	
c	Given exercise, improved abdominal strength will be achieved so patient will be able to complete 20 situps with ease; improve lower extremity strength so patient can do 15 repetitions with ease	Instruct patient in exercises to strengthen abdominal and lower extremity muscles; exercises that may be used: 1. Pelvic tilt with sliding legs: Patient supine, both knees bent; tilt pelvis backward; flatten back against mat; slowly straighten legs down to the mat to a count of 5; *must* be able to maintain pelvic tilt throughout the exercise if unable, straighten legs only to the point that the pelvic tilt can be maintained 2. Partial sit-up: Patient supine, both knees bent, arms straight in front, tuck chin in, sit up toward knees only enough to clear head and upper back from mat; hold for 5 seconds 3. Diagonal sit-up: Patient supine, both knees bent, arms straight in front; sit up toward right side enough to clear head and upper back from mat; hold for 5 seconds 4. Quad sets/straight leg raise: Patient supine, one knee bent, one leg straight; tighten thigh muscle on the straight leg to set the quadriceps muscle; while holding the set lift leg straight up about 6 inches (15.2 cm) from mat; hold for 5 seconds; return to start position; repeat with other leg 5. Hip abduction: Patient lying on one side, bottom leg slightly bent forward; lift top leg up toward ceiling; hold for 5 seconds; return; repeat with other leg	Start at 5 repetitions and increase 1 each day until reach 20 sit-ups and 15 lower extremity exercise repetitions If pain at certain level, decrease number of repetitions, and maintain at lower level for several days Cuff weight added at ankle for more resistance when patient can do 15 repetitions with ease; start patient at 10 repetitions with new weight Cuff weight added to ankle for more resistance when patient can do 15 repetitions with ease; start patient at 10 repetitions with new weight

Sample treatment plan—cont'd

E Problem	F Specific OT objectives	G Methods used to meet objectives	H Gradation of treatment
d	Given strengthening exercise of upper extremities, ability to lift weight will increase from 10 pounds (22 kg) to 20 pounds (44 kg) and increase individual weight exercises by 20%	Instruct patient in any or all of the following upper extremity strengthening exercises: 1. Curls (elbow flexion): With long-weight bar patient to stand against a wall, pelvis tilted, back flat against wall, feet 12 inches (30.5 cm) to 15 inches (38.1 cm) away from wall, arms at sides with elbows bent, on receiving the bar patient to flex arms toward chest and then slowly return arms to sides 2. Bench press (shoulder flexion and pectoralis major and minor): If bench press equipment available, use equipment, otherwise long-weight bar sufficient; patient supine on mat, arms at sides, elbows bent 90°; therapist to hand weight bar to patient, asks patient to push straight up into full elbow extension and 90° shoulder flexion; hold for 5 seconds, slowly return to starting position	PRE method of exercise used for the following strengthening exercises; determine the patient's maximal weight at 10 repetitions When patient can comfortably perform the progressive method for one maximum, ask patient to do several more repetitions at the same maximum; if can comfortably handle the increased repetitions, progress him to a new level; if cannot do 10 repetitions, have him continue at the current level
e	With activities and exercise, general endurance will improve and work tolerance will increase to 4 hours	Decide on appropriate activities; may include endurance walk, stationary bicycle, treadmill, and stair climbing Patient to start any of these activities until notices an aggravation of pain or until reaches level of endurance exhibited by shortness of breath, perspiration, flushing, or fatigue	Progress patient at own pace; use as many parameters, such as distance, time, and weight; when patient ready to progress increase only one parameter at a time; for example, all activities can be timed, to progress patient increase amount of time spent on the activity
d, f	Given education and practice, body mechanic techniques will improve so that proper body mechanics are used consistently in ADL and simulated work tasks	Occupational or physical therapist to instruct back anatomy class, provide a foundation for later body mechanics teaching Occupational therapist to instruct principles of body mechanics Occupational therapist to provide practical application of body mechanic principles by having patient try activities, such as standing, sitting, lying, lifting, carrying, and reaching posture and ADL, such as dressing, hygiene, vacuuming, sweeping, and washing windows Patient to run through a "par course" of activities, such as carrying a bag of groceries unloading the groceries on varying shelf heights sweeping a floor, and washing dishes	Provide 30- to 45-minute sessions for classes; use variety of media if possible In teaching posture techniques start with standing posture; progress to sitting and lying; instruct in dynamic postures for lifting, carrying, and reaching Start with demonstration, progress to patient participation; use as many real situations as possible

Continued.

Sample treatment plan—cont'd

E Problem	F Specific OT objectives	G Methods used to meet objectives	H Gradation of treatment
g	Given a supportive approach and environment, anger, depression, and low self-esteem will decrease and interaction with others will increase so that patient expresses less anger and displays a more positive attitude half of the time	Use a supportive, honest approach with the patient; explain procedures carefully and thoroughly Workshop activities of woodburning, leather crafts, and mosaics to improve self-esteem; socialization and expression encouraged in group situations	Simple, short-term crafts that the patient can accomplish easily and quickly; interact with patient Progress to more difficult crafts, being sure to structure the activity of success Patient to perform activities in a group situation
h	Given selected activities, physical tolerance and capabilities will be documented and aid determination of feasibility of future employment	During workshop activities or recreational therapy, sitting and standing tolerances can be observed and recorded Give patient task, such as woodburning, during workshop time; patient to stand while working on project; occupational therapist to observe patient and record amount of time standing tolerated	 Encourage patient to gradually increase standing time; patient to try using a footstool and varying work heights while standing
		While patient engaged in a craft activity and sitting, occupational therapist to observe and record the amount of time patient able to sit comfortably	Encourage patient to gradually increase sitting tolerance; patient to try different types of chairs, lumbar supports, work heights, and angles
		Occupational therapist to provide patient with variety of lifting and carrying situations; for example, carry a weighted box for a given distance and lift a weighted box to various heights	Patient to lift and carry to tolerance; amount of weight gradually increased as strength and endurance improve
		Patient to lift weighted tool box from floor to 36 inches (91.4 cm) and then to a shelf at 72 inches (183 cm)	Patient to start lifting and carrying objects that are easily manageable, progress to more awkward sizes and shapes
		Patient to carry a weighted tool box for a given period of time and set distance	
		Patient to lift and carry different sizes and shapes of wood or other objects, such as long but lightweight objects and bulky objects	

REVIEW QUESTIONS

1. List three risk factors that may contribute to the incidence of low back pain.
2. Name the major components of the spine.
3. Explain the mechanism of an intervertebral disk.
4. List the four areas of assessment that the therapist evaluates on an individual with low back pain.
5. What are some of the problems that a person with chronic low back pain encounters?
6. List five possible treatment phases for a patient suffering from low back pain.
7. How is an individual progressed when on a treatment program?
8. What is the foundation for good body mechanics?
9. List the principles of proper body mechanics for lifting, carrying, reaching, pushing, and pulling.
10. In a team environment what other disciplines might be seeing or treating the person with low back pain?

REFERENCES

1. Anderson, G.B.J., editor: Symposium: low back pain in industry, Spine **6:**52, 1981.
2. Cailliet, R.: Low back pain syndrome, Philadelphia, 1982, F.A. Davis Co.
3. Finneson, B.: Low back pain, ed. 2, Philadelphia, 1980, J.B. Lippincott Co.
4. Frymoyer, J.W., et al.: Risk factors in low back pain J. Bone Joint Surg. **65A:**213, 1983.
5. Keim, H.A.: Low back pain, vol. 2, Summit, N.J., 1973, CIBA Pharmaceutical Co.
6. Mines, S.: The conquest of pain, New York, 1974, Grosset & Dunlap, Inc.
7. Toufexis, A.: That aching back, Time **116:**30, 1980.
8. Trigiano, L.L.: Treatment of chronic pain, paper presented at the International Congress on Natural Medicine, Rome, March 25, 1983.

CHAPTER 27

Hip fractures and total hip replacement

KAREN PITBLADDO
JAN POLON
HELEN BOBROVE
ELIZABETH BIANCHI

The occupational therapist plays a key role in defining and remediating the many functional problems imposed by both acute and chronic orthopedic conditions, thus sharing in the goal of returning the orthopedic patient to optimal performance of safe and independent daily living activities.

This chapter discusses hip fractures and total hip replacement, their medical and surgical management, the psychological implications of hospitalization and disability, and the health care team approach in an acute hospital setting.

FRACTURES

It is important for the therapist working with orthopedic patients to have a good understanding of the site, type, and cause of the fracture before beginning the patient in treatment. A basic understanding of fracture healing and medical management is also necessary to appreciate risks, precautions, and complications involved.

Fractures occur in bone when the bone's ability to absorb tension, compression, or shearing forces is exceeded. Fractures are classified according to the type of fracture sustained and the direction of the fracture line[4] (Fig. 27-1).

Fracture healing[4]

Grossly, bone tissue occurs as cancellous or cortical. Cancellous or spongy bone surrounds spaces filled with bone marrow in the metaphysis of long bones and the bodies of short bones and flat bones of the pelvis and ribs. Cortical or compact bone is on the outer surface of the bone, giving it strength. It is covered with periosteum, and the inner surface is lined with endosteum.

At the time of fracture blood vessels are torn across the fracture site, causing

The authors extend their appreciation to Karen Donaldson, O.T.R., for the illustrations and Susan Sitko, R.P.T., and Annie Affleck, M.A., O.T.R., for their consultations.

bleeding then clotting; this situation is called a fracture hematoma. The repair cells or osteogenic cells form an internal and external callus from the endosteum and periosteum respectively. A fracture callus is formed from osteogenic tissue by the end of the first few weeks. Primary woven bone is formed by osteogenic cells differentiating into osteoblasts away from the fracture sites. Nearer to the fracture site the osteogenic cells differentiate into chondroblasts, creating cartilage. Clinical union occurs as this cartilage changes to bone and the callus becomes hard enough so that no movement occurs at the fracture site.[7] It is important to note that once clinical union occurs, immobilization is usually not required but the fracture should be protected from undue stress until consolidation occurs.

The fracture is consolidated many months later when excess callus is reabsorbed and the bone returns to almost its normal diameter. Remodeling of bone occurs in response to physical stress referred to as Wolff's law.[7] Bone is deposited in sites where there is stress, such as weight bearing, and reabsorbed where there is little stress.

Cancellous bone is structurally different than cortical bone, so the healing process differs. The internal callus plays a greater role in forming primary woven bone; because of greater blood supply and larger surface area, healing occurs more rapidly.

As a result of the lack of blood supply, articular cartilage cannot regenerate into hyaline cartilage but instead forms fibrous tissue and fibrocartilage. This form of scar tissue cannot withstand

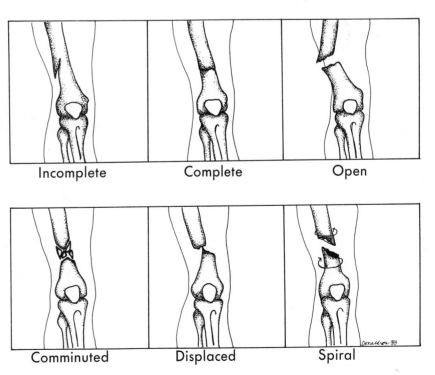

Incomplete   Complete   Open

Comminuted   Displaced   Spiral

Fig. 27-1. Types of fractures. (Adapted from Gartland, J.J.: Fundamentals of orthopaedics, Philadelphia, 1979, W.B. Saunders Co.)

normal wear-and-tear stresses. If the gap is significant, degenerative changes may develop.[4]

The time required for fracture healing varies with the age of the patient, site and configuration of the fracture, initial displacement of the bone, and the blood supply to the fragments. The fracture healing may be abnormal in one of three ways: a bony deformity develops (called a malunion), the healing process takes longer than normal (called a delayed union), or a nonunion occurs so that the fracture will not heal.[7]

Etiology of fractures[4]

Trauma is the major cause of fractures. The force may be transmitted directly or through torsion. A forceful muscle contraction may also break a bone, as in certain patella fractures. Stress fractures occur when bone fatigues from repeated loading, as seen in some metatarsal fractures. Osteoporosis, a type of metabolic bone atrophy, is a common bone disease of people over 65 years of age. It involves mostly the vertebral bodies and cancellous metaphyses of the neck of the femur, humerus, and distal end of the radius. Because the bone becomes fragile and porous, the affected bones are prone to fracture. A pathological fracture can occur because of a bone weakened by disease or tumor. This can occur in diseases, such as osteomyelitis and lytic tumors of bone caused by deposition of metastatic carcinoma.

Medical management

The aims of fracture treatment are to relieve pain, maintain good position of the fracture, allow for bony union for fracture healing, and restore optimal function to the patient.[7] Occupational therapy provides a significant role in the restoration of function of the patient; that role will be discussed later in this chapter following the discussion of medical treatment and the course and outcome.

Reduction of a fracture refers to restoring the fragments to normal alignment.[4] This can be done by a closed procedure (manipulation) or by an open procedure (surgery). A closed reduction is performed by applying a force to the displaced bone opposite to the force that produced the fracture. Depending on the nature of the fracture, the reduction is maintained in a cast, cast brace, skin traction, skeletal traction, or skeletal fixation.

With open reduction the fracture site is exposed surgically so that the fragments can be aligned. The fragments are held in place with internal fixation by pins, screws, a plate, nails, or a rod. Further immobilization by a cast or a cast brace may be necessary. Usually an open reduction and internal fixation (ORIF) must be protected from excessive forces, so weight bearing restrictions are indicated.[5] In the hip fracture the articular fragment of the hip may need to be removed and replaced by a prosthesis called an endoprosthesis. This is necessary when there are complications of avascular necrosis, nonunion, or degenerative joint disease.

Hip fractures

A knowledge of hip anatomy is necessary to understand medical management of hip fractures. The *articular capsule of the hip joint* refers to the dense connective tissue enclosing the joint. It provides stability and assists with hip motion. The capsule extends from the margins of the acetabulum downward anteriorly to the intertrochanteric ridge and posteriorly to the middle of the neck. The greater trochanter serves as the attachment of the hip abductors; gluteus minimus, gluteus medius, and external rotators; piriformis; gemellus; and obturators. The iliopsoas tendon, a hip flexor, attaches to the lesser trochanter. Blood supply to the femoral head is via the ligamentum teres, capsular vessels, and vessels from the femoral shaft (Fig. 27-2).

The levels of fracture lines are shown in Fig. 27-3. The names of the fractures generally reflect site and severity of injury. These terms are frequently indicators of which medical treatment will be used. For example, femoral neck fracture will be treated with femoral neck stabilization.

FEMORAL NECK FRACTURES. Femoral neck fractures are common in adults over 60 years old and occur more frequently in women. The bone is osteoporotic, and only slight trauma or rotational force causes the fracture.[2] Treatment of a displaced fracture in this area is complicated by poor blood supply, the osteoporotic bone that is

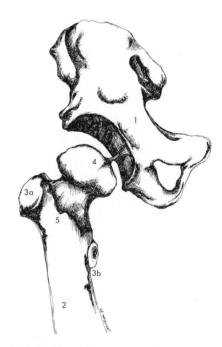

Fig. 27-2. Normal hip anatomy. *1*, Acetabulum; *2*, femur; *3a*, greater trochanter; *3b*, lesser trochanter; *4*, ligamentum teres; *5*, intertrochanteric crest. (Adapted from Crouch, J.E.: Functional human anatomy, ed. 3, Philadelphia, 1978, Lea & Febiger, and Grant, J.C.: Grant's atlas of anatomy, ed. 6, Baltimore, 1972, Williams & Wilkins.)

not suited to hold metallic fixation, and the thin periosteum limiting fracture healing. The type of surgical treatment used is based on the amount of displacement and the circulation in the femoral head.

The age and health of the patient are, of course, considered in deciding on the surgical procedure. Generally hip pinning or use of a compression screw and plate is employed when displacement is minimal to moderate and blood supply is intact. With a physician's approval a patient is usually able to begin out-of-bed activities 2 to 4 days after surgery. Weight bearing restrictions must be observed with the aid of crutches or a walker for at least 6 to 8 weeks while the fracture is healing. Limited weight bearing may be necessary beyond this time if precautions are not observed or delayed union occurs.[5]

With severe displacement or an avascular femoral head the femoral head is excised and replaced by an endoprosthesis. Several types of metal prostheses can be used; each has its own shape and advantages. Weight bearing restrictions are sometimes indicated. Because of the surgical procedure used, precautions for positioning the hip must be observed to avoid dislocation. Patients who have had a prosthesis implanted can usually begin out-of-bed activity with a physician's approval about 2 to 4 days after surgery.[5]

INTERTROCHANTERIC FRACTURES. Intertrochanteric fractures between the greater and lesser trochanter[2] are extracapsular, and the blood supply is not affected. Like femoral neck fractures, intertrochanteric fractures occur mostly in women[2] but in a slightly older age-group. The fracture usually is caused by direct trauma or force over the trochanter. ORIF is the preferred treatment. A nail or compression screw with a sideplate is used. Sometimes as long as 4 to 6 months weight bearing restrictions must be observed when a patient is ambulating. Again the patient is allowed out of bed 2 to 4 days after surgery pending the physician's approval.[5]

SUBTROCHANTERIC FRACTURES. Subtrochanteric fractures 1 to 2 inches below the lesser trochanter usually occur because of direct trauma. These fractures are most often in younger people[2] less than 60 years old. Skeletal traction followed by an ORIF is the usual treatment. A nail with a long sideplate or an intramedullary rod is used, possibly requiring further immobilization after surgery.[2]

Total joint replacement[8]

Restoration of joint motion and treatment of pain by total hip replacement is sometimes indicated in osteoarthritis, rheumatoid arthritis, and ankylosing spondylitis. Osteoarthritis or degenerative joint disease may develop spontaneously in middle age and progress as the normal aging process of joints is exaggerated. It may also develop as the result of trauma, congenital deformity, or a disease that damages articular cartilage. Weight bearing joints, such as the hip, knee, and lumbar spine, are usually affected. There are a loss of cartilage centrally on the joint surface and a build-up of cartilage peripherally, producing joint incongruity. Pain arises from the bone, synovial membrane, fibrosis capsule, and muscle spasm. The muscles can then contract further, restricting joint motion and placing further stress on limited joint surface area. The osteoarthritic hip may assume a flexed, adducted, and externally rotated position that causes a painful limp.

Ankylosing spondylitis, a chronic progressive polyarthritis, primarily involves the sacroiliac and spinal joints. The soft tissues eventually ossify, producing a bony ankylosis. The proximal joints of the extremities, particularly the hips, may be affected, which could also progress to bony ankylosis.

Rheumatoid arthritis (covered in Chapter 23) is another type of arthritis that may involve the hip joint. Surgery is often performed early in the disease process to avoid fibrotic damage to joint and tendon structures.

Total joint replacement or replacement arthroplasty may be necessary in various types of arthritis. This surgery is designed to alleviate pain and regain joint motion. There are two components to a "total hip." A high-density polyethylene socket is fitted into the acetabulum, and a metallic prosthesis replaces the femoral head and neck. Methylmethacrylate or bonelike cement

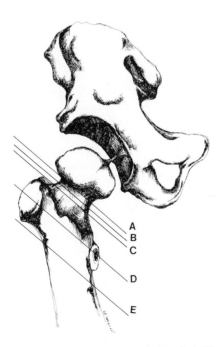

Fig. 27-3. Levels of femoral fractures. *A*, Subcapital; *B*, transcervical; *C*, basilar; *D*, intertrochanteric; *E*, subtrochanteric. (Adapted from Crow, I.: Fractures of the hip: a self study, ONA J. **5:**12, 1978.)

fixes the components to the bone. Various surgical approaches are used according to the surgical skill or technique of the orthopedist, severity of the joint, and past surgery to the hip. For example, with an anterolateral approach the patient will be unstable in external rotation and adduction of the operated hip and usually must observe precautions to prevent these movements for 6 to 12 weeks. If a posterolateral approach is used, the patient must be cautioned not to move the operated leg in specific ranges of flexion (usually 60° to 90°) and not to internally rotate or adduct the leg. Failure to maintain these precautions during the time of healing of muscles and soft tissue may result in hip dislocation. Some surgeons may advise that the patient limit weight bearing on the operated extremity because of the need for cement "seating." The restrictions on weight bearing will vary in terms of amount of pressure and length of time. A walking aid, usually a walker or crutches, is necessary for at least the first month while the hip is healing and muscles are becoming stronger.

It is important to be aware of complications or special procedures that occurred during surgery. For example, a trochanteric osteotomy may have been necessary. In this case, if the greater trochanter was removed and rewired down, active abduction would be prohibited. Patients with total joint replacements usually begin out-of-bed activity 3 to 5 days after surgery.

Total joint surface replacements are a variation of the total hip replacement.[4] The surface of the femur is capped by a metallic shell, and the acetabular cavity receives a plastic cup. Both are held in place by methylmethacrylate. This technique preserves the femoral head and neck. Weight bearing restrictions may apply because of the cement seating.

PSYCHOLOGICAL FACTORS

Psychological issues are critical considerations in the overall treatment of the orthopedic patient. A large number of patients in this population are faced with either a chronic disability (such as rheumatoid arthritis), a life-threatening disease (such as cancer), or the aging process. Therefore loss or potential loss of physical ability is a predominant problem faced by most of these patients. This is a stressful process, requiring an enormous amount of physical and emotional energy.[6] Therefore an awareness of and a sensitivity toward the orthopedic patient is critical to the delivery of optimal patient care.

When dealing with this patient population, the therapist must realize that each patient's experience of loss will depend on that patient's intrinsic makeup (personality, physical diseases, specific changes, or experience of body dissolution) and the environmental factors affecting the patient (personal losses or gains, family dynamics, or the home environment).[6] For example, the losses experienced by a young woman with rheumatoid arthritis would create an entirely different psychosocial picture than the losses experienced by an elderly man suffering from a fractured femur.

Those patients suffering from a chronic orthopedic disability often experience one or all of the following: body dissolution, deformity, disease of a body part, change in body image, decreased functional ability, or pain. The onset of these factors may occur at a relatively young age and often in rapid succession. Orthopedic patients often consider themselves prisoners of their own bodies, left with accumulated layers of unresolved grief, fatigue, and a sense of emptiness.[2] Thus when treating a patient with a chronic orthopedic disability, it is important to address these issues and provide the support needed for the mourning and grieving process to take place. Without an opportunity to resolve these conflicts, the patient becomes depressed, filled with guilt and anxiety, and paralyzed with fear. These emotions inhibit the patient's progress and enhance the development of poor self-image. Therapists can help reintegrate some of these conflicts, which will give the patient a feeling of accomplishment and pride, enhancing the treatment process.

The same holds true for the elderly patient dealing with disability. In addition to the issues just discussed, however, the elderly also face psychological issues specific to the aging process. The elderly patient often experiences the need to reflect on and review past life experiences.

This life review is conceived of as a naturally occurring universal mental process characterized by the progressive return to consciousness of past experiences, and particularly the resurgence of unresolved conflicts; simultaneously and normally, these revived experiences and conflicts are surveyed and reintegrated. It is assumed that this process is prompted by the realization of approaching dissolution and death.[1]

A second important issue experienced by the elderly, disabled individual is dependency. With the onset of a disability late in life, the patient is forced to face the realities of the aging process and let go of years of independence and self-sufficiency.[6] For some this can be a devastating experience, but others use these negative changes to acquire benefits that are satisfying to them. Examples of this are patients who remain in the hospital because they enjoy the extra attention in contrast to those who use their illness to manipulate their support systems and avoid taking responsibility for themselves and others.

A third psychosocial phenomenon experienced by the aged when hospitalized is relocation trauma. This presents itself through confusion, emotional lability, and disorientation. Older people, when removed from their familiar environment, will often decompensate cognitively. Therefore it is important that their new environment be made as familiar as possible. Decorating it with familiar objects from the patient's home and providing the patient with a calendar and current newspapers and magazines are often helpful in reducing this traumatic effect.

Learning to cope and adjust to the changes resulting from chronic disability or the aging process is a critical part of patient treatment. Therapists must realize that a great deal of a patient's functional independence has been relinquished as a result of disease or disability. For this reason it is critical that the psychosocial issues resulting from these losses be addressed while focusing on increasing a patient's functional level of independence.

REHABILITATION MEASURES[8]

Good communication and clear role delineation between members of the health care team are essential for an efficient and smooth therapy program. The health care team usually consists of a primary physician, nursing staff, a physical therapist, an occupational therapist, a discharge planner, and possibly a social worker. Regular team meetings to discuss each patient's ongoing treatment, progress, and discharge plans are necessary to coordinate individual treatment programs. Members from each service usually attend to provide information and consultation.

The role of the physician is to inform the team of the patient's medical status. This includes information regarding a previous medical history, diagnosis of the present problem, complete account of the surgical procedure performed that would include the type of appliance inserted, the anatomical approach, and any movement precautions that could endanger the patient. The physician is also responsible for ordering specific medications and therapies. Any change or progression in therapy or changes in the patient's medication regime should be approved by the physician.

The nursing staff is responsible for the actual physical care of the patient during hospitalization. Responsibilities of the nurse include administering medications, assisting the patient with bathing and hygiene, and constant monitoring of vital signs and physical status. Each patient's blood pressure, pulse, and respiratory status are checked every 1 to 2 hours. Wound and skin care, such as the changing of dressings or the sterilization of wounds, are performed by the nurse. The orthopedic nurse must have a thorough understanding of the surgical procedures and movement precautions for each patient. Proper positioning using pillows, wedges, and ski boxes is carried out by the nurse, especially in the first few days following surgery. As the patient's therapy program progresses, the patient starts to take more responsibility for proper positioning and physical care. The nurse works closely with the physical and occupational therapists to help establish a self-care program that implements skills that the patient has already learned in therapy.

The physical therapist is responsible for evaluation and treatment in the areas of musculoskeletal status, sensation, pain, skin integrity, and locomotion (especially gait). In many cases involving total hip replacements and surgical repair of hip fractures, physical therapy is initiated on the first day after surgery. The therapist obtains baseline information including range of motion (ROM), strength of all the extremities, muscle tone, mental status, and mobility, adhering to the prescribed precautions of protocol. A treatment program that includes therapeutic exercises, ROM activities, and progressive gait activities is established. The physical therapist is responsible for recommending the appropriate assistive device to be used during ambulation. As the patient's ambulation status advances, instructions in stair climbing, managing curbs, and outside ambulation are given.

The role of the discharge planner is to assure that each patient is being discharged to the appropriate living situation or facility. Usually the discharge planner is a registered nurse with a thorough knowledge of community resources and nursing care facilities available. With input from the health care team the discharge planner makes the arrangements for ongoing therapy after hospitalization, for admission to a rehabilitation facility for further intensive therapy, or for nursing home care if necessary. The discharge planner works closely with the health care team and is instrumental in coordinating the program after the patient's discharge from the hospital.

Occupational therapy role

Following a total hip replacement or surgical repair of a fractured hip, occupational therapy is usually initiated when the patient is ready to start learning the proper technique of getting out of bed. Occupational therapy is usually initiated 2 to 5 days after surgery. The average time varies depending on the age, general health, surgical events, and motivation of the individual patient. Before any physical evaluation, it is important for the therapist to introduce and explain the role of occupational therapy, establish a rapport, and then gather by interview any pertinent information regarding the patient's prior functional status, home environment, and living situation. The goal of occupational therapy is for the patient to return home independent in activities of daily living (ADL) with all movement precautions observed during activities. It is the role of the occupational therapist to teach the patient ways and means of performing ADL safely.

A brief physical evaluation is necessary to determine whether any physical limitations not related to surgery might prevent functional independence. Upper extremity ROM, muscle strength, sensation, coordination, and mental status are assessed before a functional evaluation is made. It is also important to consider the patient's pain and fear at rest and during movement. Occupational therapy is then a progression of functional activities that simulate a normal, daily regime of activity that is in accordance with all the movement precautions. The reader should refer to the Medical Management section of this chapter for a review of the different prescribed precautions.

Guidelines for training
Total hip replacement—anterolateral approach

POSITIONS OF HIP STABILITY: flexion, abduction, and internal rotation

POSITIONS OF HIP INSTABILITY: adduction, external rotation, and excessive hyperextension

Bed mobility. It is recommended that the patient lie in bed in the supine position. The appropriate wedge and ski box should be in place (Fig. 27-4). It is not recommended that a patient sleep on the side, although it is possible for a patient to roll if the wedge is in place and the operated extremity is supported by someone to maintain hip abduction. The patient is instructed in getting out of bed on both sides, although initially it may be easier to observe precautions by moving toward the nonoperated leg. Careful instruction is given to avoid adduction past midline and to maintain the operated extremity in internal rotation.

Transfers. It is always helpful for the patient to first observe the proper technique for transfers.

CHAIR: A firmly based chair with armrests is preferred. Before sitting, the patient is to extend the operated leg, reach back for the armrests, and then sit down slowly (Fig. 27-5). To stand from sitting the patient is instructed to extend the operated leg and push off from the armrests. Low-seated or sling-seated chairs should be avoided.

COMMODE CHAIR: An over-the-toilet commode chair is used initially while in the hospital. Usually by the time of discharge the patient will have enough hip mobility to safely use a standard toilet seat. It is recommended not to twist while wiping. To flush the toilet the patient should stand up and turn around to face the flusher.

SHOWER STALL: Nonskid stickers are recommended in all shower stalls and tubs.

To transfer, walker or crutches go in first, then the nonoperated leg followed by the operated leg. For patients with weight bearing precautions, the operated leg should lead.

SHOWER-OVER-TUB: The patient is instructed to stand parallel to the tub, facing the shower fixtures. Using a walker or crutches, the patient should transfer in sideways by bending one knee at a time over the tub.

CAR: A benchtype seat is recommended. The patient is instructed to back up to the passenger seat, sit down slowly with the operated leg extended, and then slide buttocks toward the driver's seat. The upper body and lower extremities move as one unit until the patient is squarely seated. Patients should avoid prolonged sitting in a car.

Lower extremity dressing. It is usually recommended to sit in a chair or on the side of the bed to dress. The patient is instructed to avoid externally rotating or crossing the legs to dress. Crossing the operated extremity over the nonoperated extremity at either the ankles or knees is avoided. Assistive devices may be necessary to observe precautions (see Fig. 27-6).

Homemaking. Heavy housework, such as vacuuming, lifting, and bed making, should be avoided. Kitchen activities are practiced with suggestions made to keep commonly used items at counter top level. Carrying items can be done by using aprons with large pockets, sliding items along the counter top, or attaching a small basket to a walker if necessary.

Family orientation. A family member or friend should be present for at least one occupational therapy treatment session so that any questions may be answered. Appropriate supervision recommendations and instructions regarding activity precautions are given at this time.

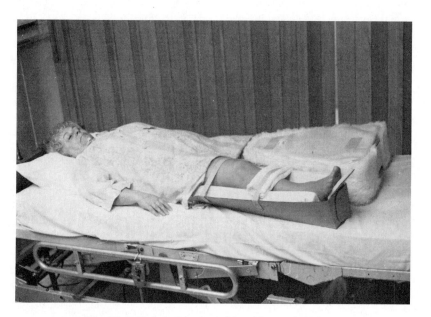

Fig. 27-4. Bed positioning with wedge and ski box.

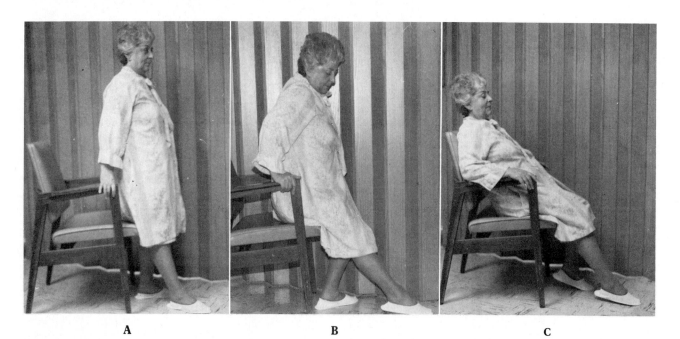

A   B   C

Fig. 27-5. Chair transfer technique. **A,** Patient extends operated leg and reaches for armrests. **B** and **C,** Bearing some weight on arms, patient sits down slowly, maintaining some extension of operated leg.

Total hip replacement—posterolateral approach

POSITIONS OF HIP STABILITY: Flexion (within limitations of precautions), abduction, and external rotation

POSITIONS OF HIP INSTABILITY: Adduction, internal rotation, and flexion greater than limitations of precautions

Bed mobility. The supine position with the appropriate wedge and ski box in place is recommended (see Fig. 27-4). It is not recommended that a patient sleep on the side. If a skin rash is present, sidelying is possible by assisting the patient to roll toward the uninvolved extremity with the wedge or larger pillows between the legs and someone holding the operated extremity to maintain hip abduction.

Transfers

CHAIR: A firmly based chair with armrests is recommended. The patient is instructed to extend the operated leg, reach back for the armrests, and sit slowly, being careful not to lean forward (see Fig. 27-5). To stand, the patient extends the operated leg and pushes off from the armrests, being careful not to lean forward. Because of the hip flexion precaution, the patient should sit on the front part of the chair and lean back. Firm cushions or blankets can be used to increase the height of chairs, especially if the patient is tall. Low chairs, soft chairs, reclining chairs, and rocking chairs should be avoided.

COMMODE CHAIR: Over-the-toilet commode chairs with armrests are to be used in the hospital and at home. The height and angle are adjusted so that the front legs are one notch lower than the back legs so that the patient's legs can touch the floor when sitting. The patient should wipe between the legs in a sitting or standing position to avoid twisting. The patient is to stand up and turn to face the toilet to flush.

SHOWER STALL: To enter, the walker or crutches go first, then the nonoperated leg followed by the operated leg. The patient is provided with a long-handled sponge to reach the feet safely. Grab bars should be installed if balance is a problem.

SHOWER-OVER-TUB: The patient is instructed to stand parallel to the tub facing the shower fixtures. Using the walker or crutches, the patient is to transfer in sideways by bending at the knees, not at the hips. For patients with weight bearing precautions or poor balance, this transfer is not recommended. They should take a sponge bath.

CAR: Bucket seats in small cars should be avoided. Benchtype seats are recommended. The patient is instructed to back up to the passenger seat, hold onto a stable part of the car, extend the operated leg, and slowly sit in the car. Remembering to lean back, the patient then slides the buttocks toward the driver's seat. The upper body and lower extremities then move as one unit to turn to face the forward direction. It is helpful to have the seat slid back and reclined to maintain the hip flexion precaution. Prolonged sitting in the car should be avoided.

Lower extremity dressing. To maintain hip precautions a dressing stick is used to aid in donning and removing pants and shoes. For pants, the operated leg is dressed first by using the dressing stick to bring the pants over the foot and up to the knee. A reacher, elastic laces, and a long-handled shoehorn are also provided. A sock aid is given if the patient lives alone. The patient is instructed to sit in a chair with arms or on the edge of the bed for dressing activities.

Homemaking. This is the same as for anterolateral approach. Reachers are provided to reach items in low cupboards or on the floor.

Family orientation. This is also the same as for anterolateral approach.

SPECIAL EQUIPMENT. The occupational therapist should be familiar with the following equipment that is commonly used in the treatment of hip fracture and total hip replacement.

NELSON BED: An adjustable bed that allows for chair or 90° vertical tilt positions in comparison with regular hospital beds may be used in some programs in the initial postoperative days to facilitate a change in the patient's position and allow a progressive tilting program before ambulation. It continues to be used until the patient has been instructed in transfer skills on and off the side of the bed.

HEMOVAC: A plastic drainage tube is inserted at the surgical site to assist with drainage of blood postoperatively. It has an area for collection of drainage and may be connected to a portable suction machine. The unit should *not* be disconnected for any activity, since this may create a blockage in the system. The Hemovac is usually left in place for 2 days following surgery.

ABDUCTION WEDGE: Large and small triangular wedges are used when the patient is supine to maintain the lower extremities in the abducted position. The large wedge is also used postoperatively to assist with stretching of hips into increased abduction.

SKI BOX: The box is fabricated by the staff in the cast room. It is a cardboard box with foam padding inside and Velcro attachments to secure the leg in place. It is used to maintain the operated extremity in a position of neutral hip rotation

BALANCED SUSPENSION: The balanced suspension device is an alternative to the use of the abduction wedge and ski box initially. It is fabricated and set up by the cast room technician and physician and is usually used for about 3 days following surgery. Its purpose is to support the affected lower extremity in the first few postoperative days. The patient's leg should *not* be taken out of the device for exercise until the device's use has been discontinued by the physician.

RECLINING WHEELCHAIR: A wheelchair with an adjustable backrest that allows a reclining position while in the chair is used for patients who have hip flexion precautions while sitting.

COMMODE CHAIRS: The use of a commode chair instead of the regular toilet aids in safe transfers and allows the patient to observe necessary hip flexion precautions. The two front legs of the commode chair may be adjusted slightly lower than the back legs to increase the patient's ability to observe hip flexion limitations and decrease the risk of dislocation.

BOLSTERS: Large, firmly folded blankets are used to assist with positioning the patient for passive hip stretching exercises.

DRESSING AIDS: Dressing aids are used to encourage independence in performing ADL while maintaining precautions against specific hip motions. These include a dressing stick, reacher, long-handled sponge, long-handled shoehorn, and sockaid (Fig. 27-6).

SKATE BOARD AND SKATES: A large, flat surface or board and a skate device to support the extremity are used to assist the patient with independent hip abduction exercises. It may be used on a bed or mat table while the patient is in the supine position.

FOOT BLOCK: A 6-inch wooden block on which to rest the foot while sitting in a chair provides a stretch to increase the range of hip flexion.

ANTIEMBOLUS HOSE: Thigh-high hosiery provides external support to the lower extremities following surgery. Their purpose is to assist circulation and prevent edema.

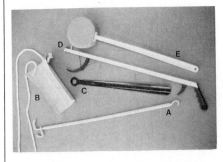

Fig. 27-6. Assistive devices useful for hip fracture. **A,** Dressing stick. **B,** Sock aid. **C,** Long-handled shoe horn. **D,** Reacher. **E,** Long-handled bath sponge.

SUMMARY. Occupational therapy is determined by the surgical procedure performed and the precautions prescribed by the physician. For patients who have an ORIF, weight bearing precautions must be observed during all ADL. Particular attention should be paid to the patient's weight bearing during bathing activities. It is often safest for the patient to bathe in the sitting position. A tub bench or shower seat may be necessary for safe and independent bathing. A simulation of the home environment is helpful to prepare the patient for potential problems that may arise when discharged. Recommendations to remove throw rugs and slippery floor coverings are made since the patient will most likely be going home using an ambulatory assistive device.

Sample treatment plan

Case study

Mr. B. is an 82-year-old man who has noticed increased right hip pain over the past year. He had a hip x-ray examination 3 months ago, and a diagnosis of degenerative arthritis was confirmed. He has been admitted to the orthopedic unit of the hospital for elective right total joint replacement using the anterolateral approach.

Mr. B. is a widower from Kentucky whose wife died shortly after moving to California 6 months ago. Mr. B. lives in his own cottage behind his son's home. Mr. B. has been independent in meal preparation, self-care, and homemaking. He enjoys gardening, walking in the neighborhood, and visiting with his two grandchildren. His increased hip pain has limited his daily activity so that he must take frequent rests during the day and use a cane.

Mr. B. has been admitted to the hospital 1 day before surgery for a preoperative assessment. Occupational therapy staff will evaluate the patient's present function, describe the rehabilitation program as it will progress following surgery, and carry out functional training after surgery.

TREATMENT PLAN

A. Statistical data.
1. Name: Mr. B.
   Age: 82
   Diagnosis: Degenerative arthritis affecting right hip; elective right total hip replacement
   Disability: Limited ROM and ambulation
   Precautions: Avoidance of right hip external rotation and adduction for 6 weeks after surgery
2. Treatment aims as stated in referral:
   Orientation of patient to rehabilitation program preoperatively
   Evaluation of patient's function preoperatively
   Instruction of patient in maintaining hip precautions for ADL postoperatively

B. Other services.
Medical: Perform total hip replacement surgery; prescribe rehabilitation therapies and medication
Nursing: Nursing care; positioning; supervise patient in activities and exercises following therapist's instruction of the patient
Physical therapy: ROM and strenghening exercises and gait training
Discharge planner: Arrange for home care follow-up
Family: Provide emotional support and physical assistance after discharge from hospital; encourage patient to observe precautions for hip movements at home

C. OT evaluation.
1. Before surgery.
   General appearance: Observe ease of movement, personal hygiene, hospital equipment in use, and patient's position and expression
   Mental and behavioral state: Observe
   Communication, vision, and hearing: Observe
   Sensation and pain: Test, observe
   Strength of extremities and trunk: Test
   Muscle tone: Test
   Posture: Observe
   Bulbar function: Screen
   Perceptual and cognitive function: Test, observe
   Avocational and vocational activities and endurance: Interview
   Home layout and accessibility: Interview
   Rehabilitation program after surgery: Orient patient
   Patient's goals from this surgery: Interview

2. Specific evaluation.
   Bed mobility: Demonstrate, interview
   Transfers (bed, chair, toilet, shower, and car): Demonstrate or interview
   Dressing: Interview
   Self-care: Interview
3. After surgery. The presurgical evaluation and evaluation of the patient's ability to observe hip precautions during functional activities and simulated work or avocational activities are repeated. The need and use of assistive devices is also assessed.

D. Results of evaluation.
1. Evaluation data.
   a. Physical resources.
      (1) Before surgery. Upper extremity (UE) active ROM was limited to 160° shoulder flexion bilaterally; right lower extremity (LE) active ROM was limited to 5° to 85° to hip flexion, 5° internal rotation, 10° external rotation, and 15° abduction; otherwise, ROM is within normal limits (WNL); strength in UE was grossly 4+ to 5 (G+ to N), LE right, 4 to 5 (G to N) and left was 4 to 5 (G to N).
      (2) After surgery. UE ROM and strength remains as stated above; right LE ROM remains as stated above, except hip flexion limited to 10° to 65°.
   b. Sensory-perceptual functions. WNL.
   c. Cognitive functions. Mr. B. reports forgetfulness (especially dates, places, and phone numbers) at times in daily activities. He describes the forgetfulness as more

Sample treatment plan—cont'd

"bothersome" than an actual problem. After surgery the patient showed slight memory deficits in names of personnel and times of therapy sessions; he required frequent review of instructions on hip precautions.

d. Psychological functions. Before surgery the patient was anxious about the hospital stay and surgery but appeared motivated to gain increased function and decreased pain. Mr. B. shows interest in the rehabilitation program by asking appropriate questions and commenting during the evaluation. After surgery the patient is highly cooperative during treatment, although he is tearful at times when discussing the loss of his wife.

e. Avocational potential. For the initial 6 weeks of recovery from hip surgery, Mr. B. will be cautioned against activities, such as gardening and heavy lifting, that may violate hip precautions. After 6 weeks he will be allowed to resume his full leisure activities with less pain and increased endurance expected.

f. Functional skills.
  (1) Before surgery. Mr. B. was able to do most ADL independently, except tying shoes and donning socks were difficult. He required frequent rests for meal preparation and homemaking because of pain. Heavier household tasks required assistance.
  (2) After surgery. Mr. B. requires use of adaptive equipment for independence in dressing. Endurance is improved for homemaking; however, assistance is required for heavier household tasks because of hip precautions. After the 6 weeks of recovery he is expected to be independent in most household tasks and in all ADL without equipment.

2. Problem identification.
  a. Before surgery.
    (1) Pain limiting present functional independence; anxiety about surgery and initial dependence after hospitalization

  b. After surgery.
    (1) For six weeks no adduction and no external rotation of the right hip allowed
    (2) Crutches required for 6 weeks for all ambulation
    (3) Supervision required for showering
    (4) Assistance required for basic homemaking and shopping
    (5) Dependent for heavy household tasks and driving for 6 weeks
    (6) Adjustment of avocational activities for initial 6 weeks to accommodate positioning precautions
    (7) Slight memory deficits

3. Assets and functions.
  a. Motivated toward independence in ADL
  b. Good understanding of rehabilitation program after surgery
  c. Supportive family
  d. Good safety judgment

E Problem	F Specific OT objectives	G Methods to meet objectives	H Gradation of treatment
a	Given explanation and illustration the patient will gain understanding of surgery and hip precautions as related to functional activity Given explanation and demonstration patient will understand progression of rehabilitation program following surgery	Describe surgery and necessary precautions; demonstrate how precautions will be carried out; have patient describe procedures to the therapist Explain OT program and progression of ADL while in the hospital	
b	Given instruction patient will be able to state hip precautions Given demonstration and instruction patient will consistently observe precautions in all hospital and simulated ADL	Give written, verbal, and demonstrated instruction of hip precautions; avoid adduction, external rotation, and excessive hyperextension Training is followed by the patient actively observing precautions for bed, chair, and toilet transfers; car and shower stall transfers; lower extremity dressing; bending and picking up objects; use of adaptive equipment; and self-care and hygiene activity following protocol for total hip replacement, anterolateral approach, described on pp. 383-384.	Patient progresses from verbally stating precautions to writing guidelines for home reference Daily ADL progresses so that on the day before discharge from hospital the patient is independent in basic ADL

Continued.

Sample treatment plan—cont'd

E Problem	F Specific OT objectives	G Methods to meet objectives	H Gradation of treatment
c	Given instruction and demonstration patient will use crutches for ADL safely and consistently	Demonstration and instruction is followed by patient's demonstrating safe use of crutches during transferring; maneuvering in room; reaching, bending, and carrying items; and preparing ADL work station	Begin with room activities progressing toward problem solving and simulated home activities
d	Given instruction and supervision patient will demonstrate good safety skills in shower transfer consistently	Correct shower procedure according to protocol is demonstrated; family member supervises shower activity with therapist standing by	
e	Given instruction and practice patient will observe hip precautions for basic home activities and recognize when assistance is needed consistently	Home activities such as tidying room, making a bed, and preparing light meal, will be simulated in clinic	Patient will be brought to clinic with a family member during latter part of hospital stay
	Given explanation and demonstration patient will identify need for assistance with activities that require lifting of objects and state needs consistently	Precautions against twisting and lifting objects greater than 10 lb are discussed (shopping, and heavy housework); patient is taught to gauge weight of common grocery and household items	
f	Through instruction and demonstration the patient will understand limitations in household tasks and avoid those that are contraindicated until precautions are removed by the physician	Patient and family are instructed in activities that must be avoided for 6 weeks after surgery (jumping down from stepstool or bus step, driving, and heavy gardening)	
g	Through instruction and demonstration the patient will state how he may modifiy gardening, visiting with grandchildren, and walking in neighborhood to ensure observance of hip precautions and safety	Simulate gardening positions (bending, reaching, and carrying items) in clinic approximating types of objects, weight, shape, and duration; discuss safety skills in ambulating with crutches around children and practice with obstacle course in clinic; discuss pacing and awareness of safe surfaces for ambulating in neighborhood with practice pacing and variable surfaces in and around the hospital	Patient is asked to problem solve through simulated situations and discussion
h	Given repetitive training patient will recall instructions and follow through with them appropriately	Increase treatment repetitions for specific skills taught; supply written guidelines for reference for both patient and family	Patient is seen twice daily for repetition of skills; patient is asked to briefly write skills taught; patient is given written instruction and pictures

I. **Special equipment**
   1. Ambulation aids.
      Crutches
   2. Assistive devices.
      Dressing stick
      Long-handled sponge
      Sock aid

REVIEW QUESTIONS

1. Why is it critical for an occupational therapist to understand hip anatomy and treatment of hip fractures?
2. When reviewing the patient's medical history, what information should be obtained?
3. Define "clinical union." How does it relate to weight bearing and activity?
4. Identify four factors that will influence fracture healing.
5. What is a pathological fracture, and in which diseases can it occur?
6. Describe the differences in approach and maintenance of closed and open reductions.
7. Femoral neck fractures are common in women greater than 60 years old. The type of surgical treatment used is based on the amount of displacement and what other factor?
8. Why would a compression screw and plate not be a surgical choice when there is poor blood supply to the femoral head?
9. Why are weight bearing precautions observed with ORIF hip pinnings?
10. Which surgical procedure is generally used with a severely displaced femoral neck fracture or with an avascular femoral head?
11. Why must hip position precautions be observed during activity in patients with total hip replacements?
12. In which diagnostic groups other than fractures will there be frequent indication for total joint replacement? What are the goals for this surgical approach in these diagnostic conditions?
13. Briefly describe the positions of instability in both the anterolateral and posterolateral approaches to hip replacement orthoplasty.
14. Briefly describe a total joint surface replacement and indications for its application.
15. Briefly describe a wedge and ski box and the indications for its use and application.
16. Following initial postoperative assessment, which functional activities are generally assessed in planning the initial treatment program?
17. Briefly describe the transfer method to a chair for a person after total hip replacement using posterolateral approach. What is the rationale applied here? What types of chairs should be avoided? Why?
18. Briefly describe a car transfer recommended for the patient with hip replacement orthoplasty using an anterolateral approach.
19. Which pieces of adaptive equipment might help a patient who has had a posterolateral total hip replacement achieve independence in lower extremity dressing?
20. What suggestions could be made concerning carrying items when ambulation aids are necessary?

REFERENCES

1. Butler, R.N.: The life review: an interpretation of reminiscence in the aged. In Kastenbaum, R., editor: New thoughts on old age, New York, 1964, Springer Publishing Co., Inc.
2. Butler, R.N.: Aging and mental health, ed. 3, St. Louis, 1982, The C.V. Mosby Co.
3. Crow, I.: Fractures of the hip: a self study, ONA J. 5:12, 1978.
4. Gartland, J.J.: Fundamentals of orthopedics, Philadelphia, 1979, W.B. Saunders Co.
5. Hogshead, H.P.: Orthopaedics for the therapist, Gainesville, 1973, University of Florida. Unpublished.
6. Lewis, S.C.: The mature years: a geriatric occupational therapy text, Thorofare, N.J., 1979, Charles B. Slack, Inc.
7. Satler, R.B.: Textbook of disorders and injuries of the musculoskeletal system, Baltimore, 1970, Williams & Wilkins.
8. Sitko, S., and Pitbladdo, K.: The total hip replacement protocol, Stanford, Calif. 1982, Stanford University Hospital, Department of Physical and Occupational Therapy. Unpublished.

CHAPTER 28

Lower motor neuron dysfunction

GUY L. McCORMACK

The lower motor neuron system[2] includes the anterior horn cells of the spinal cord, spinal nerves and their associated ganglia, and 10 pairs of cranial nerves and their nuclei, which are housed in the brainstem (cranial nerves 1 and 2 are fiber tracts in the brain).[9] The motor fibers of the lower motor neurons are divided into the somatic and autonomic components. The somatic motor components include the alpha motor neurons, which innervate skeletal (extrafusal fibers) muscles, and gamma motor neurons, which innervate muscle spindles (intrafusal fibers). The autonomic component innervates the glands, smooth muscles, and heart musculature.[10,13,33] A lesion to any of these neurological structures constitutes a lower motor neuron dysfunction.[10]

Lower motor neuron dysfunction can result from several different causes, including traumatic injury, such as bone fractures and dislocations, contusions, compression of nerve roots, lacerations, traction (stretching), penetrating wounds, and friction. Vascular deficiencies may also cause lower motor neuron dysfunction. Examples of these deficiencies include arteriosclerosis, diabetes mellitus (sensory loss), peripheral vascular anomalies, and polyarteritis nodosa.[6] Furthermore, toxic agents, such as lead, phosphorus, alcohol, benzene, and sulfonamides, can cause lower motor neuron dysfunction. Other contributing factors may include neoplasms, such as neuromas and multiple neurofibromatosis, and inflammatory processes, such as polyneuritis or mononeuritis. Degenerative diseases of the central nervous system (CNS) and congenital anomalies can also produce lower motor neuron dysfunction.[11,39]

Since the occupational therapist traditionally treats a variety of lower motor neuron dysfunctions that affect the upper extremities, this chapter will deal with the conditions most likely to be seen in clinical practice.

DISEASES OF THE LOWER MOTOR NEURON
Poliomyelitis

Poliomyelitis is a contagious viral disease that affects the anterior horn cells of the gray matter of the spinal cord and the motor nuclei of the brainstem. The cervical and lumbar enlargements of the cord are affected the most. Because of the active immunization program (Salk and Sabin vaccines) in the United States, new cases of poliomyelitis are rare. However, the recent complacency about immunization has created some new cases, and "old cases" are frequently referred to occupational therapy for rehabilitation or improvement of the quality of life.[16]

Clinically patients who have poliomyelitis initially have flaccid paralysis that may be local or widespread. The lower extremities, accessory muscles of respiration, and muscles that promote swallowing are primarily affected. Marked atrophy may be seen in the involved extremities, and deep tendon reflexes may be absent. Since poliomyelitis destroys the anterior horn cells, sensory roots are spared, and sensation is intact. Contractures can occur very early in the course of the disease. In cases of local paralysis the asymmetry of muscles pulling on various joints may promote deformity complications, such as subluxation, scoliosis, and contractures. In severe cases osteoporosis (bone atrophy) may weaken the long weight-bearing bones, and pathological fractures can occur.[26]

The medical treatment for poliomyelitis during the acute phase includes bed rest, positioning, and applications of warm packs to reduce pain and promote relaxation. Since there is no known cure for poliomyelitis, the disease must run its course. There is an incubation period of 1 to 3 weeks, and the recovery is dependent on the number of nerve cells destroyed. Paralysis may begin in 1 to 7 days after the initial symptoms. The medical aspects of rehabilitation may include reconstructive surgery, such as tendon transfer; arthrodesis; and surgical release of fascia, muscles, and tendons. Although the lower extremities are primarily affected, the hand splinting techniques were developed and codified at Rancho Los Amigos Hospital in the West and at Georgia Warm Springs Hospital in the East. Other medical procedures may include therapeutic stretching, casts, muscle reeducation, and bracing for standing or stability.[20]

OCCUPATIONAL THERAPY INTERVENTION. During the acute phase the patient receives symptomatic treatment and is confined to bed. The therapist should assist the nurse in providing good bed positioning to prevent contractures and protect weakened joints. Since the poliomyelitis virus is infectious during this stage, isolation procedures should be carefully followed. The therapist should provide gentle passive range of motion (ROM) at the patient's physical tolerance level to prevent contractures, joint stiffness, and deformities. Care should be taken not to grasp the involved muscle bellies, because they will be extremely tender and painful. The muscles may also be prone to spasms when painfully stimulated.[16]

The primary emphasis should be placed on the avoidance of muscle fatigue. Fatigue at this point can result in further residual weaknesses. If the patient has bulbar poliomyelitis, which affects the muscles of respiration, a respirator may be used to facilitate ventilation of the lungs or a tracheostomy may be performed. If the muscles necessary for swallowing are impaired, tube feeding may also be prescribed. The therapist should collaborate treatment procedures with the nursing staff to ensure proper functioning of the equipment necessary for the life support systems.[9,16,20,23]

The treatment program should include psychological support. The patient's fears and anxieties about the crippling effects of the disease should not be underestimated. The patient may need encouragement and positive experiences to promote an optimistic outlook during the rehabilitation process. The family may also need assistance in adjusting to the patient's disability.

As the rehabilitation process progresses, the precautions against physical and body fatigue continue. Assistive devices, splints, and mobile arm supports may be used to gain independence in daily activities. The long-range rehabilitation program should follow a functional course of action. After the acute medical problems have subsided, the recovery stage may last as long as 2 years.[9] Since the damage to the anterior horn cells is permanent, the therapist should assist the patient in making the best possible use of whatever muscular function remains. Before treatment is started, an evaluation of the existing disability must be obtained. A thorough manual muscle test not only provides a baseline for muscle strength but detects joint deformities caused by contracted muscles, ligaments, tendons, and joint capsules. Manual muscle tests should be repeated monthly for the first 4 months and bimonthly for the next 4 months. After 8 months of therapeutic exercises the average patient has probably responded to his or her maximal ability.[6,9,11] In short the therapeutic regime includes combinations of rest, movement, muscle reeducation, functional activities, and psychological support. Consequently the prognosis of poliomyelitis depends on the personality of the patient and the perseverance of the therapist.

Movement for the patient who is recovering from acute poliomyelitis proceeds from passive to active ROM, depending on the patient's level of voluntary control. Muscle reeducation should be preceeded by gentle stretching exercises. For the upper extremity emphasis should be placed on stretching the pectoralis major and minor and latissimus dorsi to ensure free motion of the shoulder region. All active motions should be performed under careful supervision of the therapist. Compensatory movement should be avoided. A limited but correct movement is preferred to an ampler but incorrect movement. Active movements should be

done in front of a mirror, which enables the patient to observe and correct motions accordingly.[16,20,23]

Muscle reeducation is accomplished in a graded fashion. At first the patient should learn "muscle-setting" exercises, that is, alternating contraction and relaxation of muscles without moving the joints. Isometric exercises and electromyographic (EMG) biofeedback may be beneficial at this juncture. As the patient progresses, light resistance can be applied manually by the therapist before the use of pulleys and weights. This allows the therapist to develop an empirical understanding of the patient's physical strengths and weaknesses. Weakened muscles must be protected at all times. Muscles that cannot resist the forces of gravity are supported during exercise and rest periods. As a rule of thumb, resistive exercises are not attempted until the muscle is able to carry out a complete ROM against gravity. Weakened or flaccid muscles can be splinted at night to counteract the forces of gravity or the pull of the stronger antagonist muscles. During resistive exercises the therapist should stress correct body positioning, joint alignment, and energy conservation. Periods of rest should be included in the exercise program, as well as activities that incorporate the same movements and musculature.[15]

The rationales for resistive exercises in the rehabilitation of the patient who has poliomyelitis are to cause hypertrophy of the undamaged muscle fibers and give usefulness to the slightest contraction by integrating it into the global movement that permits the performance of a given activity. Emphasis is placed on strengthening individual weakened muscles. After the 8-month period if the muscle is unable to contract completely against gravity, it is doubtful that additional muscle strength will return. At this point the emphasis should be placed on maintenance of existing muscles and functional activities of daily living (ADL). Again a self-care evaluation should be administered to achieve a baseline of function. Dressing activities may include putting on braces, prostheses, or orthoses. Assistive and adaptive devices should be tailored to the needs of the patient. The adaptation of assistive devices should

begin where the patient's functional abilities are limited. Assistive and adaptive devices should provide the patient with the most ability within the limits of the disability.[32] It may also be advantageous to begin activities for prevocational and vocational exploration. The patient's quality of life can be improved if he or she is employed and productive.

Today therapist's are seeing more "old polio" patients in rehabilitation centers. Some of the patients are experiencing additional weakness and paralysis. The phenomenon is not fully understood, but it is believed to be the normal loss of neurons in later life. Since the poliomyelitis victim has a diminished number of neurons in the anterior horn cells, further loss can be debilitating. This problem may pose some new challenges to the therapist in the future.

Guillain-Barré syndrome

Guillain-Barré syndrome, also known as either infectious polyneuritis or Landry's syndrome, is an acute inflammatory condition involving the spinal nerve roots, peripheral nerves, and, in some cases, selected cranial nerves. The Guillain-Barré syndrome often follows an afebrile illness. It is probably caused by a virus that produces a hypersensitive response that results in patchy demyelination of lower motor neuron pathways. The axons are generally spared, so recovery often follows a predictable course. In severe cases, however, wallerian degeneration of the axon results in a slow recovery process. This disease affects men and women equally from ages 30 to 50.[6,9,16,34,39]

Clinically Guillain-Barré syndrome is characterized by a rapid onset. Initially there is an absence of fever, pain and tenderness of muscles, and weakness and decrease in deep tendon reflexes. As the disease progresses, it produces motor weakness or paralysis of the limbs, sensory loss, and muscle atrophy. The prognosis is varied. In severe cases cranial nerves 7, 9, and 10 may be involved, and the patient may have difficulty speaking, swallowing, and breathing. If vital centers in the medulla are affected, the patient may experience respiratory failure.

In the majority of the cases the patient completely recovers within 3 to 8 months. Some slight exacerbation can occur, producing residual weaknesses and muscular atrophy.[20]

OCCUPATIONAL THERAPY INTERVENTION. Once the patient is medically stabilized, treatment goals should be coordinated with the nurse, physical therapist, and other members of the team to implement a comprehensive rehabilitation program. The occupational therapist should grade the activity to the patient's physical tolerance level. Physical fatigue should be avoided at all costs. Gentle, nonresistive activities can be introduced to alleviate joint stiffness and muscle atrophy and prevent contractures.[16,37]

Treatment should always begin with a thorough evaluation of the patient's level of functioning. During the early stages of recovery the evaluation process itself may be fatiguing. It is often best to spread the evaluation process over the course of a few days. For example, testing may begin by gently squeezing the muscle bellies of the large muscle groups to determine the extent of muscle tenderness and atrophy. Since the muscles of the limbs are usually affected symmetrically, this test can be grossly administered. Manual muscle testing should not be done in one session. It is best to test a few muscles at a time and allow the patient periods of rest. Particular attention should be paid to the intrinsic muscles of the hands to determine residual weakness. If swallowing or speech is impaired, a tongue depressor may be used to apply light resistance against the tongue to estimate the motor involvement in the twelfth (hypoglossal) cranial nerve.

Manual muscle testing should follow the strict definitions for grading strength. The patient's previous physical condition and occupation should be taken into account when calibrating the muscle strength.[16] It is important to establish an objective baseline for all of the clinical findings and record the progression of the affected muscles on a standardized chart.

Sensory testing should also be conducted because the sensory pathways are often affected. Sensory tests should include light touch, stereognosis, pain and temperature, proprioception, and two-point discrimination. Test findings should be recorded and deficits should be noted.

Passive ROM should begin with gentle movement of the proximal joints and should proceed only to the point of pain. As the patient's tolerance level increases, active ROM and light exercises may be introduced. The program should stress joint protection, and the therapist should look for muscle imbalance and substitution patterns. Progressive resistive exercises should be used conservatively. Throughout the course of recovery the therapist should guard against fatigue and irritation of the inflamed nerves. As the patient's strength and tolerance level increase, more resistance can be employed, but to a moderate degree. The therapist may also introduce sedentary or tabletop activities during the early stages of recovery. As the patient's strength increases, activities promoting more resistance, such as leather work, textiles, and ceramics, can be incorporated into the treatment regime. Grooming, self-care, and other ADL should be included as the need and desire arise. Slings and mobile arm supports may be employed to alleviate muscle fatigue and gain independence.

Bell's palsy

Bell's palsy is an acute inflammatory disorder that affects the seventh (facial) cranial nerve. It is commonly attributed to exposure to cold, herpes zoster of the middle ear, traumatic conditions, and in some cases there is a familial tendency.[9,15] The course of the disease is usually short in duration, lasting 2 to 8 weeks. Approximately 70% of Bell's palsy patients experience spontaneous recovery whereas 30% do not.[4] During the acute onset of the disorder one side of the patient's face is expressionless with an inability to close the eye. The patient may have difficulty eating and speaking, and the eye on the affected side may produce tears.[5,10]

OCCUPATIONAL THERAPY INTERVENTION. The occupational therapist may play an important role in the treatment of the patient with Bell's palsy.

Beals[4] developed a treatment program based on phylogenetic facial expression. Since the facial musculature is controlled by both cortical and subcortical centers, facial expression represents a reflex action of high complexity. Therefore the treatment plan should first emphasize subcortical facial reactions of a spontaneous or reflexive nature. The treatment should promote gross patterns of expression facilitated by high-intensity stimuli. For example, a small slice of lemon is used to stimulate the buccal area. This stimulus affects the maxillary portion of the trigeminal nerve and is transmitted to the brainstem where synaptic connections are made with motor neurons of the facial nerve.[2,14] In addition, strong smells, such as ammonia, cause the sensory endings of the trigeminal nerve to discharge into reflex arcs that stimulte the action of the nares and depressor septi. Thus the facial musculature can be stimulated reflexively through indirect synaptic connections via the trigeminal and olfactory cranial nerves.

The conscious component of facial expression can be activated in a graded fashion by reciting the alphabet, reading prose, or through activities that use pantomine.

Brown, et al.[7] described a successful program using EMG biofeedback for the reduction of facial paralysis. This program used visual and auditory feedback signals to allow the patient to gain functional control of facial musculature. The patients were trained to use EMG biofeedback and to practice facial expressions and verbalizations while viewing themselves in a mirror. This program reported successful results within a 3-month training period.

The occupational therapist may also work with the orthotist to fabricate a temporary facial splint to prevent stretching of the delicate muscle fibers. The affected facial muscles can also benefit from gentle, upward massage for 5 to 10 minutes 2 to 3 times a day to increase circulation and maintain muscle tone. Electrical stimulation and infrared treatments by the physical therapist may also be included in the patient's treatment regime. The therapist should assist the patient in carrying out his or her normal personal hygiene tasks. The lack of facial sensation on one side will require careful visual awareness while shaving. Brushing the teeth will require careful visual attention because food particles can collect on the affected side. Some patients may wear a patch over the affected eye, so visual awareness should be stressed to compensate for the temporary loss of sight and sensation.

Trigeminal neuralgia (tic douloureux)

Trigeminal neuralgia is characterized by sudden attacks of excruciating pain in the sensory distribution of one or more branches of the trigeminal nerve. The cause of this disorder is multifaceted. There are reports of degenerative changes in the trigeminal ganglia, aberrant arteries impinging on the nerve roots, tumors, demyelinating conditions, and mechanical causes.[9,11,15] Statistically trigeminal neuralgia affects middle-aged and elderly people. It is more common in women and frequently affects the right side of the face. In 90% of the cases it affects the second and third divisions of the trigeminal nerve distribution.[15]

At the present time it is not understood why the neurons that subserve pain sensation for the trigeminal nerve suddenly discharge. In many cases there is a "trigger zone" in the facial or oral region that is extremely sensitive to temperature changes, light touch, or facial movement. Any irritation to the trigger zone can cause paroxysmal pain of brief durations.[10]

The medical management for trigeminal neuralgia includes alcohol injections, surgery and drugs.

OCCUPATIONAL THERAPY INTERVENTION. Treatment should begin with a thorough interview and sensory evaluation to identify the location of the "trigger zones" and the stimuli that precipitate the pain attacks. In cooperation with the medical treatment prescribed by the physician, the therapist may implement one of several approaches. First the therapist may attempt to systematically desensitize the patient to the stimuli that triggers the pain attacks. This would require a carefully graded program using relaxation techniques and biofeedback. The EMG biofeedback machine can monitor muscle tightness in selected muscles, such

as the temporalis or upper trapezius, to watch for muscle tension following pain.[17] Galvanic skin resistance biofeedback may also be used, since it measures the activity of the sympathetic nervous system. The combined effects of biofeedback and relaxation techniques enable the patient to obtain information about his or her body's physiological responses and to establish some cortical control over the intensity of pain sensation. Recent studies on pain management suggest that when the patient feels he or she is able to do something to control the pain, the pain perception is decreased.[12,24,25,36] It has also been suggested that placebos may stimulate the release of endogenous opiates (enkephalins) and contribute to pain reduction.[40]

A second approach is to incorporate a consistent program of graded cutaneous stimulation. The therapist should avoid noxious stimuli, such as icing and electrical brushing, since they will activate the C and A delta size pain fibers.[28] Instead, the therapist may try stretch pressure and low frequency vibration (60 Hertz) over the facial muscles to activate the large fibers of the proprioceptive system. According to the gate control theory of pain mechanisms, pain sensation may be suppressed in the neurons of the spinal cord and the brainstem.[24] Another benefit of graded sensory stimulation is the cutaneous receptors will eventually adapt and perhaps raise their threshold to stimuli that triggers pain responses.[29]

A third and important treatment is the implementation of a daily program of purposeful activities. The therapist may want to administer an activity configuration to identify the periods in which the patient is most inactive. Most patients experience more pain sensation during the evenings or when they are inactive.[12] During these junctures the patient tends to focus on the pain experience. This is the best time to engage the patient in routine activities to direct the conscious energies toward a purposeful task. Cortical distraction during painful episodes is a proven method of alleviating pain sensation.[12,40]

Transcutaneous electrical nerve stimulation (TENS) is an effective modality for reducing acute and chronic pain.[25,36] The role of the occupational thera-

pist in the use of TENS is controversial at this time. In many settings nurses and therapists use TENS under the prescription of a physician.

INJURIES TO PERIPHERAL NERVES
Clinical signs of peripheral nerve injuries

Regardless of the origin of the injury peripheral nerve lesions produce similar clinical manifestations. The most obvious manifestation is muscle weakness or flaccid paralysis, depending on the extent of the nerve damage. Because of the loss of muscle innervation atrophy will follow, and deep tendon reflexes will be absent or depressed. Sensation along the cutaneous distribution of the nerve will also be lost. Trophic changes, such as dry skin, hair loss, cyanosis, brittle fingernails, painless skin ulcerations, and slow wound healing in the area of involvement, may also be present as clinical signs. Occasionally minute muscle contractions called fasciculations may be seen on the surface of the skin overlying the denervated muscle belly. As a result of disturbances of sympathetic fibers of the autonomic nervous system, there will be a loss of the ability to sweat above the denervated skin surfaces. The patient may experience paresthesias, that is, sensations such as tingling, numbness, and burning or pain (causalgia), particularly at night. In addition if the nerve damage was caused by trauma, edema will be a prominent clinical manifestation. EMG examinations may reveal extremely small muscle contractions called fibrillations.*

Extensive peripheral nerve damage may produce deformity if contractures, joint stiffness, and poor positioning are allowed to occur. Disfigurement of the hands is particularly noticeable and may produce some psychological complications. Other complications may include osteoporosis of the bony structures and epidermal fibrosis of the joints.

All of the clinical manifestations just discussed may not be present. The clinical findings may vary with the underlying cause of the lesion.

---

*References 2, 3, 9, 10, 14, 21.

Clinical signs of peripheral nerve regeneration

Peripheral nerve regeneration begins about 1 month after the injury occurred. The rate of regeneration depends on the nature of the nerve lesion. If, for example, the nerve has been severed, the regeneration would occur at the rate of ½ inch (1.3 cm) per month.[30] Early medical treatment may require suturing the nerve and immobilizing the involved extremity to ensure good opposition of the severed nerves: The introduction of microsurgery has brought new advancements to the process of peripheral nerve regeneration. An experimental technique of nerve grafting called the mesothelial tube promotes nerve regeneration across an extended gap.[22] The mesothelial tube is a silicone chamber that protects the severed nerve endings so the newly formed nerve has a larger diameter. Another newly developed surgical technique called direct neurotization[8] has shown that a denervated muscle will accept an implanted motor nerve, and functional innervation can be attained. This innovative surgical technique offers new hope for patients with significant muscle paralysis as a result of peripheral nerve lesions.

In most postsurgery cases the therapist may fabricate resting splints and assist in the proper positioning of the extremity to reduce edema. The therapist may also supervise the patient in active ROM to maintain the strength of the uninvolved muscles and joint mobility. Active rehabilitation begins about 7 weeks after the incision or graft has healed. In the past full recovery of muscles was not probable because regenerated fibers lose about 20% of their original diameter and conduct impulses at a slower rate.[10,28] Newer surgical techniques may improve the regenerative process.

Since peripheral nerves have the capacity to regenerate, the course of recovery can be somewhat predictable. The clinical signs of regeneration do not always abide by a specific sequence. Yet one might expect to see the following clinical signs:

Skin appearance: As the edema subsides and collateral blood vessels develop, the circulatory system should become more normalized. The skin should improve in its color and texture.

Primitive protection sensations: The first signs of cutaneous sensation will usually be the gross recognition of crude pain, temperature, pressure, and touch.

Paresthesias (Tinel's sign): Tapping along the involved nerve route will produce crude sensations. The patient may also experience pain sensations, especially at night.

Scattered points of sweating: As the parasympathetic fibers of the autonomic nervous system regenerate, the sweat glands will recover their functions.

Discriminative sensations: The more refined sensations, such as the ability to identify and localize touch, joint movements (proprioception), recognition of objects in the three dimensional form (stereognosis), speed of movement (kinesthesia), and two-point discrimination, should be returning at this juncture.

Muscle tone: As nerve fibers regenerate and tie into their respective musculature via their motor end-plates, flaccidity will decrease and tone will increase. An important principle is that paralyzed muscles must first sense pressure before tone and movement can be realized.

Voluntary muscle function: The patient will be able to move the extremity first with gravity eliminated, and, as strength increases, he or she may actively move the extremity through full ROM. At this point graded exercises can begin.

Full recovery of muscle power is not probable, because the possibility that thousands of regenerating fibers will find their previous connections is unlikely.*

Phelps and Walker[30] reported that for complete laceration of peripheral nerves, the two-point discrimination test and the wrinkle test are viable methods of monitoring sensory return. The two-point discrimination test provides a quantitative measure of sensation. An earlier study by Moberg reveals the normal distance to

discriminate one point from two points on the distal fingertip is 2 to 4 mm. A two-point discrimination of greater than 15 mm denotes tactile agnosia (absent sensation). This test can be achieved with the use of a high-quality caliper with blunted tips so that the pain sensation is not elicited. Light application of the calipers to the patient's skin in a random pattern can help the therapist map out the cutaneous, topographical areas that are innervated and denervated.

Another test that can be clinically significant is the wrinkle test. This test is performed by immersing the patient's hand in plain water at 108° F (42.2° C). The hand remains submerged for about 20 to 30 minutes until wrinkling occurs. At this point the patient's hand is dried, graded on a scale of 0 to 3, and photographed. The "0" on the scale represents an absence of wrinkling, whereas "3" represents normal wrinkling. The wrinkle test appears to provide an objective method of testing innervation of the hand with recent complete and partial peripheral nerve injuries. The actual physiological mechanism that causes the wrinkling is not fully understood, and the test is not appropriate for patients with traumatic peripheral nerve compression injuries.[30] Nevertheless, the test can be significant in determining the rate of sensory regeneration and can provide a graphic record of denervated areas.

Medical management of peripheral nerve injuries

The medical-surgical management of peripheral nerve lesions depends on the type of injury that has occurred. Lacerations may be treated with microsurgery to suture the severed nerve. Exploratory surgery (neurolysis) may be conducted to remove unwanted scar tissue from the site of the lesion. Nerve grafts and transplants are performed for severe traumatic injuries. Alcohol injections, vitamin B_{12}, and phenol are used to alleviate the pain that might accompany peripheral neuropathy. For inflammatory processes high caloric diets with liberal use of vitamin B complex is the treatment of choice.[6,9,15]

---

*References 2, 6, 9, 10, 21, 28.

Specific peripheral nerve injuries

BRACHIAL PLEXUS INJURY. The nerve roots that innervate the upper extremity originate in the anterior rami between C4 and T1. This network of lower anterior cervical and upper dorsal spine nerves is collectively called the *brachial plexus*. This very important nerve complex can be palpated just behind the posterior border of the sternocleidomastoid as the head and neck are tilted to the opposite side.[6,9,20,35]

Lesions to the brachial plexus usually result from a variety of traumatic injuries. Most brachial plexus injuries in children are caused by birth trauma. The more classic of these brachial plexus injuries are call Erb's palsy and Klumpke's paralyses. Erb's palsy is indicative of lesions to the fifth and sixth plexus roots. Paralysis and atrophy occur in the deltoid, brachialis, biceps, and brachioradialis muscles. Clinically the arm hangs limp, the hand rotates inward, and functional movement is extremely limited.

Klumpke's paralysis affects the more distal aspect of the upper extremity. The disorder results from injury to the eighth cervical and first thoracic plexus roots. Consequently there will be paralysis to the distal musculature of the wrist flexors and the intrinsic muscles of the hand.[6,9]

LONG THORACIC NERVE INJURY. The long thoracic nerve (C5-7) innervates the serratus anterior (magnus) muscle, which anchors the apex of the scapula to the posterior of the rib cage. Although injury to this nerve is not common, it has been injured by carrying heavy weights on the shoulder, neck blows, and axillary wounds. The resulting clinical picture is threefold: First, winging of the scapula occurs when the arm is extended and pressed against a stabilized object in front of the patient. Second, the patient will have difficulty flexing the outstretched arm above the level of his or her shoulder. Third, the patient will have difficulty protracting the shoulder or performing scapula abduction and adduction.

Injuries involving the long thoracic nerve are usually treated by stabilizing the shoulder girdle to limit scapula motion. The therapist must avoid using activities that promote shoulder movements. If nerve regeneration is not complete, surgery may be indicated to relieve the excessive mobility of the scapula. After medical treatment the occupational therapist encourages maximal functional independence and teahces the patient to use long-handle devices to compensate for shoulder limitations.

AXILLARY NERVE INJURY. The axillary nerve is composed from the C5-6 spinal nerves and derived from the posterior region of the brachial plexus. The motor branches of the axillary nerve innervate the superior aspect of the deltoid muscle and the teres minor muscle. Although the axillary nerve is rarely damaged by itself, it is often damaged along with traumatic lesions to the brachial plexus. As a result, the patient will experience weakness or paralysis of the deltoid muscle, causing limitations in horizontal abduction and hyperesthesia on the lateral aspect of the shoulder. In addition to the loss of muscle power, atrophy of the deltoid muscle produces asymmetry of the shoulders. If the nerve damage is permanent, a muscle transplantation may be required to provide some abduction of the arm.[6,9,34]

The occupational therapist should maintain ROM to prevent deformity and improve circulation. Passive abduction of the shoulder should be done daily. The teres minor and deltoid muscles should be protected from stretch during the manual ROM activities. The patient may be taught to use long-handle assistive divices to compensate for the abduction deficit. If a surgical transplant is performed, the therapist should be familiar with the surgical procedure and assist in muscle reeducation. An EMG biofeedback machine can be beneficial in providing the patient with visual and auditory incentives during muscle reeducation sessions. The occupational therapist may also assist the patient in dressing activities. If the asymmetry of the shoulders presents a cosmetic problem when wearing shirts or jackets, a foam rubber or Orthoplast pad can be fabricated to fill in

the space that was once filled by the deltoid muscle. The patient should be encouraged to learn self-ranging techniques and implement an exercise program to maintain the integrity of the unimpaired muscles of the involved extremity.

RADIAL NERVE INJURY. The radial nerve represents the largest branch of the brachial plexus and descends along the humerus in the musculospiral groove. Below the elbow it bifurcates into the superficial radial nerve and the deep radial nerve. The superficial radial nerve terminates in the first, second, and third phalanges, whereas the deep radial nerve descends along the posterior region of the forearm, branching out to supply the extensor-supinator group of muscles.

The sensory branches innervate cutaneous receptors along the dorsal aspect of the arm and forearm and the posterior surface of the thumb, index and middle fingers, and half of the ring finger. The motor branches innervate the triceps, brachioradialis, anconeus, extensor digitorum communis, extensor carpi ulnaris, supinator, abductor pollicis longus, extensor pollicis brevis, extensor pollicis longus, and extensor indicis proprius muscles.

The actions produced by the radial nerve are wrist extension, metacarpophalangeal (MP) extension, thumb abduction and extension, ulnar and radial deviation, and release of grasping actions.

The most common types of injury to the radial nerve are fractures of the humerus or lacerations across the dorsum of the forearm.

The most blatant clinical feature of radial nerve injury is extensor paralysis. The patient will exhibit "wrist drop" and an inability to extend the thumb, proximal phalanges, and elbow joint. In addition the patient will have difficulty pronating the hand and grasping objects.[3,9,27,28,37]

MEDIAN NERVE INJURY. The median nerve originates in the lateral and medial cords of the brachial plexus. The two cords unite, forming one nerve trunk that descends along the medial part of the arm to the anterior region of the forearm, branching out until it terminates in the hand.

The sensory branches of the median nerve supply the volar surface of the thumb, the index and middle fingers, and half of the ring finger. The motor branches innervate the pronator teres, flexor carpi radialis, palmaris longus, flexor digitorum sublimis, flexor pollicis longus, half of the flexor digitorum profundus, lumbricales 1 and 2, and pronator quadratus.

The actions produced by the median nerve are thumb opposition and abduction, interphalangeal (IP) flexion of the index finger, distal interphalangeal (DIP) flexion of the thumb, wrist flexion, forearm pronation, MP flexion of the second and third fingers, and IP flexion of the third, fourth, and fifth fingers.

The most common types of injury for the median nerve are forearm lacerations, wrist trauma, and deep lacerations to the flexor pollicis brevis muscle.[3,9,28,37]

Clinically one would expect to see loss of thumb opposition, thenar atrophy, and ape hand deformity. Furthermore the patient would have difficulty making a fist because the second and third fingers would remain extended while the fourth and fifth would flex.

CARPAL TUNNEL SYNDROME. The carpal tunnel represents a small passage in the volar aspect of the wrist formed by the concavity of carpal bones and bridged by the transverse carpal ligament. The tunnel provides a restricted space for the tendons of the long flexors of the fingers, the flexor pollicis longus, and the median nerve.[9,15] Anytime the wrist is flexed or extended the transverse ligament tightens over the wrist.[15]

The so-called carpal tunnel syndrome can result from several factors. For instance, a dislocation of the lunate bone or a malunited Colles' fracture can cause narrowing of the passage. Arthritic complications, such as tenosynovitis, following rheumatoid arthritis can cause enlargement of the tendons. Other causes would include trauma, spur formation, lipomas and hypertrophy of the wrist because of occupational hazards.[11,15,20] These conditions result in compression or entrapment of the median nerve in the carpal tunnel. Carpal tunnel syndrome may also obstruct venous return causing edema, increased

pressure, and ischemia. This may result in permanent damage to the median nerve.

Clinically the onset of carpal tunnel syndrome can be sudden or occur over a long time. The patient may feel numbness, paresthesias, or pain, especially at night. Physical examination of the hand would reveal diminished sensation on the radial half of the hand, atrophy of the thenar eminence, fasciculations in the area of wasting, and trophic changes on the first, second, and third fingertips.[9,11,15] Medical management would be contingent on the cause of the pressure or entrapment of the median nerve.

The occupational therapist can provide supportive devices, such as splinting if indicated, teaching the patient the use of assistive devices for one hand activities, and adaptive devices for daily activities. It is also important to engage the patient in purposeful activities to maintain function, joint mobility, and muscular strength in the uninvolved extremities. The patient should be instructed to visually compensate for sensory loss so further damage does not occur in the denervated tissues. For some patients prevocational exploration may be appropriate to maintain gainful employment during the period of recovery.

ULNAR NERVE INJURY. The ulnar nerve is the largest branch of the medial cord of the brachial plexus. It travels down the medial side of the arm and passes posteriorly to the medial epicondyle of the humerus. From the elbow it descends along the ulnar side of the forearm to innervate the small muscles of the hand.

The sensory branches of the ulnar nerve innervate cutaneous receptors in the little finger, half of the ring finger, and the medial portion of the hand. The motor branches innervate the flexor carpi ulnaris half of the flexor digitorum profundus, adductor digiti minimi, opponens digiti minimi, flexor digiti minimi, lumbricales 3 and 4, interossei, adductor pollicis, flexor pollicis brevis, and palmaris brevis muscles.

The actions produced by the ulnar nerve are finger adduction and abduction, wrist flexion, and MP extension. Grasp and pinch are achieved by proximal interphalangeal (PIP) flexion of the

fourth and fifth phalanges and thumb adduction and opposition.

The usual sites of injury of the ulnar nerve are the posterior elbow region and the palmar region of the hand from the MP joint of the fifth finger to the carpal joint.[3,9,37]

COMBINED ULNAR AND MEDIAN INJURY. Since the ulnar and median nerves are anatomically close to each other in the wrist region, they are often injured together. The clinical picture depends on the severity of the lesion and which nerve has undergone the most damage. If both nerves suffer a complete transection, ape hand deformity would be present, the wrist would be hyperextended, and flexor movements and abduction and adduction of the fingers would be greatly impaired.[3,9,28,37]

VOLKMANN'S CONTRACTURE. A fracture of the lower end of the humerus (supracondylar region) may result in a diminished supply of well-oxygenated blood to the muscles of the forearm. Ths phenomenon can occur when the fracture has been tightly cast and bandaged. Edema sets in near the site of the injury and shuts down the blood supply to the muscle bellies because the site of injury cannot swell outward. Ischemia will deprive tissues of oxygen and nourishment. The muscle can become necrotic, causing atrophy and contractures of the wrist, fingers, and forearm. The flexor digitorum profundus and flexor pollicis longus muscles are severely affected. The median nerve is often more impaired than the ulnar nerve.[6,20]

Shortly after a fracture of the humerus has been immobilized, the patient may have a cold, distal extremity with a smooth, glossy, or dusky appearance of the skin. If the therapist cannot detect a radial pulse, the physician should be informed immediately, and the cast should be removed. Early detection and prevention of this problem can eliminate a very severe deformity. If, for example, the ischemia lasts 6 hours, some contracture will follow. Ischemia lasting 48 hours or more will result in a permanent deformity of the forearm.

If mild ischemia has occurred, the physician may prescribe vigorous, active exercises to increase circulation, activate musculature, and prevent joint stiffness.

The occupational therapist may be involved in the treatment of acute peripheral nerve injury or may be involved later in the rehabilitation process. Treatment during the acute postoperative phase is aimed at the prevention of deformity. Initially static splints are used to immobilize the extremity and protect the site of injury.[16,37] During this phase the reduction of edema may be of primary importance. The first step in the reduction of edema is to elevate the extremity above the level of the heart. This will decrease the hydrostatic pressure in the blood vessels and promote venous and lymphatic drainage. Manual massage while the extremity is elevated may also reduce edema. The massage should entail centripetal strokes to gently force the excess fluids toward the proximal aspects of the body. Care must be taken not to disturb the healing process of the site of injury. External elastic support can also be used to alleviate the edema. Furthermore, passive ROM will assist in the prevention of edema by promiting venous return.[38]

Occupational therapy intervention for peripheral nerve injuries

The treatment goals for peripheral nerve injuries are generally similar. The aim is to assist the patient in regaining the maximal level of function. The rate of return and the residual impairments depend largely on the severity of the lesion and the quality of care during the rehabilitation process. Table 28-1 is a useful summary of the major nerve roots and clinical manifestation of their lesions.

As the patient's muscle tone returns, a mild progressive resistive exercise program can be established. Resistive activities, such as woodworking, ceramics, leather work, and copper tooling, may be used in conjunction with isometric and isotonic exercises. The therapist should not overtax the returning musculature and should protect the weaker muscle groups from stretch and fatigue.

The peripheral nerve injury may create some challenging problems in ADL that the therapist and patient must overcome. If one upper extremity is impaired (flaccid paralysis), the therapist may design a temporary "static sling" to be worn during shower activities or anytime the extremity needs to be securely positioned so that the person can move about. Static slings have some disadvantages. They should not be worn for long periods because they hold the arm in a flexed position, interfere with the postural support of the arm during some activities, limit proprioceptive feedback, and change the body image. Some therapists are fabricating "dynamic slings," designed by Farber[13] for hemiplegic patients, that can also help the patient with peripheral nerve injury. Elastic straps are used instead of webbing straps, and a cone is secured in the patient's hand to maintain a functional position. Tourniquet hosing has also been used in place of a rigid shoulder strap to allow some mobility of the joints, yet allow enough support to keep the arm flexed and close to the trunk. This elasticity allows better circulation to the extremity and better tactile, proprioceptive, and kinesthetic stimulation.

Table 28-1
Clinical manifestations of peripheral nerve lesions

Spinal nerves	Nerve roots	Motor distribution	Clinical manifestations
Brachial plexus			
C5-7	Long thoracic	Shoulder girdle, serratus anterior	"Winged scapula"
C5-6	Dorsal scapular	Rhomboid major and minor, levator, scapulae	Loss of scapular adduction and elevation
C7-8	Thoracodorsal	Latissimus dorsi	Loss of arm adduction and extension
C5-6	Suprascapular	Supraspinatus, infraspinatus	Weakened lateral rotation of humerus
C5-6	Subscapular	Subscapularis, teres major	Weakened medial rotation of humerus
C6-8, T1	Radial	All extensors of forearm, triceps	"Wrist drop," extensor paralysis
C5-6	Axillary	Deltoid, teres minor	Loss of arm abduction, weakened lateral rotation of humerus
C5-6	Musculocutaneous	Biceps brachii, brachialis, coracobrachialis	Loss of forearm flexion and supination
C6-8, T1	Median	Flexors of hand and digits, opponens pollicis	"Ape hand" deformity, weakened grip, thenar atrophy, unopposed thumb
C8, T1	Ulnar	Flexor of hand and digits, opponens pollicis	"Claw hand" deformity, interosseus atrophy, loss of thumb adduction
Lumbosacral plexus			
L2-4	Femoral	Iliopsoas, quadriceps femoris	Loss of thigh flexion, leg extension
L2-4	Obturator	Adductors of thigh	Weakened or loss of thigh adduction
L4-5, S1-3	Sciatic	Hamstrings, all musculature below the knee	Loss of leg flexion, paralysis of all muscles of leg and foot
L4-5, S1-2	Common peroneal	Dorsiflexors of foot	"Foot-drop," "steppage gait," loss of eversion
L4-5, S1-3	Tibial	Gastrocnemius, soleus, deep plantar flexors of foot	Loss of plantar flexion and inversion of foot

Assistive devices, such as long-handle reaching aids and one-handed kitchen tools used in the treatment of hemiplegia, have also been found to be beneficial.

MYASTHENIA GRAVIS

Although myasthenia gravis is not a true lower motor neuron disease, it warrants some discussion in this chapter.

Myasthenia gravis is a chronic neuromuscular condition characterized by abnormal voluntary muscle fatigue. The cause of this disease is unknown at the present time. However, the defect occurs at the myoneurojunction where the presence of IgG autoantibodies seems to block acetylcholine receptors on the postsynaptic membrane.[15] Another theory suggests that there is a defect in the resynthesis of acetylcholine in the presynaptic membrane of the myoneurojunction.[33] In addition, many patients develop concurrent complications of the thyroid and thymus glands. It is not understood how the thymus gland affects the disease, but surgical removal causes significant improvement in 70% to 80% of the patients.[9]

Statiscally this disease affects women between age 20 and 40 and men between age 50 and 70. It affects all races. The prevalence in the United States is estimated to be about 20,000 persons.[11]

Clinically myasthenia gravis produces a variety of symptoms. The disease can affect any of the striated skeletal muscles of the body. Yet it seems to have an affinity for the muscles innervated by the brainstem nuclei. Therefore the muscles most often affected are those that move the eyes, eyelids, tongue, jaw, and throat. The muscles that are used most often fatigue the earliest.[15] Therefore the patient may have double vision, drooping of the eyelids, and difficulty with speech or swallowing as the day goes on.

Medical management includes a long list of drugs, such as anticholinesterase, prednisone, and possibly corticosteroid therapy. A thymectomy is performed on patients not responding to anticholinesterase therapy. A new therapy called plasmapheresis entails filtering the blood to remove the IgG autoantibodies. This treatment may be accompanied by cytotoxic immunosuppressive therapy.[1,18,19]

Occupational therapy intervention

The prognosis for myasthenia gravis varies with each individual. Spontaneous remissions have been reported with thymectomy, but for most it is a progressively disabling disease.[9] It is important for the therapist to monitor the patient's muscle strength on a regular basis. The therapist need not evaluate all of the muscles because the evaluation will contribute to fatigue. Instead, the therapist can test the strength of a few muscles during each visit and keep a running chart to note any significant changes. If the patient is taking oral cholinergic drugs, optimal strength is expected about 1 or 2 hours after the medication has been ingested.[1] Therefore the therapist should coordinate muscle testing with the drug treatment regime so the test results are not confounded by the medication. The therapist should also record any changes in the patients physical appearance, such as ptosis of the eyelids, drooping facial muscles, or alterations of breathing or swallowing. The therapist should provide gentle nonresistive activities that are intellectually and psychologically stimulating. The activities should be graded so they do not fatigue the patient. The treatment plan should include energy conservation, work simplification, and an array of adaptive and assistive devices to reduce effort during daily activities. If appropriate, electronic communication devices can be installed in the patient's home so he or she can maintain contact with community agencies. In addition, the therapist may assist with home planning to determine architectural barriers, bathroom adaptations, and furniture rearrangements. Supportive devices can also be fabricated to prevent overstretching the weakened musculature.

The therapist should assist in educating the patient about the disease. The patient should avoid emotional stress, fatigue, and excessive heat or cold because they may exacerbate the symptoms of the disease. Women may experience an increase in symptoms during menstruation because of hormonal changes taking place. The patient may need additional rest during this time. The therapist should also follow infection control procedures, since minor infections can also exacerbate the symptoms.

Sample treatment plan

Case study

John is a 23-year-old man employed as a construction worker. He is a high school graduate, married, and has two children. Recently while working he sustained a deep laceration of the right anterior forearm. This injury resulted in a severed ulnar nerve and partial damage to the median nerve. The patient has undergone microsurgery, and the severed nerves have been repaired with moderate success.

John is an energetic young man who has difficulty adjusting to the hospital environment and to a sedentary existence.

He was referred to occupational therapy for services during the acute and rehabilitation phases of his treatment program. The goals are to prevent deformity, restore joint and muscle function to the maximal level possible, facilitate adjustment to hospital and disability, and evaluate potential for return to former employment.

TREATMENT PLAN

A. **Statistical data.**
　1. Name: John
　　Age: 23
　　Diagnosis: Laceration to right forearm, peripheral nerve injury
　　Disability: Ulnar and median nerve dysfunction; moderate to severe motor paralysis

Sample treatment plan—cont'd

2. Treatment aims as stated in referral:
   To prevent deformity
   To restore joint and muscle function to maximal level possible
   To facilitate adjustment to hospital and disability
   To evaluate potential for return to employment

B. Other services.
   Medical-surgical: Surgery, medication, supervision of rehabilitation program
   Nursing: Nursing care during acute phase of treatment, psychological support
   Physical therapy: ROM, muscle reeducation, edema control
   Social service: Financial arrangements, counseling to client and family
   Vocational rehabilitation counselor: Explore vocational potential, vocational counseling

C. OT evaluation.
   Sensation: Test (light touch, stereognosis, proprioception, two-point discrimination, pain)
   Nerve regeneration: Wrinkle test
   Muscle strength: Manual muscle test
   ROM: Measure
   Grip and pinch strength: Test with instruments
   Hand evaluation: Observation, Jebsen-Taylor Test of Hand Function; tests of speed and dexterity
   ADL: Observe performance
   Psychosocial adjustment: Observe
   Muscle function: EMG biofeedback evaluation to obtain quantitative information for baseline function

D. Results of evaluation.
   1. Evaluation.
      a. Physical resources—right upper extremity.
         (1) Muscle strength
             Wrist flexors: P
             Finger adductors: P
             Finger abductors: P
             Opposition of thumb: P
             Marked muscle atrophy of web spaces (interossei)
             Moderate atrophy of thenar muscles
             Ape hand deformity
             Grasp strength: Right 10 lb pressure, left 130 lb
             Palmar pinch strength: Right 4 lb pressure, left 24 lb

         Hand function and fine dexterity: Below standard norms for age in gross grasp, fine prehension, and movement speed
         (2) ROM: Within normal limits for wrist, thumb, and finger joints; some tightness in long finger flexors when fingers are extended actively
      b. Sensory-perceptual functions.
         (1) Light touch, proprioception, and two-point discrimination: Absent in medial half of right hand; impaired in lateral aspect of right hand, especially thenar region
         (2) Stereognosis: Impaired
         (3) Superficial pain sensitivity (pinprick):
             (a) Intact: Median cutaneous region
             (b) Absent: Ulnar nerve root distribution
         (4) Nerve regeneration: Absence of wrinkling along cutaneous sensory distribution of ulnar nerve; mild wrinkling along median nerve root distribution; photograph of results recorded for visual documentation
      c. Cognitive functions. Client's cognitive functions are considered normal for a 23-year-old man of average intelligence. During evaluation and early treatment he has demonstrated normal memory, good judgment, and problem-solving skills. He attends to the task at hand and shows ability to concentrate for long periods. Motivation for recovery and return to former life roles is very high.
      d. Psychosocial functions. John is married and has two children. The marriage is stable, and his wife is supportive. John has a high level of energy and is accustomed to being very active and moving about freely. The sedentary existence imposed by hospitalization has resulted in mild agitation, impatience, and mild depression. John's leisure interests were playing

         baseball and racquetball and racing sports cars. At home he enjoyed improving his home by painting, decorating, and light construction. John and his wife had many friends and engaged in social activities on weekends. Since John was injured on the job, his financial support and medical expenses are covered by workmen's compensation and disability insurance.
      e. Prevocational potential. If there is good to normal return of neuromuscular function, client is expected to resume his former occupation. If there is residual weakness that precludes employment as a construction worker, prevocational assessment will be undertaken to determine alternatives.
      f. Functional skills. John is independent in most self-care activities. He has adapted easily to performing essential self-maintenance skills with one hand. He demonstrated some difficulty with cutting meat, managing soap in the shower, buttoning small buttons, and carrying large heavy objects such as a carton or tray. Assistive devices were recommended to increase independence.
         Client is able to drive a standard car with power steering and automatic transmission.
   2. Problem identification.
      a. Muscle weakness, resulting in loss of normal function of right hand
      b. Sensory loss
      c. Loss of vocational role
      d. Difficulty adjusting to inactivity
      e. Changed leisure roles
      f. Changes in body image
   3. Assets.
      a. Intelligence
      b. Family support
      c. Financial support
      d. Good prognosis
      e. Good potential for reemployment
      f. Motivation
      g. Age
      h. Vocational skills

Continued.

Sample treatment plan—cont'd

E Specific OT objectives	F Methods used to meet objectives	G Gradation of treatment
Acute phase of treatment Given a hand splint deformity will be prevented and muscles will be maintained at normal length	Static resting splint in functional position to be worn at night and periods of inactivity	Decrease amount of use as hand function increases
Through positioning and passive ROM exercises edema in the hand will be prevented or will remain minimal	Overhead sling attached to headboard of bed, which supports forearm and hand in elevated position; allow some movement to increase blood circulation; gentle passive ROM exercises to thumb, fingers, and wrist after sufficient healing of nerve has occurred to allow some traction on the nerve; teach client ROM exercises and proper positioning of hand[20,31]	Decrease then eliminate use of overhead sling when active rehabilitation program commences
Through appropriate activities client will be more relaxed and less depressed, resulting in tolerance for hospital routines and social interactions	Isometric exercises for shoulder and elbow muscle groups; isometric resistive exercises for unaffected extremities; supportive approach to client, positive reinforcement for participation in activities: puzzles, games (cards, checkers, chess, dominoes, Atari television sports games), reading (sports magazines)	Decrease extrinsic motivation and initiation of activities; increase number of persons participating with client; elicit ideas on improving physical arrangement of clinic; draw up plans and material list
Given assistive devices client will perform personal hygiene and eating activities independently	One-handed rocker knife, rubber placemat for stability of plate, plate guard, suction soap holder to fix soap to wall, wash mitt, built-up handle on razor for shaving	Decrease use of assistive devices as right hand function increases
Rehabilitation phase of treatment—6 weeks after surgery Through therapeutic exercise full ROM of all joints of hand and wrist will be preserved	Passive ROM exercise to each joint motion 5 to 10 repetitions twice daily; active ROM of each joint motion	Decrease passive exercise; increase active exercise as strength improves
Through exercise and activity to affected wrist and hand muscles strength of affected muscles will increase from P to G	Active exercise to wrist flexors, thumb flexors, finger abductors and adductors; thumb abduction; opposition; construction of small jewelry box with mosaic tile top; ceramics—pinch pot or coil project; therapeutic putty exercises	Increase resistance as F+ muscle grades are attained; commence PRE program
Given adequate recovery of muscle strength and hand function feasibility for return to same or related job will be explored	Construction of a large wood chest or book shelf; client is to plan and perform all operations; activities should be performed standing; purposes are to evaluate handling and use of hand tools, safety awareness, standing tolerance, and physical endurance; engage client in construction of closet or shelves for health care facility under direction of maintenance supervisor, as a job trial; aspects of the actual construction duties can be simulated in the clinic; weighted objects similar to construction materials will be lifted, carried, and manipulated and will be graded according to gained strength and endurance	Increase weight of loads and requirements for bending, lifting, and carrying large objects

Sample treatment plan—cont'd

H. Special equipment.
1. Ambulation aids.
   None required
2. Splints.
   Static resting splint in functional position to be worn at night and during periods of inactivity in acute phase of treatment

3. Assistive devices.
   One-handed rocker knife for meat cutting
   Rubber placemat to prevent plate slipping
   Plate guard to prevent food spills
   Suction soap holder to stabilize soap in shower

Wash mitt to eliminate need to manipulate washcloth and soap
Built-up handle on razor to accommodate weak grasp
Elastic material for sling to wear while taking a shower, to support hand in elevated position while bending and reaching

REVIEW QUESTIONS

1. Describe the components of the lower motor neuron system.
2. Describe the pathology and major clinical findings of poliomyelitis.
3. Compare and contrast poliomyelitis with Guillian-Barré syndrome.
4. List some treatment strategies for Guillain-Barré syndrome.
5. List at least six clinical manifestations of peripheral nerve injury.
6. Describe the sequential signs of recovery following peripheral nerve injury.
7. Describe some evaluations to determine sensory loss.
8. Identify the classic deformities associated with the radial, ulnar, and median nerves.
9. Describe some treatment strategies for peripheral nerve injuries.
10. List some contraindications when treating peripheral nerve injuries.
11. Describe the clinical signs of Bell's palsy.
12. Discuss some treatment strategies used to rehabilitate the facial muscles.
13. Describe the clinical signs of trigeminal neuralgia.
14. List three treatment techniques that can be used for trigeminal neuralgia.
15. Describe two new surgical techniques that may improve peripheral nerve regeneration.
16. Describe the pathophysiology of carpal tunnel syndrome.
17. Discuss some treatment intervention techniques for occupational therapists.
18. Describe the pathophysiology of myasthenia gravis.
19. Discuss the clinical signs of myasthenia gravis.
20. Describe the role of occupational therapy for patients who have myasthenia gravis.

REFERENCES

1. Barone, D.: Steroid treatment for experimental autoimmune myasthenia gravis, Arch. Neurol. 37:663, 1980.
2. Barr, M.L.: The human nervous system, ed. 2, New York, 1974, Harper & Row, Publishers, Inc.
3. Bateman, J.: Trauma to nerves in limbs, Philadelphia, 1962, W.B. Saunders Co.
4. Beals, R.: A study of occupational therapy in Bell's palsy, Am. J. Occup. Ther. 5:185, 1951.
5. Bickerstaff, E.: Neurology, ed. 3, London, 1978, Hodder & Stoughton, Ltd.
6. Brashear, R.H., and Raney, R.B.: Shands' handbook of orthopaedic surgery, ed. 9, St. Louis, 1978, The C.V. Mosby Co.
7. Brown, M.D., et al.: Electromyographic biofeedback in the reeducation of facial palsy, J. Am. Phys. Ther. Assoc. 57:183, 1978.
8. Brunelli, G.: Direct neurotization of severely damaged muscles, J. Hand Surg. 7:572, 1982.
9. Chusid, J.G.: Correlative neuroanatomy and functional neurology, ed. 18, Los Altos, Calif., 1982, Lange Medical Publications.
10. Clark, R.G.: Clinical neuroanatomy and neurophysiology, ed. 5, Philadelphia, 1975, F.A. Davis Co.
11. Drupp, M.A., and Chatton, M.J.: Current medical diagnosis and treatment, ed. 16, Los Altos, Calif., 1977, Lange Medical Publications.
12. Evans, F.J.: Placebo response in pain reduction, Adv. Neurol. 4:289, 1974.
13. Farber, S.: Neurorehabilitation: a multisensory approach, Philadelphia, 1982, W.B. Saunders Co.
14. Gardner, E.: Fundamentals of neurology, ed. 6, Philadelphia, 1975, W.B. Saunders Co.
15. Gilroy, J., and Meyer, J.: Medical neurology, ed. 3, New York, 1979, Macmillan Publishing Co., Inc.
16. Hopkins, H.L., and Smith, H.D.: Willard and Spackman's occupational therapy, ed. 5, Philadelphia, 1978, J.B. Lippincott Co.
17. Jacobs, A., and Felton, G.S.: Visual feedback of myoelectric output to facilitate muscle relaxation in normal patients and patients with neck injuries, Arch. Phys. Med. Rehabil. 50:34, 1969.
18. Khana, E., et al.: Creutzfeldt-Jakob disease: focus among Libyan Jews in Israel, Science 183:90, 1974.
19. Kornfeld, P.: Plasmapheresis in refractory generalized myasthenia gravis, Arch. Neurol. 38:478, 1981.
20. Larson, C.B., and Gould, M.: Orthopedic nursing, ed. 9, St. Louis, 1978, The C.V. Mosby Co.
21. Laurence, T.N., and Pugel, A.V.: Peripheral nerve involvement in spinal cord injury: an electromyographic study, Arch. Phys. Med. Rehabil. 59:209, 1978.
22. Lundborg, G., et al.: Nerve regeneration across an extended gap: a neurobiological view of nerve repair and the possible involvement of neuronotrophic factors, J. Hand Surg. 7:500, 1982.
23. Melville, I.D.: Clinical problems in motor neurone disease. In Obeham, P., and Rose, F.C., editors: Progress in neurological research, London, 1979, Pitman Publishing, Ltd.
24. Melzack, R., and Wall, P.D.: Psychophysiology of pain, Int. Anesthesiol. Clin. 8:3, 1970.
25. Moore, D.E., and Backer, M.M.: How effective is TENS for chronic pain, Am. J. Nurs. 83:1175, 1983.
26. Morrison, D., Pathier, P., and Horr, K.: Sensory motor dysfunction and therapy in infancy and early childhood, Springfield, Ill., 1955, Charles C Thomas, Publishers.
27. Nichols, H.F.: Manual of hand injuries, Chicago, 1955, Year Book Medical Publishers, Inc.

28. Noback, C.R., and Demares, R.J.: The nervous system: introduction and review, ed. 2, New York, 1977, McGraw-Hill, Inc.

29. Pertovaara, A.: Modification of human pain threshold by specific tactile receptors, Acta Physiol. Scand. **107**:339, 1979.

30. Phelps, P.E., and Walker, C.: Comparison of the finger wrinkling test results to establish sensory tests in peripheral nerve injury, Am. J. Occup. Ther. **31**:465, 1977.

31. Rathenberg, E.: Dynamic living for the long term patient, Dubuque, Iowa, 1962, Wm. C. Brown Co., Publishers.

32. Robinault, I.: Functional aids for the multiply handicapped, New York, 1973, Harper & Row, Publishers, Inc.

33. Schmidt, R.F.: Fundamentals of neurophysiology, ed. 2, New York, 1978, Springer-Verlag New York, Inc.

34. Schumacher, B., and Allen, H.A.: Medical aspects of disabilities, Chicago, 1976, Rehabilitation Institute.

35. Smith, B.: Differential diagnosis in neurology, New York, 1979, Arco Publishing, Inc.

36. Taylor, A.G., et al.: How effective in TENS for acute pain, Am. J. Nurs. **83**:1171, 1983.

37. Trombly, C.A., and Scott, A.D.: Occupational therapy for physical dysfunction, Baltimore, 1977, Williams & Wilkins.

38. Vasudevan, S., and Melvin, J.L.: Upper extremity edema control: rationale of the techniques, Am. J. Occup. Ther. **33**:520, 1979.

39. Walter, J.B.: An introduction to the principles of disease, Philadelphia, 1977, W.B. Saunders Co.

40. West, A.: Understanding endorphins: our natural pain relief system, Nursing '81 **12**:50, 1981.

CHAPTER 29

Spinal cord injury

LORRAINE WILLIAMS PEDRETTI

Spinal cord injuries are caused by trauma from automobile accidents, gunshot and stab wounds, falls, sports, and diving accidents. The most common cause is the automobile accident that results in forced flexion and hyperextension of the neck or trunk, causing fracture and dislocation of the vertebrae.[22] Spinal cord functions may also be disturbed by diseases, such as tumors, myelomeningocele, syringomyelia, multiple sclerosis, and amyotrophic lateral sclerosis. Some of the treatment principles outlined in this chapter may have application to these conditions. However, the emphasis will be on rehabilitation of the individual with traumatic injury.

RESULTS OF SPINAL CORD INJURY

Spinal cord injury results in quadriplegia or paraplegia. Quadriplegia is the paralysis of the four limbs and trunk musculature. There may be partial upper extremity (UE) function, depending on the level of the cervical lesion. Paraplegia is paralysis of the lower extremities and possibly of some trunk musculature, depending on the level of the lesion.

Spinal cord injuries are referred to in terms of the regions (cervical, thoracic, and lumbar) of the spinal cord in which they occur and the numerical order of the neurological segments. The level of spinal cord injury designates the last fully functioning neurological segment of the cord, for example, C6 refers to the sixth neurological segment of the cervical region of the spinal cord as the last fully functioning neurological segment. Thus in this instance all muscles innervated by segments below the C6 neurological level will be paralyzed.

Complete lesions result in total dysfunction of the spinal cord below the level of the injury. Incomplete lesions may involve several neurological segments, and some spinal cord function may be partially or completely intact, which allows for some function below the level of the injury.

A lower motor neuron lesion that results in flaccid paralysis is present in muscles innervated at the level of the lesion. An upper motor neuron lesion that results in spastic paralysis is present below the level of the lesion. The reason for this is the destruction of the anterior horn cells and reflex arc at the level of the lesion, although these remain intact but are divorced from higher centers of control below the level of the lesion. Therefore the person who has quadriplegia usually has predominantly flaccid paralysis of the upper extremities and spastic paralysis of the lower extremities.[25]

After spinal cord injury the victim enters a stage of spinal shock that may last as long as 3 months but usually lasts less than 24 hours. This spinal shock phase is a period of areflexia, the cessation of all reflex activity below the level of the injury.[17] During this phase there is loss of all sensation and voluntary motor function below the level of the injury, which results in a complete flaccid paralysis. Bladder, bowel, and sexual functions are no longer under voluntary control. The bladder and bowel are atonic or flaccid. Deep tendon reflexes are decreased, and sympathetic functions are disturbed. This disturbance results in decreased constriction of blood vessels, low blood pressure, slower heart rate, and absence of perspiration.[11,26]

As spinal shock declines, the after shock phase commences and reflexes return to a hyperactive state. There is continued loss of motor function, but muscles that are innervated by the neurological segments below the level of injury usually develop spasticity. Deep tendon reflexes become hyperactive, and clonus may be evident. Sensory loss continues, and the bladder and bowel usually become spastic in patients whose injuries are above T12. The bladder and bowel usually remain flaccid or atonic in lesions at L1 and below. Sympathetic functions become hyperactive. Spinal reflex activity (mass muscle spasms) becomes evident in the

limbs. Reflex erections may develop in patients with thoracic and cervical injuries but usually do not occur in clients with lumbar and sacral injuries, since the essential reflex arc is usually interrupted in these individuals.

Prognosis for recovery

Prognosis for significant recovery of neuromuscular function after spinal cord injury is generally poor. In complete lesions if there is no sensation or return of motor function below the level of lesion 48 hours after the injury occurs, then no motor function return is expected. Return of function to one spinal nerve root level below the fracture is the usual gain and occurs in the first 6 months after injury.

In incomplete lesions progressive return of motor function is possible.[11,26] Perianal sensation, toe flexion, and sphincter control are evidence of an incomplete lesion where there is some neural transmission across the site of injury. With incomplete lesions prognosis is uncertain. When improvement begins immediately and return of muscle function appears consistently, prognosis for recovery is better than if return of motor function occurs sporadically and inconsistently several months after the injury occurred.[17,26]

MEDICAL AND SURGICAL MANAGEMENT OF THE PERSON WITH SPINAL CORD INJURY

After a traumatic event in which spinal cord injury is a possibility, the conscious victim should be carefully questioned about cutaneous numbness and skeletal muscle paralysis before being moved, if possible. Careful palpation of the spinal axis should also take place before moving the victim. The victim should be moved from the accident site with extreme caution. Flexion of the spine must be prevented during the transfer procedures. A firm stretcher or board to which the victim's head and back can be strapped should be procured before moving the victim.

After transferring the victim to the stretcher or board, while maintaining axial traction on the neck and preventing any flexion of the spine and neck, the victim is strapped to the board or stretcher and transferred carefully, avoiding bumping, to the hospital emergency room.

Careful examination, stabilization, and transportation of the person with spinal injury may prevent a temporary or slight spinal cord injury from becoming permanent or more severe.

Initial care in the hospital is directed toward preventing further damage to the spinal cord and reversing neurological damage if possible by stabilization or decompression of the injured neurological structures.[13,17] A careful neurological examination is carried out to aid in determining site and type of injury. This is done with the patient in a supine position with the neck and spine immobilized. A catheter is placed in the patient's bladder for drainage of urine. Anteroposterior and lateral x-ray films may be taken, with the patient's head or spine immobilized, to obtain a rough idea of the type of injury. A myelogram may be required for further evaluation.

In early medical treatment the goals are to restore normal alignment of the spine, maintain stabilization of the injured area, and decompress neurological structures that are under pressure. Spinal relignment and stabilization can be achieved through rest on a well-padded frame or a hospital bed with a fracture board and positioning pillows and rolls, in some cases. In more severe fractures traction is applied to the spine while the patient rests in bed or on a Stryker frame. In recent years the halo and halo brace have been widely used with success for cervical spine injuries that require skeletal traction and immobilization. If on a bed or frame the patient's position must be changed every 2 hours to prevent pressure sores.

Open surgical reduction with plating, wiring, and spinal fusion or laminectomy is sometimes carried out. The goals of surgery are to decompress the spinal cord and achieve spinal stability and normal bony alignment. The laminectomy has been performed much less frequently in recent years and only under special circumstances, as outlined by Pierce and Nickel.[17]

Complications and concomitant problems

PRESSURE SORES OR DECUBITUS ULCERS. Sensory loss enhances the development of pressure sores. The patient cannot feel the pressure of prolonged sitting or lying in one position or pressure from splints or braces. Pressure causes loss of blood supply to the area, which can ultimately result in necrosis. The areas most likely to develop pressure sores are bony prominences over the sacrum, ischium, trochanters, elbows, and heels. It is important for rehabilitation personnel to be aware of the signs of developing pressure sores. At first the area reddens and blanches when pressed. Later the reddened area becomes blue or black and does not blanch when pressed. This indicates that necrosis has begun. Finally a blister or ulceration appears in the area and it may become infected. If allowed to progress, these sores may become very severe, and bony prominences may become uncovered and may eventually be destroyed.

Pressure sores can be prevented by relieving and eliminating pressure points and protecting vulnerable areas. Turning in bed, special mattresses, foam "booties" to protect the heels, and shifting weight when sitting are some of the methods used to prevent pressure sores.

The use of hand splints and other appliances can also cause pressure sores. The therapist must inspect the skin, and the patient must be taught to inspect the skin, using a mirror, to watch for signs of developing pressure sores. Reddened areas can develop within 30 minutes, so frequent shifting, repositioning, and vigilance are essential if pressure sores are to be prevented.[17,26]

DECREASED VITAL CAPACITY. Decreased vital capacity will be a problem in persons who have sustained cervical and high thoracic lesions. Such individuals will have markedly limited chest expansion and decreased ability to cough. This can result in proneness to respiratory tract infections. The reduced vital capacity will affect energy, tolerance level for activity, and dressing potential. This problem may be alleviated by methods of assisted breathing and by teaching the client glossopha-

ryngeal, or "frog," breathing. Strengthening of the strenocleidomastoids and the diaphragm and deep breathing exercises are helpful. Manually assisted coughing and mechanical suctioning of chest secretions may be required if there are excess secretions or respiratory tract infection. These measures are usually carried out by physical therapy, respiratory therapy, and nursing services.[17,26]

OSTEOPOROSIS OF DISUSE. Because of disuse of long bones, particularly of the lower extremities, osteoporosis is likely to develop in patients with spinal cord injuries. A year after the injury the osteoporosis may be sufficiently advanced for pathological fractures to occur. Pathological fractures usually occur in the supracondylar area of the femur, proximal tibia, distal tibia, intertrochanteric area of the femur, and neck of the femur. Pathological fractures are not seen in the upper extremities. Daily standing helps to prevent or delay the osteoporosis that underlies these fractures by placing the weight load on the long bones of the lower extremities.[17,26]

POSTURAL HYPOTENSION. Postural hypotension results in fainting or blackouts. It is due to the pooling of blood in the abdominal and lower extremity (LE) vasculature from lack of movement and poor venous return of blood to the heart. It occurs when the patient is brought to the upright position following a period of bed rest. It is a normal reaction and should be dealt with immediately in a matter-of-fact manner by locking the wheelchair brakes and tilting the chair back to elevate the feet above the level of the heart. If the patient is on a tilt table, it should be returned to the horizontal position. Abdominal binders, corsets, and leg wraps may relieve or eliminate this problem by giving support to paralyzed abdominal muscles and can aid in breathing as well.[26]

AUTONOMIC DYSREFLEXIA. Autonomic dysreflexia is a phenomenon seen in persons whose injuries are above the T4 to T6 levels. It is caused by reflex action of the autonomic nervous system in response to some stimuli, such as a distended bladder, fecal mass, bladder irrigation or rectal manipulation, thermal and pain stimuli, and visceral distention. The symptoms are perspiration, especially of the forehead; goose bumps; nasal congestion and obstruction; paroxysmal hypertension; pounding headache; and fast, then, slow pulse. Autonomic dysreflexia is a *medical emergency*. If any of these symptoms appear, the patient should be returned to the nursing station at once, and the physician should be alerted for the administration of appropriate prophylactic measures and medication. The patient should not be left alone.

Autonomic dysreflexia is treated by placing the patient in an upright position to reduce blood pressure. The bladder should be drained by unclamping the catheter or tapping over the bladder if there is an automatic bladder. Any person with a spinal cord injury who complains of headache should have a blood pressure reading to determine if there is autonomic dysreflexia.[1,17,26]

SPASTICITY. Spasticity is an increase of stretch reflexes below the level of injury that results from lack of inhibition from higher centers. Patterns of spasticity change over the first year, gradually increasing in the first 6 months and reaching a plateau about 1 year after the injury. A moderate amount of spasticity can be helpful in the overall rehabilitation of the patient with a spinal cord injury. It helps to maintain muscle bulk, assists in joint ROM, and can be used to assist during wheelchair and bed transfers and mobility. During the first year spasticity should be controlled by maintaining joint ROM; icing the skin, followed by stretching contractures; and using relaxant drugs.

Severe spasticity that interferes with function must be treated more aggressively. Surgical procedures that involve cutting or lengthening spastic muscles and peripheral and spinal nerve blocks designed to paralyze the spastic muscles may be used to eliminate problems of severe and disabling spasticity.[17,26]

HETEROTOPIC OSSIFICATION. Heterotopic ossification is the deposition of osseous material, usually in the muscles around the hip and knee but also at the elbow and shoulder. The first symptoms are heat, pain, swelling, and decreased joint ROM. The ossification may progress to ankylosis of the affected joint. Treatment is the maintenance of joint ROM during the early stage of active bone formation to keep breaking up the depositions of new bone and develop pseudoarthroses in the ossified area.

If the ossification progresses to ankylosis and severely limits function because of joint immobility, surgical intervention may be pursued if necessary criteria and conditions are met.[17]

SEXUAL FUNCTION

At the time of injury there is a complete loss of sexual function for any level of injury. As spinal shock subsides, variable degrees and types of sexual function may be recovered by a significant number of persons with spinal cord injuries. In clients with thoracic and cervical lesions the reflex arc from the penis or glans clitoris to the spinal cord is intact.[9] Therefore reflexogenic erections are possible in approximately 60% to 90% of persons with lesions at these levels.[7] The ability to effect erections often correlates with bladder function. Persons with upper motor neuron or spastic bladders usually have reflexogenic erections without ejaculations, while persons with lower motor neuron or atonic bladders are unable to have erections. This is most likely in lesions below the L1 level. There are exceptions in both instances, however.

Persons with incomplete injuries, especially those who have sacral function, may have psychogenic erections. For these men, ejaculation may accompany the erection and thus they may be capable of siring children.[26]

Reflexogenic erections may be effected by tactile and thermal stimuli or manipulation.[2] In men the quality and duration of the erection is variable and may not always be useful for sexual activity.[17] Spontaneous reflexogenic erections from exteroceptive stimuli may occur when not desired.[2,9] Successful sexual intercourse is usually possible for men who have reflexogenic erections. Alternate modes of sexual activity, described in explicit detail by Mooney, Cole, and Chilgren,[15] can be used by these persons as well as those in whom reflexogenic erections do not occur.

Fertility is disturbed in most men with spinal cord injuries because of urinary tract infections, retrograde ejacula-

tions, testicular atrophy, and temperature changes that affect viability of sperm.[23] In women there is no appreciable decrease in fertility. The menses will not be significantly disturbed or changed after the spinal cord injury and will usually return to normal within a few months after the injury occurred. Normal pregnancy and childbirth are possible, although urological clearance should be obtained before pregnancy is considered. The distention of pregnancy may evoke autonomic dysreflexia, and labor may not be perceived by the pregnant woman. Appropriate precautions are necessary to deal with these possibilities. Birth control counseling is important for those sexually active persons who do not desire pregnancy.[17]

Women who have spinal cord injuries experience essentially the same physical and psychological reponses that men who have spinal cord injuries experience. However, women possibly make a better and more rapid psychological adjustment and acceptance of changed sexual function than do men.[9]

Sensation is absent in persons with complete spinal cord transection and may be partial in persons with incomplete lesions. Sexual satisfaction is largely on a psychological level and is derived from pleasure given to the partner, full participation in intimate relationships, intimate communication with a significant partner, and development of a sense of personal worth and significance as a sexual being. These are important reasons for engaging in sexual activity that are above and beyond the sensual pleasures that can be derived. Finally, although not the least important reason for engaging in sexual activity, is the sexual expression of affection and love.[21]

Physically disabled individuals quickly sense the attitudes of professional helpers toward their sexuality. Traditionally professionals have viewed disabled persons as asexual and often communicated a sense that it was not all right to discuss sexual functioning. Professionals tended to put the topic off, whereas their clients waited for them to bring it up, granting permission for this important concern to be aired. Fortunately these tendencies and attitudes are changing, and sexual counseling and education are becoming a regular part of many rehabilitation programs for all types of physical disabilities.

Because occupational therapists are concerned with the functional aspects of their clients' lives, they are in an excellent role to provide information and counseling on sexual functioning. Staff education and attitude assessment are critical preliminaries to initiating sexual counseling and education.[16]

Some clients lack basic sex education. Others feel asexual because of their disabilities and are isolated from peers; thus they may fear any type of sexual interaction. Therefore sexual counseling must be geared to the needs of the individual client. In some instances social interaction skills will need improvement before sexual acitivity can be considered. Occupational therapy can play an important part in improving social skills.

It is important for the professional worker to introduce the topic and give an opening for the discussion. The disabled person and the partner should be counseled together if possible. A sense of trust must develop between the client and the counselor. It is important to use terminology that the client is accustomed to and comfortable with when discussing sexual matters and to maintain confidentiality. When counseling is introduced, safe or relatively superficial topics can be discussed first and then, as trust and comfort develop, deeper and more intimate and sensitive topics can be broached.

Sexual counseling and education may be carried out in a variety of ways. One-to-one counseling with audiovisual aids and literature is useful. Group discussions with partners and experienced disabled persons present may be a useful method. Neistadt and Baker[16] describe a sexual counseling program using counseling by the occupational therapist and literature. Clients opted for one or both methods, depending on individual interests and needs.

Finally clients need a time and place and permission to explore and experiment with the sexual options open to them. Home visits on weekend passes are an appropriate means to this end.

OCCUPATIONAL THERAPY FOR SPINAL CORD INJURY

The general treatment program is directed primarily to the quadriplegic client with a C5-6 level of injury because this is the most common level of injury. It may be modified for higher or lower levels of injury, using the information in Table 29-1 as a guide.

The long-range goals in the rehabilitation of the person with a spinal cord injury are (1) to achieve the maximal level of self-care independence possible; (2) accept the disability; and (3) resume meaningful family, social, community, vocational, and leisure roles.[22] Occupational therapy can make a significant contribution in assisting the client to move toward the achievement of these goals.

Evaluation

The client's muscle strength should be evaluated using the manual muscle test. This evaluation will help to determine areas of strength and weakness; establish a baseline for progress; determine need for special equipment, such as splints, MASs, and assistive devices; and determine the level of injury. The client's muscle strength is a critical factor in determining functional potential.

During the bed phase, when the client is still in traction or is wearing a cervical collar, resistance should not be applied to shoulder musculature. The client should not move the shoulders actively any further than the individual thinks possible. No rotary or flexion and extension movements of the spine are permitted until medical clearance is obtained.[24] During this phase of rehabilitation muscle strength testing may be limited to hands and forearms, and gross rather than specific manual muscle testing may be used to estimate strength while not jeopardizing stability of the spine. The occupational therapist should obtain the physician's approval before proceeding with a complete UE manual muscle test during the early phases of rehabilitation.[25] The muscle test should be repeated monthly during the early stages of rehabilitation for up to 6 or 8 months after the injury occurred.

Passive range of motion (ROM) should be measured with the same precautions for shoulder motions just described in the early stages. This evaluation is to determine potential or present contractures that could limit functional potential and suggest the need for preventive or corrective splints and positioning.

Sensation is evaluated for light touch, superficial pain (pinprick), temperature, proprioception, and stereognosis. This aids in denoting areas of lost, impaired, and intact sensation. It may be helpful in establishing the level of injury. It provides information for precautions that must be taken by the therapist and the client and provides a baseline for measuring progress.

Spasticity in UE muscle groups innervated below the level of lesion is estimated by the degree of resistance to passive movement. This can often be determined during the passive ROM measurements. Spasticity is mild if stretch reflexes and clonus are evoked during passive motion, but the part moves easily through the full ROM. Spasticity is considered moderate if resistance can be felt through the entire ROM, but it is still possible to complete the ROM. Spasticity is considered severe if resistance is felt through the ROM, and it is not possible to complete the full ROM because of strong hypertonicity in the muscles.

Performance of activities of daily living (ADL) is an important part of the occupational therapy evaluation. The client must have adequate balance and neck stability before complete ADL training can be accomplished. The purpose of the evaluation is to determine present and potential levels of functional ability. The evaluation may begin during the bed phase with light activities, such as oral hygiene and feeding. In later stages it may progress to bed mobility, wheelchair mobility, transfers, toileting, bathing, dressing, and then driving.[24] Before driving evaluation is attempted, the client must meet certain criteria. These are the ability to (1) lock the elbow in extension with a substitution pattern if triceps is absent; (2) depress the shoulders; (3) flex, abduct, and externally and internally rotate the shoulders; (4) manage adapted driving equipment; and (5) maintain lateral and forward trunk stability. It is helpful if the client can transfer self and the

Text continued on p. 411.

Table 29-1
Functional potential in spinal cord injury

Level*	Muscles innervated	Movements possible	Pattern of weakness	Functional capabilities and limitations
C1-3 (8, 10, 13)†	Sternocleido-mastoids Trapezius (upper) Levator scapulae	Neck control	Total paralysis of arms, trunk, lower extremities Dependence on respirator	Total ADL dependence Can drive electric wheelchair equipped with portable respirator with chin or breath controls Communication devices and environmental control systems with mouths-tick control. Require full-time attendant care
C3-4 (4, 5, 10, 13, 14)	‡Trapezius (superior, middle and inferior) ‡Diaphragm (C3-5) Cervical and paraspinal muscles	Neck movements, scapula elevation Inspiration	Paralysis of trunk and lower extremities Difficulty in breathing and coughing	Confined to wheelchair and essentially dependent Only head-neck and some scapula movement Respiratory assistance may be required at least part time Assistance with skin inspection (patient cannot position mirrors but should inspect himself) Some activities can be accomplished through use of head wand or mouth stick (for example, typing, page turning, and manipulation of checkers, chess, and cards) Can operate electric wheelchair with mouth, chin, or breath controls Rancho electric arm can be operated by tongue microswitches to allow limited self-feeding with swivel utensils and other activities mentioned above Require full-time attendant care
C5 (4, 5, 10, 12, 14, 17, 24)	All muscles of shoulder at least partially innervated except latissimus dorsi and coracobrachialis ‡Partial deltoids	Shoulder extension and horizontal abduction (weak) Shoulder flexion (weak) Shoulder abduction to 90°	Weakness of shoulder movements, elbow flexion, and spuination Absence of elbow extension, pronation and all wrist and hand movements Total paralysis of trunk and lower extremities	Confined to wheelchair and still essentially dependent Unable to roll over or to come to sitting position independently and has no independent hand functions Need assistance in transfers If good muscle power, may be able to perform UE dressing with some success Dependent for skin inspection
	‡Biceps brachii Brachialis Brachioradialis Levator scapula, diaiphragm, and scaleni now fully innervated Rhomboid (major and minor) Serratus anterior (C5-7)	Elbow flexion and supination Scapular adduction and downward rotaton (weak) Scapular abdution and upward rotation (weak)	Endurance low because of paralysis of intercostals and low respiratory reserve	Manual wheelchair with handrim projections or electric wheelchair with joystick or adapted arm controls Cannot apply own hand splints, but with standard mobile arm support (MAS) or elevating proximal arm with outside powdered hand splint some functional activities are possible, such as feeding, light hygiene, applying makeup, and shaving; handwriting (sufficient for legal signature); telephoning (push-button telephone); and typing (five WPM), if set up and placed on a lapboard by an attendant

From Reedy, J.: Spinal cord level chart, unpublished paper presented in partial fulfillment of the requirements for the course O.T. 135, San Jose, Calif. November 1974, Department of Occupational Therapy, San Jose State University.
*Each level includes the muscles and functions of the preceding levels.
†The number in parentheses are references.
‡Key muscles.

Continued.

Table 29-1—cont'd
Functional potential in spinal cord injury

Level*	Muscles innervated	Movements possible	Pattern of weakness	Functional capabilities and limitations
C5—cont'd	Teres major (C5,6) Subscapularis (C5,6)	Shoulder internal rotation (weak)		Require at least part-time attendant care
	Pectoralis major (C5-8, T1)	Shoulder horizontal adduction (weak)		
	Infraspinatus Supraspinatus Teres minor (C5,6)	Shoulder external rotation		
C6 (8, 10, 12, 14, 24)	All partially innervated C5 muscles now fully innervated except serratus and pectoralis major	Full (or nearly full) strength to shoulder flexion and extension, abduction and adduction, internal and external rotation, and elbow flexion	Functions of shoulder prime movers still not fully developed Absence of elbow extension Radial wrist extension possible	Still confined to wheelchair and essentially dependent, although may be able to perform many activities on own with equipment. Flexor hinge splint or universal cuff aid in self-feeding with regular utensils; personal hygiene and grooming (oral and upper body); UE dressing; handwriting; typing (15-20 WPM); telephoning; light kitchen activities; possibly driving, with equipment Roll from side to side in bed with aid of bed rails and assist in rolling over Sit up independently in bed by using elbow flexors to pull on rope looped about forearms and attached to foot of bed or trapeze bar
	Partial but significant innervation to serratus anterior (C5-7)	Scapular abduction and upward rotation		Independent in wheeling wheelchair on level terrain and 6° ramps
	Latissimus dorsi (C6-8)	Shoulder extension and internal rotation	Endurance low because of reduced respiratory reserve	Propel standard wheelchair with adapted rims (projections or friction tape) Relieve pressure independently when sitting
	‡Pectoralis major (C5-8, T1)	Shoulder horizontal adduction and internal rotation		Independent in managing communication devices with adapted equipment Assist in transfers by substituting shoulder adduction and rotation for elbow extension and may be independent with aid of transfer board Drive with adaptations Independent skin inspection May manage bladder and bowel care Employment possible Some assistance required for bathing May require attendant care mornings and evenings only
	Coracobrachialis (C6, 7)	Shoulder flexion		
	Pronator teres (C6, 7)	Forearm pronation		
	Supinator	Complete innervation for forearm supination		
	Flexor carpi radialis (C6, 7 sometimes)	Radial wrist flexion	Absence of wrist flexion usually (may be present on radial side)	
	‡Extensor carpi radialis longus and brevis (C6, 7)	Radial wrist extension	Absence of hand functions Total paralysis of trunk and lower extremities	

Table 29-1—cont'd
Functional potential in spinal cord injury

Level*	Muscles innervated	Movements possible	Pattern of weakness	Functional capabilities and limitations
C7-8 (4, 5, 10, 13, 14, 17, 22)	Shoulder prime movers now fully innervated, as well as the rest of the partially innervated C6 muscles	Full strength of all shoulder movements, radial wrist flexors and extensors, and strong pronation	Full strength of shoulder muscles but lack of trunk fixation for the origins of the shoulder prime movers	Essentially confined to wheelchair, but many attain complete wheelchair independence Can come to sitting position in bed Can perform transfers to and from bed and wheelchair independently or with minimal assistance
	‡Triceps brachii Extensor carpi ulnaris (C6-8)	Elbow extension Ulnar wrist extension		
	‡Flexor carpi radialis	Radial wrist flexion	Weakness of pronation and ulnar wrist flexion	Can roll over, sit up, and move about in sitting position
	‡Flexor digitorum superficialis and profundus (C7-8, T1)	Proximal interphalangeal and distal interphalangeal flexion	Limited grasp, release, and dexterity because of incomplete innervation of hand intrinsics	Can dress independently and perform personal hygiene activities except changing catheter Self-feeding (usually with no assistive devices) Wrist-driven flexor hinge splint may still be helpful for some patients because of weakness of grasp
	‡Extensor digitorum communis (C6-8)	Metacarpophalangeal (MP) extension		Can propel standard wheelchair (may need friction tape on handrims for long distances; may need assistance on rough ground)
	Extensor pollicis longus and brevis	Thumb extension (MP and interphalangeal [IP])	Total paralysis of lower extremities	Drive with adaptations
	Abductor pollicis longus	Thumb abduction	Weakness of trunk control Limited endurance because of reduced respiratory reserve	Independent bladder and bowel care and skin inspection Employment at home or outside home possible Light housework possible but best in assistant or supervisory role
C8-T1 (4, 5, 8, 10, 12, 24)	All muscles of upper extremities now fully innervated			
	Pronator quadratus	Forearm pronation	Paralysis of lower extremities	Independent in bed activities, wheelchair transfers, and self-care and personal hygiene
	Flexor carpi ulnaris	Ulnar wrist flexion	Weakness of trunk control	Can manage standard wheelchair up and down curb
	‡Lumbricales and ‡interossei dorsales and palmares	MP flexion	Endurance reduced because of low respiratory reserve	Can move from wheelchair to floor and return Nonfunctional ambulation for standing or exercise may be possible but still not a practicable mode of mobility
	‡Interossei dorsales and abductor digiti minimi	Finger abduction		Can get up and down from standing in stall bars independently Independent bladder and bowel care and skin inspection Homebound work or work in a wheelchair-accessible environment possible
	‡Interossei palmares	Finger adduction		Light housekeeping can be done independently Drive with adaptations
	Flexor pollicis longus and brevis	Thumb flexion (MP and IP)		Independent in management of communication devices

Continued.

Table 29-1—cont'd
Functional potential in spinal cord injury

Level*	Muscles innervated	Movements possible	Pattern of weakness	Functional capabilities and limitations
C8-T1—cont'd	Adductor pollicis ‡Opponens digiti minimi ‡Opponens pollicis	Thumb adduction Opposition of fifth finger Thumb opposition		
T4-T6 (8,24)	All muscles of upper extremities plus partial innervation of intercostal muscles and long muscles of the back (sacrospinalis and semispinalis)	All arm functions Partial trunk stability Endurance increased because of better respiration	Partial trunk paralysis and total paralysis of lower extremities	Self-care independence Independence in standard wheelchair and transfers May stand with braces and crutches and ambulate for short distances but not practical for mobility Can work at sedentary occupations and do some heavy lifting from sitting position Driving Wheelchair sports possible Independent in light housekeeping
T7-L2 (8,24)	Intercostal muscles fully innervated Abdominal muscles partially to fully innervated (rectus abdominis, internal and external obliques)	Partial to good trunk stability Increased physical endurance	Paralysis of lower extremities	Independence in self-care, personal hygiene, sports, work, and housekeeping activities possible in well-designed environment Ambulates with difficulty using braces and crutches, but wheelchair is ambulation of choice for speed and energy conservation
L3-L4 (8, 24)	Low back muscles Hip flexors, adductors, quadriceps	Trunk control and stability Hip flexion Hip adduction Knee extension	Partial paralysis of lower extremities; hip extension, knee flexion, and ankle and foot movements	Independent in all activities outlined above Can ambulate with short leg braces, using crutches or canes May still use a wheelchair for convenience and energy conservation
L5-S3 (4,8)	Hip extensors—gluteus maximus and hamstrings Hip abductors—gluteus medius and gluteus minimus Knee flexors—hamstrings, sartorius, and gracilis Ankle muscles—tibialis anterior, gastrocnemius, soleus, and peroneus longus Foot muscles	Partial to full control of lower extremities	Partial paralysis of lower extremities, most notable in distal segment	Independent in all activities No equipment needed if plantar flexion is sufficiently strong for push off in ambulation

wheelchair to and from the car.[26] Specially equipped vans require less function for independent driving.

In addition to these specific assessments the occupational therapist should assess the client's stage of adjustment to the disability and psychosocial functioning skills. The therapist should obtain the medical, social, educational, and vocational histories of the client. These can be obtained from the medical record and from interviews with paraprofessionals, the client, and family members and friends.[17] The occupational therapist should communicate with the client initially and continuously during the early phase of the evaluation process regarding needs, interests, aspirations, feelings about the disability and the hospital and its personnel, and frustrations.[22] This is an important time to establish rapport and mutual trust, which will facilitate participation and progress in later and more difficult phases of rehabilitation.

Establishing treatment objectives

It is important to establish treatment objectives in concert with the client and with the rehabilitation team. The primary objectives of the rehabilitation team are often not those of the client. Fuller participation can be expected if the client's priorities are respected to the extent that they are possible and realistic.

The general objectives of treatment for the person with a spinal cord injury are to (1) increase strength of all innervated and partially innervated muscles of the shoulders, elbows, and wrists; (2) maintain or increase joint ROM and prevent deformity; (3) increase physical endurance; (4) train in the use of special equipment, such as the MAS and flexor hinge splint and assistive devices; (5) develop maximal independence in the performance of ADL; (6) explore vocational and avocational potential; and (7) aid in the psychosocial adjustment to physical disability.

Treatment methods

Medical clearance should be obtained before occupational therapy is initiated. During the acute or bed phase of the rehabilitation program the client is still in traction or is wearing a neck stabilization device, such as a cervical collar or halo brace, to achieve stability of the neck. Precautions against resistive exercises and extremes of ranges of shoulder motions must be in force during this period. Flexion, extension, and rotary movements of the spine and neck are contraindicated. The therapist may provide gentle passive ROM to all UE joints to tolerance and within precautions. Active and active-assisted ROM to all joints within strength, ability, and tolerance levels should also be performed. Muscle reeducation techniques to wrists and elbows should be employed. Resistive exercises to wrists may be carried out. Some gentle resistance to elbows may be given with caution regarding resistance to the shoulders.[24] The client should be encouraged to engage in light self-care activities, such as feeding, writing, and light hygiene, if possible, using simple devices, such as wash mitt and universal cuff with a wrist cock-up splint. The occupational therapist can provide splints and overhead slings as needed and may introduce avocational activities, such as reading or watching television, and provide the electric page turner and prism glasses so that these activities may be enjoyed while in a supine position.[22,24]

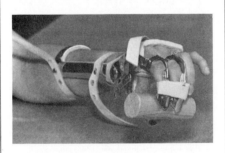

Fig. 29-1. Wrist extension is used to effect prehension through the mechanism of flexor hinge hand splint.

During the convalescent or wheelchair phase of the rehabilitation program, when the client can sit upright in a wheelchair, has achieved some sitting tolerance, and has stability of the neck and spine, the client can participate in a fuller and more active rehabilitation program. Progressive resistive exercise and resistive activities, such as woodworking, can be applied to innervated and partially innervated muscles. Shoulder musculature may be exercised with emphasis on the shoulder depressors, rotators, and adductors needed to perform sliding or loop and trapeze transfers.[2,24] The biceps needed for transfers and for shifting weight to relieve pressure when in the wheelchair should be strengthened. Wrist extensors need to be exercised to power the flexor hinge splint in clients who have wrist function and will be using the splint to aid prehension (Fig. 29-1).

Active and passive ROM exercises should be continued regularly to prevent undesirable contractures. Stretching may be indicated to correct contractures that are becoming established. In clients who have wrist extension, which will be used to substitute for absent grasp through tenodesis action of the long finger flexors, it is desirable to develop some tightness in these tendons to give some additional tension to the tenodesis grasp. This will allow some clients to discard the splint and use natural tenodesis action for functional grasp. The desirable contracture is developed by ranging finger flexion with the wrist fully extended and finger extension with the wrist fully flexed, thus never allowing the flexors or extensors to be in full stretch over all of the joints that they cross[14,22] (Fig. 29-2).

A 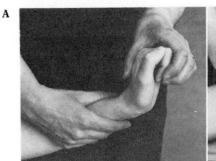 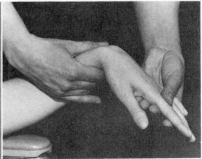 B

Fig. 29-2. A, Wrist is extended when fingers are passively flexed. **B,** Wrist is flexed when fingers are passively extended.

The ADL program may be expanded to include independent feeding with devices; oral hygiene and upper body bathing; bowel and bladder care, such as suppository insertion and application of the urinary collection device; UE dressing; and transfers using the sliding board. Communication skills in writing and using the telephone, tape recorder, and electric typewriter and personal computer with devices should be an important part of the treatment program.[22] Training in the use of the MAS, flexor hinge splint, and assistive devices is also part of the occupational therapy program.

The occupational therapist should continue to provide psychological support by allowing and encouraging the client to express frustration, anger, fears, and concerns. The occupational therapy clinic could provide an atmosphere where clients can establish support groups with more advanced clients and rehabilitated individuals who can offer their experiences and problem-solving advice to those in earlier phases of their rehabilitation.

The treatment program should be graded to increase the amount of resistance required in exercise and activity as muscle power improves, increase the amount of time spent in sitting and in activity to improve sitting tolerance and endurance, and increase the number and complexity of ADL while reducing the time it takes to perform them.

There are many assistive devices and pieces of special equipment that can be useful to the person with a spinal cord injury. The universal cuff for holding eating utensils, toothbrushes, pencils, paintbrushes, and typing sticks is a simple and versatile device that offers increased independence (see Fig. 12-28). A plate guard, cup holder, extended straw with straw clip, and non-skid table mat can facilitate independent feeding (see Fig. 12-26). The wash mitt and soap holder or soap on a rope can make bathing possible (see Fig. 12-8). Many persons with quadriplegia can use a buttonhook (see Fig. 12-4) to fasten clothing. A transfer board is essential for transfers. A wrist cock-up splint to stabilize the wrist during use of the universal cuff can be useful for persons with little or no wrist extension. Clients who have quadriplegia

with high cervical injuries may benefit from an externally powered flexor hinge splint or the myoelectric arm. A wheelchair lapboard may be helpful during early wheelchair use for training in feeding while using MASs (see Chapter 19), reading, and performing communication and avocational activities, such as sketching, painting, or writing. An overhead trapeze may be used by some for transfers to and from bed. A special wheelchair cushion to prevent pressure sores is essential.

During the extended phase of the rehabilitation program driving evaluation and training and home management activities may be introduced and added to the activities just mentioned. Avocational possibilities should be further explored. Activities, such as checkers, chess, Scrabble, and mosaic tile work, may be used. The MAS or flexor hinge splint (see Chapter 20) may be needed by some to perform these skills. The use of table-based power tools, such as the jigsaw, drill press, printing press, and hand electric sander, may be feasible for many clients if they are adapted with extended handles and positioned properly. Weaving, painting, and sketching are also feasible activities if used with devices or special adaptations.[22]

The client should be introduced to home and community by the occupational and physical therapists before discharge from the treatment facility. The therapists can offer recommendations for major and minor modifications in the home, such as installation of grab bars, bathtub seats, and guardrails around the toilet. The therapists can assist in family education and adjustment by training family members that provide care or attendants in proper techniques of skin care and inspection, use of special equipment, bed mobility, positioning, transfers, dressing, and toileting activities that require supervision or assistance.

Occupational therapy services can offer valuable evaluation and exploration of vocational potential of persons who have quadriplegia. By the sheer magnitude of the physical disability vocational possibilities for these persons are limited. Clients with high intelligence have greater potential for employment than clients with low intelligence.

Many clients with spinal cord injuries must change their vocation or alter former vocational goals. Lack of intelligence, poor motivation, and lack of interest and perseverance on the part of many clients make vocational rehabilitation extremely difficult.

The occupational therapist, during the process of the treatment program and through the use of craft and work sample activities, can help to assess the client's level of motivation, functional intelligence, aptitudes, attitudes, interests, and personal vocational aspirations. The occupational therapist can observe the client's attention span, concentration, manual ability with splints and devices, accuracy, speed, perseverance, work habits, and work tolerance level. This information can be provided to the vocational counselor, who can counsel the client regarding vocational potential and future possibilities, perform specialized vocational testing, and suggest feasible educational and vocational training possibilities.[17]

The occupational therapy service can offer a work adjustment program in which work tolerance level and work habits can be developed while specific job testing and trials are under the direction of the vocational counselor.

For the person with quadriplegia who is of adequate intelligence and motivation, further education is often the solution to the vocational future. Such individuals may perform successfully in occupations, such as teaching, engineering, business management, research, psychology, counseling, and sales. Adaptive equipment and a barrier-free environment may be essential to the performance of these jobs.[17]

When suitable vocational objectives have been selected, they may be pursued in an educational setting, at the treatment facility if it is equipped for vocational training, or in a work setting. This phase of rehabilitation is beyond the scope of occupational therapy.

Maximal self-care independence, personal satisfaction through avocational activities, and socialization should be the end goals of the rehabilitation program for those persons who have high-level injuries or those who lack the intelligence for further education or vocational training and essential personal skills and habits for good work adjustment.[17]

Sample treatment plan

Case study

John is 17 years old. He is a C7 quadriplegic who sustained the disability in a swimming accident. He was a bright and active high school senior who had planned to go to college within a year. He enjoyed sports, art and popular music. He was not sure what his career would be, but he was interested in forestry or the technical aspects of radio and television studio operations.

Medical problems related to bladder and bowel control are stabilized, and all precautions are in force to prevent pressure sores. He is able to sit in a wheelchair with support of a body brace and special cushion for periods up to 4 hours per day. Nursing service has reported that the client made little effort to help with daily hygiene and dressing activities.

John has demonstrated a rather flip, carefree attitude toward his problems, which seems to be an effort to cover up a deep anxiety about his physical condition and the future. Occupational therapy was ordered for this patient with aims to increase muscle strength and functional independence and aid with adjustment to disability.

TREATMENT PLAN

A. Statistical data.
1. Name: John
   Age: 17
   Diagnosis: Traumatic injury to cervical area of the spinal cord
   Disability: Quadriplegia, C7 level
2. Treatment aims as stated in referral:
   Increase muscle strength
   Increase functional independence
   Aid with adjustment to disability

B. Other services.
Medical: Maintenance of general health, prescription and supervision of rehabilitation program, evaluation of physical status and progress, management of bladder and bowel problems
Nursing: Administration of medications, bed positioning, supportive care, management of bladder and bowel training
Social service: Family and client counseling, discharge planning, liaison with community agencies
Physical therapy: LE ROM exercises, tilt table tolerance, transfer training, UE exercises

Vocational counselor: Vocational and aptitude evaluation, vocational counseling, arrangements for vocational or educational training
Psychology-psychiatry: Facilitation of adjustment to disability, sexual counseling, psychometric evaluation
Community social groups: Provision of peer group interaction and opportunities for socialization
Recreation therapy: Provision of recreational and diversional activities, building of physical endurance, socialization, community outings
Spiritual counselor: Supportive counseling, aid in acceptance of disability

C. OT evaluation.
Strength: Test
ROM: Test
Physical endurance: Observe
Involuntary movement and spasticity (spasms, clonus): Observe
Equilibrium and protective mechanisms: Observe
Coordination-Muscle control: Observe and test
Sensory-perceptual functions: Test
   Touch
   Pain
   Temperature
   Stereognosis
   Proprioception
Cognitive functions: Observe
   Judgment
   Safety
   Motivation
Psychosocial skills: Observe
   Maturity
   Interpersonal skills
   Adjustment to disability
   Reality functioning
Prevocational potential: Observe
   Work habits
   Potential work skills
   Work tolerance level
Functional skills: Observe and test
   Feeding
   Self-care
   Homemaking
   Community travel (public-private transportation)

D. Results of evaluation.[6]
1. Evaluation data.
   a. Physical resources.
      (1) Strength
          Shoulder: All muscles G
          Scapula: All muscles G
          Elbow: Triceps P+, biceps G

Forearm: Supinator F+, pronator F
Wrist: Flexors P, extensors F
Fingers: O
Thumb: O, except for extensors: T and abductors: T
      (2) Passive ROM: All joints within functional to normal range, no contractures
      (3) Physical endurance: Endurance is fair; sitting and activity tolerance level up to 4 hours
      (4) Involuntary movement and spasticity: No involuntary movements observed; mild spasticity in lower extremities, no spasticity in upper extremities
      (5) Equilibrium and protective mechanisms: Trunk balance is weak; sufficient arm strength to right self
      (6) Coordination-muscle control: UE muscle control and coordination of innervated muscles is within normal limits
      (7) Hand function: Lateral prehension with difficulty, weak with tenodesis grasp
   b. Sensory-perceptual functions. All sensation below lesion (trunk and lower extremities) is absent. Touch, pain, and temperature absent from T1 dermatome down and posterior and anterior ulnar side of arm and fifth finger. Stereognosis and proprioception are within normal limits.
   c. Cognitive functions. John appears to use good judgment during wheelchair exercise and transfer training. He can anticipate results of behavior and actions. He needs some instruction in safety precautions necessary to guard desensitized areas from injury. He has a low level of motivation because of stage of adjustment to disability.

Continued.

d. Psychological functions. John's adjustment to disability is poor. He expresses a flip, carefree attitude. His expectations for recovery are demonstrated by denial of the reality and permanency of the disability. Therefore he is poorly motivated in treatment modalities that emphasize a lifelong disability, expressing interest in activities that involve lower extremities and that suggest the possibility of a total recovery.

e. Prevocational potential. Potential work skills are limited by weakness of grasp and poor finger dexterity. Training and adaptations will increase potential. Vocational pursuits are limited because of wheelchair ambulation. Work habits are immature at present. Client needs to improve responsibility, concen-tration, and perseverence. Work tolerance level is potentially good. Physical endurance and sitting tolerance level should improve to allow a full day of activity. Following psychological adjustment vocational potential is good because of interests and intelligence.

f. Functional skills. John is able to accomplish light hygiene activities independently but is poorly motivated and dependent in bathing and dressing. He currently requires moderate assistance in feeding. He relies excessively on staff and family. His potential for independence is good. John is currently unable to perform any home-making activities independently because of poor balance, weak grasp, and poor motivation. His potential for homemaking skills is fair. He will always require moderate assistance. John has not participated in a community mobility evaluation yet but is a candidate for driving evaluation and for reaching independence in a wheelchair mobility.

2. Problem identification.
   a. Muscle weakness
   b. Limited endurance
   c. Poor trunk balance
   d. Weak prehension with tenodesis grasp
   e. Sensory deficits
   f. Low motivation
   g. Poor adjustment to disability
   h. ADL dependence
   i. Limited vocational possibilities
   j. Redirection of educational goals
   k. Need for avocational outlets
   l. Restricted mobility
   m. Family adjustment

E Problem	F Specific OT objectives	G Methods used to meet objectives	H Gradation of treatment

a	Through a program of enabling exercise the client's muscle grades will increase by at least ½ to 1 grade
	Shoulder: G to N
	Scapula: G to N
	Elbow
	  Flexors: G to N
	  Extensors: P to P+
	Wrist
	  Extensors: F to G
	  Flexors: P to F
	  Thumb extensor: T to P
	  Thumb radial abductor: T to P
		Skateboard exercises for both upper extremities; in a gravity-eliminated position the client will perform the following movement patterns:
		Scapula abduction-horizontal and adduction-elbow flexion
		Scapula adduction-horizontal and abduction-elbow extension
		Shoulder flexion-elbow extension
		Shoulder extension-elbow flexion
		Work for 10 repetitions of each pattern and add resistance when possible
		Active exercises for wrist extension; begin active exercise of wrist against gravity; stabilize the forearm to isolate motion to the wrist; client extends the wrist against gravity for 10 repetitions; when F+ grade is achieved, progress to resistive exercises against gravity using a handcuff with wrist weight attachment; work toward three sets of 10 repetitions with short rest between each set
		Active exercises for wrist flexion in a gravity-eliminated plane; forearms are stabilized on a low platform just above the table surface; client performs wrist flexion for 5 to 10 repetitions; progress to active exercise against gravity as strength improves
			Increase resistance
			Increase number repetitions of all exercises

E Problem	F Specific OT objectives	G Methods used to meet objectives	H Gradation of treatment
		Muscle reeducation to long thumb extensor and abductor; active-assisted exercise, graded to active exercise	
d	Given a wrist-driven flexor hinge splint and training the client will be able to use the splint for some self-care and recreational activities	Practice application and removal of splint, using arm motions and teeth to fasten straps Grasp and release practice using blocks, pegs, or common objects	Progress to holding fork for feeding and use of splint for table games such as chess or checkers
c	Through a program of activity and exercise trunk balance will increase so client can achieve maximal independence in ADL	Beach ball toss (patient to therapist), with trunk stabilization through corset, wheelchair support, or manual assistance	Vary position of therapist and client to catch ball, increase distance of toss, and increase number of repetitions
g	Through the use of therapeutic relationships, the therapeutic environment, group experiences, and activities the client will increase acceptance of physical disability so that his motivation for rehabilitation procedures and his social interactions will increase	Through patient-therapist interaction: Assist client in orientation to rehabilitation center; allow client to give up denial gradually (therapist not to condone or condemn denial); encourage ventilation of feelings and verbalization of problems; foster client therapist relationship of warmth, responsiveness, empathy, individuality, and perception; purposeful conversation during all treatment sessions, allowing patient to consider alternatives and possibilities for the future; involve the patient in goal setting and treatment planning; encourage pride, individuality, independence, and self-esteem; facilitate problem-solving skills and needs gratification	Reintroduction to family and social life should be a gradual process progressing from family to groups of friends (outside) to public situations
		Through social interaction: Social, recreation, special interest, and expressive groups with other disabled individuals; group work focusing first on adjustment and secondly on acquisition of skills needed for success in the community;[6] group painting project with other clients with spinal cord injuries to encourage mutual sharing, accomplishment, and success experience; community outings to restaurants or public buildings first with therapist and one or two other clients	Outings with family members and therapist; outings with nondisabled friends
h	Given instruction, daily practice, and assistive devices the client will be able to feed himself without assistance and with a minimal number of assistive devices	Eating aids and assistance: Initially a suction mat stabilizing a plate with plate guard and a universal cuff may be used (progress to use of the flexor hinge splint for holding utensils); plate with plate guard is still used and regular utensils are used, if tenodesis grasp is developed and client chooses not to use flexor hinge splints	Patient progresses from easy-to-eat to more difficult-to-eat foods; eating speed increases

Continued.

E Problem	F Specific OT objectives	G Methods used to meet objectives	H Gradation of treatment
	Given instruction, daily practice, and assistive devices dressing will be performed in 45 minutes or less	Teach dressing techniques described in Chapter 12 　Donning and removing: 　　Shirts 　　Trousers and undershorts 　　Socks 　　Shoes	Practice UE dressing first, progress to LE dressing if feasible
	Given instruction and daily practice the client will protect his own skin from pressure sores so that there is no evidence of their development	Shifting weight in wheelchair: 　Every 10 minutes client leans to one side, then the other side of the wheelchair by flexing elbow around wheelchair handle on that side and pulling body weight, using elbow and shoulder muscles or client pushes himself up on the wheelchair armrests to relieve ischial pressure 　Every morning and every evening, in bed, in side lying position, client inspects skin over buttock, trochanters, and heels with long handle skin inspection mirror; while sitting in bed or in wheelchair, client inspects elbows and knees	Reminders, supervision, and assistance are gradually decreased as client becomes more responsible for his own self-care
j	Through appropriate experiences, trials, and exploration the feasibility of attending college will be determined by the client in concert with occupational therapy and vocational counselor	Writing training; training in use of electric typewriter with typing sticks if necessary; training in use of tape recorder for recording and transcribing; wheelchair mobility practice, indoors and outdoors; trial in an adult education class	
k	Through a program of activity the client will explore avocational interests so that adaptive skills and personal satisfaction will increase	Painting and sketching—watercolor, oil, charcoal, or pencil—using flexor hinge splint or universal cuff or tenodesis grasp; practice and assistance in handwriting skills with splint Games, using flexor hinge splints: 　Cards 　Chess 　Backgammon 　Jigsaw puzzles 　Crossword puzzles[6] Music (collecting and listening to records); spectator sports	Reduce reliance on assistive devices when appropriate; increase length of time spent working on projects

I. **Special equipment.**
　1. Ambulation aids.
　　Active duty lightweight wheelchair with pneumatic tires and handrim projections for easy maneuverability and transfer of wheelchair into car and on soft, sandy, or rough surfaces. For energy conservation an electric wheelchair may be more practical.
　2. Splints.
　　Wrist-driven flexor hinge splint

　3. Assistive devices.[20]
　　a. Soap holder
　　b. Bath bench
　　c. Hand-held shower
　　d. Razor holder
　　e. Sliding transfer board
　　f. Button hook
　　g. Zipper pull
　　h. Suppository insertion device
　　i. Electric typewriter
　　j. Tape recorder
　　k. Dressing sticks
　　l. Skin inspection mirror
　　m. Long-handle bath sponge

REVIEW QUESTIONS

1. List three causes of spinal cord injury. Which is most common?
2. Describe the patterns of weakness in quadriplegia and paraplegia.
3. Describe the functional and prognostic differences between complete and incomplete lesions.
4. When reference is made to "C5" in quadriplegia, what is meant in terms of level of injury and functioning muscle groups?
5. What are the characteristics of spinal shock?
6. What physical changes occur following the spinal shock phase?
7. What is the prognosis for recovery of motor function in complete lesions and incomplete lesions?
8. What are the purposes of surgery in management of spinal injury?
9. What are some medical complications, common to patients with spinal cord injuries, that can limit achievement of functional potential?
10. How should postural hypotension be treated?
11. How should autonomic dysreflexia be treated?
12. What is the role of the occupational therapist in the prevention of pressure sores?
13. Why is vital capacity affected in patients with spinal cord injuries?
14. What effect will reduced vital capacity have on the rehabilitation program?
15. Which level of injury has full innervation of rotator cuff musculature, biceps, and extensor carpi radialis and partial innervation of serratus anterior, latissimus dorsi and pectoralis major?
16. What additional muscle power does the patient with C6 quadriplegia have over the patient with C5 quadriplegia? What is the major functional advantage of this additional muscle power?
17. What are the additional critical muscles that the patient with C7 quadriplegia has, as compared to the patient with C6 quadriplegia?
18. What additional functional independence can be achieved because of this additional muscle power?
19. What is the first spinal cord lesion level that has full innervation of UE musculature?
20. Which evaluation tools does the occupational therapist use to assess the patient with a spinal cord injury? What is the purpose of each?
21. List five goals of occupational therapy for the patient with a spinal cord injury.
22. How is wrist extension used to effect grasp by the patient with quadriplegia?
23. How does the patient with C6 quadriplegia substitute for the absence of elbow extensors?
24. What is the "contracture" that is encouraged in patients with spinal cord injuries? Why? How is it developed?
25. What is the splint that allows the C6 quadriplegic to achieve functional grasp?
26. What are some of the first self-care activities that the patient with a C6 spinal cord injury should be expected to accomplish?
27. List four assistive devices commonly used by persons with quadriplegia, and tell the purpose of each.
28. Describe the role of occupational therapy in the vocational evaluation of the client with a spinal cord injury.

REFERENCES

1. Autonomic dysreflexia for staff, San Jose, Calif., 1969, Santa Clara Valley Medical Center. Mimeographed.
2. Bors, E., and Comarr, A.E.: Neurological disturbances of sexual function with special reference to 529 patients with spinal cord injury, Urol. Surv. **10**:191, 1960.
3. Bromley, I.: Tetraplegia and paraplegia: a guide for physiotherapists, ed. 2, New York, 1981, Churchill Livingstone, Inc.
4. Chusid, J.G.: Correlative neuroanatomy and functional neurology, ed. 15, Los Altos, Calif., 1973, Lange Medical Publications.
5. Daniels, L., and Worthingham, C.: Muscle testing, ed. 3, Philadelphia, 1972, W.B. Saunders Co.
6. Fodera, C., and Olsen, K.: Treatment plan for spinal cord injury, unpublished paper presented in partial fulfillment of the requirements for the course O.T. 167, San Jose, Calif., May 1979, Department of Occupational Therapy, San Jose State University.
7. Freed, M.: Traumatic and congenital lesions of the spinal cord. In Kottke, F.J., Stillwell, G.K., and Lehmann, J.F., editors: Krusen's handbook of physical medicine and rehabilitation, ed. 3, Philadelphia, 1982, W.B. Saunders Co.
8. Functional goals in spinal cord lesions, Downey, Calif., Physical Therapy Department, Rancho Los Amigos Hospital. Mimeographed.
9. Geiger, R.: Sexuality in the handicapped, lecture to Crippled Children's Services Conference, Oakland, Calif., March 1973.
10. Greb, M., and Mueller, J.M.: Functional goals at specific levels of spinal cord injury, Denver, Colo., Craig Hospital.
11. Hamilton, R.: Spinal cord injury: medical and surgical management, lecture in course O.T. 135, San Jose, Calif., 1973, Department of Occupational Therapy, San Jose State University.
12. Long, C., and Lawton, E.: Functional significance of spinal cord lesion level, New York, 1954-58. Mimeographed.
13. Malick, M.H., and Meyer, C.M.H.: Manual on management of the quadriplegic upper extremity, Pittsburgh, 1978, Harmarville Rehabilitation Center.
14. McKenzie, M.W.: The role of occupational therapy in rehabilitating spinal cord injured patients, Am. J. Occup. Ther. **24**:257, 1970.
15. Mooney, T.O., Cole, T.M., and Chilgren, R.A.: Sexual options for paraplegics and quadriplegics, Boston, 1975, Little, Brown, & Co.
16. Neistadt, M., and Baker, M.F.: A program for sex counseling the physically disabled, Am. J. Occup. Ther. **32**:646, 1978.
17. Pierce, D.S., and Nickel, V.H.: The total care of spinal cord injuries, Boston, 1977, Little, Brown & Co.
18. Reedy, J.: Spinal cord level chart, unpublished paper presented in partial fulfillment fo the requirements for the course O.T. 135, San Jose, Calif., November 1974, Department of Occupational Therapy, San Jose State University.
19. Runge, M.: Self-dressing techniques for patients with spinal cord injury, Am. J. Occup. Ther. **21**:367, 1967.
20. Sammons, F.: Be OK: self-help aids, professional and institutional catalog for 1984, Brookfield, Ill., 1984, Fred Sammons, Inc.
21. Sidman, J.M.: Sexual functioning in the physically disabled adult, Am. J. Occup. Ther. **31**:81, 1977.

22. Spencer, E.A.: Functional restoration. In Hopkins, H.L., and Smith, H.D., editors: Willard and Spackman's occupational therapy, ed. 6, Philadelphia, 1983, J.B. Lippincott Co.

23. Talbot, H.S.: The sexual function in paraplegia, J. Urol. **73:**91, 1955.

24. Trombly, C.A., and Scott, A.D.: Occupational therapy for physical dysfunction, Baltimore, 1977, Williams & Wilkins.

25. Venegas, N., and Del Pilar-Christian, M., editors: Proceedings of the workshop "Occupational therapy for patients with physical dysfunction," Puerto Rico, 1967, Occupational Therapy Department, University of Puerto Rico.

26. Wilson, D.J., Mckenzie, M.W., and Barber, L.M.: Spinal cord injury: a treatment guide for occupational therapists, Thorofare, N.J., 1974, Charles B. Slack, Inc.

CHAPTER 30

Cerebral vascular accident

LORRAINE WILLIAMS PEDRETTI

Cerebral vascular accident (CVA), commonly referred to as a stroke or shock, is a complex dysfunction caused by a lesion in the brain. It results in an upper motor neuron dysfunction that produces hemiplegia or paralysis of one side of the body, limbs, and sometimes the face and oral structures that are contralateral to the hemisphere of the brain that has the lesion. Thus a lesion in the left cerebral hemisphere will produce hemiplegia on the right side of the body and vice versa. When referring to the client's disability as *right* hemiplegia, however, the reference is to the paralyzed body side and *not* to the locus of the lesion.[20]

Accompanying the motor paralysis may be a variety of other dysfunctions. Some of these are sensory disturbances, perceptual dysfunctions, visual disturbances, personality and intellectual changes, and a complex range of speech and associated language disorders.[24]

EFFECTS

The outcome of the CVA will depend on which artery supplying the brain was involved in the vascular disease process.

Involvement of the *middle cerebral artery* (MCA) is the most common cause of CVA.[15] The general symptoms caused by occlusion of the MCA include contralateral hemiplegia with greater involvement of the arm, face, and tongue, sensory and perceptual disturbances; contralateral homonymous hemianopsia; and aphasia, if the lesion is in the dominant hemisphere.[9,20,22] Occlusion of the *anterior cerebral artery* (ACA) usually results in contralateral hemiplegia, with leg involvement greater than arm involvement; sensory deficits; mental confusion; apraxia; and aphasia, if the lesion is in the dominant hemisphere. Signs of *posterior cerebral artery* (PCA) occlusion include contralateral hemiplegia and homonymous hemianopsia; hemisensory deficits; and receptive aphasia, if the dominant hemisphere is involved. Ataxia, rigidity, tremors, and choreiform movement may also result less often.[9,20]

The cerebellar and basilar arteries may also be involved in vascular disease that produces stroke. *Cerebellar artery* occlusion results in ipsilateral ataxia, contralateral loss of pain and temperature sensitivity, ipsilateral facial analgesia, and contralateral hemiparesis.[9] If the *basilar artery* is involved, results could include dysfunction of cranial nerves 3 to 12, cerebellar dysfunction, loss of proprioception,[20] hemiplegia, quadriplegia, and sensory disturbances.[9,22]

ETIOLOGY

CVA is caused by an interruption of the blood supply to the brain because of thrombus, embolus, or hemorrhage.[5,6,13,20] Cerebral anoxia and aneurysm can also result in hemiplegia.[5,6,20] Some of the treatment approaches outlined in this chapter may be applicable to hemiplegia that results from causes other than CVA or stroke, such as head injuries, neoplasms, and infectious diseases of the brain.[5]

Vascular disease of the brain can result in a completed CVA with the full clinical picture just described or can cause transient ischemic attacks (TIAs) because of temporary vascular insufficiency. These attacks result in temporary neurological symptoms (less than 24 hours duration) that disappear. They signal the probability of complete CVA sometime in the future.[20] If they are caused by extracranial vascular disease, surgical intervention to reestablish patency of arteries may be effective in preventing the CVA and the resultant disablity.

PREDISPOSING FACTORS

Some of the factors that predispose an individual to the possible onset of CVA are arteriosclerosis, hypertension, obesity, diabetes, smoking, or congenital vascular weakness that results in aneurysm.[20]

MEDICAL MANAGEMENT[5]

It is the physician's responsibility to make the diagnosis and apply the early lifesaving measures. These may include ordering appropriate nourishment and hydration and establishing an airway.

The physician also prescribes medication to treat or prevent infection or concomitant medical problems.

During the acute illness the need for urinary drainage should be determined and catheterization carried out, if necessary. The physician should also order early mobility, adequate diet and fluids, and use of suppositories and medication to prevent or treat fecal impaction.

The physician should see that appropriate measures are instituted to prevent contractures. This means writing orders for appropriate positioning, splints, and passive exercise in the early phases of rehabilitation. Pressure sores should be vigilantly guarded against through early mobilization, frequent repositioning in bed or chair, excellent hygiene, and skin inspection. The physician is responsible for ordering these measures, seeing that they are carried out, and inspecting the patient's skin on a regular basis.

It is important for the physician to not overlook the possibility of disability of unaffected parts because of disuse and immobility. The physician should see to it that the patient is involved in physical activities and exercises that are commensurate with his or her medical status and abilities as early as possible in the rehabilitation program.

Evaluating the residuals of the CVA, writing orders for the rehabilitation therapies, and reevaluating the patient's progress are the responsibilities of the physician, who supervises the rehabilitation program.

MOTOR DYSFUNCTION AFTER CVA

Bobath[4] outlines four major factors that interfere with normal motor performance in an adult hemiplegia: sensory disturbances, spasticity, disorder of the normal postural reflex mechanism, and loss of selective movement patterns.

The degree of sensory involvement will have a profound influence on the degree of spontaneous motor recovery and the results of treatment. All movement is in response to some sensory stimuli acting on the central nervous

419

system (CNS) from the external and internal environments.[4,7] These sensory stimuli progress through the CNS and are integrated at the cortical level, where they produce an effective, coordinated motor response to meet the demands of the environment. Sensations arising from the movement response serve to guide it through its course,[4] determine its effectiveness, and give cues for the need for any revision of the movement response. Fig. 30-1 shows a schematic diagram of the sensorimotor process.

Because of this critical sensory-motor relationship and interdependence, it is important to think of the sensorimotor cortex as one functional unit of the brain.[4] The sensory disturbance in patients with hemiplegia aggravates the motor dysfunction even in the absence of severe spasticity. The patients lack the urge to move[4] probably in part because they cannot sense and interpret the environmental stimuli that normally evoke movement.

Characteristics of the motor disturbance after CVA

After CVA there is upper motor neuron paralysis that follows a one-sided distribution and includes musculature of the trunk and limbs on the affected side. The muscles of the face and mouth may also be involved. The paralysis is usually characterized by increased muscle tone or spasticity. There may, in some cases, be apparent hypotonicity of flaccidity. Even in these instances some spasticity may be evoked in the finger and wrist flexors and the ankle extensors, if prolonged and strong stretch stimuli are applied. In cases where apparent flaccidity persists indefinitely, it is usually combined with severe sensory loss, and active motion is impossible.[4]

Coordination or control of smooth, rhythmical movement is lost. Rather the spasticity occurs in gross patterns of flexion and extension called *synergies* (Chapter 15). Synergies are released when cortical control of motion is interrupted. All muscles in the synergy are neurophysiologically linked, and when one of the movement components of the synergy is performed, some or all of the movement components are likely to occur simultaneously.[6,13]

Normal postural reflex mechanisms are disturbed after CVA. Normal righting, equilibrium, and protective reactions (Chapter 8) are lost on the hemiplegic side.[4] This affects the client's ability to maintain and recover balance and make the normal postural adjustments that accompany movement and activity. Primitive reflexes (Chapter 8) may be released so that changes of the position of the head and body in space will have an abnormal influence on muscle tone.

Bobath[4] describes the loss of "adaptive changes of muscle tone as a protection against the forces of gravity." This is the ability to control slow, unresisted movements in the direction of gravity. For example, in lowering the upraised arm the antigravity muscles contract and hold while their antagonist muscles relax. The person with hemiplegia has lost this mechanism of automatic control on the affected side. He or she will tend to compensate for the loss with the automatic reactions of the unaffected side. The patient will not initiate movement with the affected side, will not support him or herself on the affected arm and hand, and will bear little weight on the affected leg.

Because of the spasticity and release of abnormal synergistic movement patterns, there is a loss of selective, discriminative, and isolated movement after CVA. This loss is most apparent in the arm and hand,[4] probably because of

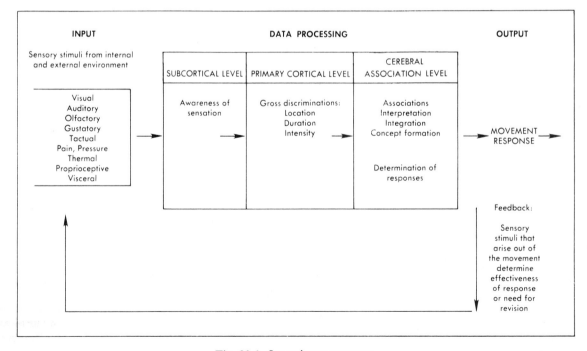

Fig. 30-1. Sensorimotor process.

the nature of the normal function of this part. However, selective movement is also lost in the leg and foot and is evident in the inability to dorsiflex the ankle and toes regardless of the position of the hip and knee or in the inability to flex the knee while the hip is extended.[4] In function this is evidenced by the gait pattern, which is usually performed with the leg held in stiff extension or in the extensor synergy pattern. The individual with hemiplegia lacks ability to perform a wide variety of movement combinations to effect normal motor performance.[4]

Characteristics of synergistic movement

The flexor synergy dominates in the arm, and the extensor synergy dominates in the leg. Performance of synergistic movement, either reflexly or voluntarily, may be influenced by the primitive postural reflex mechanisms. When the client performs the synergy, the strongest of its components are often most apparent, rather than the entire classic patterns, as discussed in Chapter 15. By the same token the resting posture of the limb, particularly the arm, is usually characterized by a position that represents the strongest components of both flexor and extensor synergies, that is, shoulder adduction, elbow flexion, forearm pronation, and wrist and finger flexion. However, with facilitation or voluntary effort the more classic synergy pattern can usually be evoked.[6]

The recovery process

The stages of recovery described by Brunnstrom[6] were outlined in Table 15-1. The recovery follows an ontogenetic process. It is usually proximal to distal so that shoulder movement can be expected before hand movement. Flexion patterns occur before extension patterns in the upper limb. Reflex motion occurs before controlled, volitional movement, and gross movement patterns can be performed before isolated, selective movement.

Recovery may cease at any stage, and the amount of recovery attained varies widely from person to person. Motor recovery is influenced by many factors, such as sensation, perception, motivation, affective states, and concomitant medical problems or general health.[13]

Few patients make a very good recovery of arm function, and the greatest loss is usually in the wrist and hand.

It should be noted that no two patients are exactly alike. There will be much individual variation on the characteristic motor disturbances and the recovery process among patients. The motor behavior and recovery process described represent common characteristics that may be observed in a majority of persons after CVA occurs.[6]

PROGNOSIS FOR RECOVERY OF ARM FUNCTION.[23] The physician and therapist may wish to estimate the potential for recovery of arm function for planning rehabilitation goals. Some of the factors that are considered to be good prognostic signs are (1) good sensation and perception, (2) intact body scheme, (3) minimal spasticity, (4) functional ROM, (5) attempts at spontaneous use of the affected arm in bilateral activities, and (6) development of some isolated motion. Conversely, poor prognostic signs include such factors as (1) severe sensory and perceptual impairments, (2) moderate to severe spasticity, (3) body scheme and motor planning deficits, (4) limited ROM, (5) no attempts at spontaneous use of the affected arm during bilateral activities, and (6) inability to perform controlled movement.

RECOVERY PERIOD. Spontaneous neurological recovery that results in improvement of motor performance occurs primarily in the first 3 months after the onset of the CVA. Recovery may continue to the sixth or seventh month after the onset.[13] Slight, continued recovery is sometimes seen up to 1 year and in rare instances is seen somewhat longer. This does not imply that motor behavior cannot be influenced by appropriate therapy after a year, however.

FUNCTIONAL USE OF THE AFFECTED ARM. Therapy aimed to improve arm function is often frustrating to the client and the therapist unless realistic goals and expectations have been set. Progress should be judged by the amount of spontaneous use of the affected arm, rather than by comparing it to the normal one as a standard for progress or as a goal to be reached. Realistically few clients will recover full function of the arm. The client may use the hand and arm only when needed and perhaps then not by choice. He or

she may use the affected arm only to assist the unaffected arm in activities that require stabilization of objects. The stage of recovery limits how the affected arm can be used. The arm that has little or no voluntary motion but has good sensation may be used as a passive stabilizer. If there is voluntary control of the flexion synergy with gross grasp and good sensation, the arm can be used for grasping and pulling. Voluntary control of the flexor synergy, elbow extension, grasp, active release, and good sensation may render enough function for grasping, pushing, pulling, and releasing. If isolated movements or gross movement combinations that deviate from the synergy patterns are possible and there is good sensation, the arm can be used to perform some gross movements and activities with combined movements. If the highest recovery stages are achieved and there is normal shoulder, elbow, and forearm movement, good sensation, and limitations only in fine hand movements, the arm can be used to perform all normal daily activities except for those that require fine manipulation and motor speed.[25]

CONCOMITANT DYSFUNCTIONS

Therapists have placed much emphasis on the evaluation and treatment of the motor dysfunction. They should also be aware of and be able to evaluate and treat the total disability. On the basis of a comprehensive evaluation realistic rehabilitation goals, considering all aspects of the disability, may be planned with the client.[24]

Sensory disturbances

Disturbances in the senses of touch, pain, temperature, pressure, and vibration may occur as a result of CVA. Such disturbances prohibit the sensory feedback that is so important to the perceptual-motor functioning of the individual and thus may be one cause of disuse of the affected extremities, even when motor recovery is apparently good.[24]

Somatic perceptual dysfunctions

LOSS OF PROPRIOCEPTION. The loss of the ability to perceive position and motion of body parts[1] will affect use of those parts. Impaired proprioception is a common deficit seen in patients who have CVA. Such patients are likely to leave the affected arm in a state of disuse, drop things, and not be aware of the position and movement of the arm. The arm may have a sensation of heaviness.[24]

TACTUAL PERCEPTION. Tactual perception is the ability to recognize, localize, and make discriminations about touch stimuli to the skin surface. It includes the ability to recognize and localize light touch stimuli, ability to recognize symbols "written" on the skin (graphesthesia), ability to recognize two stimuli in close proximity (two-point discrimination), ability to recognize two simultaneous stimuli, and ability to identify common objects and geometric forms through manipulation without the aid of vision (stereognosis). The inability to perceive the tangible properties of an object tactually (astereognosis) interferes with perceptual-motor functioning of the patient in that he or she receives no sensory feedback about the objects he or she is manipulating unless vision is used to compensate for the sensory loss. This compensation is often ineffective, since it is difficult to visually supervise the hand performing an activity while trying to watch the activity and focus on its goal.[24]

BODY SCHEME DISORDERS. Body scheme disorders are disturbances in the neurological function that include knowledge of body construction, its anatomical elements, and spatial relationships; ability to visualize the body in movement and its parts in different positional relationships; ability to differentiate right from left; and ability to know body health or disease.[1] Body scheme disorders are found frequently enough in patients with hemiplegia to make routine evaluation for the presence of this dysfunction advisable. Since knowledge of the body scheme is basic to all motor function, a disturbance in body scheme will have a profound effect on the success of the patient's rehabilitation. Patients with body scheme disturbances will have difficulty with ADL, especially self-care and

dressing activities that require a good knowledge of the body. They may have difficulty following directions related to their own bodies. They may be unable to correctly localize body parts, recognize right and left, or visualize and plan how to move their bodies to accomplish a given activity.[24]

APRAXIA. The disturbance in praxis, or the ability to plan motor acts, is often intimately associated with the body scheme disorder.[1] To dress, for example, one must not only have a good knowledge of the body scheme but must also be able to plan the motions necessary to put the garment on the body. When there is apraxia, the individual often cannot formulate a plan of movement to accomplish an act.[24] He or she may be unable to imitate movements of the therapist in demonstrated instructions. The patient is unable to carry out a purposeful movement on command even if he or she understands the concept of the task, although he or she may be able to carry out the act automatically.[13,19] These problems characterize ideomotor apraxia. If there is ideational apraxia as well, the patient will not be able to carry out routine activities, such as combing his or her hair automatically or on command because he or she no longer understands the concept of the task.[19]

Visual-perceptual dysfunctions

VISUAL FIELD DEFECT—HOMONYMOUS HEMIANOPSIA. Homonymous hemianopsia is blindness of the medial half of one eye and the lateral half of the other. The affected side of the vision corresponds to the paralyzed side of the body. A patient with left hemiplegia with left homonymous hemianopsia cannot see things in the left visual field unless the patient turns his or her head toward the affected side to compensate for the deficit. In practical activity he or she may not see things placed on the left side. Instructions, demonstrations, and conversation given from the left side may be ignored. Objects moving toward the patient from the left may startle him or her. The patient may bump into things on the left when walking. Many patients with hemiplegia compensate for this deficit quite automatically, whereas others do not seem to make this adjustment and

must be trained to use the intact visual field to compensate for the visual loss.[24]

VISUAL INATTENTION. Visual inattention refers to defect in reception of and reaction to visual stimuli. It manifests itself in defective scanning of the visual field, difficulty in shifting gaze from one object to another, slowed eye movements, loss of the fixation point, and difficulty in shifting attention.[24]

SPATIAL RELATIONSHIPS. The ability to recognize the relationship between one form and another in spatial areas[12] may be lost as a result of CVA. Disturbances in the perception of visual-spatial relationships are particularly common among patients with left hemiplegia. The result is a disorganization of constructional abilities such as in drawing or constructing three-dimensional objects and designs. The patient with this deficit will have difficulty or failure with tasks involving spatial analysis. Dressing failures are common.[24] Problems in body scheme and apraxia may be severe enough to prohibit the learning of dressing skills, but the problem may be compounded by the patient's inability to perceive the shape and relationship of the clothing to his or her body. Tasks such as matching parts in a sewing or woodworking project are impossible, as is matching puzzle parts or block designs.

VERTICALITY. The perception of vertical lines and elements in the environment is verticality. Patients with hemiplegia often have difficulty making visual judgments of what is vertical or horizontal. Patients with left hemiplegia tend to misjudge verticality in a counterclockwise direction. Since visual orientation to verticality is important to the optical righting reactions that help in the maintenance of upright posture, directional disturbances in perception of vertical and horizontal may interfere with balance and ambulation.[24]

FIGURE-BACKGROUND PERCEPTION. Figure-background perception is the recognition of forms hidden within a gestalt[12] and the ability to attend to a relevant visual stimulus while separating it from and ignoring background stimuli. Some patients with hemiplegia have difficulty distinguishing a figure from its background. The result is that they cannot always select the most relevant visual cue to which to respond.[24]

The patient may appear distractible when, in truth, he or she is responding to many irrelevant visual stimuli. The patient may have difficulty selecting items from a cabinet or refrigerator because he or she cannot perceive the desired object as separate from the surrounding objects that constitute its background.

VISUAL SEQUENCING. Visual sequencing is the ordering of visual patterns in time and space and involves temporal concepts, such as first, second, and third, and spatial ordering, such as top to bottom, left to right, and around.[2] A disturbance in sequencing skills may affect the patient's ability to plan steps and anticipate consequences of tasks and activities that require ordering of objects and steps in a procedure.

Intellectual and cognitive dysfunctions

Since CVA may interfere with integrative processes of the brain, and intelligence and cognitive abilities depend on the integrative functions of the brain, some patients with hemiplegia will show impairment of specific intellectual functions. These may be demonstrated by a drop in intelligence test scores and an overall change in organization, mental abilities, and ability to do abstract reasoning.[13]

MEMORY. The ability to recall various details of recent and past visual and auditory stimuli[2] may be disturbed as a result of CVA. Memory disturbance will retard rehabilitation efforts. The patient may have difficulty recalling persons, objects, and procedures learned from day to day.

Retrieval of information may be reduced, and learning ability may be impaired. Patients with right hemiplegia are likely to have impaired memory for language and numbers, whereas patients with left hemiplegia have impairments involving tasks of position and movement.[22]

Patients with deficits in memory will require much repetition of activity before training can be retained. The therapist needs to discover each patient's best mode of sensory learning and provide the necessary sensory and perceptual cues and methods of instruction to suit the individual.

JUDGMENT. Poor judgment may be easily detected or may be masked by good social or verbal skills. The patient may be unable to abstract the future and make judgments about the consequences of certain behaviors. The patient may not be able to judge, for example, that not locking his or her wheelchair may have grave consequences.

ABSTRACT THINKING. Abstract thinking and reasoning may also be impaired. These patients will be very concrete, dealing best with the realities of concrete objects and situations than with ideas and speculations about them. They may not be able to generalize learning from one situation or therapist to another and may be unable to comprehend the abstract ideas conveyed in humor or idioms.[24]

Personality and emotional changes

REGRESSION. In regression the patient does not appear to use his or her full adult capacities to deal with personal difficulties. The patient seems to regress to a lower level of emotional maturity. This is not an uncommon reaction to illness and may be due in part to sensory loss.[3]

RIGIDITY. Rigidity is an inability to be flexible or adapt to change. The patient seems to feel most secure in a familiar and unchanging environment. This phenomenon manifests itself in the inability to function in a changed time schedule, disturbance at lack of symmetry or change in personnel, and a tenacity to old and familiar methods of performing familiar activities.[24]

DENIAL. Denial is an unawareness of the hemiplegia and a denial of the defective performance of the paralyzed side. It manifests itself when the patient neglects the affected side. The patient may move the normal side and claim he or she is moving the affected arm or leg. The client may declare that his or her arm belongs to someone else or may regard it as an object. This phenomenon may be a psychological reaction to an unbearable truth or may be due to sensory and perceptual dysfunctions.[3]

PERSEVERATION. Perseveration is the meaningless, nonpurposeful repetition of an act. The patient does not stop unless someone or something intervenes. It becomes particularly apparent during activities that are repetitive by nature, such as sanding wood, but can manifest itself in ADL as well. Perseveration may be exhibited in buttoning, stirring foods, and sponge bathing, for example.

DEPRESSION. Depression is usually a reaction to a catastrophic illness. The patient may feel inadequate in dealing with his or her problems and may be overwhelmed by them. He or she has a sense of loss and must mourn for the loss. The patient may feel rejected and out of control of his or her own affairs as well as his or her own body. The depression usually lifts and rehabilitation progresses as the patient rediscovers his or her assets and gains confidence and self-esteem.[3]

EMOTIONAL LABILITY. The patient with CVA may lose the cortical control of emotional responses and thus may manifest loss of emotional control more easily than he or she did formerly. Emotional lability may exhibit itself in automatic laughing or crying that seems inappropriate. Situations of stress often provoke crying. The patient is embarrassed by these outbursts and requires the reassurance and understanding of family and rehabilitation workers.[3]

REDUCTION IN BEHAVIORAL AND EVALUATIVE STANDARDS. The patient demonstrating a reduction in behavioral and evaluative standards may exhibit a reduced level of aspiration. He or she may seem satisfied with shoddy performance. His or her pride and perseverance in working toward goals may be poor. Inadequate performance and poor products may be acceptable to the patient in contrast to his or her standards before the illness occurred. This problem may be organic in origin but is enhanced by inactivity and the psychological trauma of the illness.[10]

MOTIVATION. Many patients with hemiplegia manifest an apparent defect in "intrinsic" motivation, or the inner drive to act spontaneously. This is likely to be organic in origin and should not be regarded as something the patient can modify at will. This lack of motivation may cause rehabilitation workers to overestimate the disability.

It may cause workers to regard the patient as "stubborn" or "unwilling to try" and may reduce their motivation to help the patient. The problem may be related to the patient's readiness to deal with the overwhelming problems of the disability and to the tremendous amount of energy it takes every day for these patients to put their all into everything they attempt to do. Therapists must approach this problem with patience and perseverance. Patients need encouragement, reassurance, praise for success, and a lot of "extrinsic" motivation in prodding, cuing, and the planning of activities by therapists and caretakers.

FRUSTRATION TOLERANCE. Patients with hemiplegia are likely to have a reduction in ability to tolerate stress and frustration.

Speech and language disorders

CVA may result in a wide variety of speech disorders and disturbances in the ability to deal with symbols and may vary from mild to severe. These dysfunctions occur most frequently in right hemiplegia, or damage to the left hemisphere of the brain, but may also occur in left hemiplegia. All persons with CVA should be evaluated by the speech pathologist for the presence of speech and language disorders. The speech pathologist can provide valuable information to other members of the rehabilitation team regarding the best ways to communicate with a particular client. The occupational therapist should carry over the work of the speech therapist in the treatment sessions, as it is appropriate. This may occur in reinforcing communication techniques that the client is learning; presenting instruction in ways that the client is able to integrate; and instructing and practicing writing, which often is the responsiblity of the occupational therapist.

When reading the descriptions of the specific speech and language dysfunctions that follow, the reader should remember that they can exist in mild to severe form and in combination with one another.

APHASIA. The loss of ability to speak or understand the spoken word is known as *aphasia*. If there is greater difficulty with expression than with comprehension, the patient is said to have *expressive aphasia*. If there is greater difficulty with comprehension than with expression of speech, the patient is said to have *receptive* or *sensory aphasia*. Aphasia is a dysfunction in the ability to deal with spoken or written symbols. Patients with expressive aphasia may be able to produce automatic speech, such as singing, praying,[22] or using profanity. It is rare for an aphasic patient to be completely speechless. A few words can usually be produced.[5]

DYSARTHRIA. Patients with dysarthria can understand and express symbolic language.[22] However, there is an articulation disorder because of a dysfunction of the CNS mechanisms that control speech musculature. This results in paralysis and incoordination of the organs of speech that make it sound thick, sluggish, and slurred.[5,22]

ASSOCIATED DYSFUNCTIONS. Associated dysfunctions include *anomia*, or the inability to remember the names of persons or objects; *agraphia*, or the loss of the ability to write, which is often associated with expressive aphasia; *alexia*, or the inability to read;[21] and *acalculia*, or the loss of the ability to deal with mathematical calculations and symbols.

COMMUNICATION WITH PATIENTS. Horwitz[14] describes principles for communication with aphasic patients. She states that they respond best to intelligent and sympathetic understanding from professional staff and family members who are interacting with them. Here are some useful principles for facilitating communication and meaningful interaction with aphasic patients.*

1. Talk to the patient naturally, using short, simple, and concrete sentences.
2. Encourage, but do not pressure, the patient to respond in whatever way he or she can.

---

*Adapted from Horwitz, B.: An open letter to the family of an adult patient with aphasia, Chicago, 1964, National Society for Crippled Children and Adults, Inc.

3. Never ridicule the patient or insist that he or she respond accurately and articulately.
4. Do not increase volume of voice when speaking to aphasic patients. They are *not* deaf.
5. Do not talk about the patient in his or her presence. The patient can understand part or all of what you say. Include the patient in conversations about him or her if he or she is present.
6. Create an air of relaxation by your mannerisms, patience, and attitude of acceptance.
7. Include the patient in family activities and help him or her maintain his or her former role in the family.
8. Professional staff may explain to the patient what has happened to him or her, carefully and simply.
9. Keep instructions and explanations simple. The best way to know that the patient has understood you is by observing the way he or she carries out instructions.
10. Do not confuse the patient with rapid, complicated speech or too many people speaking at once. Do not use esoteric and abstract words.
11. Ask direct questions requiring one-word answers. Some patients may say "yes" when they mean "no" and vice versa.
12. Do not answer for the patient if he or she is capable of responding independently.
13. Use routine daily living activities (for example, eating and dressing) as opportunities to encourage simple speech.
14. Encourage the use of words of greeting and simple social exchanges.
15. If the patient can write and spell, he or she should be encouraged to write responses.
16. Encourage the use of gestures to communicate.
17. Accept bizarre, inaccurate use of language and profanities without amusement or anger.
18. Aphasic patients often cannot remember the names of people and objects. Reassure the patient that this is part of his or her disability and does not mean he or she is "losing his mind."

Contrast between right and left hemiplegia

There is an apparent difference between the performance and learning styles of persons with right hemiplegia and those with left hemiplegia. This contrast is related to the difference in hemispheric function.

The right cerebral hemisphere (left hemiplegia) is responsible primarily for perception. It discriminates form, position, weight, distance, and visual-spatial relationships.[22] Left hemiplegia may be characterized by (1) disorganization of tasks, such as construction or drawing, (2) failures on tasks that involve spatial analysis, (3) frequent failures on tasks that require maintenance of spatial orientation, and (4) apraxia for dressing. There is a significant correlation between extremely poor performance on perceptual organization tasks and failures in dressing and grooming.[16] The patient with left hemiplegia may retain good verbal skills, which may tend to mask the perceptual dysfunction and give the impression of good performance. The therapist needs to require performance evaluation of self-care skills and not rely on the interview as a means of determining the patient's ability to function.

The primary responsibilities of the left cerebral hemisphere (right hemiplegia) are analysis, logic, understanding of symbolic language, and conceptualization. Even in the absence of aphasia problems in these functions may exist. The patient with right hemiplegia has little or no difficulty with visual-spatial tasks but may have difficulty with written or oral instructions. Demonstrations and pantomime may be necessary to convey information and instruction. The patient may perform very slowly and methodically in an effort to be correct.[22] He or she is usually more successful in achieving self-care independence earlier than the patient with left hemiplegia.

Conclusion

When the patient has some or all of the perceptual and psychological problems discussed, the traditional rehabilitation goals for motor and functional retraining may be more than he or she can master. Rehabilitation goals cannot be based on the motor evaluation alone.

Rather, the total scope of the disability must be considered, including sensory, perceptual, psychological, emotional, and intellectual impairments and the patient's social and family situation. If evaluation of the patient is inadequate and inappropriate goals are set for him or her, the result will be frustration for the therapist, patient, and family.

Therapists must evaluate for and observe the effect of all of the concomitant dysfunctions as well as the motor dysfunction. If the limitations of the patient are clearly recognized and identified, realistic rehabilitation goals may be set. Retraining to the degree possible can be achieved, and the therapist, patient, and family will feel a sense of achievement rather than failure in the rehabilitation program.[24]

OCCUPATIONAL THERAPY FOR CLIENTS WITH CVA

The role of the occupational therapist in the treatment of CVA that results in hemiplegia revolves around facilitating symmetrical motor function, use of the affected side, and restoring the client to his or her maximal level of independence.

Each client must be evaluated for his or her residual abilities and disabilities. A treatment program must be especially tailored to the client's particular needs, since the range of possible motor, sensory, perceptual, and cognitive dysfunctions after CVA is wide. The selection of treatment objectives and treatment methods will depend on factors, such as stage of motor recovery, sensory perceptual status, cognitive functions, age, date of onset, concomitant illness, social and economic factors, and potential for further recovery.

The occupational therapist may be involved in the acute care of the client and the early mobilization aspects of treatment. Later occupational therapy may be a primary service in extended rehabilitation when the emphasis is on achieving self-care independence and performance skills for work or leisure activities.

The role of occupational therapy

EVALUATION.[5,23,26] The occupational therapist begins the program with a thorough evaluation of the client's deficits and assets to establish a baseline for progress. The evaluation process is continuous, beginning with the evaluation of motor and sensory status and simple self-care skills and progression to perceptual, cognitive, and more complex performance evaluations.

Motor functions. Degree of spasticity is estimated by evaluating the amount of resistance to passive movement (Chapter 7). This is usually performed by passively moving the elbow, wrist, and fingers through their ROMs. Quick motion is more likely to elicit the stretch reflex in clients who appear to have predominantly flaccid limbs. The stage of motor recovery can be estimated using Brunnstrom's test (Chapter 15). Abnormal movement patterns, presence of primitive reflexes, and equilibrium reactions should be evaluated. These may be the responsibility of or performed in conjunction with the physical therapist. Joint ROM is measured or estimated for limitations. Ability to perform isolated movement should be evaluated and coordination should be observed when the client has some control of voluntary movement.

Sensory-perceptual functions. Senses of touch, superficial pain, temperature, and pressure should be tested. Olfactory and gustatory sensation may be tested, since these senses are disturbed in some clients and are often overlooked. Stereognosis, proprioception, body scheme, and motor planning should be routinely evaluated. Visual perception, including tests for hemianopsia and visual-spatial relationships, should be included in the battery of evaluation procedures. Tests for these functions are found in Chapter 9.

Cognitive functions. Memory, attention span, judgment, reasoning, abstract thinking, ability to follow instructions, motivation, and affect should be observed or tested (Chapter 9).

Psychosocial factors. Through observation and interview of the client, family members, friends, or other rehabilitation team members, the occupational therapist should ascertain the client's vocational and recreational histories, role in the family and community, amount of family support, adjustment to disability, and frustration tolerance and coping skills.

Performance skills. Performance skills should be evaluated by interview and, more importantly, by actual performance of test items. Self-care and home management skills, mobility and transfer techniques, physical endurance, and work-related activities, if appropriate, should be included in the performance evaluation. It may take several weeks to complete the performance evaluation, which is an ongoing part of the treatment program.

Observation and periodic reevaluation should be carried out to record objective evidence of progress.

TREATMENT

Motor dysfunction. The occupational therapy program may include one or a combination of the sensorimotor approaches to treatment for the purposes of facilitating movement and use of the affected side, developing more normal postural reflex mechanisms, and inhibiting abnormal reflexes and movement patterns.

Therapists who do not use these approaches may use more traditional forms of therapeutic exercise, adapting them to the level of skills and movement of the client. Skateboard exercises are commonly used and can be adapted to use some of the patterns of motion suggested by Brunnstrom.[6]

The maintenance of joint ROM and prevention of deformity is an important early goal in the treatment program and should be continued indefinitely if a substantial amount of spontaneous voluntary movement is not regained. This is achieved through positioning techniques, such as those recommended by Bobath[4] and passive, assistive, and self-administered ROM procedures (Fig. 30-2). Both Bobath[4] and Brunnstrom[6]

caution against the traditional passive ROM exercises to the shoulder in the absence of good scapular mobility. Passive flexion, abduction, and rotation of the glenohumeral joint to extreme ranges can be more harmful than helpful.

Normal abduction and upward rotation of the scapula are prevented by spasticity of scapula musculature when the glenohumeral joint is flexed or abducted. Shoulder joint motion without the normally associated scapula movement results in faulty mechanics and can cause joint trauma. Bicipital tendinitis, coracoiditis, brachial plexus traction, or supraspinatus tendinitis caused by compression of the tendon between

the humeral tuberosities and the acromion can result from joint trauma.[8] Inappropriate exercise and incorrect handling of the upper extremity during transfers, ambulation, and bed mobility activities are some causes of trauma to the shoulder joint.

Reciprocal pully exercises, frequently used for maintenance of shoulder ROM, are usually contraindicated, since they are forced passive exercise[6] and can cause joint pain and possibly damage if there is inadequate scapular mobility.[18]

Subluxation of the humerus from the glenoid fossa is a common problem in hemiplegia. The rotator cuff muscles are probably of primary importance in

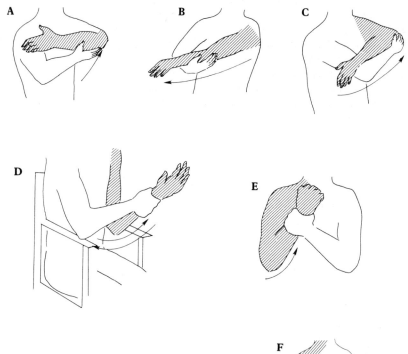

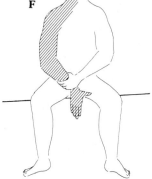

Fig. 30-2. Self-administered ROM procedures for person with hemiplegia. **A,** Affected arm is supported by unaffected arm and lifted into shoulder flexion to touch forehead. **B,** Affected arm is supported by unaffected arm to achieve adduction. **C,** Affected arm is moved to side to achieve shoulder abduction. **D,** Upper part of affected arm is stabilized between chest and wheelchair armrest. Unaffected arm moves affected arm into external and internal rotation. **E,** Unaffected arm flexes affected elbow. **F,** Unaffected arm brings affected arm down between legs to achieve elbow extension. **G,** Unaffected arm turns affected forearm into supination. **H,** Unaffected hand turns affected forearm into pronation. **I,** Unaffected hand flexes affected wrist. **J,** Unaffected hand extends affected wrist. **K,** Affected fingers are passively flexed into palm to achieve full flexion of MP and IP joints. **L,** Fingers are gently extended. If resistance is felt, they should be flexed once more and again extended, avoiding sudden stretch of finger flexors if there is spasticity.

the maintenance of joint stability. The function of the supraspinatus muscle is especially important to the prevention of subluxation. Brunnstrom[6] recommends procedures to activate the muscles surrounding the shoulder joint as a means of preventing subluxation. Occupational therapists have often applied arm slings to the client for wear when the arm is in a dependent position. The benefits of such a sling are questionable for the reasons outlined in Chapter 16. Bobath[4] maintains that subluxation cannot be prevented if the muscles are weak and that slings contribute to poor positioning, pain, and swelling.

Flexor spasticity in the hand musculature can result in wrist flexion and a fisted position, which can progress to contracture and deformity if not prevented. Resting splints in the functional position have been used to avoid the position of deformity. However, there is a lack of agreement about the benefits of various types of splints. Volar splints are thought to provide cutaneous stimulation to the flexor muscles, thus contributing to an increase of spasticity.

Constructing splints that are applied to the dorsal surface of the forearm and hand provide sensory stimulation to the extensor surface and thereby are thought to enhance extensor tone, which is a desirable effect.[22] Techniques to facilitate relaxation of spastic wrist and finger musculature followed by gentle passive ROM, which is done to avoid stretch of the relaxed musculature, may be adequate to prevent the flexion deformity of the hand if done regularly.

Some occupational therapists use a broad wheelchair armrest to support the arm when the client is inactive and is sitting or moving about in the wheelchair. These armrests are commercially available or may be custom made at the treatment facility. They fit on the regular wheelchair armrests and are removable. The client's arm should be stabilized in the trough of the armrest by straps, or the trough should have a fence on the lateral side to prevent possible injury to the arm and hand if they bump into walls and furniture. These armrests are usually padded and some

have positioning devices to maintain the hand in a functional position. Rubber balls or other soft objects, such as a wadded washcloth, should *not* be used for this purpose. Soft objects tend to increase flexor spasticity, which is an undesirable effect, whereas it is thought that firm pressure over tendons has an inhibitory effect. Therefore grasping a hard object may have a more beneficial effect in inhibiting spastic muscles. A cone made of a thermoplastic material or from a large spool of yarn can be used to enhance the functional position of the hand. It should be positioned with the wide end on the ulnar side of the hand (Fig. 30-3).

The occupational therapist should use therapeutic activities as early as possible. These will enhance development of alertness, interest, and motivation and will provide opportunities for socialization and communication. In addition they should be selected to accommodate for use of the affected extremities. In the earliest phases of recovery the affected arm may be used as a passive stabilizer of objects or materials. As recovery progresses, the affected arm can take an increasingly active role in bilateral activities. Examples of some therapeutic activities that have been used effectively to include the affected upper extremity are weaving, leather lacing, braid weaving, sanding and other woodworking processes, and letterpress printing. When planning therapeutic activities the therapist needs to take into account the client's sensory, perceptual, and cognitive dysfunctions. It is important for the client to

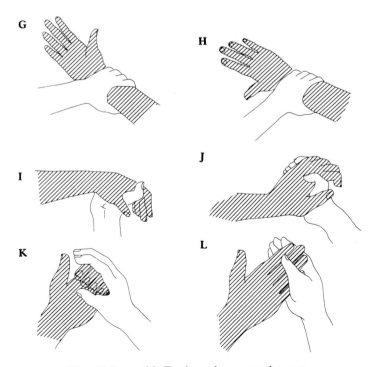

Fig. 30-2, cont'd. For legend see opposite page.

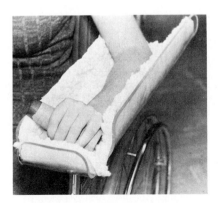

Fig. 30-3. Wheelchair armrest with yarn spool positioned in hand.

be successful at accomplishing the tasks. This can only be achieved if the tasks chosen are within his or her capabilities.

Performance skills. Training in ADL is a primary function of the occupational therapy service. Specific procedures are described in Chapters 12 and 16. Early in the rehabilitation process this may include wheelchair mobility and transfer skills (Chapter 18) and simple self-care activities, such as feeding and oral hygiene. Training in more complex bathing and dressing skills might be added later. As the client progresses in independent performance of the skills of self-maintenance, evaluation and training in appropriate home management activities should be included in the ADL program.

Unless there is adequate function of the affected arm, these skills should be learned using one-handed methods. Activities that require skill and safety, such as ironing and using the stove and appliances, and those that should be relaxing and pleasurable, such as eating, should be performed with the unaffected arm.

Coordination and skill training in one-handed performance is an important part of both the therapeutic activities and ADL programs. This is especially valuable if it is the dominant upper extremity that has been affected and if a change in dominance must be accomplished.

The client must learn methods of stabilizing objects and equipment for one-handed performance. He or she must learn to use assistive devices and equipment adapted to ease functioning with one hand. It is the role of the occupational therapist to acquire the necessary assistive devices and train the client in their use.

Some activities that can be adapted to one-handed performance and that can train in coordination are leather crafts, oil painting, mosaic work, minor woodworking, and some needlecrafts (Fig. 30-4).

In some cases one-handed performance may be necessary as a temporary measure, and in many others it will be a permanent mode of functioning. Usually the unaffected extremities will perform the primary and more complex motor functions required in activities,

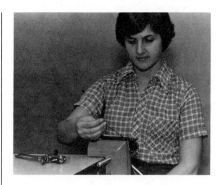

Fig. 30-4. Leather lacing is craft that can be one-handed skill if small bench vise is used to stabilize project.

and the affected limbs will play an assistive role.

Sensory retraining. Occupational therapy may include sensory reeducation and techniques to compensate for sensory, perceptual, and cognitive dysfunctions.

Techniques of sensory retraining have met with limited success. Therapists have used increased sensory stimulation in the form of cutaneous stimulation to the affected parts with terry cloth,[13] proprioceptive stimulation in the form of joint approximation, and weighting of the extremities to increase the proprioceptive feedback. A technique to improve stereognosis is described by Ferreri[11] for adults with hemiplegia resulting from cerebral palsy. This involved comparing two dissimilar objects or forms, first with the unaffected hand and then with the affected hand. The therapist verbalized about the characteristics of the objects or forms during the manipulation process. The same training item was used for each session until the subject achieved five successive correct responses in the test portion of the session. Then a new training object was substituted. The investigator met with some success in improving stereognostic function of the subjects of the study.[11] This technique could be applied to adult clients with CVA. Visualization of the training objects could be used to facilitate the perception of tactual and proprioceptive qualities of the training objects.

Teaching compensation for sensory losses through vision is a common approach to dealing with sensory deficits.

The client must be trained to monitor the location and position of the extremities. The therapist may do this by frequently reminding the patient to watch for the position of the limbs and helping him or her to include this visual monitoring as a regular part of the routine of moving and by adjusting position.[22] Success in teaching visual compensation may be limited. If the client has disturbances, such as homonymous hemianopsia, denial of the affected side, body scheme disorder, or memory deficits, it may not be possible for him or her to compensate in these ways. In addition, even for those who are alert enough and who do not have the added disturbances, it is difficult to watch out for a sensory-deficient limb when actively engaging in an activity and focusing on its goal. For example, it is not possible to watch the hand to see that it is holding a spoon and also to focus on the goal of eating.

Another method used to deal with sensory, perceptual, and cognitive deficits is adapting the environment. Using color or auditory cues, working in a nondistracting environment, and special methods of instruction may be employed.[22] Instructions must be broken down into very simple and small steps and presented one at a time. The number of steps the client is expected to perform is gradually increased. Repetition of instruction is necessary. As tasks are mastered in a completely nondistracting environment, the client may be asked to perform in increasingly stimulating environments until he or she can perform adequately in the clinic or home environment.

Perceptual retraining. Treatment of perceptual problems can be difficult and complex. The best results are obtained if the treatment is done on a daily basis.[19] Siev and Frieshtat[19] described three approaches that are used for perceptual training of the hemiplegic client. These are the sensory-integrative approach, the transfer of training approach, and the functional approach.

The sensory-integrative approach is based on neurophysiological and developmental principles and was described by A. Jean Ayres as a treatment approach for children with sensory-integrative dysfunction. It assumes that controlled sensory input can be used to elicit specific motor responses. Thus the sensory-integrative functions of the brain can be influenced by selected activities that provide the necessary input and evoke the desired motor responses. This approach may be impractical for adults because it takes years of treatment to be effective and because it is likely that the adult's CNS does not have the same capacity for learning as a child's CNS, since it does not have the same degree of plasticity. Some therapists use modifications and selected techniques from this approach with adults and report some success.[19]

The transfer of training approach assumes that practice in a particular perceptual task will carry over to performance of similar tasks or practical activities requiring the same perceptual skill. For example, practice in reproducing pegboard designs for spatial relations training could carry over to dressing skills that require spatial judgment (for example, matching blouse to body and discriminating right from left shoe). This is a common approach to the treatment of perceptual problems in occupational therapy clinics. There are conflicting reports of its effectiveness, and further research is needed to determine its benefits.[19]

The repetitive practice of particular tasks that will help the client become more independent in the performance of ADL characterizes the functional approach. This is probably the most common approach to dealing with perceptual problems. The therapist does not do specific perceptual training. Rather, the therapist helps the client to adapt to or compensate for his or her perceptual deficits. The client is made aware of the problem and taught to compensate for it. For example, if the client has an homonymous hemianopsia, the therapist may cue him or her to turn his or her head to see the blind visual field. Adaptation of environment or methods is another way to compensate for a perceptual deficit. If the client is distractable because of visual or auditory figure-ground deficits, the therapist may arrange for treatment or training to take place in a quiet and uncluttered room to minimize distractions and create the best environment for learning.[19]

Suggestions for treatment of specific perceptual deficits are offered by Siev and Frieshtat.[19] A few of these are outlined here.

BODY SCHEME DISORDER. Using the transfer of training approach, the therapist may touch the client's body parts and have him or her identify them as they are touched. Practice in assembling human figure puzzles and quizzing the client on body parts are other methods in this approach.

UNILATERAL NEGLECT. In a unilateral deficit the therapist engages the client in activities that focus his or her attention on the neglected left side. Examples are giving tactile stimulation to the affected extremities, using precautions for not increasing spasticity, placing work materials to the left side, and approaching the client from the left side for conversation and during treatment. To use adaptation or compensation the therapist may place food, utensils, and work materials on the unaffected side and give all instructions from that side.

SPATIAL RELATIONS. Using a transfer of training approach the therapist might have the client copy parquetry block design, matchstick designs, or pegboard patterns that the therapist arranges; connect dots to make a design using a stimulus design to follow; or construct puzzles.[19] To compensate for a spatial deficit the therapist might use colored dots to mark the route to a specific location.

DRESSING APRAXIA. To overcome dressing apraxia the therapist teaches a set pattern for dressing and gives cues that help the client to distinguish right from left or front from back. Some of the methods that are helpful are to have the client position the garment the same way each time, such as a shirt with the buttons face up and pants with the zipper face up. Labels can be used as cues to differentiate the front from the back of the garment. The garment may be color coded with small buttons or ribbons for front and back or right and left side.

IDEATIONAL AND IDEOMOTOR APRAXIA. Treatment of ideational and ideomotor apraxia disorders is difficult. Use of short, clear, concise, and concrete instructions is necessary, since this is usually the result of a dominant hemisphere lesion, and there is often aphasia as well. The task should be broken down into its component steps, and each step should be taught separately. Verbal and demonstrated instructions may be ineffective, and it can be helpful to guide the client through the correct movements, giving tactile and proprioceptive input to the instruction. This can be done while also giving brief verbal instruction. Once the client has performed each step of the task separately, the therapist can begin to combine the steps, grading to the complete task.[19] An example is hair combing. The therapist can break the task into steps: lift comb; bring comb to hair; move comb across top of head, down left side, down right side, down back; and replace comb on table. Much repetition is necessary if this is to be effective.

Psychosocial adjustment. An important role of the occupational therapist is to aid in the client's adjustment to hospitalization and, more importantly, to disability. A patient and supportive approach by the therapist is essential. The therapist must be emphathetic to the fact that the client has experienced a devastating and life-threatening illness. Sudden and dramatic changes in life roles and performance have resulted. The therapist must be cognizant of the normal adjustment process (Chapter 2) and gear approach and performance expectations to the client's stage of adjustment. Frequently the client is not ready to engage in rehabilitation measures with whole-hearted effort until several months after the onset of the disability.

Many clients will dwell on the possibility of full recovery of function and will need to gradually be made aware that some residual dysfunction is very likely. The therapist may approach this by discussing what is known about prognosis for function recovery from CVA in objective terms. This may need to be reviewed many times with the client before the client begins to apply the information to his or her own recovery. This should be done in a way that is honest, yet does not rob the client of all hope. The therapist can present the information about the usual period for spontaneous recovery. He or she should indicate that the final outcome, in terms of function, cannot be accurately determined until at least 1 year after the CVA onset.

The occupational therapy program should focus on the skills and abilities of the client. The client's attention should be focused, through the performance of activity, on his or her remaining and newly learned skills. Therapeutic group activities for socialization and sharing common problems and their solutions can be included.

The discovery that there are residual abilities and perhaps new abilities and success at performing many daily living skills and activities that were initially thought to be impossible can have a beneficial effect on the client's mental health and outlook. The occupational therapy program can be thought of as a laboratory for real living in which skills are learned and practiced and abilities are recovered or discovered.

Home evaluation. As the client nears discharge to home and community, the occupational therapist should be involved in a home evaluation (Chapter 10), and vocational or leisure skills potential should be explored. A living situation should be recommended that accommodates the client's needs. The occupational therapist, having evaluated self-care and home management skills performance, should be the most qualified to estimate the client's potential for independent living. Clients with hemiplegia will range from those who can resume living independently to those who require continuous supervision and assistance. The outcome depends on the severity of the CVA, success in rehabilitation, mental status, and social factors.

Gradation of treatment. Treatment of the motor dysfunction is directed toward the reintegration of the postural reflex mechanism and the recovery of controlled, coordinated movement. The manner and speed with which treatment is graded will depend on the client and the treatment approach. In general, inhibition and facilitation techniques should be decreased as voluntary control of motion is improved. The amount of assistance in exercise and activity should be decreased as control and coordination are gained. The diffi-culty of performance skills demanded can be increased as synergistic movement subsides, and isolated voluntary motion is possible.[17]

Treatment time and time spent in standing and ambulation activities can be gradually increased to improve endurance. The complexity and number of ADL can be increased as physical, perceptual, and cognitive functioning improves. The amount of assistance given during transfers and for all activities should be decreased as independence is increased.

Conclusion. The reader should consider that the degree to which the client achieves treatment goals will depend on the CNS recovery and the facilitation and utilization of that recovery by therapists, client, and family. Some clients will remain severely disabled in spite of the noblest efforts of rehabilitation workers, and others will recover quite spontaneously with minimal help in a short period of time.

Sample treatment plan

Case study

Mr. S. is a 59-year-old man who worked as a trucker until he suffered a CVA 6 weeks ago. He lives with his wife and teenage daughter in a modest, three-bedroom suburban home. He is their sole support.

Before the onset of CVA Mr. S. was a very hard worker and enjoyed working around the house doing repairs and gardening. Cooking and furniture refinishing were his hobbies.

His wife and teenager daughter are very loving but are exhibiting signs of oversolicitiousness and denial of Mr. S.'s limitations and the potential residual disability. Mr. S. is depressed and is expressing feelings of worthlessness because of the loss of his role as worker and breadwinner. He is beginning to sense his family's unrealistic attitude and feels he has to "play along" with them. He resents this and would prefer to be open and get on with the business of dealing with life adjustments.

The CVA resulted in right hemiplegia and mild expressive aphasia. Mr. S. is now able to ambulate with a quadruped cane under supervision. He walks slowly and occasionally loses his balance. He tolerates standing and walking activities up to 10 minutes. His right upper extremity exhibits beginning spasticity and some evidence of the flexor and extensor synergies, which can be elicited reflexly.

Mr. S. has been in the occupational therapy program since the first week of hospitalization for maintenance of ROM, development of sitting balance, and training in simple self-care skills. He is now referred for improvement of the function of the right upper extremity, improvement of standing balance and tolerance, increased performance of self-care skills, and aid with adjustment to the disability.

TREATMENT PLAN*

A. Statistical data.
  1. Name: Mr. S.
     Age: 59
     Diagnosis: CVA, 6 weeks after onset
     Disability: Right hemiplegia, expressive aphasia
  2. Treatment aims as stated in referral:
     Improve function of right limbs and body
     Improve standing balance and tolerance
     Improve performance of ADL

---

*Adapted from Abrams, E., et al. (1978), Loewi, J., Mungai, A., (1982), Dent, P., and Shimeall, M. (1983): Treatment plans for CVA, Papers presented in partial fulfillment of the requirements of OT 132, San Jose, Calif., Department of Occupational Therapy, San Jose State University.

Sample treatment plan—cont'd

B. Other services.

Physician: Supervision of rehabilitation team and provision of care

Nursing: Provision of nursing and supportive care; follow through in self-care skills

Social service: Assistance in family and social adjustment

Speech therapy: Treatment of expressive aphasia

Physical therapy: Gait training and improvement in LE function

C. OT evaluation.

Stage of motor recovery: Test

Standing tolerance: Observe

Standing balance: Observe

Walking tolerance: Observe

Touch: Test

Pain: Test

Temperature: Test

Stereognosis: Test

Proprioception: Test

Body scheme: Test

Visual fields: Test

Visual-spatial relationships: Test

Memory: Test and observe

Motivation: Observe

Judgment and reasoning: Observe

Problem solving: Test and observe

Expression: Observe

Adjustment to disability: Observe

Self-care: Test

Homemaking: Test

Attempts at use of involved extremity: Observe

D. Results of evaluation.

1. Evaluation data.
   a. Physical resources.
      (1) ROM: Right shoulder flexion and abduction limited by spasticity and scapula fixation to 90°; all other joints within normal limits
      (2) Standing tolerance and balance: Moderate impairment; unable to stand without cane and fatigues after 10 minutes
      (3) Sitting balance: Trunk stability sufficient to maintain sitting position
      (4) Walking tolerance: With assistive devices patient walks slowly for short distances
      (5) Stage of recovery—stage 2: Beginning spasticity upper extremity flexion synergy; slightly stronger than extension synergy; extension synergy stronger in lower extremity; exhibits proximal traction response; prone

positioning elicits flexor tone because of the influence of tonic labyrinthine reflex

   b. Sensory-perceptual functions.
      Touch: Intact
      Pressure: Intact
      Pain: Intact
      Temperature: Intact
      Stereognosis: Mildly impaired
      Proprioception: Mildly impaired
      Body scheme and praxis: Intact
      All visual tests: Within normal limits, except 60° homonymous hemianopsia

   c. Cognitive functions.
      Memory: Intact visual memory and follows demonstrated instructions well; auditory memory and ability to follow verbal instructions slightly impaired
      Motivation: Patient discouraged, shows a lack of motivation, responds well to praise and encouragement
      Judgment and reasoning: Observed to be intact
      Problem solving: Intact
      Reading: Seems to be intact
      Writing: Difficult because of inability to use dominant hand
      Expression: Mild expressive aphasia, speech limited but comprehensible for communication of basic needs, opinions, and some abstract ideas; with cues, questioning, and some use of pictures, can elicit expression of Mr. S.'s ideas

   d. Psychosocial functions. The client was a trucker and sole provider for his wife and teenage daughter. He exhibits depression and feelings of worthlessness related to loss of this role. His family denies his limitations and is overanxious to help. Before his stroke the client was a kindly, placid man, as described by his family, who enjoyed working around the house, cooking, and furniture refinishing.

   e. Prevocational potential. Mr. S. is considering the possibility that he will be forced

into early retirement because of his age and disability and the nature of the work he did. He has a pension plan that includes disability benefits, and he hopes to take advantage of this. He wants to explore the possibility of performing more cooking, home maintenance, gardening, and furniture refinishing skills at home to use his retirement purposefully.

   f. Functional skills.
      Self-care: The client feeds himself independently and helps with grooming. He needs assistance with dressing and transfer skills. His mobility is limited for walking because of limited tolerance and balance. He can walk with supervision, using a quadruped cane, for short distances.
      Home management skills: Mr. S. is able to prepare a cold meal while sitting but is unable to use the range safely or perform household tasks that require standing and walking about. He can use some one-handed assistive devices and techniques for tasks, such as cutting and spreading jam.
      Attempts at use of the affected upper extremity: The client exhibits attempts at use of the right arm about 50% of the time when confronted with bilateral activities. However, limited voluntary control renders most of these unsuccessful at this time. The client is being encouraged to use the right arm whenever possible. He anticipates the improved motor function will make it possible to use the arm more effectively in the future.

2. Problem identification.
   a. Limited standing balance and tolerance
   b. ADL dependence
   c. Depression
   d. Lack of scapula mobility and shoulder ROM
   e. Lack of voluntary control of motion

Continued.

Sample treatment plan—cont'd

f. Spasticity and decreased postural reflex mechanism
g. Visual field defect
h. Lack of skill and coordination in left hand (the unaffected, nondominant member)

i. Changed role as financial provider
3. Assets.
   a. Realistic outlook about limitations, potential disability, and employment future

b. Supportive and strong family unit
c. Leisure interests
d. Previous demonstration of good coping skills
e. Financial security
f. Homeowner

E Problem	F Specific OT objectives	G Methods used to meet objectives	H Gradation of treatment
h	Through instruction and practice left hand coordination will improve to the degree that Mr. S. can write his name and address legibly, with ease, and in no more than twice the time it takes to write with the dominant hand	Small leather lacing projects, stabilized in a table vise, requiring manipulation of needles and lacing with the left hand	Increase the complexity of the lacing stitch
		Writing practice, beginning with various sequences of lines, circles, and curves, as in the Palmer method, then progressing to series of letters and numerals[22]	Progress to words and then sentences
d	Given appropriate positioning and mobilization techniques spasticity will decrease and scapula mobility will increase so that 120° shoulder flexion and abduction will be possible	Bobath positioning techniques during sitting; clasps hands together with affected thumb on top and unaffected arm guides affected right arm into a position of full elbow extension with shoulder flexion and scapula protraction;[4] arms on wheelchair lapboard or on table in this position when client not engaged in activity	
d,g		Following scapula mobilization by the therapist, client's arm gradually brought into the reflex inhibiting pattern of scapula protraction, shoulder abduction, flexion, and external rotation, elbow extension, forearm supination, wrist and finger extension, and thumb abduction[4] (Chapter 16)	Decrease facilitation and assistance as spasticity declines and active motion improves
		Self-administered ROM; with hands positioned as described previously, client to bring both arms down between knees; then move arms from side to side, rotating trunk, and gradually elevating arms to 90° shoulder flexion with elbows extended	Grade from passive to active ROM techniques as voluntary control of isolated motion is gained
		Participation in activity group; using pegboard checkers and oversized checkerboard, will play with another client using the bilateral arm positioning pattern described previously; will move the checkers by grasping them between the palms of his hands; also facilitates trunk rotation and looking over the entire visual field	

Sample treatment—cont'd

E Problem	F Specific OT objectives	G Methods used to meet objectives	H Gradation of treatment
f,g,h	Given appropriate activity, will spontaneously compensate for visual field defect 80% of the treatment time	Client to cover small (2 feet × 2 feet or 6.096 mm × 6.096 mm) table top with mosaic tiles (1 inch or 2.5 cm); tiles placed directly to right side of client's body; table placed in front and slightly to left of client's body; glue placed on left side of body; client to reach across body to obtain tiles for placement on tabletop; affected arm positioned forward, used for weight bearing on edge of wide chair; as right arm function improves, client to reach for tiles with right hand; facilitates trunk rotation and visual attention to affected side Room arranged so client must look to affected side to get belongings, look to doorway for staff and visitors Therapist to stand on affected side when talking to client or giving instructions	
b	Through instruction and practice the client will be able to dress himself independently in no more than three times the time it takes a nondisabled adult to dress	Teach dressing techniques for pants, T-shirt, shirt, shoes, socks, and shorts, using Bobath methods for dressing (Chapter 16)	Begin with one garment, T-shirt; progress to shirt, then shorts, socks, pants, and shoes; progress to normal bilateral techniques as function improves
a	Through participation in activities that require standing and walking the client's balance will improve and standing tolerance will increase to 20 minutes	While working on leather lacing activities, client will be positioned in the stand-up table Client will begin to engage in light homemaking activities that require walking for short distances: meal preparation, table setting, and dusting Client will perform grooming activities in a standing position under supervision	Amount of support from the table will be decreased Later, client will stand at a high worktable without support Supervision is decreased as balance and stability are gained
c,i	Given twice weekly participation in an activity-oriented support group, the client will exhibit increased openness in communication of his feelings about disability and changed life roles, within the group	A group of 5 to 8 clients will meet biweekly for one and one half hours; the therapist will act as group facilitator; the group will initially be task oriented; activities such as exercises to music, simple crafts, and cooperative meal preparation will be used The group will move from the activity into discussion of the problems encountered during the activity, feelings about these, and solutions; the therapist will facilitate expansion of the discussion to include problems encountered beyond the activity and the treatment facility	Clients take increasing responsibility for planning the activities As group support and cohesiveness grows, discussion can include deeper feelings, and group members can act as facilitators

Continued.

Sample treatment plan—cont'd

I. **Special equipment.**
1. Ambulation aids.
Cane: Quadruped then regular cane to provide support and balance during ambulation
Wheelchair: For early mobility before walking is feasible
2. Splints. None required
3. Assistive devices.
Rocker knife: For one-handed meat cutting

Long-handle shoehorn: to facilitate donning shoes in a sitting position
Elastic shoelaces: To eliminate the need to tie shoes
Clip-on neckties: To eliminate the need to tie knots in necktie
Suction brushes: One for washing left hand and fingernails, one for scrubbing vegetables

One-handed cutting board: For slicing and peeling foods, spreading butter on bread, and making sandwiches
Zim jar opener: For opening jars with one hand
Pan holder: To stabilize pans on range while stirring
Long-handle scrub sponge: For washing back and feet while bathing

---

REVIEW QUESTIONS

1. Define "hemiplegia."
2. List three other dysfunctions that could accompany the motor dysfunction in hemiplegia.
3. List the disturbances that are likely to result from occlusion to the ACA, MCA, PCA, and basilar artery.
4. Which artery is most frequently affected in CVA?
5. Define "transient ischemic attack."
6. Describe the dependence of motion on sensation in the normal sensorimotor process.
7. Besides the upper motor neuron paralysis of limbs and trunk after CVA, what other important motor disturbances can result?
8. Describe or draw a picture of the typical "resting posture" of the spastic upper extremity in hemiplegia.
9. List three poor prognostic signs for functional recovery of the arm, and tell how they inhibit function.
10. If recovery has progressed so that there is voluntary control of the flexion synergy and grasp, what can be expected in terms of functional use of the affected arm?
11. If recovery has progressed so that synergies no longer dominate and grasp and release can be performed, what can be expected in terms of functional use of the affected arm?
12. In which direction does return of function usually progress in the motor recovery after CVA?
13. What differences in performance can be expected between persons with right and left hemiplegia? What accounts for these differences?
14. What is the importance of comprehensive occupational therapy evaluation of clients with hemiplegia?
15. Describe two methods that are used to maintain ROM.
16. Which synergy predominates in the arm? Which predominates in the leg?
17. List three good prognostic signs for functional recovery of the arm.
18. Describe what is meant by "lability." How can it be dealt with during a treatment sesion?
19. Why is it contraindicated for the client to grasp a ball or another soft object?
20. How does body scheme disorder interfere with rehabilitation?
21. How would training be approached if there is a memory loss?
22. Describe apraxia. Give examples of apraxic behavior. How would it interfere with rehabilitation, and what training techniques would be useful with an apraxic patient?
23. How does aphasia differ from dysarthria?
24. Describe four suggestions for more effective communication with an aphasic client.
25. List four major elements of the occupational therapy program for hemiplegia. Describe the purposes of each.
26. How can occupational therapy assist with the psychosocial adjustment of the hemiplegic client?

REFERENCES

1. Ayres, A.J.: Perceptual motor training for children. In Approaches to the treatment of patients with neuromuscular dysfunction, Proceedings of study course IV, Third International Congress, World Federation of Occupational Therapists, Dubuque, Iowa, 1962, Wm. C. Brown Co., Publishers.
2. Banus, B.S., editor: The developmental therapist, Thorofare, N.J., 1971, Charles B Slack, Inc.
3. Bardach, J.L.: Psychological factors in hemiplegia, J. Am. Phys. Ther. Assoc. **43**:792, 1963.
4. Bobath, B.: Adult hemiplegia: evaluation and treatment, ed. 2, London, 1978, William Heinemann Medical Books, Ltd.
5. Bonner, C.: The team approach to hemiplegia, Springfield, Ill., 1969, Charles C Thomas, Publisher.
6. Brunnstrom, S.: Movement therapy in hemiplegia, New York, 1970, Harper & Row, Publishers, Inc.
7. Buchwald, J.: General features of nervous system organization, Am. J. Phys. Med. **46**:89, 1967.
8. Cailliet, R.: The shoulder in hemiplegia, Philadelphia, 1982, F.A. Davis Co.
9. Chusid, J.: Correlative neuroanatomy and functional neurology, Los Altos, Calif., 1973, Lange Medical Publications.
10. Delacato, C., and Doman, G.: Hemiplegia and concomitant psychological phenomena, Am. J. Occup. Ther. **11**:186; 196, 1957.
11. Ferreri, J.A.: Intensive stereognostic training: effect on spastic cerebral palsied adults, Am. J. Occup. Ther. **16**:141, 1962.
12. Gilfoyle, E., and Grady, A.: Cognitive-perceptual-motor behavior. In Willard, H., and Spackman, C., editors: Occupational therapy, ed. 4, Philadelphia, 1971, J.B. Lippincott Co.
13. Hopkins, H.L.: Occupational therapy management of cerebral vascular accident and hemiplegia. In Willard, H.S., and Spackman, C.S., editors: Occupational therapy, ed. 4, Philadelphia, 1971, J.B. Lippincott Co.
14. Horwitz, B.: An open letter to the family of an adult patient with aphasia, Chicago, 1964, National Society for Crippled Children and Adults, Inc.
15. Larson, C.B., and Gould, M.: Orthopedic nursing, ed. 9, St. Louis, 1978, The C.V. Mosby Co.

16. Lorenze, E., and Cancro, R.: Dysfunction in visual perception with hemiplegia: relation to activities of daily living, Arch. Phys. Med. Rehab. **43:**514, 1962.

17. Perry, C.: Principles and techniques of the Brunnstrom approach to the treatment of hemiplegia, Am. J. Phys. Med. **46:**789, 1967.

18. Sharpless, J.W.: Mossman's a problem-oriented approach to stroke rehabilitation, ed. 2, Springfield, Ill., 1982, Charles C Thomas, Publisher.

19. Siev, E., and Frieshtat, B.: Perceptual dysfunction in the adult stroke patient, Thorofare, N.J., 1976, Charles B. Slack, Inc.

20. Spencer, E.A.: Functional restoration. In Hopkins, H.L., and Smith, H.D.: Willard and Spackman's occupational therapy, ed. 5, Philadelphia, 1978, J.B. Lippincott Co.

21. Taber, C.: Taber's cyclopedic medical dictionary, Philadelphia, 1959, F.A. Davis Co.

22. Trombly, C.A., and Scott, A.D.: Occupational therapy for physical dysfunction, Baltimore, 1977, Williams & Wilkins.

23. Venegas, N., and Del Pilar-Christian, M., editors: Occupational therapy for patients with physical dysfunction, Peurto Rico, 1967, University of Puerto Rico Press.

24. Williams, L.A.: Some non-motor aspects of cerebral vascular accidents, unpublished paper in partial fulfillment of the requirements for the master of science degree, San Jose Calif., 1964, San Jose State College.

25. Wilson, D.: Hemiplegia, paper presented to the annual conference of the Combined Northern and Southern California Occupational Therapy Association, Moro Bay, Calif., 1969.

26. Wilson, D., and Caldwell, C.: Occupational therapy treatment guide, adult hemiplegia, Downey, Calif., 1968, Department of Occupational Therapy, Rancho Los Amigos Hospital. Mimeographed.

CHAPTER 31

Head injury in adults

BARBARA B. ZOLTAN
DIANE MEEDER RYCKMAN

During the evolution of rehabilitation medicine various metabolic, systemic, or traumatic injuries have come into focus. Sociological occurrences or changes in lifestyles can have a major effect on the types of disabilities that prevail. For example, with the advent of war an increased number of gunshot wounds or amputations could occur. In recent years changes in diet and exercise regime altered the attention of medical and allied health professions to cardiac and stroke management. As society became more mobile, and the automobile developed into a necessity of life, again the focus of medical care was altered. Recently statistics on the occurrence of spinal cord injury and head trauma have forced those involved in acute and rehabilitation medicine to deal with a whole new set of concerns. The material presented in this chapter will deal only with head trauma.

The mechanism and occurrence of head injury, surgical management, and a description of the levels of recovery are briefly outlined. The patient's clinical picture, including the physical, cognitive, perceptual, functional, and psychosocial aspects, is described. The occupational therapy evaluation and treatment of these problems are also provided.

In 1975 10 million people, or 3.68% of the U.S. population, sustained a head injury significant enough to require medical attention.[11] In 1976 7.56 million Americans sustained a head injury.[14] A breakdown of the place and occurrence and severity of these injuries is presented in Tables 31-1 and 31-2. The occurrence and severity of head injury are sufficient to warrant the attention of medical and allied health personnel working in acute and rehabilitation medicine.

MECHANISM OF HEAD INJURY

Most head injuries are "blunt injuries caused either by the moving head striking a static surface . . . or by the head being struck by a moving object."[26,27] The degree of deformation and damage sustained by the brain after the injury depends on the amount of acceleration or deceleration of the skull and its contents.[33,35] *Deceleration* refers to the sudden, rapid slowing of the moving head when it strikes a solid surface. *Acceleration* refers to the movement of the brain inside the skull when the stationary head is struck. An additional type of head injury is a penetrating injury, which may be a result of "low-velocity agents" or sharp objects or to high-velocity ballistic missiles. Low-velocity penetrating injuries generally result in local damage, whereas high-velocity and acceleration-deceleration injuries will usually result in diffuse damage.

Forces can injure the brain by (1) compression (pushing the tissues together, (2) tension (tearing the tissues apart), or (3) shearing (sliding of portions of tissues over other portions). These three types of injuries can occur simultaneously or in succession.[35] Damage can occur where the blow was sustained (coup lesion) or to the intact skull opposite to where the blow was applied (contrecoup lesion).[27]

In addition to the primary damage sustained on impact, secondary events often follow that may develop a few hours or days after the onset, for example, hemorrhage, infection, and brain swelling.

For a detailed analysis and description of the mechanism and pathology of head injury, including primary and secondary damage, anoxia, and infectious encephalitis, the reader is referred to the references.* Although it is not vital that the reader have a detailed knowledge of the mechanisms of head injury, the concepts and terms used should be understood.

MEDICAL AND SURGICAL MANAGEMENT

The medical and surgical management of a person who sustains a severe head injury begins when the victim is rescued and brought into the emergency room. The patient with a severe head injury may experience many complications. Some of the major complications are increased intracranial pressure,

The valuable contributions of Liane Michael and Linda Panikoff for their editorial assistance in the preparation of this chapter are greatly appreciated.

Table 31-1
Head injuries, 1976 (total 7,560,000)

Place of occurrence	No. of injuries
Motor vehicle accident	1,202,000
At home	3,828,000
At play, in school, or in public domain	2,472,000
At work	196,000

Based on data from Caveness, W.: Incidence of craniocerebral trauma in the United States with trends from 1900 to 1975, Adv. Neurol. **22:**1, 1979.

Table 31-2
Types of injury sustained, 1976 (total 7,560,000)

Types of injuries	No. of injuries	
Superficial or minor		6,305,000
Lacerations of head	4,686,000	
Contusions of scalp, face, and neck, except eye	1,619,000	
Major		1,255,000
With concussion	644,000	
With skull fractures, extradural, subdural, or subarachnoid hematomas	611,000	

Based on data from Caveness, W.: Incidence of craniocerebral trauma in the United States with trends from 1970 to 1975, Adv. Neurol. **22:**1, 1979.

*References 8, 13, 21, 26, 35, 37, 41.

wound infection or osteomyelitis, pulmonary infections, hyperthermia, shock, and associated injuries or fractures.[15]

When the patient arrives at the hospital, the first concern is to establish an unobstructed airway, and this may require suctioning, intubation, or tracheostomy. The patient may be in shock and may require intravenous fluids, plasma, blood transfusions, or vasopressor agents. The neurosurgeon then performs a neurological examination to determine the extent and severity of the head injury. The neurosurgeon may need to perform an emergency craniotomy after arteriography to reduce increased intracranial pressure and any demonstrated hematoma.[21]

Because of the patient's decreased level of awareness and decreased oral-bulbar status, nasogastric tube feedings or a gastrostomy procedure may be required to ensure that the patient gets adequate nutrition. This, compounded with a tracheostomy, will make it difficult to establish the patient's oral-bulbar training as the patient's overall level of awareness improves.

Posttraumatic seizures are also complications. These may begin as early as 1 week after sustaining a head injury in some patients and as late as 1 week to 10 years or more after injury in others.[21] In some cases seizures following head injury may never occur at all or may be controlled by medication prescribed by the physician. The patient may often be incontinent and may require catheterization; later in the rehabilitation phase, as these functions start to return, a bowel and bladder program may need to be established.

Once the patient has been medically stabilized and cleared by the physician, the occupational therapist may begin the evaluation and treatment program. It will be important for the therapist to be aware of the medical and surgical management problems and precautions before establishing a treatment plan. Usually a patient with an open head injury will require a helmet before getting up for the first time to protect the open skull from further brain injury in case the patient falls. Treatment should start as early as possible while the patient is in the intensive care unit but should be closely coordinated with the physician and nursing staff.

DESCRIPTION OF THE DYSFUNCTION
Recovery stages

The recovery of an individual from a severe brain injury can be extensive and involve the physical, cognitive, visual-perceptual, psychosocial, and behavioral functions. The adult with head injury can regain lost functions rapidly, over a period of many years, or not at all. Moving out of coma through the rehabilitation stages to reenter the community is often a complicated and difficult process. No two patients will have the same clinical picture, problems, needs, or family support systems. There are many different methods for analyzing the stages of recovery or the changes in level of awareness that lead to a higher level of functioning. The following is an overview of some of the different methods of rating recovery in patients with head injury.

NEUROLOGICAL EXAMINATION. In general the neurological examination performed by the physician describes the states of awareness as follows[21]:

Head injury with loss of consciousness
COMA : No response to painful stimuli
SEMICOMA : Withdrawal of a body part from a painful stimulus
STUPOR : Spontaneous movement and groaning in response to various stimuli
OBTUNDITY : Arousal by stimuli and response to a question or command; confusion and disorientation with poor judgment
FULL CONSCIOUSNESS : Recovery of orientation and memory; full recovery

Glasgow Coma Scale.[48] The Glasgow Coma Scale is the method most frequently used by the physician to categorize the levels of consciousness following a traumatic injury to the brain. This test is an attempt to quantify the severity of the brain injury and establish a baseline from which to predict the outcome of the patient. The physician using this scale assesses consciousness by three major areas: (1) motor responses, (2) verbal responses, and (3) eye opening. The patient is then rated and assigned the corresponding number of points for the best response elicited.

Levels of awareness. Still another system used for evaluating a patient's level of awareness is one that was developed at Rancho Los Amigos Hospital in Downey, California. The Rancho Los Amigos scale uses the following eight levels: (1) no response; (2) generalized response; (3) localized response; (4) confused-agitated; (5) confused, inappropriate, nonagitated; (6) confused-appropriate; (7) automatic-inappropriate; and (8) purposeful-appropriate.[39]

The mechanism of a traumatic head injury and the resulting neurological impairment vary so much that it is extremely difficult to label or categorize the individual with brain damage. Whereas general trends for recovery can be seen in patients with head injuries, no two individuals have the same set of problems, rate of recovery, environment, disposition, or neurological deficits.

THE PATIENT AT THE PRIMARY LEVEL. The term *primary* is a classification used in the Head Injury Unit at the Santa Clara Valley Medical Center in San Jose, California, to describe the patient who is functioning at a very basic or low level, such as the comatose patient. The patient at the primary level may be at a low level in any one or a combination of the following areas:

1. *Severe motor impairment.* The patient may have severe spasticity, abnormal reflexes, and loss of motor control in any or all four limbs. Head and trunk control are severely impaired, and the patient is generally dependent in all self-care activities.
2. *Severe impairment of perceptual-motor skills.* The patient may have poor gross visual skills and perceptual-motor skills that prevent the individual from being involved in any self-care or higher level functional activities, that is, severe motor planning problems prevent the patient from self-feeding or dressing and/or poor visual attentiveness and visual tracking prevent performance of the simplest ADL.
3. *Decreased functional cognition and behavior.* The patient with cognitive-behavioral deficits has extremely poor judgment, safety awareness, problem-solving abilities, and memory, which make the patient dependent in most functional tasks even though the individual may be physically intact.

Generally the patient at the primary level is very dependent or requires maximal assistance either physically, cognitively, perceptually, or in all three ways. A person may have severe motor involvement with perceptual and cognitive abilities intact. It is very frustrating for the patient at the primary level who has severe motor deficits, because the patient is "locked in" to a body and cannot communicate or control any aspect of the environment. On the other hand, the patient who has severe cognitive or perceptual deficits, but who has good motor skills, that is, can ambulate, may still be considered at the primary level because that individual cannot perform self-care activities or function safely witout verbal cues and constant supervision. Memory may be so impaired that the patient shows limited carry-over in therapy from day to day. This patient is often referred to as the "walking wounded," that is, good motor function but poor cognitive abilities.

THE PATIENT AT THE ADVANCED LEVEL. The term *advanced* is applied to the patient who may have cognitive, perceptual, motor, and behavioral deficits, but they are not significant enough to cause total dependence in activities of daily living (ADL). The occupational therapist working with the patient at the advanced level must be able to correlate the underlying neurological problems with the functional ones at this stage. The patient at the advanced level, unlike the patient at the primary level, has the potential to make an adaptive motor response and carry over learning in therapy toward achieving a functional goal. For example, the patient may now have sufficient equilibrium reactions and upper extremity (UE) function to work on UE dressing while sitting with legs over the edge of the bed.

The overall level of awareness of the patient at the advanced level is higher, and such a patient has a better ability to control more aspects of the environment and participate in the program. The patient still may have significant cognitive, perceptual, or motor deficits, but therapy can now be structured toward working on a functional goal, such as feeding or dressing. It is important to assess whether the patient at the advanced level has sufficient memory and understanding to benefit from repetitive, structured training. The general aims of treatment for a patient at

the primary level are discussed later in this chapter and should help to clarify the distinguishing characteristics of the two levels.

Clinical picture

PHYSICAL ASPECTS. The physical deficits encountered in patients with head injury can be quite severe and complex. The therapist may encounter patients with motor involvement of one to four extremities; decreased total body function, oral-bulbar status, sensation, coordination, balance, endurance, and range of motion (ROM); abdnormal reflexes, motor patterns, and muscle tone; muscle weakness; and poor isolated muscle control. The occupational therapist must have a good theoretical knowledge of these physical deficits to remedy them during sensorimotor and functional activities.

An injury to the brain from a traumatic insult has a different clinical picture from that typically seen in cerebral vascular accident (CVA). Bilateral motor involvement is frequently seen in head injury because the insult may occur at the brainstem or midbrain level, thus blocking impulses from being sent to the higher brain centers, or from lesions occurring in both the right and left hemispheres.[19]

Limitation of joint motion. Loss of ROM that results in contractures is a frequent problem. During the coma or acute rehabilitation phase patients can develop decorticate or decerebrate rigidity or posturing.[9] The failure of the brain to control or inhibit abnormal postural reflexes and hypertonicity may cause joint deformities and contractures. The prolonged immobilization of the comatose patient with severe spasticity can lead to the development of possible joint ossification and calcification. It is extremely important in the early period after the onset to become aware of and start to control potential loss of ROM. In head injury a patient may start out with flaccid muscles and may very rapidly develop severe spasticity and deformities.

Muscle weakness. Most adults with head injury do not have muscle weakness. Rather, there is severe spasticity or excessive abnormal muscle tone. The patient without close to full isolated muscle control cannot have the muscle

tested, for resistance applied to a spastic muscle would only set off the stretch reflex and would not truly test muscle strength.

Abnormal reflexes and tone. Abnormal postural reflexes are a common problem after head injury. Postural reflexes regulate the degree and distribution of muscle tone. The brain, depending on the site of the lesion, can no longer inhibit certain reflexes that were integrated at an earlier developmental stage.[7] The most common abnormal reflexes and reactions found are asymmetric tonic neck reflex (ATNR), symmetric tonic neck reflex (STNR), and tonic labyrinthine reflex (TLR); associated reactions; positive support reaction; extensor thrust; and decreased equilibrium, righting, and protective reactions. These abnormal reflexes and reactions affect ROM, muscle tone, and selective movements. Unless prevented or controlled, they may prevent the patient from making even basic physical and functional gains. Table 31-3 was developed to help define the abnormal postural reflex mechanism by giving (1) an observation of the problem, (2) the reflex underlying the problem, (3) the reflex-inhibiting posture or treatment, and (4) the possible functional implications. Specific reflex testing must be performed to establish which abnormal reflexes are present. This table is not meant to imply that a mere observation of an abnormal pattern means that the abnormal reflex is present.

Patterns and isolated muscle control. The components of the flexor and extensor patterns have been described in Chapters 15 and 16. Patients with head injury will usually have severe flexor patterning of the upper extremities and extensor patterning of the lower extremities. Often a patient has a combined flexor-extensor pattern in the upper or lower extremities. The patient, for instance, may have spasticity in both the triceps and biceps. The muscle group with a greater degree of hypertonicity has the stronger action. Until gross motor skills develop, the patient will not perform well in fine motor activities. Development of controlled movement usually progresses from proximal to distal, although at times it can occur distal to proximal or concurrently. For example, without good, selective

Table 31-3
Abnormal postural reflex mechanisms

Observation	Reflex	Reflex-inhibiting posture and treatment	Functional implication
Severe plantar flexion, clawing of toes, inversion of ankle	Positive supporting reaction—extensor tone predominates	Dorsiflexion of toes to shift weight to heel (hips and knees will want to flex) Foot wedge and inhibitive foot plate for dorsiflexion of toes	Cannot bear weight without facilitating extensor pattern; poor balance reactions with rigid limb, small base of support for foot
Neglect of one side and head off to right or left	ATNR—increased extensor tone on jaw (preferred) side and increased flexor tone on skull (neglected) Rule out visual-perceptual deficits	Head and neck in midline; turning and tracking to skull side Head devices, neck devices, turning to auditory stimulus or getting neck rotating during feeding training.	Prevents reach, grasp, and midline activity; imbalance of muscle tone, decreasing selective movement, mostly in upper extremities
Severe flexor spasticity of upper extremities, severe extensor tone of lower extremities	STNR—flexed head increases flexor tone of upper extremities and extensor tone of lower extremities and vice versa	Extend head-neck to increase extensor tone of upper extremities and flexor tone of lower extremities. Consider key points of control to decrease spasticity, not just reflex Other methods—heat, cold, casting	Will affect coordination, reciprocal movements, total body function; can develop contractures; decreased ability to bear weight on upper extremities in transfers
Severe extensor spasticity and adduction of lower extremities when supine in bed	TLR—extensor tone predominates in supine and flexor tone in prone (depends on position of head in space)	Key points of control In supine position abduct hips and flex knees In sitting position hip flexion works to break pattern Knee abductor, seat wedge	Cannot roll over, that is, bend leg to roll or bring shoulder forward to roll; decreased mobility, sitting, and transfers; cannot bear weight on lower extremities
Increased spasticity in arm while ambulating	Associated reactions—increased spasticity in some part of the body produced by forceful activity of another part	Must take care in using resisted activity in spastic conditions even of sound limb, as it can cause associated reaction Neurodevelopmental treatment (NDT) inhibition techniques during mat, functional, and ambulation activities	Functional activities, such as writing and dressing, and other purposeful movements of sound hand can increase flexor spasticity of affected hand

shoulder control, hand function and coordination will be limited. Gross grasp and release usually return in the adult with head injury before prehension.[7]

Many patients may have deficits in coordination at the trunk, head, and hips in addition to that typically seen in the upper and lower extremities. The origin of the incoordination must be analyzed to establish an effective treatment plan.

Ataxia. Ataxia is an abnormality of movement and disordered muscle tone that is seen in patients with damage to the cerebellum or the sensory pathways to result in a cerebellar or sensory ataxia. A patient may have ataxia of the total body, trunk, or upper or lower extremities or may have gait ataxia. The normal flow of a smooth voluntary movement is destroyed by errors in the direction and speed of movement.[31]

Ataxia ranges from mild to severe and can be a significant impediment to achieving a functional goal. The therapist must carefully assess the joints most affected by ataxia to control it and reduce its limitation on function.

Spasticity. Spasticity is one of the most frequent and damaging physical problems encountered in head injuries. Spasticity is the activation of a hyperactive stretch reflex with resultant hypertonicity.[50] It ranges from minimal to severe in any particular muscle or muscle group. Spasticitiy may occur in combined flexor and extensor patterns, thus making its inhibition more complicated. Usually flexor spasticity predominates in the upper extremities, and extensor spasticity predominates in the lower extremities.

Loss of sensation and perception. The most common sensory and perceptual

losses seen are decreased proprioception, response to deep pain, superficial pain, touch, and stereognosis; and diminished temperature sense, two-point discrimination, and kinesthesia. The patient may also have impaired senses of taste and smell, depending on the cranial nerves involved. The primary-level patient's response to pinprick or deep pain can help to establish a level of awareness. Evaluation of a patient at the primary level is discussed later in this chapter.

Abnormal posturing. Along with the abnormal reflexes and hypertonicity, postural problems can develop (Table 31-3). The nature of the abnormal patterns can be much more severe than those seen in the patient with CVA. Abnormal postures frequently exhibited in adults with head injury are as follows:

Head: Forward flexion or hyperextension may rotate to preferred side because of the influence of the ATNR. Lateral flexion of the neck often accompanies lateral flexion of the trunk.

Trunk: Lateral flexion and retraction of one side, kyphotic posture, scoliosis, or extension are exhibited.

Scapula: Humeral depression is common with either protraction and elevation or retraction patterns.

Upper extremities: Bilateral involvement with asymmetry between sides or unilateral involvement may be seen, depending on the areas of brain damage. A strong flexor pattern usually predominates; however, patients may exhibit a UE extensor pattern or a combination flexor-extensor pattern.

Pelvis and hip: Usually a posterior pelvic tilt exists, causing too much sacral sitting. Some patients tend to slide forward in the wheelchair when sitting and have the appearance of extending over the backrest. Pelvic obliquity is often a problem because of asymmetry of muscle tone. Aside from these problems, hip flexors or adductors are often contracted.

Lower extremities: Knee flexor contractures are frequently present. On the other hand, there can also be an extensor pattern in the lower extremity. The pattern is usually affected by a change in position, for example, supine versus sitting.

Feet: Inversion, plantar flexion, with a downward clawing of the toes. A positive supporting reaction is present in some cases.

It is important to know the biomechanics of the body and prevent deformities rather than try to deal with them after the poor posture has developed.

Decreased physical capacity. Decreased vital capacity, endurance, and general tolerance for an exercise or activity are common problems of head injury. Having gone through medical complications, such as pneumonia, prolonged bed rest, or immobilization, the patient with head injury who suddenly starts getting up in a wheelchair will be easily fatigued or overloaded. The comatose patient or patient at the primary level must be closely monitored for changes in blood pressure and vital signs the first few times he or she gets up.

Loss of total body function control. Total body function skills include head and trunk control, sitting and standing balance, reaching, bending, stooping, and functional ambulation. At the acute phase of the patient's recovery, decreased head and neck, trunk, and hip control are encountered along with the upper and lower extremity losses. Sitting balance and the ability to support oneself with the legs over the edge of the mat or the bed are poor. The patient at the primary level has a tendency for excessive forward flexion of the neck or too much hyperextension. The patient at the advanced level exhibits such problems as poor sitting or standing balance and difficulty bending and stooping and reaching to high and low areas. Total body function skills are necessary for performing higher level funtional skills, such as functional ambulation during a kitchen activity.

COGNITIVE-BEHAVIORAL ASPECTS. As previously described, there are several levels of awareness that the patient with head trauma may exhibit. As the patient begins to progress out of a semicomatose state, more formal cognitive testing can be tolerated. At this stage the therapist may begin to realize how severely impaired the patient may be. In most rehabilitation facilities the speech pathologist or psychologist performs the structured cognitive evaluations. It is necessary, however, for all members of the rehabilitation team to have a working knowledge of the cognitive problems that may appear and how to deal with these problems in the most effective way for the patient.

The occupational therapist should direct attention to areas that may affect the patient's functional status. Some problems that are frequently seen may be disorientation; decreased level of attention, safety awareness, and insight into disability; impaired memory, sequencing, judgment, and problem-solving skills; and decreased ability to process information accurately and think abstractly.

Reduced attention level and concentration ability. Individuals may have problems with attention to task, attention to control of their behavior, and the attentional aspects of memory. Reduced level of attention and the ability to concentrate may seriously affect functional independence. Most normal individuals find it difficult to concentrate on reading while the radio or television is on or people are talking nearby. An individual must be able to tune out nonessential stimuli in the environment and attend to stimuli that are important to the task at hand. Patients with head trauma may be unable to distinguish those stimuli that are pertinent to successful performance. The patient with head injury often loses not only the ability to filter out distraction but also the ability to concentrate for any length of time.

Impaired sequencing. Sequencing is the ability to accurately process information in steps or sequentially. One does this automatically primarily through the visual and auditory modes. Because of the extensive disruption of central nervous system (CNS) functions, these skills may be severely disturbed in the patient with a head injury. The patient may be able to process information presented visually but not information presented auditorily. The patient may be able to process the information through both systems, but with extreme delay. For example, the patient may understand a request even though there may be significant time lag before the message has been processed and a response is made. At times the patient may be able to process information only when it is presented in the simplest manner. Instructions involving long explanations, specific sequence of direction, or complex, unfamiliar vocabulary may hinder performance. It is vital for the occupational therapist to know exactly what the patient's processing abilities are to establish an appropriate treatment approach.

Decreased safety awareness. The patient with head injury often displays unsafe behavior. This may be a result of impulsiveness, decreased insight into the disability, impaired judgment, or a combination of all of these. Decreased insight, disorientation, and impaired memory can contribute to the patient's inability to recognize his or her limited abilities for specific situations or analyze the consequences of his or her actions. It is therefore imperative that all members of the treatment team assist the patient in structuring the environment and understanding the limitations to maximize relearning of appropriate, safe behavior.

Impaired memory. Impaired memory is probably one of the most devastating problems that the patient with head injury must face. There are several types of memory impairments, ranging from the inability to recall a few words just heard to remembering events that occurred a few months or years before the injury. Although the degree of severity differs with each patient, the majority of patients with head injuries will have some level of impaired memory. This manifests itself in the inability to learn and carry over new tasks and contributes to confusion and inability to participate in the environment.

Impaired intellectual functions and abstract thinking. An additional aspect of impaired cognition is that of reduced intellectual functioning. The patient has lost the ability to solve problems, analyze information presented, and come up with appropriate solutions. The patient is unable to structure thoughts or formulate a good cognitive strategy. Relearning these skills may require external structure from staff and family. The patient may be able, with some assistance, to recognize errors but may be unable to resolve the errors without external cuing. Patients with head injury tend to analyze problems in concrete terms, interpreting all information at the most literal level. The ability to think abstractly and generalize knowledge and experience is usually significantly impaired. Functional independence demands the mastering and manipulation of basic cognitive and academic skills, such as categorizing, calculating, and generalizing experiences. The occupational therapist must consider and incorporate these critical cognitive skills into the treatment plan.

Behavior disorders. Common aberrant behavior that the patient with head injury displays includes distractibility, agitation, combativeness, emotional lability, inappropriate affect, and socially unacceptable behavior. The patient who is unable to filter distractions will become agitated in a noisy environment. The patient with limited insight will become frustrated and at times combative when unable to perform simple tasks. Most patients with head injury are unable to process and respond to excessive stimulation, and as a result, a turning off, or shutdown of systems, occurs. When this happens, the patient

is no longer able to participate effectively.

Depending on the area of the brain affected, the patient may show an inability to control emotions. The patient may show inappropriate outbursts of anger, tears, or laughter and may be socially inappropriate in behavior, shouting obscenities, or making indiscriminate sexual advances. At the other extreme the patient may display flat affect or passivity or may lack initiative, interest, or participation in the environment. This lack of participation may be interpreted as poor motivation on the patient's part when in fact this apparent lack of responsiveness is the result of organic damage. It is important to recognize that the behavior exhibited by the patient with head injury correlates significantly with the level of cognitive function.

Cognitive and behavioral aspects of head injury are vast and complicated. This constitutes an overview of areas that pertain to occupational therapy. For a detailed analysis of cognitive functions as they relate to head injury, the reader is referred to the references.[23,30] Practical remediation techniques are discussed in the treatment section of this chapter.

PERCEPTUAL-MOTOR ASPECTS. The ability to accurately perceive and respond to people and objects within the environment is necessary for successful, independent function. Disruption of various pathways within the CNS can cause the patient with head injury to have difficulty with a multitude of perceptual-motor skills that were previously taken for granted. Depending on the nature and extent of damage, the impairment may involve gross visual-perceptual or perceptual-motor skills.

Impaired gross visual-perceptual skills. Gross visual skills involve basic abilities, such as visually attending to a task or effectively scanning the environment. The patient with head injury is often unable to focus on an object for more than a few seconds. When asked to follow a moving object by moving the eyes, incomplete scanning and jerky eye movements may be present. Inattentiveness and impaired scanning may be further complicated by the presence of either homonymous hemianopsia or visual-spatial neglect. Homonymous

hemianopsia can be described as "blindness of right-sided or left-sided fields of both eyes."[44]

Extinction phenomenon is also quite common in the adult patient with head injury. Extinction is defined as a "process in which a sensation disappears or a stimulus becomes imperceptible when another sensation is evoked by simultaneous stimulation elsewhere in the visual field."[25] Frequently the adult with brain injury has other types of field losses aside from a homonymous hemianopsia, such as a scotoma. A scotoma is an area of partial or complete blindness within the confines of a normal or relatively normal visual field. A central scotoma, which is commonly seen, is a central blind spot.

Apraxia. The ability to determine the appropriate type and sequence of movement to perform a task is praxis or motor planning. Despite intact sensation, motor power, or coordination, the patient with head injury may exhibit impaired motor planning skills, or apraxia. One or more types of apraxia may be apparent. The patient may be able to carry out tasks that involve one limb and at the same time may be unable to perform tasks that involve total body movement. The patient may be unable to blow out a match but can cut paper with scissors. If asked to pantomime, some patients are unable to demonstrate how a task is performed unless allowed to use the necessary objects. For example, at the most concrete level a patient may be unable to demonstrate taking a drink of water from a glass unless provided with a full glass of water when he or she happens to be thirsty.

Categories of motor planning skills generally include four areas of possible body involvement. These are Buccofacial, unilateral limb, bilateral limb, or total body movements. Each of these four areas of the body may be tested with five classes of actions. These actions can be defined as follows[46]:

Transitive: Gestures and actions demonstrating the use of a missing object
Conventional: Gestures that are representative or symbolic of culturally specific concepts, for instance, a salute
Natural: Gestures that are nonculturally specific, for instance, a stomach ache

Real object: Actions demonstrating the use of a real object (same as transitive only with object)

Nonrepresentative: Actions that convey no message, for example, puffing cheeks

The presence of any of these motor planning impairments, combined with additional cognitive problems, can be a source of extreme frustration for the patient. Apraxia is often unjustly interpreted by members of the team as uncooperative behavior. It is vital therefore for the occupational therapist to accurately assess the patient's motor planning abilities to avoid unrealistic expectations and mislabeling of the patient's behavior.

Constructional apraxia is "the inability to produce designs in two or three dimensions by copying, drawing or constructing, upon command, or spontaneously."[44] The patient with a head injury with damage to the right side of the brain may show a lack of perspective and poor spatial relations. Those patients with damage to the left side of the brain may show a tendency toward simplicity of design and difficulty in the execution of the requested tasks. There has been considerable documentation on the relationship between constructional praxis abilities and the ability to dress.[29,55] Because of this high correlation between abilities the occupational therapist must include a constructionnal praxis evaluation in the perceptual-motor testing.

Impaired body scheme. Impaired body image and impaired body scheme are related but are not identical perceptual disorders. Body image is the "visual and mental memory image of one's body."[44] A patient's body image, often tested by the Draw a Man test, reveals that individual's feelings and perceptions about himself or herself. Body scheme relates to the ability to perceive one's body position and the relationship of body parts. To deal effectively with objects within the environment, the patient must develop an internal awareness of the body and its parts.[41] The patient with impaired body scheme will not know how to move around in the environment effectively.[1]

Impaired figure-ground perception. The ability to distinguish an object from its background visually is figure-ground perception. The patient with figure-ground impairment may have difficulty locating an item on a supermarket shelf or finding an item in a cluttered drawer. A white facecloth placed on the white sheets of the bed may be missed. Severe figure-ground impairment can obviously have a dramatic effect on function.

Impaired position-in-space perception. Position-in-space perception is the "ability to understand and deal with concepts of spatial position such as up-down, in-out, right-left, before-behind."[44] The therapist who is treating the patient with impaired position-in-space perception must carefully analyze how to instruct the patient to follow commands. For example, the patient may not be able to conceptualize a command, such as "Get your toothbrush, which is behind your comb." Taken at its extreme the patient with severely impaired perception of position in space may be unable to make a sandwich, because he cannot place the lunchmeat "in between" two slices of bread.

Some remaining areas of impaired perception that may appear in the patient with head injury are form and size discrimination, part-whole visualization, and depth perception. A classic example of impaired form perception is the patient who mistakes a water pitcher for a urinal.[44] The patient with impaired part-whole perception, when presented visually with only part of an object, may not be able to synthesize the parts to identify the object correctly. A hair dryer may be mistaken for a telephone. Impaired depth perception will affect the patient's ability to ambulate on stairs or on uneven surfaces, such as the ground.

From this summary of perceptual problems found in patients with head injury, the reader may be led to believe that impairments occur in an isolated manner. This is rarely the case. Rather, the therapist is usually presented with a patient who has a constellation of problems. The therapist's job is to carefully observe the patient's behavior and interpret the reasons or impairments underlying abnormal responses.

It is also important to formulate an awareness of the cognitive functions and their relationship to perceptual-motor abilities. Essentially it is impossible to separate cognition from language, perception, or behavior, because all these areas are instrumental to learning. The significance of the interaction between cognition and perception is that "the object of perception does not come to us as a given, but rather, that it must actively be sought after and constructed through cognitive processes."[10] For example, the therapist who is evaluating praxis via a block design test can at the same time be assessing the cognitive strategy the patient uses to duplicate the design. Aside from analyzing only the perceptual skills, the cognitive functions of sequencing and problem solving should also be assessed.

Many clinicians have found that cognitive-perceptual-motor skills involve the integration of sensory, motor, perceptual, and cognitive modalities into a meaningful mode to create successful interactions with the environment. Perceptual motor skills should be considered as building blocks or significant components of cognition.[33] On the other hand, it can also be stated that cognitive skills are significant components of perception. For example, during a task the patient might be able to visually discriminate the correct object (perceptual skill) from a set of pictures but have no memory (cognitive skill) for what that object or person was in the past or is in the present. Cognition, language, and perception are integrated for function. They cannot be separated or treated in a deficit-specific approach lest the patient develop splinter skills without integration. Without the integration of perceptual and cognitive skills the individual will fail to function optimally in any environment.

Psychosocial factors. The psychosocial aspects of head injury are frequently overlooked but can be key components to the success of the patient's recovery process. It is important to know the family and social history along with previous personality characteristics, because as the patient's level of awareness improves, these traits will start to appear again, possibly in an exaggerated way.

Family support is an important concept when dealing with head injury. It can be a determining factor in the patient's level of motivation to achieve functional independence. Family and friends are an integral part of the rehabilitation process, especially in the beginning stages, since they may be able to elicit a response from the patient when no one else can.

Family role alterations and the patient's coping mechanisms for dealing with these role changes must be considered. The patient may go from being an extremely independent individual to being totally dependent, and this is very frustrating and degrading. It will be difficult for both the patient and the family members or significant others to cope. No matter how cognizant the family and the patient are of the disability, it disrupts the family structure. It is often difficult for family members to understand the uncontrolled behavior they observe in their loved one.

Mood and affect can have frequent swings, with the patient being unable to control these variations in emotion. The patient may be inappropriately friendly and indiscriminate in showing affection. As the patient becomes more aware of self and the environment again, the patient may be depressed by a sense of loss and may suddenly start to perceive the confinements of the current world and begin to face the fact of no longer being the same.

The alteration of sexual functioning and the ability to deal with sexual needs and feelings can occur. The patient may lack the impulse control to keep from making sexual advances toward others. These impulsive advances may be coupled with verbal abuse, and often the patient is not cognitively aware of this behavior. Memory deficits further complicate this problem. The patient may not remember that the woman he is making advances toward is his therapist or nurse.

Previous eduational status and values play an important part in the patient's progress toward independence. These factors must be incorporated into the long-term treatment plan. Eventual discharge plans must be set up to meet the needs of the patient. For example, a patient who had a learning disability before the head injury and always had difficulty in school may not benefit from a traditional college program but rather from a disabled students' program, directed toward the specific problem areas, at a community college.

A lack of insight into the disability can be a serious problem affecting adults with head injury. The patient may not even be aware of the deficits or the necessity of working on a certain functional activity or exercise. The patient may be embarrassed by performing a certain task or may simply refuse to do it. In general the psychosocial aspects of the patient with head injury go hand in hand with the cognitive and behavioral aspects and contribute to or retard recovery throughout the overall rehabilitation process.

FUNCTIONAL LIMITATIONS. A patient with head injury may have problems in all performance skills. Possible areas of deficit are listed as follows:

Self-care
  Feeding
  Dressing
  Hygiene
  Grooming
  Bathing
  Toileting
Mobility
  Bed
  Wheelchair
  Transfer skills
  Functional ambulation
Home management
  Kitchen tasks
  Housekeeping
  Child care
  Marketing
Communication
  Speech
  Symbolic language
Transportation
  Public modes
  Driving ability
Community function
  Shopping
  Street safety
  Community facilities
Work skills
  Prevocational activities
  Work activities
Leisure activities
  Social activities
  Sports and games
  Hobbies

The functional disabilities cannot be separated from the cognitive, perceptual, sensory, motor, or behavioral problems. A problem in one of these areas can cause or contribute to the functional deficit. In other words, visual perception, sensation, motor ability, cognition, and psychosocial skills are all the basic building blocks to ADL, each playing an integral part at various levels of task performance. For instance, a kitchen activity requires a combination of skills, such as UE function, wheelchair mobility, figure-ground and form perception, scanning, sequencing, direction following, memory, safety awareness, and judgment. It is easy to forget how complex such a task is and take for granted the skills required, because it has become automatic to the nondisabled person. The individual with head injury struggles to put even the most basic components of the process together in some meaningful and ordered fashion.

Another example of a functional task that can be analyzed for areas of function that interact for effective performance is feeding ability. If there is decreased feeding ability, improvement in some or all of the following areas is necessary to independent functioning: oral reflexes, level of awareness, oral sensation such as hypersensitivity, head and trunk control in sitting, UE function, and cranial nerve functions.

It becomes extremely important, then, for the therapist to identify the underlying components that relate to the functional deficit so that the best treatment approach can be established. The therapist must have good observational skills and the ability to do formal testing to help pinpoint how the functional task should be broken down into steps and structured to gain optimal results in performance.

EVALUATION

Joint measurement, muscle testing, evaluation of reflexes and equilibrium reactions, sensory testing, ADL, home management, and home evaluations are described in Chapters 5, 6, 8, 9, and 10. Evaluation for degree of spasticity is described in Chapter 7. All of these assessments may be applicable to the patient with head injury.

Guidelines for evaluation of the patient at the primary level
Position and posture
TEST POSITION: Note whether the patient is supine, sitting, or upright in a wheelchair. The response may vary with proprioceptive, kinesthetic, labyrinthine, and

visual input. The best response usually occurs when the patient is optimally positioned and sensory input is more normalized.

POSTURAL REFLEXES: Note symmetry between the two sides of the body and check for any abnormal postural reflexes. Note tonus changes and differences from one position to another, and estimate ROM and spasticity. Note if there is decorticate or decerebrate posturing or rigidity.

DECEREBRATE RIGIDITY: Note clenching of the jaw and extension of all four limbs (upper extremities more than lower extremities). Upper extremities are adducted and internally rotated, shoulders elevated, and feet plantar flexed. Basically it is a postural extensor synergy. Wrists and fingers are flexed.[9]

DECORTICATE RIGIDITY: Note triple flexion of upper extremities, that is, they are adducted, elbows and wrists severely flexed, and fists clenched. Lower extremities are hyperextended. Simultaneous hyperactivity of extensor muscles in upper extremities can also occur.[9]

Motor picture

Observe ROM, spasticity, flaccidity, and contractures. Note if there is no movement response or if there are any spontaneous movements. If there is a response, is it (1) to a stimulus, (2) with sensory input and imitation, (3) to imitation only, or (4) on command? Note also if the movement is (1) reflexive, (2) generalized, or (3) localized and voluntary.

Sensorimotor picture

PAIN: Evaluate for response to pinprick on upper and lower extremities and face. Is the response generalized or localized? Assess whether the response is away from, toward, delayed or absent.

DEEP PAIN: Either pinch the patient on the leg, arm, or neck and note response (same as for pain), or put pressure on fingernail with a hard object like a pen.

ORAL AREA: Refer to testing of oral reflexes. If patient is prone to seizures, placing ice on lips can set off seizures.

OLFACTORY: See if the patient can be aroused with noxious odors. Watch out for rebound phenomenon. Noxious stimuli have an arousing effect, whereas pleasant odors have a calming effect. Various smells may be used to arouse the patient before a treatment session (refer to olfactory stimulation on p. 448).

GUSTATORY: Check out response to taste. This can be used as a stimulation technique or for working on the oral feeding mechanisms, for example, sour tastes help with lip pursing, which in turn helps with sucking. This area is mentioned because the patient may need to be aroused to truly assess level of awareness (refer to gustatory stimulation on p. 448).

AUDITORY: Use a bell, jingle keys, clap hands, or simply talk to see if the patient responds to sound. Note if the patient turns the head or eyes toward the sound or if there is merely a startle response. Note if there is a generalized, localized, delayed, or absent response. Abnormal postural reflex mechanisms may prevent the patient from responding. Positioning should be optimal.

TACTILE: Note if there is any response to touch, rubbing, vibration, or different textures. Response could be the same as for auditory. Fine tactile discrimination cannot be assessed with the patient with head injury at the primary level, but responses can be observed to combine with observations of other responses to come up with a clinical picture.

Gross visual skills

TEST POSITION: Patient should be sitting with the head upright for testing visual skills.

ATTENTIVENESS: See if the patient can attend to a bright object or to the therapist. Be sure to measure attentiveness in terms of the amount of time it takes for response so that future tests can be measured against this baseline to show progress. Keep a flow sheet record, noting the time that it takes to respond.

TRACKING: See if the patient can track a large, bright object of side-to-side or up-down. Note the specific quality of the movement, that is, jerkiness, nystagmus, convergence, completeness, or delay. Also note and be aware of any other clues the therapist is giving to the patient to encourage tracking of the object, such as verbal or by standing on one side of the patient. Keep a flow sheet of the kind of cuing used and the length of the delay from introduction of stimulus to the response. Tracking requires attentiveness.

NEGLECT: It is difficult to test specifically for field deficits or visual-spatial neglect in a patient with a head injury at the primary level, but generally it can be noted if the patient tends to neglect one side or responds better on the other side. The therapist may want to work initially on the more responsive side and then on the neglected side to facilitate head turning and body awareness.

FORM AND COLOR PERCEPTION: The therapist may want to evaluate basic perceptual skills, such as color discrimination and form perception. Color perception may be assessed by asking the patient to select a color from two colored objects, such as blocks or pegs. A higher level of color discrimination can be demanded by asking the patient to match colored cubes to design cards. Form perception can be evaluated with a form board that uses basic shapes, such as the circle, square, triangle, and diamond.

RESPONSES: Before commencing any evaluation, it is important to establish some system of responses with the patient. For tasks that require simple yes or no responses or the choice of one object over another, signals such as eye blinks, gazing toward the correct answer, hand signals, or shaking of the head in different directions may be used. The therapist must establish beforehand which means is the easiest for the nonverbal patient to give an optimal response.

Head and total body control

TEST POSITION: Evaluate the patient with another person to assist the patient over the bed edge.

BALANCE AND CONTROL: Check for sitting balance, trunk control, head control, and any balance reactions. After looking at all these areas together, evaluate head and trunk control separately in the wheelchair after hips and lower exremities are properly positioned. Head and neck control will develop along with visual skills. Measure head control by the amount of support required. This will help determine the type of device needed to support the head. The length of time that the head can be held erect by itself or during an activity, number of times per day without head device, and length of time without head device are also important to note for assessing improvement. Set up a flow sheet to keep a record of progress.

Summary

In general it is important to provide consistent sensory input to evaluate the quality of the motor output. It is best to structure the environment or task to demand a motor response after sensory stimulation. Keep track on a flow sheet of which sensory stimulation is being used, its frequency, duration, sequence, and combinations. Then on the flowsheet, note the response after specific stimulation techniques. Keep track of progress by consistency (how often) and by timing (how long) the various responses. Most of all, record observations to note the quality of the response. Is the response to a specific stimulus, with sensory input and imitation, to imitation only, or to command?

For the patient with head injury at the primary level note if there is a delay in processing, and be sure to allow time for the delay. The patient needs times to make the adaptive response and therefore increase the level of awareness.

Oral reflexes

Oral functions of the adult with head injury may be affected and have an influence on the ability to eat, drink, swallow, and speak. The oral reflexes and procedures for their evaluation are outlined in Table 31-4.

Table 31-4
Oral reflexes

Area evaluated	Age	Function	Stimulus	Response
Face	Birth to life	Appropriate level of sensitivity allows for touch awareness Motor component allows for food handling and expression	Pressure to perioral area and temples Functional muscle test; coordination evaluation	Appropriate toleration of pressure; isolated muscle function
Tongue	Birth 4-6 mo 10-12 mo	Tongue elevation Lateralization Tip elevation; moves and locates food in mouth; directs food back in mouth to be swallowed	Feeding cortical command; manually palpate with index finger or rubber seizure stick	Elevation; lateralization; tip elevation; rapid lateralization
Soft palate	Birth to life	Elevation; allows food to escape nasal cavity	Light touch on lateral portion of soft palate	Soft palate elevation
Rooting	Birth to 3-5 mo	Assists in locating food source	Touch on corner of lip or cheek	Rooting reflex can cause possible impedance of normal or motor function; head turned toward stimulus, open mouth, and tongue slightly protracted
Bite	Nonreflexive after 3-5 mo	Allows introduction of food and leads to chewing	Padded tongue blade or rubber seizure stick on patient's tongue, gum, and tooth surfaces	Sustained reflexive clamping
Sucking and swallowing	Birth to 3-5 mo	Initial intake of food; sucking followed by swallowing	Nipple; straws of various diameters	Sucking with buccinator and orbicularis oris compressing; subsequent swallow
Swallowing	Birth to life	Food intake of solids and fluids; nutrition	Stretch digastric and geniohyoid muscles; depress spoon or tongue blade half way back on tongue; introduce eye dropper full of fluid	Swallowing
Coughing	Birth to life	Prevents aspiration	Observe for voluntary or spontaneous coughing	Coughing
Gag	Birth to life	Prevents aspiration, triggers swallowing mechanism	Apply pressure on posterior third o tongue	Simultaneous head and jaw extension with rhythmical protrusion of tongue and contraction of pharynx

Perceptual-motor evaluation

In evaluating perceptual-motor impairments in head injuries, care must be taken to do so in an orderly, progressive, and complete manner. Gross visual skills must be assessed before higher level visual-perceptual skills, such as figure-ground or position in space. Motor planning skills must be evaluated early to ensure that problems noted in higher level skills are not a result of apraxia but are truly difficulties in the function being tested.

In assessing perceptual-motor functions the clinician should evaluate the patient both quantitatively (with a numerical score) and qualitatively (with

good observations). The quantitative assessment enables the therapist to more accurately assess the level of impairment and measure progress over time. The observations recorded during the evaluations will provide vital information necessary for goals in treatment planning.

A valid and reliable comprehensive perceptual-motor evaluation is used in the Occupational Therapy Department at the Santa Clara Valley Medical Center.[56,57] The areas assessed in this battery of tests include body scheme, total body and buccofacial movements, praxis (ideational, ideomotor, and constructional), gross visual skills, and

higher level visual discrimination skills. These skills include attentiveness; scanning; visual fields; visual neglect; depth, form, size, and figure-ground perception; position in space; and part-whole integration. For additional examples of complete, progressive cognitive-perceptual-motor evaluations, the reader is referred to the references.[41,51,55]

Cognition

In many facilities it is the role of the occupational therapist to administer functional cognitive evaluations. It is fundamental to the occupational therapist's role to observe, interpret, and apply methods of treatment to ameliorate or retrain various facets of cognition and behavior relevant to the patient's performance. The Occupational Therapy Department at Santa Clara Valley Medical Center is presently developing a structured functional cognitive evaluation. The evaluation encourages a dynamic process of rating the patient on specific skills throughout an entire functional task. The areas that are assessed during the evaluation are orientation, attention and memory, cognitive strategy or integration (for example, following directions, sequencing, problem solving, planning, and initiating), and behavior.

Hand function

After muscle tone, ROM, muscle strength, and selective movements have been assessed, hand function can be examined. The therapist must analyze first if the hand has isolated control for (1) gross grasp and release, (2) lateral pinch, (3) palmar prehension, and (4) fingertip prehension. A good test used for this purpose is the Quantitative Test of Upper Extremity Function by Carrol.[12] Higher level skills are assessed only if full isolated muscle control is possible. Manipulation of objects and fine finger dexterity are examples of these skills.

It is also important to assess speed of movement and any other complicating clinical signs, such as ataxia or shoulder weakness, because these will affect hand function. A test frequently used is the Jebsen-Taylor Test of Hand Function.[26] This test assesses speed and coordination by timing the patient's performance of a variety of simulated functional tasks, such as writing, feeding, and fine prehension activities. It is extremely important for the occupational therapist to assess hand function through the application of standardized tests, because then the therapist can begin to correlate objective improvement with that seen in gains made in performance of daily living skills.

Total body function

It is important for the occupational therapist to assess total body function to relate it to ADL. For the patient with head injury at the primary level,

one of the first things the therapist should evaluate is head and trunk control when the patient is sitting over the edge of the bed, along with total body patterning to see what kind of wheelchair is appropriate. Next the therapist should assess sitting balance when unsupported, noting equilibrium and protective reactions. As the patient progresses, the therapist will need to assess standing balance when unassisted and standing balance while performing a UE activity, such as bending or reaching for an item in a kitchen cupboard. It is one thing to ambulate, for instance, forward and backward in the parallel bars, but it is much more complex to maneuver in tight spaces when peforming an activity. Functional ambulation needs to be assessed in various settings, such as kitchen, bathroom, and community. It is essential that the therapist know what perceptual-motor skills are significant to total body function to break them down and work on the deficit areas. A patient may be able to climb stairs, but the coordination, speed, and perception needed to step on a city bus or get on an escalator in a shopping center are considerably more complex.

Kitchen evaluation

The patient's ability to be safe and independent in the kitchen may determine a future living place. In evaluating the patient with head injury in the kitchen, that individual's cognitive status is of the utmost importance. Adapting utensils and equipment and adapting and structuring the environment may be necessary to improve the patient's safety, judgment, and problem-solving skills. The components of the kitchen evaluation used for the patient with head injury are not very different from those used with other patient populations. The major difference is the need for the occupational therapist to closely evaluate the amount and type of supervision and structuring and the degree of physical assistance required in these tasks.

Prevocational evaluation

Before a formal prevocational evaluation is administered, it is important to assess the patient's overall physical capacity. This evaluation will reveal areas

that may pose problems in future job training and placement. The wheelchair-bound patient should be assessed for indoor and outdoor mobility, reaching height, ability to retrieve items from the floor, and sitting tolerance. The ambulatory patient must be evaluated for the ability to alternately stand and sit, stoop, crouch, carry objects, and maintain standing balance. Patients classified at either primary or advanced levels should be evaluated in communication skills, unilateral and bilateral strength and coordination, and overall endurance. Some tests that can be used for measuring hand function and coordination and speed in performance are the Purdue Pegboard,[40] the Bennett Hand Tool Test,[5] and the Minnesota Rate of Manipulation Test.[36]

After the occupational therapist has completed a comprehensive disability evaluation, including overall physical capacity, structured prevocational evaluations can be administered when appropriate. Possible tools for evaluation are the TOWER,[49] Micro-TOWER,[2] and Valpar[51] systems. Although these and other standardized systems of evaluation are extremely useful, the patient with head injury is often unable to follow the exact test procedures. When this happens, it is the evaluating therapist's responsibility to modify and structure the test for optimal success. By doing so the therapist will be unable to use the standardized methods of scoring but instead can describe the patient's performance and how the testing was altered to get a general picture of the patient's skills. It is also advisable that the patient with head injury be evaluated separately from other patient populations. In this way the therapist can provvide special guidance, structure, and support, which the patient may require, without causing the patient embarrassment and frustration.

Driving evaluation

The first step in the driving evaluation of the patient with head injury is a complete disability evaluation. The patient's visual, cognitive, and perceptual status is extremely important, because the task of driving requires complex visual functions and vision influences more than 90% of the decisions of the individual while driving.[3]

In addition to the previously mentioned perceptual tests, it is helpful to use specific visual-perceptual exercises that depict various street scenes and driving situations. These can be indicative of a previous driving style and can demonstrate some problem-solving abilities.

Before the patient attempts the actual driving task, in addition to the complete disability evaluation, the therapist must have a complete patient history and information about previous driving record, medication, seizure history, and the type of car the patient may drive. The Department of Motor Vehicles in California does not have a specific ruling regarding a time period to be seizure free, since one case differs from the next. (Section 2572 of California Administrative Code Title 17 defines the policy of the Department of Motor Vehicles regarding this issue.) Therapists should check for similar regulations in each state.

After the history and disability evaluations are completed and it has been determined that the patient is a candidate for driving, then an "on-the-road" evaluation is initiated. Ideally this should be done by both the occupational therapist and an adaptive driving instructor. The actual driving phase should progress from a quiet residential area to a more congested areas, including highways. It should be noted that there is very little training done at this stage. It is more observational, with minimal instruction given on problem areas to determine the patient's rate of relearning and degree of compensation. Level of alertness and ability to concentrate in varied driving situations are carefully assessed. Conversing with the patient may occur during this assessment to examine abilities to maintain simultaneous attention to the driving task. Although the patient with visual field defect or visual neglect may demonstrate lane positioning difficulties, such an individual is assessed in the potential to compensate with some cuing from the instructor.

Various pieces of adaptive equipment can also be used to improve vehicle control, such as a steering device for one-handed steering, signal level extensions, left foot accelerator, or hand controls, if necessary.

Each problem is assessed separately during the evaluation and in training. Sometimes it may prove to be too early for a client to drive. If so, the client should be seen for a reassessment at a later time.

Although each patient is different, the fundamental principle behind the evaluation and training is the ability to drive defensively. No matter what the major problems are, the patient must be able to compensate for them by planning ahead, maintaining good vehicle control, and driving defensively.

GENERAL PRINCIPLES OF OCCUPATIONAL THERAPY INTERVENTION

The occupational therapist who will be working with patients with head injury must be committed to improving the quality of life for a difficult, complicated, and, more often than not, frustrating patient population. Since there are no clear-cut localized lesions, as seen in stroke patients or patients with spinal cord injury, the therapist is often dealing with unknown long-term expectations for level of recovery and prognosis. Additionally, the therapist will come to realize that each patient has a different set of problems that forces the therapist to use clinical observation and creative problem-solving skills and make unique judgments and treatment plans in each case.

Although there is no set of magic answers to the treatment of patients, certain priniples and guidelines for occupational therapy intervention can be generalized for most patients with head injury. All patients require structured, normalized sensory input from their environment. For example, the semicomatose patient must not remain indefinitely in bed but must be placed upright and positioned to inhibit abnormal muscle tone. As a result, the patient can begin to perceive the environment from the proper perspective and consequently may display an increased level of awareness. During treatment of the patient at the primary level the therapist should assume that at least some information is getting through. In approaching all patients with head injury, the therapist should not relate to them in a condescending manner. They are adults and as such deserve respect.

They will not respond any better if they are yelled at or patronized.

The occupational therapist treating patients with head injury must constantly observe, reevaluate, interpret behavior and response, and alter treatment accordingly. This patient population demands a great deal of flexibility and astute observation skills from the treating therapist.

When establishing a treatment plan, the therapist is faced with a long list of problems regarding the patient's physical, cognitive, perceptual, psychosocial, and ADL functioning. The therapist must place these problems in order of priority and set up realistic goals for the patient. The therapist must analyze the treatment tasks and activities that were chosen and structure the treatment sessions to facilitate maximal function. Treatment strategies for each problem can vary, and one must be chosen that is best for the therapist and the patient. Common impairments already discussed can be treated functionally with table-top activities for perceptual retraining or using sensorimotor approaches. However most therapists who treat this population feel that any combination of methods may be the most beneficial. To minimize patient confusion and agitation and facilitate carry-over of learned tasks, there must be constant communication among team members. If the nursing staff is instructing a patient in one type of transfer and the occupational therapist is instructing in another type, the patient will become confused and show limited progress. A consistent, repetitive, and appropriately structured approach to the patient by all members of the treatment team will yield optimal results.

General aims and methods of treatment

PATIENTS WITH HEAD INJURY AT THE PRIMARY LEVEL. The general aims of treatment for the patient at the primary level are fundamental to increasing the patient's level of response and overall awareness. Input must be well structured, timed, and broken down into simple steps, and enough time must be allowed for a response, since response will often be delayed during this phase of treatment.

Sensory stimulation program. After the

patient has been evaluated, a baseline for treatment is established. Treatment of the patient at the primary level should start as soon as the patient is medically stable. Often the patient may still be comatose or semicomatose. The goal of treatment is to increase the patient's level of awareness by trying to arouse the patient with controlled sensory input. The occupational therapist needs to provide visual, auditory, tactile, olfactory, and gustatory stimulation. In addition to these, it will be important to start getting the patient up in a wheelchair to normalize sensory input through the kinesthetic and labyrinthine systems.

Many patients who appear semicomatose when lying supine in bed suddenly respond when sitting erect in a wheelchair. The therapist is changing the position of the body in space and placing the patient in a position to start to visually perceive the environment. Once the patient is up, the therapist will start to work on gross visual skills, starting first with visual attentiveness. The goal is that the patient attend to an object and people in the environment. Next it will be important to try to elicit visual tracking by using a bright object and sometimes the additional input of an auditory stimulus. The different levels or ways and analysis of the patient's response should be noted according to guidelines given in the preceding section on evaluation.

AUDITORY AND TACTILE STIMULATION. Auditory and tactile stimulation are used to see if the patient can localize the specific stimulus given. Even when working with a comatose patient with head injury, the therapist should talk as if the patient can understand. Even if the patient is not responsive, verbal commands that are clear and simple should be given. Examples of auditory stimuli are ringing a bell, clapping hands, cassette tape recordings of familiar sounds, or the therapist's voice. The goal is to get the patient to localize the sound or respond to it voluntarily. Usually the automatic responses, such as turning the head toward a loud noise, will occur before the voluntary responses. Tactile stimulation includes superficial pain (pinprick), deep pain (pressure on the fingernails),

rubbing an affected limb with cloths of various textures, and stroking body parts while giving verbal cues to increase overall body awareness.

OLFACTORY STIMULATION. Olfactory stimulation may be done with a relatively "pure" olfactory stimulants, such as musk ketone, exaltolide (musk perfume), linalyl acetate, and coumarin (floral). Common odors that are trigeminal nerve stimulants should not be used when evaluating olfactory nerve impairment; these include ammonia, camphor, anisole, menthol, cloves, and peppermint.[22,37] A 30-second delay is recommended between each stimulus. A positive, neutral, or negative response to stimuli and specific observations of behavioral response are noted.

GUSTATORY STIMULATION. Taste stimuli can include sodium chloride solution (salt), sucrose solution (sweet), quinine (bitter), and vinegar or lemon juice (sour).[53] Containers should be coded, and stimuli should be given in a water solution. Salty and sweet stimuli are usually recognized within 2 or 3 seconds. Sour takes a little longer, and recognition of bitter could take as long as 5 seconds.[54] As with olfactory evaluation, the therapist should note positive, negative, or no response and observe specific behaviors.

VESTIBULAR STIMULATION. The use of vestibular stimulation and sensory-integrative therapy for the adult with head injury is essential to the patient's progress. The vestibular system, that is, the vestibular pathways running throughout the brainstem and cerebellum,[4] has a major influence on posture and equilibrium responses. By providing vestibular stimulation via slow spinning, rocking, or inverting the head during developmental activities on the mat, tone in the antigravity muscles can be reduced, followed by muscle cocontraction.

There are three major roles of the vestibular reflexes: (1) the body acts to oppose or compensate for changes in the direction of the force of gravity (negative geotrophic movement); (2) through kinetic action the muscles cocontract to maintain equilibrium and ocular stability during movement; and (3) the vestibular reflex activity helps maintain posture and regulate muscle tone.[4] Therefore the vestibular system

can be used to reduce or inhibit abnormal muscle tone or spasticity, facilitate equilibrium and righting reactions, and enhance gross visual skills. "The maintenance of body equilibrium and posture and appreciation of spatial orientation in everyday life are complex functions involving multiple receptor organs and neural centers in addition to the labyrinths. Visual and proprioceptive reflexes in particular must be integrated with vestibular reflexes to ensure postural stability."[4]

It is important that the occupational therapist use a neurophysiological basis for the treatment of head injury. The goal is not to develop specific or splinter skills or simply learn to compensate for a visual or motor problem but to try to reintegrate or redevelop the impaired function. For example, asking a patient to lift the foot may be ineffective, because it is a cortical level approach to treatment. The problem must be approached from a lower level of the brain for its integration there, if the skill is to be mastered. Rood stated that the cortex is not the highest control center of motor activity. Rather, she believed that treatment should be aimed at the cerebellum and basal ganglia to gain effective and long-lasting results.[41]

An example of vestibular stimulation is through the use of a scooterboard up and down inclines to get an inverted position of the head. It is important to monitor the patient's vital signs closely during mat activities that provide vestibular stimulation, such as when the patient is inverted over a bolster while bearing weight on the upper extremities or is rocking on an equilibrium board. In some cases continued vestibular stimulation can cause seizures, nausea, fatigue, dizziness, blood pressure changes, and associated reactions. The patient's level of awareness is an important factor. The patient at the primary level may not be able to voluntarily give cues to the therapist as to when enough stimulation has been given. The therapist should communicate closely with the physician, nursing staff, and other members of the rehabilitation team before, during, and after vestibular stimulation has been initiated in the treatment program to determine and monitor its effects on the patient.

Rood stated that once cocontraction has been established through the use of the inverted position, stability in space is gained, and this is the basis for kinesthetic figure-ground perception. Kinesthetic figure-ground perception serves as a foundation for orientation of the body in the dimensions of space and time. Once a person can separate figure from ground internally, then the person can begin to deal with the external environment and begin to gain bilateral integration and proper body image.[41]

The use of vestibular stimulation in conjunction with NDT is an important tool for changing and maximizing the patient's response. Ayres stated that the primary cerebellar function is that of an integrating and regulating servomechanism whose action has been frequently linked to motor output.[41] As in any type of sensorimotor stimulation, it is important to demand a motor response, after giving the stimulation, to help facilitate CNS integration. It is important in the treatment of the patient with head injury to provide stimulation in a structured and goal-oriented way and help regulate the response toward the desired outcome. At all times during treatment application, precautions and contraindications to specific treatment modalities should be kept in mind.

The use of vestibular stimulation in the treatment of adults with head injury is important to the patient's recovery. However, this area of treatment is complex and requires specific study and training before it is used. The beginning therapist *should not* attempt to incorporate vestibular stimulation into the treatment program unless supervised by an experienced therapist.

ORAL-BULBAR PROBLEM FACILITATION. Treatment of oral-bulbar problems should follow a sequence similar to that outlined in Table 31-4. The therapist should have special training in appropriate facilitation-inhibition techniques for improving oral-bulbar status before attempting to treat a client. The following section briefly describes some oral-bulbar deficits and a few treatment techniques for these deficits. It is meant to serve as an orientation to these problems. The reader is referred to the references for more detailed information.[17,18,41,53]

The most common problems found in the patient's oral-bulbar status can stem from the presence of abnormal reflexes. The problems can fall into any of the areas outlined in Table 31-4. Reactions in any of these components can be hypoactive and/or hyperactive.

Tongue control in protraction, retraction, and lateralization is a necessary function for moving and locating food in the mouth and stabilizing food for chewing. Tongue position and function should be tested while resting, exercising, feeding, and speaking. At rest, the normal tongue lies symmetrically on the floor of the oral cavity with the tip behind the lower teeth.[17,18] Tongue lateralization can be facilitated by pressure applied to the sides of the tongue with the index finger or a padded seizure stick. This pressure is applied gently but quickly, pushing toward the other side of the mouth. Repeated bilateral application is the most appropriate method.[17,18] The patient can also work on tongue movements by trying to lick jelly or peanut butter off the corners of the mouth.[17]

Sucking occurs before swallowing and may be impaired or absent in the patient with head injury. Sucking can be encouraged by manual vibration or ice used around the mouth area. It should be kept in mind that ice around the mouth, or for that matter any "novel" stimuli, may set off a seizure in the individual with a seizure disorder. As sucking is facilitated, the individual can try to suck on ice Popsicle. As sucking improves, thicker liquids may be used to increase resistance.[18]

Facilitation of swallowing can also be done in conjunction with sucking patterns. The "laryngopharyngeal musculature is digitally vibrated starting under the chin and progressing down to the sternal notch. Stretch pressures are then applied to the same muscles in the direction of their fibers."[18] When working on swallowing, it is best to start with pureed foods, since they are safer and easier to swallow. The therapist may start with a small amount of food on a nonbreakable spoon, depending on how depressed the swallowing ability is.

A hypoactive gag reflex is one of the more dangerous feeding problems encountered, since the patient can aspirate his food. Stimulation of the gag reflex is facilitated by pressure applied with a padded seizure stick two-thirds of the way back on the tongue. Gentle tapping of the tongue, inner cheek surfaces, and the palatopharyngeal arches with a soft toothbrush can also be done. This procedure should be performed with extreme care to avoid damaging intraoral tissues.[18] The patient with a hypoactive gag reflex should never be given chunks of food that require chewing or should never be left unsupervised.

Since the patient's mouth and gums may be hypersensitive, the therapist may start with desensitization techniques, such as rubbing the gums with a cotton swab. Generally, facilitation of a delayed oral mechanism can be done through a quick stretch to the muscle controlling that movement, such as the orbicularis oris for lip control or sucking. The patient's oral reflexes and basic feeding mechanisms must be closely analyzed to set up the most effective treatment program. Once the patient can start to put together in sequence the mechanisms required for feeding, that individual can generally start to take in food of a thicker consistency. Once the patient has progressed from an oral facilitation-inhibition program to a self-feeding program, then the aspects of UE function and feeding devices can be incorporated into the training sessions.

Positioning. With the release of abnormal postural reflexes, abnormal muscle tone, and decreased isolated muscle control, it becomes very difficult for the adult with head injury to control the body or maintain good posture (Fig. 31-1). The parts of the body that are usually affected were previously described in the section on abnormal posturing. The occupational therapist must help inhibit this abnormal muscle tone and facilitate voluntary movement through proper wheelchair positioning. (Fig. 31-2).

PELVIS. Wheelchair positioning should generally be initiated at the pelvis, because poor hip placement will alter head and trunk alignment and influence tone in the extremities. A padded seat roll or a seat insert that is slightly wedged (the downward slope pointing toward the back of the wheelchair) with a recess at the perianal region can be used to flex the hips, if needed. A solid seat wedge placed underneath a stan-

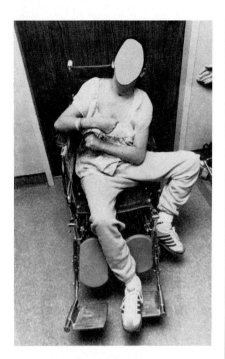

Fig. 31-1. Abnormal reflexes and postural tone result in poor control of posture in wheelchair.

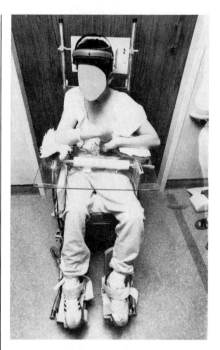

Fig. 31-2. Improved posture and trunk alignment is achieved with positioning devices.

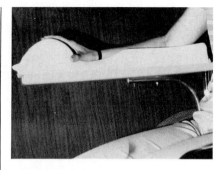

Fig. 31-3. Arm through maintains functional position of the hand.

dard wheelchair cushion can be used to facilitate anterior pelvic tilt. A lumbar roll can also be used, if needed, in conjunction with a solid seat insert. A knee abductor, side wedges, or a seat cushion with the sides slightly sloped toward or away from center, depending on the pattern of abnormal tone, can be beneficial in controlling lateral hip placement.

TRUNK. Once the pelvis is properly positioned, then trunk positioning can follow. Lateral trunk supports or a chest strap can be employed to decrease kyphosis or scoliosis. Generally a three-point pressure system is used for a scoliosis in which the pressure is applied to the apex of the curve on the one side and then distributed to two points above and below the curve on the opposite side. A solid seat (homemade or commercially made) or a firm wheelchair cushion (for example dense cell foam) may be all that is needed to facilitate a more erect posture of the spine. If a great deal of difficulty in positioning the trunk remains, it may prove helpful to recheck hip placement.

LOWER EXTREMITIES. Lower extremity (LE) positioning is done to

break up the abnormal postural patterns or reflexes that affect the lower extremities and trunk, such as excessive plantar flexion and inversion of the ankle. To inhibit this pattern a foot cast with an inhibitive toe plate is used. For an abnormal positive supporting reaction a foot wedge is attached to the wheelchair footrest to equally distribute the weight throughout the foot, taking the pressure off the ball of the foot.

UPPER EXTREMITIES. After good trunk and LE alignment are accomplished, an effort to gain UE control can be made. The application of a lap tray may support the upper extremities for those patients with only a slight problem. The upper extremities should be placed in positions opposite to reflex or spastic patterns. Using cones or straps as needed, the positioning can be done on a lap tray, on a one-half lap tray, or with an arm trough made out of a rain gutter pipe or Kydex (Fig. 31-3).

To position the arms out of a flexor pattern the shoulders must be protracted and slightly flexed with some external rotation, elbows extended, forearms in neutral, and wrists and

fingers extended to submaximal stretch with thumb abducted.[28] A stretch splint or a bivalved elbow cast (Figs. 31-4 to 31-6) can be used in conjunction with the positioning device, such as the arm trough on the wheelchair, to break up the total pattern. It is important to maintain both upper extremities on the same height surface so as not to disturb trunk alignment.

HEAD. Head positioning is one of the most difficult tasks for the therapist. The patient with poor head control usually needs to be in a recliner wheelchair that is in the upright or slightly reclined position. The standard head extension found on the recliner wheelchair is a good base from which to work when making the head device. If possible, without causing resistance, the head should be kept in midline, and the force used to keep the head erect is best applied around the occipital region of the skull and at the forehead. A circumferential (bicycle-helmet shape without the outer helmet) or a U-shaped device that extends around the occipital areas and has a forehead strap can be fabricated out of Kydex and fastened to the headrest bars. The traditional neck collars do not seem to work for head positioning. In head positioning caution must always be taken to avoid overstressing the cervical area or causing excessive resistance to spastic neck musculature. It is essential to look at the placement of the shoulders and upper trunk when working on correct positioning, because they can influence neck muscle tone.

Positioning the patient is a key factor to normalizing sensory input from the environment. Positioning is in concert

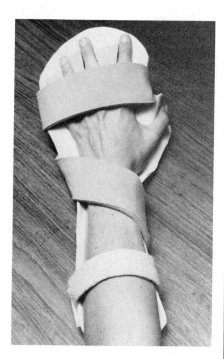

Fig. 31-4. Stretch splint.

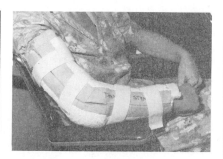

Fig. 31-5. Bivalved elbow cast worn by patient.

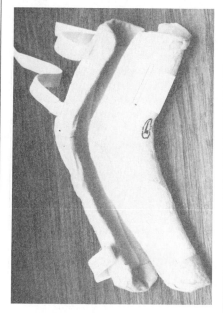

Fig. 31-6. Bivalved elbow cast.

with neurodevelopmental techniques done on the mat and with other sensorimotor integration techniques. Wheelchair positioning is a dynamic process necessitating constant reassessment. The devices should be removed gradually as the patient starts to actively control the body and manipulate more aspects of the environment. A patient may not require the devices while engaged in therapy, such as during wheelchair mobility or when increasing head control. It is critical to make a schedule for the use of the head device. The patient can then learn to control the head and not merely rely on the static device for support. Positioning is done in a graduated sequence; the devices are slowly phased out or made less complicated, offering less support. Positioning needs change rapidly, for example, and a patient discharged from the hospital may no longer require positioning devices a month later. This constant change in status warrants close monitoring, especially after discharge from the hospital.

Functional cognition. One fundamental aspect of functional cognition retraining is to reacquaint the disoriented patient to the environment. With the disorientation, confusion, and decreased

memory that the patient may experience, the therapist must consistently provide structure and familiarize the patient with the environment, self, and current events. A reality orientation group is held every morning at the same time for patients with head injury at the Santa Clara Valley Medical Center and provides a good means to assess improvement. Little benefit will come from such a group unless the patient has sufficient attentiveness, level of awareness, controlled behavior, and potential for carry-over of learning from day to day. As in all treatment techniques used with patients with head injury, the treatment plan must be structured and the patient must start on the next phase of treatment only when it is appropriate and when true benefit can come from it.

Supplementing the reality orientation group, additional group or individual treatment is given for functional cognitive skills. A retraining program developed at Santa Clara Valley Medical Center is administered in learning modules and sequenced by the level of skill required to complete a task.

Splinting and casting. Splinting and casting for the spastic upper or lower extremities are effective means of reducing muscle tone, preventing contractures, increasing ROM and coordination, and complementing mat activities. The most frequently used splints and casts for the upper extremity are the elbow cast (Fig. 31-5), stretch splint, stretch splint-cast, cock-up splint, and cock-up cast. For the lower extremities the posterior knee shell, foot splint, foot cast, and inhibitive foot-toe plate are used. The elbow cast is usually fabricated to break up an upper extremity flexor pattern and increase ROM. Serial casting of the elbow should be done every 24 to 48 hours to progressively stretch out the flexor muscles.

The stretch splint is used to break up the UE flexor pattern by placing wrist and fingers in maximal extension with the thumb radially abducted (Fig. 31-4). A stretch splint can also be used during weight-bearing activities, such as mat work or bed mobility. Maintained stretch accomplished through splinting or casting changes the muscle bias and therefore facilitates muscle relaxation.[50] If a patient's wrist and finger flexors are so tight that ROM is severely limited, the therapist may begin with a resting hand splint that is changed or adjusted for progressive stretching. For cases of severe spasticity a bivalved stretch splint-cast was developed at Santa Clara Valley Medical Center to provide equal pressure over the dorsal and volar surfaces to minimize skin breakdown and maintain a fuller static stretch. *Bivalved* means that a cast is sawed in half and the edges are lined with moleskin so that it may be strapped on and taken off easily at any time (Fig. 31-6).

Once selective hand movements have started to develop, a cock-up splint or cast can be used to promote hand skills, such as prehension. A cock-up splint is also useful in cases where ataxia or intention tremors are present at the wrist.

It has a stabilizing effect, thus giving finer motor control.

LE splinting or casting is usually done to break up an extensor pattern or a positive support reaction. The goal is to extend the knee and place the ankle in midline with the foot dorsiflexed to neutral. In cases where there is severe plantar flexion, serial casting should be used in conjunction with foot wedges to distribute the weight equally from the ball of the foot to the heel. LE casts may also be bivalved.

It is important to establish a splint schedule for the nursing staff to follow, with regular splint checks for any potential pressure areas. In cases of severe spasticity the initial splint schedule may only be 2 hours on and 2 hours off until the patient can tolerate it for longer periods. The patient should never be locked up in the splints, casts, or positioning devices all the time, because they are only static tools to help the patient become more mobile. Splinting and casting for patients with head injury and severe spasticity must at all times be done in a progression, from initially breaking up the abnormal pattern to eventually aiding the individual to improved UE function and coordination.

Communication systems. As a result of head trauma, there may be severe language impairment (Chapter 30) and inability to communicate.[21,24] Communication involves many different modalities, such as speech, writing, and sign language. There are several communication systems available to the adult with head injury to compensate for nonfunctional speech.

Communication systems range from simple to complex. There are three major approaches to consider when developing a nonoral communication system: direct selection, scanning, and encoding.[45] By direct selection a patient would directly select the desired choice. For example, the patient might directly select pictures or letters to spell a word on a communication board. The occupational therapist must work closely with the speech pathologist in adapting the communication system to allow for a maximal response based on perceptual and motor abilities.

When a scanning system is used, the patient signals when a desired choice is present or directs an indicator toward the choice.[45] Various control systems, such as the puff and sip mechanism, may be adapted to be a scanner system so that a light scans across a row of letters or symbols until the desired choice is reached. At that time the patient signals the light to stop.

The third kind of system is the encoding system in which the patient indicates a choice by a code of input symbols.[45]

The inability to communicate needs to others is one of the most frustrating problems that the adult with head injury faces. It is extremely important for the therapist to assess the patient's level of awareness, gross visual skills, visual perception, and motor status before working on adapting a communication system. The communication system allows the patient to interact again with the environment and should be geared to the patient's level of function. For example, a patient who could respond yes and no to questions by nodding may not be able to do so until good head control is developed or proper head positioning is provided.

It is essential that the therapist uses good observational skills along with the evaluation to help solve the communication problem. There was one dramatic example of a patient examined at Santa Clara Valley Medical Center 5 years after the head injury occurred who had severe motor impairment involving his whole body, except for his head. He did not orally communicate nor interact with his environment at all on admission because of severe motor deficits. A mouth stick set was fabricated for the patient, and he was able to type, pick up small objects, draw, and engage in avocational activities. He learned to type, and the first thing he wrote was that he loved his wife. It cannot be emphasized enough that the potential for communication may be lying dormant within the patient and can be used, if only it can be tapped.

PATIENTS WITH HEAD INJURY AT THE ADVANCED LEVEL. The patient at the advanced level has progressed to a point to tolerate formal evaluations and full treatment sessions. Obviously the evaluation results, specific to each patient, will outline which areas are priorities for treatment. Usually the patient will have some degree of deficit in all major categories. The following is a description of the areas that may require treatment and the general principles of occupational therapy interventions for these.

Self-care. When the patient begins to enter a more advanced stage, the therapist can begin to analyze the patient's ability to manipulate and effectively use familiar objects. With this in mind, light hygiene and early dressing activities can be initiated. Not only is this an effective means of identifying possible difficulty in motor planning, but it is also an avenue to increase the patient's functional independence and improve body image.

Because of the patient's cognitive status, hygiene or dressing activities must be broken down into segments and done repetitively in the same way. Depending on the patient's balance and total body function, training in dressing should progress from in bed to the wheelchair to the bed edge to standing. During training it is necessary to decide which techniques to use. The therapist must be aware of techniques that increase functional independence but cause the reinforcement of abnormal motor patterns. The therapist must constantly assess the techniques at each stage in recovery with other team members and decide if the goal is normalization or compensation. For example, teaching the patient to place the unaffected leg under the affected leg to enable removing the legs from the bed improves functional independence but reinforces an abnormal pattern of movement. Incorporation of normal movement patterns in ADL is important to the patient's recovery. Specific techniques for this are described in Chapter 16.

Feeding. To reinforce the neuromuscular facilitation techniques used in oral-bulbar training and increase the patient's functional independence, training in feeding is initiated when appropriate. There are numerous factors to consider when feeding the patient who has CNS dysfunction. The following are just suggestions that will assist in feeding patients with a few specific types of impairments. The reader is referred to the references for additional resources.

The patient should be upright with head and neck in the neutral position or slightly flexed. A small spoon and small amounts of food should be used; a plastic spoon should not be used with patients who have a bite reflex. The spoon is removed as soon as lip closure has occurred, being careful to avoid scraping the teeth. If the patient with a bite reflex clamps down on the spoon, no attempt should be made to pry the mouth open. The therapist must wait until the patient relaxes or push up on the jaw to facilitate opening. Swallowing must occur before presenting the next bite.

When feeding the patient who has tongue thrust or lack of lateralization of the tongue, food should be deposited in the corners of the mouth. Place the food in the molar region of the mouth, applying pressure on the tongue as the food is deposited. As the patient improves with increasing lateralization and decreasing thrust, food can be placed in the more frontal, midposition of the tongue.

Milk and sweet fluids will increase the flow of saliva; therefore when working with the patient who has difficulty swallowing secretions, liquids such as beef broth are preferred, because they will thin the saliva.

Mobility. Mobility training can be subdivided into bed mobility and transfer training, including functional ambulation and wheelchair mobility.

When working on *bed mobility* the occupational therapist must aim for improving independence while using the sensorimotor approaches to improve sensory and motor function. It is of little benefit to simply teach the patient to compensate for a loss of function or develop splinter skills. The bed mobility skills that the patient with head injury may need to work on include scooting in supine position, rolling, bridging, moving from supine to sitting position, long leg sitting, sitting over the bed edge, and sitting balance.

The occupational therapist must have a good theoretical knowledge of treatment to reduce spasticity, for example, in the upper extremities, to incorporate this goal into a gross motor activity such as bed mobility. The following example of using a Bobath (NDT) technique when working with the patient

sitting over the edge of the bed is provided to clarify the application of theory to practice. The affected spastic arm and hand are extended, outwardly rotated, and used for support. It is important to decrease flexor spasticity and use protective extension to prevent falling. The shoulder girdle should be held back. Wrist and fingers should be extended with thumb abducted. A stretch splint is good for this bed mobility activity. It is important to keep the shoulder girdle level and practice weight shifts from side to side with the upper extremities back slightly behind the patient. Joint approximation can be given to the shoulder in this position, or the patient can bear weight on an elbow by leaning on it to the side. The patient should learn how to go from supine to sitting position by pushing up from the affected elbow, with the therapist applying approximation to reduce muscle tone and ultimately improve function.[7]

Transfer training has been described in Chapter 18. Cognitive, perceptual, and physical status will affect the type of transfer used in training. Memory and limited carry-over mandate that training be consistent in type and sequence among all staff members treating the patient. When the patient has begun to master the mechanics and sequence of the bed-to-chair transfer, toilet, bathtub, and car transfers can be initiated. At this stage the therapist becomes involved with evaluating the need for equipment. Bathroom dimensions and layouts are discussed with the family, and a home visit is planned. Architectural barriers, which are a constant issue for the wheelchair-bound individual, are considered at this time. It is preferable, if possible, that transfers be practiced moving in either direction. Often a patient becomes proficient in a transfer with an approach to one side and is dismayed when entering a public bathroom only to discover that the particular approach is not possible. An additional reason for encouraging transfers to both sides is that by doing so, more normal sensory input is provided by encouraging the patient to bear weight on the affected leg and use the trunk muscles of the affected side. Thus the therapist is encouraging normalization of tone and movement, rather than compensation.

Bathtub transfers are practiced with both a dry surface and the more realistic wet surface. Generally it is safer to have the patient in the bathtub before filling it with water. On the same note the water should be emptied, and the patient should be dry before attempting to get out of the bathtub. Bathtub mats can aid in safety by making the bathtub surface less slick. There is a variety of bathtub, shower, and toilet equipment that is commercially available. Although this equipment is often necessary, the therapist should remember that the ultimate goal is to eliminate the need for as much equipment as possible without creating a safety hazard for the patient or family.

The car transfer is one of the most important transfers to the patient. Patient motivation for this area is rarely a problem, because this is the patient's ticket out for a day or a weekend. The patient and an appropriate family member should be cleared by the occupational therapist in car transfers before the patient is allowed out on a weekend pass. This depends on the patient's *functional* level and may take more than one session for the necessary arrangements, which should be made in advance. Teaching the family member car transfers is only one of the many areas with which the therapist and family are involved. This ongoing communication will alleviate many of the family's and patient's fears and lessen the chance of failure during the initial visits home.

Although ideally not a common occurrence, the patient may at some time fall to the floor. It is therefore necessary that the occupational therapist instruct the patient and his family in wheelchair mobility techniques, for example, getting from the floor back to the wheelchair. The patient will need sufficient gross motor skills and balance to be able to accomplish this task. Generally, if lying on the side, the patient will need to get in the all fours or kneeling position. The patient can use the wheelchair, if stabilized, or a sturdy piece of furniture to assist. Next the patient must prop both elbows on the seat of the wheelchair and bring one or both legs into position as if to stand.

Then, pushing up into a bent stand–pivot position, the patient will reach for an armrest, pivot, and sit. Floor-to-wheelchair transfers can only be done with a patient who is advanced in motor skills. Any abnormal patterns that the patient might have should be kept in mind. The method described is only one general technique, and each transfer should be worked out for the individual's unique set of problems and assets.

UE function. The types of motor impairment present in the patient with head injury are numerous. Weakness, synergistic movement, spasticity, rigidity, ataxia, primitive reflexes, and impaired sensation affect the patient's ability to perform UE activities. Treatment techniques for the patient with synergistic movements, spasticity, or the presence of primitive reflexes are described. The general aims of treatment for the upper extremity of the primary-level patient and the CVA patient were presented earlier.

The key to designing a treatment program that increases UE function is the analysis of normal movement. The amount of UE selective control a patient displays usually relates closely to the degree of tone and postural reflexes present, which affect the head, trunk, and lower extremities. For example, normalization of tone in the trunk before working with the upper extremity often yields optimal results. Although the UE program for each patient with head injury is individualized the common principles of treatment are to analyze the degree of selective control that is present and inhibit and/or facilitate specific movements or combinations of movements as appropriate (for example, to decrease abnormal movement patterns and subsequently facilitate normal movement). For example, to initiate beginning hand function the patient must have the ability for controlled alternating flexion and extension of the fingers. These controlled alternating movements will facilitate a light controlled grasp and release rather than the uncontrolled primitive grasp usually seen.

During the treatment session the therapist is continually evaluating the patient's response and altering techniques, depending on the patient's response. The therapist must observe and feel for the patient's reaction to the treatment. Specific modalities and techniques used to obtain normal upper extremity movement are limited only by the therapist's creativity.

Ataxia is a common and frustrating problem that often develops early, persists into the late rehabilitation phase, and may remain permanently. Although various treatment methods have been tried, it is difficult to assess their ultimate long-term value. Weighting of body parts and use of resistive activities appear to improve control during performance of tasks but show inconsistent carry-over of control when the weights are removed. When applying weights to the patient, the therapist must carefully evaluate at which joint or joints the tremor originates. Applying weights to a patient's wrists when the tremor originates in the trunk or shoulder is ineffective. The amount of weight applied will also affect results. Generally 2 to 2½ pounds (0.91 to 1.14 kg) is the optimal weight that can be applied without causing additional tremor. Resistive bracing, in which resistance is applied at each joint throughout the ROM, has been tried at Santa Clara Valley Medical Center with some success. By adding continued resistance throughout the ROM, muscle groups are forced into cocontraction, and therefore tremor decreases. Unfortunately, bracing is expensive and often is not cosmetically acceptable to the patient.

Perceptual training.[42] Most occupational therapy literature on the treatment of cognitive-perceptual-motor dysfunction pertains to remediation of these deficits in adults with CVA and children. The following four treatment approaches, however, can be applied to the treatment of cognitive-perceptual-motor deficits in adult patients with head injury:

1. Neurodevelopmental or sensorimotor[1,44]
2. Transfer of training[44]
3. Behavioral or social
4. Functional[44]

The sensorimotor approach is based on neurophysiological and developmental principles. A major assumption of this approach is that controlled sensory input followed by facilitation and demand of a specific motor response increases integration of the sensorimotor functions of the brain.[1] The premise of the NDT approach is the facilitation of more normal movement patterns on a subcortical-automatic level to gain the desired motor response or integration. Neurodevelopmental principles can be applied to both the performance of functional activities and the development of perceptual skills, since most of the patient's performance requires movement as part of the response. The assistance given by the therapist in the NDT approach is primarily manual rather than by verbal command, thus putting less stress on the patient and encouraging a more automatic response.

The transfer of training approach[44] assumes that repeated practice of a perceptual training task will affect the patient's performance on similar tasks. For example, practice in doing simple shape matching during a tabletop or computer activity may carry over to performance skills requiring similar perceptual skills, such as matching clothing shape to body parts. However, unless closely monitored and structured, this may result in the development of splinter skills that are isolated and have no functional carry-over.

Behavioral techniques are an integral part of the perceptual training program. Some factors that lead to behavioral problems in patients with head injury are fatigue, low frustration tolerance, sensory overloading, lack of control of the environment, defective cognitive processing, perseveration, lack of insight, and poor memory. A classical conditioning approach can be used in which the therapist pairs a neutral stimulus with the stimulus that elicits the desired response. For example, a patient refused to get out of bed and became extremely agitated when anyone tried to get the patient up and take the individual to the clinic for therapy. As a solution, the rehabilitation team started to provide meals for the patient only in the therapy clinic. The original problem of the refusal to get out of bed was resolved in 5 days. A system of token economy or positive reinforcement can also be incorporated into the perceptual training program.

The last major approach to the treatment of perceptual deficits is the functional approach. In this approach there is repetitive practice of specific functional skills, such as transferring from a wheelchair, cooking a meal, or making change. The functional approach can include compensatory training that involves making the patient aware of the problem and teaching the patient to work with the deficit. It can also involve adaptation of the environment to compensate for the patient's symptoms, or it can involve adaptation of the patient's behavior. In other words, the patient can formulate a new scheme or strategy for performing the task.

Probably the best way to handle functional treatment is to incorporate NDT, transfer of training, and behavioral approaches into the process. For example, when working on dressing or transfer skills, the patient can also be prompted to improve sequencing, following directions, and memory for steps of the task and to decrease visual spatial neglect. The incorporation of kinesthetic, proprioceptive, visual, and tactile information through total body movement and weight bearing can facilitate the development of visual discrimination skills, for example, position in space and depth perception.

The use of computers in cognitive-perceptual training programs has become popular in recent years. The computer primarily uses visual and auditory stimulation and feedback. It does not provide adequate tactile and proprioceptive stimulation, which are vital sensory stimuli for training. Computers have an integral place in cognitive-perceptual training but should be used in conjunction with the approaches described previously.

There are no prescribed formulas for the treatment of perceptual deficits associated with head injury. Rather, the therapist must work to improve specific skills on an individual basis and subsequently combine these skills for application in functional situations. In this way learning is carried over from treatment to the real environment.

Home management. As the patient gains increased skills and independence in dressing, feeding, and functional mobility, treatment is expanded to include kitchen and homemaking tasks. As in other areas of treatment, kitchen training is graded to suit the patient's progress. Beginning tasks might include

simple sandwich preparation. Depending on the patient's cognitive status, the therapist may place all food items on the table and have the patient verbally review the task before doing it for the first time. At the end of the session the following day's activities can be discussed. A session such as this requires simple sequencing, organizing, and memory for the task. As the patient improves, more demands are made until the patient reaches the final stages in the progression. Then the patient should be able to plan and cook a complete meal with no verbal cuing or structure given by the therapist.

Total body function and endurance are also important aspects of kitchen activities. Standing endurance and ability for bending to low shelves or reaching for high shelves are measured. Safety becomes a key issue in this setting. The patient's judgment in handling sharp utensils and using the stove can become key issues in selecting a living place after discharge.

Homemaking activities can include light housekeeping, such as dusting, vacuuming, or making the bed. As in other functional training, energy conservation and work simplification are stressed.

Child care is an area of treatment that is often overlooked. Family involvement is vital if a woman is to return effectively to her role as wife and mother. Sensory overload is a common problem that must be handled. Most people would agree it is a problem even for the mother who has not sustained a head injury. One-handed diapering techniques or commercially available strollers, cribs, and child care equipment that can be handled more easily by the handicapped woman are examples of the areas that might be covered by occupational therapy services.

Community reintegration. Often in the rehabilitation process the patient with the head injury reaches a maximal level of independence in the protected and structured atmosphere of the hospital and, when discharged into the community, is faced with people, situations, and problems that have not yet been encountered and resolved. It is therefore vital that the occupational therapist initiate a community reintegration program before discharge. The training can

begin with the basic skills involved in a simple purchase, that is, handling money or communicating needs. As the patient's cognitive, perceptual, and physical status changes, the therapist can help the patient progress to a more demanding activity or setting. Table 31-5 illustrates sample settings and the skills demanded for these. The transition of treatment from an initial setting, such as a hospital gift shop to a community store, not only demands skills in the areas listed but also presents new psychosocial issues with which the patient must deal. It is often of benefit for an appropriate family member to accompany the therapist and patient on a community trip. The family member can gain increased insight into the individual's level of functioning and into how the outside world views the disability. The therapist must be aware of the patient's and family's attitudes toward a community reintegration program. The therapist may become frustrated when a cooperative patient suddenly refuses to participate in the program. The patient may not feel ready for the outside world to view the handicap, and it is the therapist's responsibility to give the patient the support and guidance needed for the easiest transition possible.

Prevocational training and placement. Vocational training and placement of the patient with head injury are extended processes that require the involvement of an occupational therapist, vocational evaluator, and other allied health professionals usually under the coordination of a vocational counselor. Each professional brings to the case a different expertise that is essential to successful job placement. Many patients with head injury are not immediately ready for sheltered workshop or competitive employment, therefore it may be more appropriate for them to be involved in an adapted learning program at a local university or community college. Regular follow-up and reevaluation of the patient by the therapist and counselor will ensure changes in placement as the patient improves. When assessing different alternatives for placement, it should be considered that workshops geared for mentally retarded persons are often not the best choice for patients with head injury. They are unable to identify with retarded persons, and the workshop staff is usually not trained to deal with the memory, cognitive, and behavioral problems that are specific to head injury.

One of the most exciting ways for

occupational therapist to use problem-solving skills is environmental and equipment modification at the patient's job site. Employers are extremely receptive and pleased when the employee with head injury is no longer a liability

but is a competitive, successful employee.

Family training and follow-up. The participation of the family members in the recuperation of the patient with head injury is extremely important. Frequently, the familiar faces of the patient's relatives are among the first that the patient is able to remember when coming out of coma. Education of family members starts from the first time the professional meets them; however, the information provided should be given in gradual steps.

Family involvement in treatment should occur throughout the patient's rehabilitation. Constant communication between the therapist and the patient's family aids in appropriate follow-through of the newly acquired skills the patient has learned. Constant communication also provides feedback to the therapist and enables the family to show the unique ways they solve a given problem. This often happens after a patient has been home and returns for an assessment or for outpatient therapy. The family often discovers methods the therapist has never considered. For example, because of memory loss a patient repeatedly asked the same questions, such as, "When do I eat?" Once the patient was discharged, the family constructed a set of index cards with the frequently asked questions and their answers and kept them on the patient's lap tray. In a very short period of time the patient stopped asking the questions.

Table 31-5
Community reintegration program

Setting	Skills demanded
Vending machines	Wheelchair mobility
	Physical handling of money
	Simple computation
	Decision making
Hospital gift shop	*Above skills plus:*
	Use of elevators
	Orientation to location in hospital
	Social skills—communication of needs
	Exchanging money
Hospital cafeteria	*Above skills plus:*
	Mobility in crowds
	Handling food
	Eating etiquette
	Social behavior in groups
Fast-food restaurant	*Above skills plus:*
	Architectural barriers
	Safety crossing streets
	Use of telephone
Drug store	*Above skills plus:*
	More complex money management
	Orientation to complex spaces (store and parking lot)
Grocery store	*Above skills plus:*
	Nutrition
	Long-term planning
Shopping center (department store)	*Above skills plus:*
	Greater complexity in physical, perceptual, cognitive, and social skills

Based on a program developed at Santa Clara Valley Medical Center, San Jose, Calif.

Sample treatment plan

Case study

K.B. is a 24-year-old male who sustained a gunshot wound to the head during an altercation 4 months ago. The bullet entered the left occipital area and traversed to the right temporal-parietal area. An emergency craniotomy and decompression were performed 1 week later. Craniotomy and debridement with removal of devitalized brain tissue, foreign bodies, and bone chips were performed 3 weeks after the injury.

K.B. was living in a city about 30 miles from the rehabilitation facility and had been married for 4 years. Presently he is divorced. He has a high school education and has worked as a bricklayer for 6 years. When initially interviewed by the occupational therapist, he stated that he would be returning to work "in a couple of weeks."

K.B. was referred to occupational therapy for evaluation and appropriate treatment to facilitate maximal function and independence.

TREATMENT PLAN

A. Statistical data.
   1. Name: K.B.
      Age: 24
      Diagnosis: Traumatic injury to the head
      Disability: Motor, sensory-perceptual-cognitive dysfunction
   2. Treatment aims as stated in the referral:

Evaluation
Facilitate maximal function and independence
B. Other services.
Physical therapy: Ambulation, mat mobility, strengthening exercises
Nursing: Nursing care, reality orientation
Speech: Cognitive skills, language retraining
Psychology: Intelligence, memory testing
Social service: Counseling, community placement, financial arrangements
Educational program: Academic skills retraining

Sample treatment plan—cont'd

C. OT evaluation.

ROM: Measure
Spasticity: Test, observe
Abnormal movement: Test, observe
Selective movement: Test
Sensation: Test
Hand function: Test
Perceptual-motor skills: Test, observe
Self-care, mobility: Test, observe
Functional cognitive skills: Test, observe
Behavior: Observe
Home management: Test, observe
Community skills: Test, observe
Prevocational: Test, observe
Driving evaluation: Test, observe
Physical capacities: Test, observe

D. Results of evaluation.

1. Evaluation data.
   a. Physical resources.
      (1) Strength: There is isolated motion and normal strength in the right upper extremity. In the left upper extremity there is a mild flexor pattern, with moderate spasticity in horizontal adduction, elbow extension, pronation, and finger flexion. Minimal spasticity is present in the wrist and elbow flexors.
      (2) Selective movement: With the left upper extremity the patient is able to perform the following selective movements with difficulty: shoulder flexion to 90°, hand behind back, and hand to opposite shoulder. Incomplete motion is possible when performing hand behind head and wrist flexion and extension with the elbow relaxed.
      (3) ROM: ROM is within normal limits for both upper extremities.
      (4) Hand function: The right hand functions normally. With the left hand the patient can perform gross grasp and lateral prehension, but these are weak. The patient is unable to put the prehension patterns to functional use. He is also unable to perform any fine manipulative skills with the left hand.
   b. Sensory-perceptual functions. All sensory modalities are intact in the right upper extremity. In the left upper extremity there is impairment of superficial pain (pinprick) sensation. Proprioception and stereognosis in the left upper extremity are absent. Visual attentiveness is intact. Visual scanning is impaired, that is, slow, jerky, and decreased to the left. There is no apparent left homonymous hemianopsia or neglect of the left visual field, but it is difficult to assess. There is a severe impairment in praxis, visual figure-ground perception, and perception of position in space. There is an impairment in right-left discrimination, body scheme, and three-dimensional spatial orientation. There is also a unilateral neglect of the left side of the body.
   c. Cognitive functions. K.B. is generally cooperative, in spite of his difficulty in following simple commands. Impaired safety awareness, judgment, and limited insight into his disability are apparent. He becomes extremely frustrated when unable to perform simple tasks.
   d. Functional skills.
      (1) Self-care: K.B. requires minimal physical assistance for all dressing, hygiene, and grooming activities. He has a severe dressing apraxia, that is, he would put on his shirt upside down or backwards or put his shoes on the wrong foot, unless given cues by the therapist. He requires assistance with all fastenings. For feeding he requires assistance for opening containers and cutting meat.
      (2) Transfer skills: Bed, chair, and toilet transfers require moderate physical assistance and verbal cues to compensate for apraxia, difficulty with sequencing the steps of the transfer, and decreased perception of position in space.
      (3) Bed mobility: Moderate physical assistance and verbal cues are required for rolling over, coming to sitting from supine position, scooting, and managing legs. The cues are required because of decreased motor planning skill (praxis) and impaired perception of position in space.
      (4) Wheelchair mobility: The patient is dependent for wheelchair propulsion and management of footrests and armrests because of sensory dysfunction, decreased coordination of the left arm, and perceptual-motor impairments just outlined.

2. Problem identification.
   a. Self-care dependence
   b. Dependence for functional mobility transfers, that is, bed mobility and wheelchair management
   c. Sensory impairments
   d. Lack of selective control of the left upper extremity
   e. Decreased hand function on left side
   f. Deficit in postural mechanism and equilibrium
   g. Visual perceptual dysfunction
   h. Apraxia
   i. Body scheme disorder
   j. Cognitive deficits

3. Assets.
   a. Good function of right upper extremity
   b. Good motivation
   c. Intact memory
   d. Supportive family
   e. Supportive employer and possibility for reemployment
   f. Intact functional communication skills

Continued.

Sample treatment plan—cont'd

E Problem	F Specific OT objectives	G Methods used to meet objectives	H Gradation of treatment
a	Through appropriate cues, structure, and training independence for dressing and hygiene will be increased	Daily practice in dressing and hygiene activities with structure and cues from therapist Sensory stimulation before dressing activities to increase awareness of left side Try use of a mirror for visual feedback of performance Avoid print garments to compensate for visual figure-ground deficit	Increase number of activities; decrease structure and cues as independence increases
b	Through training in hemiplegia transfer techniques, patient will perform them with increased independence, until verbal cues from therapist are no longer required	Daily training in bed, chair, and toilet transfer techniques Use consistent type and sequence of transfer Patient is to explain each step of the transfer before it is performed, until verbal cues from the therapist are no longer required	Progress to bathtub and car transfers Decrease verbal cuing and structure as there is improvement
	Through NDT training independence in bed mobility will increase	Bed mobility training Rolling side to side Supine to sitting position Sitting to supine position Sitting on edge of bed NDT (Bobath) techniques to normalize sensory input and inhibit abnormal movement patterns Weight bearing on affected arm Reflex-inhibiting patterns Equilibrium reactions in sitting	Decrease supervision, assistance, and verbal cues Decrease use of techniques of facilitation and inhibition
	Ability to use a wheelchair will improve so that patient can use the chair independently in the hospital ward	Wheelchair propulsion practice, bilateral method	Functional ambulation on ward
c	Through sensory stimulation awareness of the left upper extremity will be increased	Self-applied cutaneous stimulation with rough washcloth and application of cream to left upper extremity Weight bearing activities for increased proprioceptive input Tactile box for identification of common objects, using manual form perception without the aid of vision	
d	Ability to perform controlled, selective movement of the left upper extremity will be increased	Unilateral and bilateral reaching in all planes incorporated in coordination activities Weight bearing on left upper extremity while performing activities with right upper extremity during kitchen and other functional activities	
e	Through activities, training, and practice, function of the left hand will improve so that the patient uses it spontaneously in bilateral activities	Use of alternating distal and proximal stabilizing techniques Card turning Grasp and release of blocks Manipulative activities—paper collation, opening jars, and containers	Grade from large to small Grade gross to fine

Sample treatment plan—cont'd

E Problem	F Specific OT objectives	G Methods used to meet objectives	H Gradation of treatment
f	Through exercises and activities that involve the total body the patient's postural integration, equilibrium, and protective reactions will improve	Bending Reaching Functional ambulation Obstacle courses made with chairs and tables to maneuver during ambulation Scooterboard activities—prone lying, push off walls, up or down inclines	
g	Through appropriate activities and supervised practice the patient's visual-perceptual deficits, that is, visual scanning, visual figure-ground, and position in space, will decline	Using magazine pages have client scan from left to right and cross out a given letter each time it appears in every line Spread out playing cards in random order, call out a card, and have patient select it from the group In a real or simulated market have patient select specific items from among others on the shelves Practice finding items in a cluttered drawer Figure-ground tabletop perceptual activities using cards or pictures with hidden figures to be identified Leather craft	
h	During performance of activities to meet objectivities outline above, motor planning skill will be improved	Scooterboard activities Structuring tasks Obstacle course All functional tasks Practice imitation of postures	
i	Given activities and sensory stimulation, body scheme awareness will increase	Use a mirror when performing self-care, craft, and tabletop exercises for visual feedback Cutaneous and proprioceptive sensory stimulation to the left arm Gross motor activities—rolling, supine, sitting	
j	Through structure, support, supervision, and education functional cognition will improve ability to follow directions, insight into deficits, frustration tolerance, and ability to recognize and correct errors	Educate patient about his deficits through discussion and pointing out problems as they occur Videotape patient's performance, play back, and discuss evidence of cognitive problems Support patient when he is frustrated Structure treatment session and supervise to minimize frustration and aid in compensating for cognitive deficits	Reduce structure and supervision

I. **Special equipment.**
   1. Ambulation aids.
      Wheelchair: Primary mobility
      Walker: Early ambulation
   2. Splints
      None required
   3. Assistive devices.
      None required

REVIEW QUESTIONS

1. Describe what is meant by acceleration and deceleration injuries.
2. When is a gastrostomy performed?
3. Describe the major clinical signs of the primary and advanced levels in recovery from head injury.
4. What are the three major assessment areas of the Glasgow Coma Scale?
5. Name five major physical impairments that may be present in the patient with head injury.
6. What are the seven most common primitive reflexes present in the patient with head injury? How does each one function?
7. Define "spasticity" and "ataxia."
8. How does the patient's cognitive status affect the patient's function?
9. Define the following: visual neglect, hemianopsia, praxis, constructional praxis, body scheme, figure-ground, and position in space.
10. List four psychosocial variables that will influence the patient's behavior.
11. What are the major clinical areas that will affect function?
12. Which areas are covered in the primary-level evaluation?
13. How are gross visual skills evaluated?
14. What is included in a physical capacity evaluation?
15. What type of approach do all patients with head injury require?
16. Give examples of auditory, visual, and olfactory stimulation.
17. Describe the most common oral-bulbar problems seen in patients with head injury and the methods of intervention for these problems.
18. Where should the therapist start with wheelchair positioning? Why?
19. What are some examples of methods of reality orientation?
20. What would be the splinting-casting plan for the patient with decorticate posturing?
21. When in the treatment progression are kitchen activities appropriate?
22. How can the Bobath theory of treatment be incorporated in bed mobility tasks?
23. What are the three treatment approaches to perceptual impairment?

REFERENCES

1. Ayres, A.J.: Sensory integration and learning disorders, Los Angeles, 1972, Western Psychological Services.
2. Backman, M.E.: The development of the Micro-TOWER, New York, 1977, I.C.D. Rehabilitation and Research Center.
3. Ballard, S.S., and Knoll, H.A., editors: The visual factors in automobile driving, National Research Council, Pub. No. 574, Washington, D.C., 1958, National Academy of Sciences.
4. Baloh, R.W., and Honrubia, V.: Clinical neurophysiology of the vestibular system, Philadelphia, 1979, F.A. Davis Co.
5. Bennett, G.K.: Hand tool dexterity test, manual of directions, New York, 1965, Psychological Corp.
6. Bliss, C.K.: Semantography (Blissymbolics), ed. 2, Sydney, Australia, 1965, Semantography (Blissymbolics) Publications.
7. Bobath, B.: Adult hemiplegia: evaluation and treatment, London, 1978, William Heinemann Medical Books, Ltd.
8. Brain, L., and Walton, J.N.: Brain's diseases of the nervous system, ed. 7, New York, 1969, Oxford University Press, Inc.
9. Bricolo, A., et al.: Decerebrate rigidity in acute head injury, J. Neurosurg. 47:680, 1977.
10. Brown, J.: Aphasia, apraxia and agnosia: clinical and theoretical aspects, Springfield, Ill., 1972, Charles C Thomas, Publisher.
11. Bruce, D., Gennarelli, T., and Langfitt, T.: Resuscitation from coma due to head injury, Crit. Care Med. 6:254, 1978.
12. Carroll, D.: A quantitative test of upper extremity function, J. Chron. Dis. 18:479, 1965.
13. Cave, E., Burke, J.F., and Boyd, R.J.: Trauma management, Chicago, 1974, Year Book Medical Publishers, Inc.
14. Caveness, W.: Incidence of craniocerebral trauma in the United States with trends from 1970 to 1975, Adv. Neurol. 22:1, 1979.
15. Chusid, J.G.: Correlative neuroanatomy and functional neurology, ed. 15, Los Altos, Calif., 1973, Lange Medical Publications.
16. Denny-Brown, D.: The nature of apraxia, J. Nerv. Ment. Dis. 126:9, 1958.

17. Farber, S.: Sensorimotor evaluation and treatment procedures for allied health personnel, 1974, Indiana University Foundation.
18. Farber, S.: Neurorehabilitation: a multisensory approach, Philadelphia, 1982, W.B. Saunders Co.
19. Gatz, A.J.: Manter's essentials of clinical neuroanatomy and neurophysiology, ed. 4, Philadelphia, 1970, F.A. Davis Co.
20. Geschwind, N.: Disconnexion syndromes in animals and man, Brain 88:237, 1965.
21. Gilroy, J., and Meyer, J.S.: Medical neurology, New York, 1969, Macmillan, Inc.
22. Gordan, C.: Practical approach to the loss of smell, Am. Fam. Physician 26:192, 1982.
23. Groher, M.: Language and memory disorders following closed head trauma, J. Speech Hear. Res. 20:212, 1977.
24. Halpern, H., Darley, F.L., and Brown, J.R.: Differential language and neurological characteristics in cerebral involvement, J. Speech Hear. Disord. 38:162, 1973.
25. Harrington, D.O.: The visual fields, ed. 4, St. Louis, 1976, The C.V. Mosby Co.
26. Jebsen, R.H., et al.: An objective and standardized test of hand function, Arch. Phys. Med. Rehabil. 50:311, 1969.
27. Jennett, B.: An introduction to neurosurgery, ed. 3, London, 1977, William Heinemann Medical Books, Ltd.
28. Johnstone, M.: Restoration of motor function in the stroke patient, New York, 1978, Churchhill Livingstone, Inc.
29. Lorenze, E., and Cancro, R.: Dysfunction in visual perception with hemiplegia: its relation to activities of daily living, Arch. Phys. Med. Rehabil. 43:514, 1962.
30. Luria, A.R.: Higher cortical functions in man, New York, 1966, Basic Books, Inc.
31. Marsden, C.D.: The physiological basis of ataxia, Physiotherapy J. 61:326, 1965.
32. McLaurin, R.: Head injuries, proceedings of the second Chicago Symposium on neural trauma, New York, 1975, Grune & Stratton, Inc.

33. Meeder, D.: Cognitive perceptual motor evaluation research findings for adult head injuries. In Trexler, L.E., editor: Cognitive rehabilitation, conceptualization and intervention, New York, 1982, Plenum Publishing Corp.

34. Meyer, J.S.: An orientation to chronic disease and disability, New York, 1965, Macmillan, Inc.

35. Meyer, J.S.: Medical neurology, New York, 1969, Macmillan, Inc.

36. Minnesota Rate of Manipulation Tests: examiner's manual, Circle Pines, Minn., 1969, American Guidance Service, Inc.

37. Pinching, A.J.: Clinical testing of olfaction reassessed, 1977.

38. Plum, F., and Posner, J.: Diagnosis of stupor and coma, Philadelphia, 1966, F.A. Davis Co.

39. Professional Staff Association of Rancho Los Amigos Hospital: Rancho Los Amigos Hospital Head Trauma Rehabilitation Seminar, Downey, Calif., 1977.

40. Purdue Pegboard: examiner's manual, Chicago, 1968, Science Research Associates, Inc.

41. Randolph, S., and Heineger, M.: A psychoneurologically integrated model for learning capacity, lectures on the Rood Treatment Approach, White Plains, N.Y., May 1975, Burke Rehabilitation Foundation.

42. Ryckman, D.M.: Various approaches to cognitive re-training, Paper presented at the Sixth and Seventh Annual Post Graduate Head Trauma Rehabilitation Courses, Williamsburg, Va., June, 1982 and 1983, Medical College of Virginia.

43. Shires, T.G.: Care of the trauma patient, ed. 2, New York, 1979, McGraw-Hill, Inc.

44. Siev, E., and Frieshtat, B.: Perceptual dysfunction in the adult stroke patient, Thorofare, N.J., 1976, Charles B. Slack, Inc.

45. Sinatra, K.: Nonoral communication systems, lecture given at Santa Clara Valley Medical Center, San Jose, Calif., Feb. 8, 1980.

46. Solet, J.: The Solet test for apraxia, Boston, 1975, Copyright by author.

47. Sterno-occipital mandibular immobilizer: United States Manufacturing Co., Glendale, Calif. Commercially available head device.

48. Teasdale, G., and Jennett, B.: Assessment of coma and impaired consciousness, Lancet 2:81, 1974.

49. TOWER system: evaluator's manual, New York, 1967, I.C.D. Rehabilitation and Research Center.

50. Trombly, C.A., and Scott, A.D.: Occupational therapy for physical dysfunction, Baltimore, 1977, Williams & Wilkins.

51. Valpar Component work sample series 1-16: Tucson, Ariz., 1974-1977, Valpar Corp.

52. Wall, N., et al.: Hemiplegia evaluation, Boston, 1979, Massachusetts Rehabilitation Hospital.

53. Weiffenbach, J.M.: Variation in taste thresholds with human aging, JAMA 247:775, 1982.

54. Westerman, T.: How I do it—head and neck: an objective approach to subjective testing for sensation of taste and smell, Laryngoscope 91:301, 1981.

55. Williams, N.: Correlation between copying ability and dressing activities in hemiplegia, Am. J. Phys. Med. 46;1332, 1967.

56. Zoltan, B., et al.: Perceptual motor evaluation for the neurologically impaired adult 1983, Copyright by Santa Clara Valley Medical Center, may be purchased through Santa Clara Valley Medical Center, 751 South Bascom Avenue, San Jose, Calif., 95128.

57. Zoltan, B.: The establishment of reliability and validity of a perceptual motor evaluation on a sample of adult head injured patients, Am. J. Occup. Ther., 1985. (In press.)

Index